Computers and Medicine

Helmuth F. Orthner, Series Editor

Springer
New York
Berlin
Heidelberg
Barcelona
Budapest
Hong Kong
London
Milan
Paris
Santa Clara
Singapore
Tokyo

Computers and Medicine

(continued after index)

Virginia K. Saba
Dorothy B. Pocklington
Kenneth P. Miller
Editors

Nursing and Computers
An Anthology, 1987–1996

With 45 Illustrations

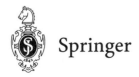 Springer

Virginia K. Saba, EdD, RN, FAAN, FACMI
2332 South Queen Street
Arlington, VA 22202, USA

Dorothy B. Pocklington, MSN, RN
10061 Century Drive
Ellicott City, MD 21042, USA

Kenneth P. Miller, PhD, RN, FAAN
8014 Crabtree Place
Gaithersbury, MD 20879, USA

Series Editor:
Helmuth F. Orthner, PhD
Professor of Medical Informatics
University of Utah Health Sciences
  Center
Salt Lake City, UT 84132, USA

Library of Congress Cataloging-in-Publication Data
Nursing and computers: an anthology, 1987–1996 / [edited by] Virginia
  K. Saba, Dorothy B. Pocklington, Kenneth P. Miller.
      p.   cm.—(Computers and medicine)
    An anthology of selected classical articles and published papers on nursing informatics.
    Includes bibliographical references.
    ISBN 0-387-94955-0 (hardcover: alk. paper)
    1. Nursing informatics.   2. Nursing–Data processing.   I. Saba, Virginia K.
II. Pocklington, Dorothy B.   III. Miller, Kenneth, 1948– .   IV. Series: Computers and
medicine (New York, N.Y.)
    [DNLM: 1. Nursing—collected works.   2. Medical Informatics—collected works.
WY 26.5 N9735   1997]
RT50.5.N863   1997
610.73′0285—dc21

97-12462

Printed on acid-free paper.

Production coordinated by Chernow Editorial Services, Inc., and managed by Terry Kornak;
manufacturing supervised by Joe Quatela.
Typeset by Best-set Typesetter Ltd., Hong Kong.
Printed and bound by Maple-Vail Book Manufacturing Group, York, PA.
Printed in the United States of America.

9 8 7 6 5 4 3 2 1

ISBN 0-387-94955-0 Springer-Verlag New York Berlin Heidelberg   SPIN 10552813

Series Preface

This monograph series intends to provide medical information scientists, health care administrators, physicians, nurses, other health care providers, and computer science professionals with successful examples and experiences of computer applications in health care settings. Through these computer applications, we attempt to show what is effective and efficient, and hope to provide guidance on the acquisition or design of medical information systems so that costly mistakes can be avoided.

The health care provider organizations such as hospitals and clinics are experiencing large demands for clinical information because of a transition from a "fee-for-service" to a "capitation-based" health care economy. This transition changes the way health care services are being paid for. Previously, nearly all health care services were paid for by insurance companies after the services were performed. Today, many procedures need to be pre-approved and many charges for clinical services must be justified to the insurance plans. Ultimately, in a totally capitated system, the more patient care services are provided per patient, the less profitable the health care provider organization will be. Clearly, the financial risks have shifted from the insurance carriers to the health care provider organizations. In order for hospitals and clinics to assess these financial risks, management needs to know what services are to be provided and how to reduce them without impacting the quality of care. The balancing act of reducing costs but maintaining health care quality and patient satisfaction requires accurate information of the clinical services. The only way this information can be collected cost-effectively is through the automation of the health care process itself. Unfortunately, current health information systems are not comprehensive enough and their level of integration is low and primitive at best. There are too many "islands" even within single health care provider organizations.

With the rapid advance of digital communications technologies and the acceptance of standard interfaces, these "islands" can be bridged to satisfy most information needs of health care professionals and management. In addition the migration of health information systems to web-based client/ server computer architectures allows us to re-engineer the user interface to become more functional, pleasant, and also responsive. Eventually, we hope, the clinical workstation will become the tool that health care providers use interactively without intermediary data entry support.

Computer-based information systems provide more timely and legible information than traditional paper-based systems. In addition, medical information systems can monitor the process of health care and improve quality of patient care by providing decision support for diagnosis or therapy, clinical reminders for follow-up care, alerts about adverse drug interactions, alternatives to questionable treatments, or warnings to deviations from clinical protocols, and more. The complexity of the health care workplace requires a rich set of requirements for health information systems. Further, the systems must respond quickly to user interactions and queries in order to facilitate and not impede the work of health care professionals. Because of this and the requirement for a high level of security, these systems can be classified as very complex and, from a developer's perspective also as "risk" systems.

Information technology is advancing at an accelerated pace. Instead of waiting for three years for a new generation of computer hardware, we are now confronted with new computing hardware every 18 months. The forthcoming changes in the telecommunications industry will be revolutionary. Within the next five years, and certainly before the end of this century, new digital communications technologies, such as the Integrated Services Digital Network (ISDN), Asynchronous Data Subscriber Loop (ADSL) technologies, and very high speed local area networks using efficient cell switching protocols (e.g., ATM), will not only change the architecture of our information systems but also the way we work and manage health care institutions.

The software industry constantly tries to provide tools and productive development environments for the design, implementation, and maintenance of information systems. Still, the development of information systems in medicine is an art, and the tools we use are often self-made and crude. One area that needs desperate attention is the interaction of health care providers with the computer. While the user interface needs improvement and the emerging graphical user-interfaces form the basis for such improvements, the most important criterion is to provide relevant and accurate information without drowning the physician in too much (irrelevant) data.

To develop an effective clinical system requires an understanding of what is to be done and how to do it, and an understanding of how to integrate information systems into an operational health care environment. Such knowledge is rarely found in any one individual; all systems described in this monograph series are the work of teams. The size of these teams is usually small, and the composition is heterogeneous, i.e., health professionals, computer and communications scientists and engineers, statisticians, epidemiologists; etc. The team members are usually dedicated to working together over long periods of time, sometimes spanning decades.

Clinical information systems are dynamic systems; their functionality constantly changing because of external pressures and administrative changes in health care institutions. Good clinical information systems will and should change the operational mode of patient care which, in turn, should affect the functional requirements of the information systems. This interplay requires that medical information systems be based on architectures that allow them to be adapted rapidly and with minimal expense. It also requires a willingness by management of the health care institution to adjust its operational procedures, and, most of all, to provide end-user education in the use of information technology. While medical information systems should be functionally integrated, these systems should also be modular so that incremental upgrades, additions, and deletions of modules can be done in order to match the pattern of capital resources and investments available to an institution.

We are building medical information systems just as automobiles were built early in this century, i.e., in an ad-hoc manner that disregarded even existing standards. Although technical standards addressing computer and communications technologies are necessary, they are insufficient. We still need to develop conventions and agreements, and perhaps a few regulations that address the principal use of medical information in computer and communication systems. Standardization allows the mass production of low cost parts that can be used to build more complex structures. What exactly are these parts in medical information systems? We need to identify, classify, and describe them; publish their specifications; and, most importantly, use them in real health care settings. We must be sure that these parts are useful and cost effective even before we standardize them.

Clinical research, health services research, and medical education will benefit greatly when controlled vocabularies are used more widely in the practice of medicine. For practical reasons, the medical profession has developed numerous classifications, nomenclatures, dictionary codes, and thesauri (e.g., ICD, CPT, DSM, SNOMED, LOINC, COSTAR dictionary codes, BAIK thesaurus terms, and MESH terms). The collection of these terms represents a considerable amount of clinical activities, a large portion of the health care business, and access to our recorded knowledge. These terms and codes form the glue that links the practice of medicine with the business of medicine. They also link the practice of medicine with the literature of medicine, with further links to medical research and education. Since information systems are more efficient in retrieving information when controlled vocabularies are used in large databases, the attempt to unify and build bridges between these coding systems is a great example of unifying the field of medicine and health care by providing and using medical informatics tools. The Unified Medical Language System

(UMLS) project of the National Library of Medicine, NIH, in Bethesda, Maryland, is a prime example of such an effort.

The purpose of this series is to capture the experience of medical informatics teams that have successfully implemented and operated medical information systems. We hope the individual books in this series will contribute to the evolution of medical, nursing, or health informatics as a recognized professional discipline. We are at the threshold where there is not just the need but already the momentum and interest in the health care and computer science communities to identify and recognize the new discipline called Medical Informatics.

I would like to thank Springer-Verlag New York for the opportunity to edit this series. Also, many thanks to the present and past departmental chairmen who allowed me to spend time on this activity: William S. Yamamoto, MD and Thomas E. Piemme, MD, of Department of Computer Medicine at The George Washington University Medical Center in Washington, DC, and Homer R. Warner, MD, PhD, and Reed M. Gardner, PhD, of the Department of Medical Informatics at the University of Utah Health Sciences Center in Salt Lake City, Utah. Last but not least I thank all authors and editors of this monograph series for contributing to the practice and theory of Medical Informatics.

Salt Lake City, Utah   HELMUTH F. ORTHNER

Preface

This anthology consists of selected classical articles and published papers on nursing informatics and is a compendium for maintaining and expanding the knowledge base of computer technology in nursing. It serves as one example of the transition of nursing knowledge of computer literacy as it developed for the profession.

The first edition contained articles, published between 1981 and 1986, from nursing journals and proceedings from computer conferences that highlighted the entry of nursing informatics into the technological era. However, this second volume represents landmark documents in the development and progress of nursing informatics, nursing information systems, and other applications using computer technology.

This volume contains 87 articles from approximately 20 published sources, such as proceedings, that have not been indexed in the major computer-based health-related bibliographic retrieval systems. As a result, these published papers are not compiled from a computer search of the systems and therefore are not readily available or used to advance nursing informatics and nursing knowledge.

The articles encompass a ten-year period from 1987 through 1996. The majority of papers are primarily derived from proceedings, conferences, and workshops, specifically:

- Nursing Informatics: NI' 88, NI' 91 & NI' 94 conferences:
  (*Proceedings of the Third, Fourth, & Fifth Conference on Nursing Use of Computers and Information Science* sponsored by International Medical Informatics Association, Nursing Informatics (IMIA-NI-Special Interest Group)
- SCAMC: 1987–1990
  (*Proceedings of the Eleventh, Twelfth, Thirteenth, & Fourteenth Annual Symposium on Computer Applications in Medical Care*) sponsored by the American Medical Informatics Association (AMIA).
- AMIA/SCAMC: 1991–1996
  (*Proceedings of the Fifteenth, Sixteenth, Seventeenth, & Eighteenth*

Annual Symposium on Computer Applications in Medical Care) sponsored by the American Medical Informatics Association (AMIA).
- Medical Informatics: MEDINFO' 89, MEDINFO' 92, & MEDINFO' 95 congresses:
(*Proceedings of the Sixth, Seventh, & Eighth World Congress on Medical Informatics* sponsored by the International Medical Informatics Association (IMIA).
- Medical Records Institute: 1988–1996
(*Proceedings of the Annual Symposium entitled Toward an Electronic Patient Record* sponsored by the Medical Records Institute.
- Selected papers from other sources and conferences that focused on Nursing Informatics such as *Annual National Nursing Computer Conference* sponsored by Rutgers, the State University of New Jersey College of Nursing Continuing Education Program.

Initially all nursing articles in the above publications were selected for review by the three editors who were responsible for:

- Categorizing the articles into one of five topical areas: (1) general informatics, (2) clinical practice, (3) nursing administration, (4) nursing research, and (5) nursing education.
- Identifying the specific focus and topic for each article.
- Evaluating and prioritizing each article.
- Presenting, discussing, and reviewing each article in a group forum.
- Selecting and assigning each article to one editor for an introduction to one of the five sections of the book.

The articles represent milestones as new nursing experts entered the field of nursing informatics. This book will help to ensure that the effort expended in the preparation of the articles is used to enhance and advance nursing knowledge of nursing informatics.

This second volume is divided into five major sections: (1) General Informatics, (2) Clinical Practice, (3) Nursing Administration, (4) Nursing Research, and (5) Nursing Education; each with its own introduction that highlights its selections, authors, and focus.

VIRGINIA K. SABA
DOROTHY B. POCKLINGTON
KENNETH P. MILLER

Contents

II. Clinical Practice

IV. Nursing Research

V.   Nursing Education

Contributors

Jos Aarts
Causa, Fontys Hogescholen, 5600 AH Eindhoven, The Netherlands

Ivo L. Abraham
University of Virginia Medical Center, Charlottesville, VA 22903, USA

Brockenbrough S. Allen
San Diego State University, San Diego, CA, 92182, USA

Joyce Arcus
Surgical Intensive Care Unit, Duke University Medical Center, Durham, NC 27710, USA

Myrna L. Armstrong
Health Sciences Center, School of Nursing, Texas Tech University, Lubbock, TX 79430, USA

Rita Axford
Department of Nursing, La Trobe University, Melbourne, Victoria 3083, Australia

Judith G. Baggs
University of Rochester School of Nursing, Rochester, NY 14642, USA

A.R. Bakker
BAZIS, 2316XA Leiden, The Netherlands

Christine Bolwell
Diskovery: Computer-Assisted Healthcare Education, Saratoga, CA 95070, USA

June E. Bonk
Department of Internal Medicine, University of Nebraska Medical Center,
Omaha, NE 68198-3333, USA

Johnetta Bowen
Surgical Intensive Care Unit, Duke University Medical Center, Durham,
NC 27710, USA

Patricia Flatley Brennan
University of Wisconsin-Madison, Madison, WI 53706, USA

Ruth Brenner

Carole Brigham
School of Nursing, Ball State University, Muncie, IN 47306, USA

James R. Campbell
Department of Internal Medicine, University of Nebraska Medical Center,
Omaha, NE 68198-3333, USA

P. Catford
Information Services Department, Mount Sinai Hospital, Toronto,
Ontario, M5G 1X5, Canada

Betty L. Chang
School of Nursing, University of California, Los Angeles, CA 90095-6918,
USA

June Clark
Department of Community Nursing, University of Wales Swansea, Wales
SA2 8PP, UK

M. Conrick
School of Nursing, Griffith University, Nathan, Queensland, 4111 Australia

Sheila A. Corcoran
School of Nursing, University of Minnesota, Minneapolis, MN 88455, USA

J. Crossley
University Hospitals of Cleveland, Cleveland, OH 44106, USA

Janet E. Cuddigan
School of Nursing, Creighton University, Omaha, NE 68178, USA

J. Curry
Faculty of Medicine, University of Calgary, Calgary, Alberta T2N 1N4,
Canada

P. Czar
Clinical Systems, St. Francis Medical Center, Pittsburgh, PA 15201, USA

Connie Delaney
College of Nursing, University of Iowa, Iowa City, IA 52242, USA

L. Delesie
School of Public Health, Catholic University of Leuven, 3000 Leuven, Belgium

Anne M. Devney
Naval Hospital Corps School, Great Lakes, IL 60088, USA

Sandra J. Engberg
Primary Health Care Nursing Program, University of Pittsburgh, Pittsburgh, PA 15261, USA

Steven Evans
Department of Research, Creighton University, Omaha, NE 68178, USA

Joyce J. Fitzpatrick
Case Western Reserve University and University Hospitals of Cleveland, Cleveland, OH 44106, USA

Kevin Fitzpatrick
Surgical Intensive Care Unit, Duke University Medical Center, Durham, NC 27710, USA

J. Foster
School of Nursing, Queensland University of Technology, Red Hill, Queensland, 4059 Australia

Lynette Fredericksen
Fleming Associates, Portland, OR 97201, USA

Carole A. Gassert
University of Maryland, Baltimore, MD 21202, USA

Stephan Gilbert
School of Nursing, University of California, Los Angeles, CA 90024-1702, USA

B. Glica
Beatrice Renfield Division of Nursing Education and Research, Beth Israel Medical Center, New York, NY 10003, USA

Judith R. Graves
Virginia Henderson Nursing Library, Indianapolis, IN 46202 , USA

Ruby Grewal
The Frankel Group, Inc., New York, NY 10017, USA

Susan J. Grobe
Professor of Nursing, University of Texas at Austin School of Nursing,
Austin, TX 78701, USA

Camille Grosso
The Catholic University of America, Washington, DC 20064, USA

J. Grzymala-Busse
Departments of Computer Science and Electrical Engineering, University
of Kansas, Lawrence, KS 64055, USA

Betty Hagen

William E. Hammond
Department of Medical Informatics, Duke University Medical Center,
Durham, NC 27710, USA

Kathryn J. Hannah
Faculty of Nursing, University of Calgary, Calgary, Alberta T2N 1N4,
Canada

Ann C. Hanson
School of Nursing, Ball State University, Muncie, IN 47306, USA

Bennie E. Harsanyi
SMS, Pittsburgh, PA 15220, USA

T. Hebda
Department of Nursing, Waynesburg College, Waynesburg, PA 15730,
USA

Barbara R. Heller
University of Maryland, Baltimore, MD 21201, USA

Suzanne B. Henry
School of Nursing, University of California, San Francisco, CA 94143-0608,
USA

Liza Hickey
Surgical Intensive Care Unit, Duke University Medical Center, Durham, NC 27710, USA

Kay Hodson
School of Nursing, Ball State University, Muncie, IN 47306, USA

Helen Hoesing
Nebraska Methodist Hospital, Omaha, NE 68101, USA

William L. Holzemer
School of Nursing, University of California, San Francisco, CA 94143-0608, USA

Evelyn J.S. Hovenga
Faculty of Health Science, University of Central Queensland, Queensland, 4702 Australia

Carole Hudgings
Office of the Forum for Quality and Effectiveness in Health Career, Rockville, MD 20852, USA

Marianne Hujcs
Latter Day Saints Hospital, Salt Lake City, UT 84112, USA

Marsha Kelly
Director, Public Policy Analysis, National Council State Boards of Nursing, Inc., Chicago, IL 60601, USA

Clyde E. Kelsey
Texas Tech University, Lubbock, TX 79409, USA

Wendy King

Vicki Klemm
School of Nursing, University of California, San Francisco, CA 94143-0608, USA

Norma M. Lang
School of Nursing, University of Pennsylvania, Philadelphia, PA 19104-6096, USA

Linda L. Lange
Clinical Nursing Informatics Program, College of Nursing, University of Utah, Salt Lake City, UT 84112, USA

Donna E. Larson
Department of Nursing, Grand Valley State University, Allendale, MI 49401, USA

Jane S. Leske

Susan Logan
Nebraska Methodist Hospital, Omaha, NE 68101, USA

Philip Lohman

Mary Ann Lubno
School of Nursing, Texas Tech University Health Sciences Center, Lubbock, TX 79409, USA

Salah H. Mandil
Advisor on Informatics, World Health Organization, CH-1211 Geneva 27, Switzerland

D.J. Mason
Beatrice Renfield Division of Nursing Education and Research, Beth Israel Medical Center, New York, NY 10003, USA

Kathleen A. McCormick
Office of the Forum for Quality and Effectiveness in Health Career, Rockville, MD 20852, USA

Susan McDermott
Nursing Service, Department of Veterans Affairs Medical Center, Washington, DC 20422, USA

Bill McGuiness

Mary L. McHugh
Wichita State University School of Nursing, Wichita, KS 67260-0041, USA

L. McQueen
Office of the Forum for Quality and Effectiveness in Health Career, Rockville, MD 20852, USA

N.K. Meehan
Department of Nursing, College of Nursing, Clemson University, Clemson, SC 29634-1703, USA

M. Mehmert
Mercy Hospital, Davenport, IA 52801, USA

S.L. Meintz
Department of Nursing, College of Health Science, University of Nevada, Las Vegas, NV 89514, USA

Kathleen J. Mikan
School of Nursing, University of Alabama, Birmingham, AL 35394-1210, USA

D. Kathy Milholland
American Nurses Association, Washington, DC 20024-2571, USA

Emmy Miller
Department of Neurosurgery, University of Texas Medical School at Houston, Houston, TX 77006, USA

D.T. Mirque
School of Nursing, University of Colorado Health Sciences Center, Denver, CO 80262, USA

L.M. Nagle
Gerald P. Turner Department of Nursing, Mount Sinai Hospital, Toronto, Ontario M5G 1X5, Canada

Lois Nauert
University Hospital and Clinics, Columbia, MO 65201, USA

Susan K. Newbold
University of Maryland at Baltimore, Baltimore, MD 21201, USA

J.P. O'Donnell
Directorate of Health Care Studies and Clinical Investigation, U.S. Army Medical Department Center and School, Ft. Sam Houston, TX 78234-6100, USA

Barbara Palmer

Steven M. Paul
Office of Research, School of Nursing, University of California, San Francisco, CA 94143-0604, USA

Eileen Grow Perciful
Department of Nursing, West Chester University, West Chester, PA 19383, USA

Connie L. Pinkley
University Hospitals of Cleveland, Cleveland, OH 44106, USA

Lucille M. Pogue
Nursing Staff Development, Medical College of Georgia Hospital, Augusta, GA 30912, USA

Richard E. Pogue
Pogue Associates, Augusta, GA 30912, USA

C.J. Portillo
School of Nursing, University of California, San Francisco, CA 94143-0608, USA

Rosa Portus
Nursing Administration, Royal North Shore Hospital, St. Leonards, New South Wales, 2065 Australia

Colleen M. Prophet
Department of Nursing, University of Iowa Hospitals and Clinics, Iowa City, IA 52242, USA

N.S. Redeker
College of Nursing, Rutgers, State University of New Jersey, Newark, NJ 07102, USA

Cheryl A. Reilly
School of Nursing, University of California, San Francisco, CA 94143-0608, USA

W. Roelofs
BAZIS, 2316XA Leiden, The Netherlands

Carol A. Romano
National Institutes of Health, Bethesda, MD 20892, USA

Judith S. Ronald
Nursing Informatics, State University of New York, Buffalo, NY 14214, USA

J.A. Rossi
Clinical Nursing Informatics Program, College of Nursing, University of Utah, Salt Lake City, UT 84112, USA

Sheila A. Ryan
University of Rochester School of Nursing, Rochester, NY 14642, USA

Virginia K. Saba
Clinical Associate Professor, Georgetown University School of Nursing, Washington, DC 20007, USA

L. Sakerka
Clinical Manager, Information Services, Sewickley Valley Hospital, Sewickley, PA 15301, USA

Maureen Scholes
The London Hospital White Chapel, London E1 1BB, UK

K.A. Seipp
Directorate of Health Care Studies and Clinical Investigation, U.S. Army Medical Department Center and School, Ft. Sam Houston, TX 78234-6100, USA

Walter Sermeus
School of Public Health, Catholic University of Leuven, 3000 Leuven, Belgium

Judith Shamian
Department of Nursing, Mount Sinai Hospital, Toronto, Ontario M5G 1X5, Canada

David M. Sharpe
Learning Resource Center, San Diego State University, San Diego, CA 92182, USA

Vaughn G. Sinclair
Vanderbilt University School of Nursing, Nashville, TN 37240, USA

Diane J. Skiba
School of Nursing, University of Colorado Health Sciences Center, Denver, CO 80262, USA

Patricia K. Sommer
University Hospitals of Cleveland, Cleveland, OH 44106, USA

Laura G. Spranzo
School of Nursing, University of Maryland, Baltimore, MD 21201, USA

William W. Stead
Duke University Medical Center, Durham, NC 27710, USA

Robin Stoupa
Department of Internal Medicine, University of Nebraska Medical Center, Omaha, NE 68198-3333, USA

Mary Anne Sweeney
The University of Texas Medical Branch, Galveston, TX 77555, USA

Linda Q. Thede
School of Nursing, Kent State University, Kent, OH 44242-0001, USA

Cheryl Thompson
University of Rochester School of Nursing, Rochester, NY 14642, USA

C. Tsatsoulis
Departments of Computer Science and Electrical Engineering, University of Kansas, Lawrence, KS 64055, USA

John P. Turley
School of Nursing, University of Texas—Houston, Houston, TX 77030, USA

M. VanDyne
Departments of Computer Science and Electrical Engineering, University of Kansas, Lawrence, KS 64055, USA

E.M.S.J. van Gennip
BAZIS, 2316XA Leiden, The Netherlands

William Verbrugge
School of Nursing, Ball State University, Muncie, IN 47306, USA

Ann Warnock-Matheron
Nursing Systems, Calgary General Hospital, Calgary, Alberta T2N 1N4, Canada

Judith J. Warren
Department of Internal Medicine, University of Nebraska Medical Center, Omaha, NE 68198-3333, USA

Charlotte A. Weaver
Fleming Associates, Portland, OR 97201, USA

Harriet H. Werley
Distinguished Professor, University of Wisconsin–Milwaukee, Milwaukee, WI 53201, USA

Joyce E. White
Primary Health Care Nursing Program, University of Pittsburgh, Pittsburgh, PA 15261, USA

Gregory K. Whymark
Faculty of Health Science, University of Central Queensland, Queensland, 4702 Australia

Linda K. Woolery
School of Nursing, University of Missouri, Columbia, MO 65211, USA

E.M. Wykpisz
Robert Wood Johnson University Hospital, New Brunswick, NJ 08903, USA

J. Yensen
Nursing Faculty, Langara College, Vancouver, BC V6P SN3, Canada

Marianne E. Yoder
Nursing Software Development, Flagstaff, AZ 86001, USA

Rita D. Zielstorff
Partners HealthCare Systems, Inc., Brookline, MA 02167, USA

Part I
General Informatics

This first section of *Nursing and Computers: An Anthology* provides a general overview and focuses on critical issues in the field of nursing informatics. It includes several articles related to nursing data and their structure as well as nursing taxonomies, classifications, and nomenclatures. Other papers focus on telecommunications and the use of the electronic information superhighway and Internet to advance the practice of nursing.

In the first triad of articles, nursing informatics is described as a new science by Ryan and Nagle. Mandil operationalizes this concept by focusing on the interaction among health informatics, the individual, and society. A third article by Nagle, Shamian, and Catford hones in on information technology developments and issues as they impact on nursing. These three articles set the stage for this introductory section of the book.

The second set of articles highlights nursing vocabularies and the major activities of the American Nurses Association's (ANA) Database Steering Committee on Databases to Support Clinical Practice. The article by Zielstorff and others provides a description of the nursing minimum data set (NMDS) and the four nursing classification schema (vocabularies) that have been recognized by the ANA as appropriate for computer-based systems requiring nursing data. These schema have been incorporated in the National Library of Medicine's (NLMs) Unified Medical Language System (UMLS) and are retrievable using GratefulMed on the Internet. Saba's article focuses on the Home Health Care Classification (HHCC) System, which is one of the four approved ANA schemes, while the article by Grobe describes a natural language lexicon of interventions.

The next set of articles on telenursing begins with Clark's article on the development of the International Classification of Nursing Practice (ICNP) project by the International Council of Nurses.

An article of special interest is devoted to the practice guidelines. The article by McQueen, McCormick, and Hudgings describes the Agency for Health Care Policy and Research's (AHCPR) development of practice

1

guidelines in order to promote the quality, appropriateness, and effectiveness of health care services.

The next set of articles in this section is on telecommunications. Several articles describe how telecommunications is used to provide patient care and distance learning education. Brennan's article focuses on the use of "ComputerLink" as an innovative method of providing home care nursing services. On the other hand, an article by Sweeney and Skiba highlights the uses of telecommunication and interactive multimedia health information on the electronic superhighway. Skiba and Mirque's article discusses the electronic community as an alternative approach to providing health care services. The article by Woolery and Yensen provides information on the uses of the Internet for nursing collaboration.

Another group of articles focus on data security. Bakker and Scholes describe data protection and how security creates an organizational challenge to nursing. McHugh then describes the structuring of nursing data for the computer-based patient record. On the other hand, Hebda and others, indicate that the best means to safeguard privacy and confidentiality is through education. Next, Kelly presents the uses of a data bank as a model for assuring public health safety and welfare. Finally, Miller describes a conceptual model for information and data requirements for professional organizations.

The next set of articles delineate the design and development of nursing information systems. Hujcs describes the uses of computers in health care and the integration of nursing within nursing information systems. Axford highlights the role of the nurses in implementing nursing information systems, while Pinkley and Sommer provide an historical perceptive of the issues confronting nursing in the development of information systems. The article by Grosso addresses knowledge and knowledge acquisition for the development of expert systems for nursing. In a final article, Saba presents a new nursing vision for nursing in the twenty-first century.

In general, the articles in this section demonstrate the wide range of topics that comprise nursing informatics. Each provides a different perspective of this topic. The remainder of the book addresses specific areas of nursing informatics and nursing information systems.

1
Nursing Informatics: The Unfolding of a New Science

SHELIA A. RYAN and L.M. NAGLE

1. Introduction

In the 80s, the term *"information* society" was used to describe the disposition of the modern world [1]. The preponderance of activities directed to the management of unwieldy volumes of data and information warranted this characterization. More recently, Toffler [2] described the transformational effects of *knowledge*, the breakdown of conventional disciplines, and resulting power shifts:

> With the help of the computer, the same data or information can now easily be clustered or "cut" in quite different ways, helping the user to view the same problem from quite different angles, and to synthesize meta-knowledge [p. 427].

An essential and core function of nursing, the ability to purvey, process, and manage information is largely determining the future of nursing as a practice discipline. The evolution of nursing informatics has provided nurses with opportunities to influence the design and selection of technologies to support practice. New tools for the manipulation of data and information beyond better management are rapidly becoming accessible to nurses in clinical settings throughout the world. The ability to electronically integrate and analyze data and information from diverse settings and populations provides an opportunity to enrich nursing science and generate nursing knowledge in ways heretofore unknown. Nursing informatics is rapidly emerging as the vehicle by which the science of "nursing" information will be elucidated for the discipline and vendor community.

Reprinted from *Nursing Informatics: An International Overview for Nursing in a Technological Era*, Grobe, S.J., Pluyter-Wenting, E.S.P. (Eds.). 1994. Pp. 443–447, with kind permission from Elsevier Science—NL, Sara Burgerhartstraat 25, 1055 KV Amsterdam, The Netherlands.

2. What Is a Science?

A discipline science is "a field of scholarly inquiry which expresses the entire domain of problems studied by that scholarly community" [3]. This is a metaterm mapping out the broad theoretical domain of problems and ideas which are unique to that particular discipline.

Nursing science has been described as a subset of the discipline of nursing [4] and distinguished from nursing research [5]. Nursing research is the systematic process of inquiry into the phenomena of interest and concern to nurses whereas nursing science has been defined as a representation of:

> our currently limited understanding of human biology and behavior in health and illness, including the processes by which changes in health status are brought about, the patterns of behavior associated with normal and critical life events, and the principles and laws governing life states and processes [5, p. 180].

Distinguished from nursing practice and nursing knowledge, the science of nursing is purported to provide an empirical substantiation for nursing practice. Nursing knowledge is derived from the conduct of nursing science.

Refinetti [6] described the two predominant modes of knowledge development espoused by philosophers: analytical and dialectical. Proponents of the analytical approach support Cartesian notions and suggest that knowledge development is a cumulative process. Where as supporters of the dialectical view advance the position that knowledge development is a wholistic and integrative process. Historically, nursing science has been dominated by the tenets of logical positivism thus the analytical view. Within the context of this paradigm, knowledge development is a gradual process and based on the movement from simple to complex concepts. A majority of nurse researchers have attempted to develop nursing knowledge on the basis of findings from *multiple* studies, across *multiple* populations, using *multiple* measures of *multiple* concepts. Although the contributions of analytic nursing science have been substantial, the advancement of nursing knowledge from these cumulative studies has been limited.

An indepth discussion of philosophy of science and knowledge development in nursing is beyond the scope of this paper, but will be necessary in determining modes of information processing. New views of nursing science have emerged and multiple methods of knowledge discovery are being advocated by nurse scientists [7,8,9,10]. Acknowledging the philosophical and methodological diversity in nursing science will be fundamental to the design of knowledge yielding systems in the future.

It has been suggested that although divergent views of knowledge development might be complementary, convergence would not be practical in terms of information processing [6]. These authors suggest that in light of new technologies an intersection of analytic and dialectic modes of knowledge development should be quite possible. Furthermore, the responsibility for unfolding nursing knowledge need not be limited to the nurse scientist, but extended to nurses in all roles. New modes of knowledge generation well need to be based upon a reconceptualization of the requirements for data and information processing in nursing—an articulation of nursing's "science of information".

3. Information as Science

The concept of information is derived from the Latin *information* which means a process to communicate or the communication of something. According to Yuexiao [11], information may refer to messages, news, data, knowledge, documents, literature, intelligence, symbols, signs, hints, tips. The process and phenomenon of information exists in the realm of human societies, but can also be described in relation to philosophical concepts (e.g. time and space) and the mechanical and animal world [12]. In fact there is a multiplicity of definitions and classifications of information, each of which may have particular meaning and import to nursing.

Examining information schemes such as that described by Mikhailov [13] may provide direction for defining the nature and boundaries of nursing information. Subsequent to an analysis of the definitions and sciences of information, Yuexiao [11] concluded that consensual definitions within professions or sciences is important and necessary for precise communication and scientific progress. This appeal for concordance may be likened to the case for a minimum data set in nursing but expands the notion from data to information.

Information related fields such as cybernetics, semiotics, library science, computer science, cognitive science abound in academia. Many disciplines have identified the science of information as it relates to the particular practice or knowledge base of the practitioners: Information Sociology, Information Economics, Information Politics, Information Psychology. Further examination of these disciplines may provide insights to the process of explicating a "nursing" science of information.

4. Science of Nursing Information: Nursing Informatics

The science of information has been named *Information Science, Informatics, Informatistics, Informology, and Informatology* [14]. Informatics has been described as the convergence of information science, computer science, and discipline-specific science [15]. Applying this definition to the study of nursing informatics, Graves and Corcoran [16] discussed the interface of computer science, information science, and nursing science. A recent discussion of the interface added the notion that this merging of sciences allows for "informatization" to occur within the discipline [17]. Informatization is defined as the "synergistic use of computer, information, and discipline-specific science resulting in the generation of new knowledge that could be used as expert decision support" [17, p. 977].

Scarrott [18] described the need for a "science of information" and its ultimate value in leading to the development of a conceptual framework to guide system design at every level. He identified six criteria which could be used to ascertain the existence of a credible "science of information". The necessity and centrality of a "science of information" to all other dimensions of nursing science becomes apparent when examined in the context of these criteria. For the purpose of illustration, each criterion will be briefly discussed as directly relates to the practice and science of nursing.

- *Should be derived from observation of the functions, structures, dynamic behavior, and statistical features of information and the symbols used to represent information.*

In nursing, data and information are derived from the practice of nurses, their observations, interactions, and their knowledge representations. Nursing information arises from the compilation of many data elements for one or several patients. The capability to accrue patient data and information over time, across multiple settings and populations from multiple sources (e.g. patient databases, monitors) should be the goal of systems to support knowledge development.

- *Should respect the distinction between limited symbol combinations and the rich human understanding they are used to represent.*

Increasingly, nurse scientists are enhancing or moving away from the traditions of the empiricist paradigm. This shifting of paradigms, in the Kuhnian sense [19], can be partially attributed to the need for methods of inquiry which capture the richness of human experience. Data and information as collected by nurses has limited capacity for quantification. Nurse scientists have begun to recognize the limited utility and generalizability of codified information. Nurse informaticists have begun to identify the need for information systems which allow for the capture of unique human experience.

- *Must fit with our established understanding of nature including the existence of complex living organisms, together with social groups of such organisms.*

To date, applications of information science and technology have been largely designed on the basis of the interdepartmental complexity of health care organizations. Accommodation of complex discipline-specific needs for information management is less apparent in the realm of current clinical information systems. However, nurse informaticists are providing vendors with insights to those complexities more than ever before.

- *Must offer a context into which established but hitherto isolated theoretical aspects of information engineering (e.g. automation theory) can be fitted.*

The science of nursing informatics supports the integration of information engineering principles into the context of nursing practice, administration, research, and education. As a matter of course, information engineering is being embraced and advanced by nurse informaticists as a mechanism to engineer new nursing knowledge.

- *Should offer useful guidance to those engaged in the design of information systems to serve organized groups of people in the most cost-effective way.*

Nurse informaticists have directed energy to the evaluation of existing system designs and components. Numerous studies report the impact of nurse involvement in the selection, implementation, and evaluation of information systems in practice and education. Evaluations of efficiency and effectiveness outcomes have largely focused on the potential cost-savings associated with hospital information systems and not direct consequences for nursing practice.

- *Should offer useful and verifiable evidence regarding the scope and limitations of AI and consequently should offer useful guidance to those engaged in selecting, supporting, and undertaking exploratory enterprises in the field of information engineering.*

Nurse researchers have investigated the potential benefits to be derived from the development of expert systems to support nurses in practice settings. Several nurse authors have acknowledged the limitations to developing and using expert systems in nursing [20,21,22]. Nevertheless, there are many opportunities for further research in understanding the nature of information processing among nurses.

5. Conclusion

New modes of knowledge generation will need to be based upon a reconceptualization of the requirements for data and information processing in nursing—an articulation of nursing's "science of information." Delineating a science of information is a challenge for all professions and disciplines, not just nursing. Nursing informatics is rapidly emerging as the vehicle by which the science of "nursing" information will be elucidated. The development of a schema for the identifying the dimensions of nursing information will provide a foundation for further explication of what and how knowledge engineering can evolve in nursing. Ideally, a science of information for nursing will evolve over the next decade such that technological opportunities can be used to illuminate the unique and essential role of the nursing profession.

References

[1] Naisbitt J. *Megatrends: Ten new directions for transforming our lives.* New York: Warner Books, 1984.

[2] Toffler A. *Powershift.* New York: Bantam Books, 1990.

[3] Schrader A M. In search of a name: Information science and its conceptual antecedents. *Library and Information Science Research* 1984, 6:227–271.

[4] Donaldson S K and Crowley D. The discipline of nursing. *Nurs Out* 1978, 26:113–120.

[5] Gortner S. Nursing science in transition. *Nurs Res* 1980, 29:180–183.

[6] Refinetti R. Information processing as a central issue in philosophy of science. *Information Processing & Management* 1989, 25:583–584.

[7] Tinkle M B and Beaton J L. Toward a new view of science: Implications for nursing research. *ANS Adv Nurs Sci* 1983, 5:27–36.

[8] Allen D, Benner P, and Diekelmann N L. Three paradigms for nursing research: Methodological implications. In *Nursing Research Methodology.* Chinn P (ed.), Rockville, MD: Aspen, 1986:23–38.

[9] Davidson A W and Ray M A. Studying the human-environment phenomenon using the science of complexity. *ANS Adv Nurs Sci* 1991, 14:73–87.

[10] Coward D. Critical multiplism: A research strategy for nursing science. *Image* 1990, 22:163–167.

[11] Yuexiao Z. Definitions and sciences of information. *Information Processing & Management* 1988, 24:479–491.

[12] Weiner N. *Cybernetics, or control and communication in the animal and the machine* 2nd ed. Cambridge, MA: MIT Press, 1984.

[13] Mikhailov A J et al. *Scientific communications and informatics* (English version translated by R H Burger). Arlington, VA: Information Resources Press, 1984.

[14] Wellisch H. From information science to informatics: A terminological investigation. *Journal of Librarianship* 1972, 4:157–187.

[15] Gorn, S. Informatics. In: *The Study of Information Interdisciplinary Messages.* Machlup F and Mansfield U (eds.). New York: Wiley, 1983:121–140.

[16] Graves J R and Corcoran S. The study of nursing informatics. *Image* 1989, 21:227–231.

[17] Shamian J, Nagle L M, and Hannah K J. Optimizing outcomes of nursing informatization. In *MEDINFO 92* Lun K C, Degoulet P, Piemme T E, and Rienhoff O (eds.). Amsterdam: North Holland, 1992:976–980.

[18] Scarrott G. The need for a "Science" of information. *J of Info Tech* 1986, 1:33–38.

[19] Kuhn T S. *The Structure of Scientific Revolutions.* Chicago: University of Chicago Press, 1962.

[20] Sinclair V G. Potential effects of decision support systems on the role of the nurse. *Comput Nurs* 1990, 8:60–65.

[21] Ozbolt J G. Developing decision support systems for nursing: Theoretical bases for advanced computer systems. *Comput Nurs* 1987, 5:105–111.

[22] Brennan P F and McHugh, M J. Clinical decision-making and computer support. *App Nurs Res* 1988, 1:89–93.

2
On the Interaction Between Health Informatics, the Individual, and Society

SALAH H. MANDIL

Introduction

In my son's first ever contact with a microcomputer he was asked to provide his name, whereupon he said to it: "My name is Basil. What is your name?" No response. He concluded that it is "NOT a clever machine." This reminds us that today's computing tools are not as "powerful" as we think they are because they are not oriented to our natural ways of teaching, comprehending, using, and testing things.

This audience is the right one to recall that computing had its origins in, and had been initially driven by, the need to determine fast, repeated, and numerous calculations. But what if computing had its origins in a socioeconomic field such as medicine? It would have certainly evolved differently, maybe in a more "natural" manner! Just compare the evolution of "informatics technology" to the evolution of a "child's capacity." They are the exact reverse of each other. A child, first, recognizes voice and facial expressions, then learns to draw, then to write, and then to calculate. Computing enabled numerical data processing first, then text processing, then graphics, and more recently imaging and voice recognition. Great care needs to be exercised on how informatics can be introduced to an individual, a group or a whole society. A few good lessons have already been learned.

Significant Informatics Development

There is wide recognition of significant developments in the informatics methodology and technology. For example, increasing computing power at

Reprinted with permission from *Nursing Informatics '91: Proceedings of the Post Conference on Health Care Information Technology: Implications for Change*, Marr, P.B., Axford, R.L. & Newbold, S.K. (Eds.). 1991. Pp. 3–6, Heidelberg-Berlin, Germany: Springer-Verlag.

still decreasing costs; robustness of the hardware, thus requiring lesser and lesser repair and maintenance; and, availability of wide ranges of generalized and special-purpose software packages which enable uses such as:

- word processing and desktop publishing
- spreadsheets
- databases and
- graphics.

Equally significant, relevant developments in computer networking and in computer-based telecommunications enable wider, more popular, and less costly services such as those provided today by:

- digital telephony
- facsimile (FAX) and
- public data networks.

The exponential rise in the uses of FAX services within and between institutions and countries and the fact that there are today at least 118 public data networks (that are compliant with the X.25 international standard) in 66 countries, including many developing countries, are testimony to the present and near-future uses of local and wide area communications networks in the health sector. At a minimum, they avail needed information services to the individual health worker, professional groups, and the public at large. They also enable those with relevant data bases to reach a wider audience with related services.

Other, relatively more recent developments are enhancing the relevance of informatics to medical and health care and, possibly, making it more directly relevant. Two leading developments are:

- Knowledge-Based Systems, such as Consultation systems; Critiquing systems and Instructional systems whereby nearly the same knowledge-base could be used for any of these purposes; and
- Imaging and signal analysis: that is, the uses of computer-supported storage and retrieval, analysis and interpretation of signals and images.

Both areas marshal the beginning of the development and uses of advanced decision support systems in medical and health care. The next few years, and for a long period to come, will witness the varied ways with which such support systems will be accepted by the health community, particularly medical groups, and nothing will aid this more than a thorough screening and validation of such systems.

In short, the dramatic and relevant developments in informatics and telematics, and the significant ways with which these are being, and will be, applied in the health/medical sector, are pointers to the need for a more profound (not less as it is sometimes claimed by the "automation prophets") interaction between the providers of the health care, and the consumers and the informatics products/producers.

Issues Affecting the Individual

In informatics, the "user" has always been and still is king. The technology has to be relevant, readily absorbed by, and friendly to the user. That is, and should remain, fundamental and uncontested. Less is said about the users' obligations towards the services that informatics technology enables and toward the technology itself.

The individual's training/education: increasingly, informatics applications, services and products provide users' training tools, often as an integral part of these tools. The typical user benefits from these only to the minimum extent needed to carry out the chore at hand. Sometimes, he/she cannot be blamed! But, the importance of informatics services to health/medical care is such that it should be an obligation on the user to influence those services which, in turn, puts an obligation on the user to be trained enough to be constructively critical. In other words, because of the impact of informatics support to health/medical care, the user has an obligation to self-inform, self-train, and self-educate.

Self-Health-Care Systems

Increasingly informatics-supported services for the individual's health care are becoming available. Whilst an individual user may or may not get the appropriate services from such systems, it is his/her obligation to the society at large to contribute to the evaluation, or even re-conception and re-design, of such services by responding to users' polls which, increasingly, are an integral part of these services.

Health Records

The obligations of the doctor and the medical institution for keeping an individual's health record and to use it in the interest of the individual concerned and society at large—and with due confidentiality and security—are well known and largely appreciated. The individual too has an obligation: to provide information for the health record and to ascertain its accuracy and currency. The individual has also another form of obligation: to authorize where necessary the use of the health record for mass analysis such as epidemiological surveillance. These obligations of the individual will become even more acute if and when the health record takes the form of a "smart card."

The individual medical/health worker should not only use the parts of the system related to his/her work but, being aware of the overall purpose of the system, he/she should realize the obligation to influence the whole systems (e.g., the nursing component of a hospital management information system). Florence Nightingale is famous and largely remembered for her dedication and pioneering nursing contributions to health care.

In fact, one of her most significant contributions was to display the power of information in influencing decisions affecting health care. With the use of figures and graphics, she showed that the mortality of British soldiers was due more to preventable public health problems than to the war!

The use of informatics methods and tools has given a significant upward boost to the levels of work satisfaction. Among other things, computing is also fun! It has contributed to making it possible for individuals to honour their obligations to their work, their work colleagues, and their workplace. The early myth that informatics will de-humanize health care, especially those functions with direct contact with patients such as nursing, has been gradually fading away. The real challenge is how the health care provider and consumer should influence and humanize the informatics serving them.

Issues Affecting Society

Major issues affecting society include confidentiality and security of medical information; legal and ethical issues, not only regarding "medical information" but also regarding the practice of medical/health care with informatics support; and organizational changes: the trauma that the introduction and uses of informatics is always accompanied by ("uncertain") organizational changes, and that any level of "automation" would lead to reduction in the work force.

Further, there is the issue of communications with others. Invariably, and increasingly, public services are carried out with the aid of an informatics tool; "the computer tells me . . . ," "but according to the computer . . ," "can't do anything now, the computer is down . . ." are examples of how the ordinary member of a society may be introduced to informatics and as such views it as a potential impediment to communications (contrary to its purpose). This must be totally averted when it is a communication between a health care provider and the recipient of such care.

Issues at the more international level include:

1. Input/output in local languages. Informatics applications in non-Latin languages such as Arabic, Thai, Chinese, and Korean were either costly and relatively difficult, or not possible, when the necessary technical means were a mixture of hardware and software. In recent years, technology evolved to provide total software solutions to the needs for computing in non-Latin languages. This reality is percolating to and affecting the designers and producers of end-user applications rather slowly. Few of these are done with a view to also cater to non-Latin multi-language input/output.

2. Technical standards for efficient and economic interface among applications, devices, and networks are essential and vastly lacking, and a lot

of effort is being carried out at the international level to fulfill these. Is such a requisite having a negative effect on society, as some claim? Is the standardization of our data and our verbiage leading to a loss of the colour and variety of our societies? To a certain extent it may be, but it is also sure that the informatics technology can support colorful and varied means of doing the same thing!

Conclusion

A great deal has been said, written, and demonstrated on how relevant and timely information is power for a business endeavor. Information is also power for social and personal transformation. Informatics technology offers a variety of means: to contribute to information bases; to access and use these; and to influence their development and evolution. Further, it offers these means to the individual (a citizen, worker, professional); to groups, such as professional groups; and to institutions (private, public, or governmental). The term "information society" is also a challenge to us all to think in terms of not only what can I use a certain service for, but also what my obligations are to it.

3
Information Technology Developments: Issues for Nursing

L.M. Nagle, Judith Shamian, and P. Catford

1. Introduction

In literature of recent years, nurse authors have used the term "*information technology*" synonymously with automation and computerization. The phrase "nursing information system" has been used by many to generically describe systems which support nursing activities in administration, practice, research, and education. According to Saba and McCormick [1], a nursing information system is:

"a computer system that collects, stores, processes, retrieves, displays, and communicates timely information needed to do the following: administer the nursing services and resources in a health care facility; manage standardized patient care information for the delivery of nursing care; link the research resources and educational applications to nursing practice" (p. 120).

The conceptual elements of a nursing information system have been described by several nurse authors [2,3,4]. Moreover, models have been proposed to assist organizations in defining their nursing information system requirements [5,6]. Although these conceptualizations and designs have served nursing well in advancing an understanding of nursing's needs for informational support, the time has come to move into a new era of technological possibilities.

Health care has lagged behind other industries in the adoption of new information technologies, but hospital administrators and government officials have demonstrated an increased interest in having access to quality clinical and financial information. In fact, the demands of current and future health care delivery models are dictating a new era of information management support.

Reprinted from *Nursing Informatics: An International Overview for Nursing in a Technological Era*, Grobe, S.J., Pluyter-Wenting, E.S.P. (Eds.). 1994. Pp. 3–7, with kind permission from Elsevier Science—NL, Sara Burgerhartstraat 25, 1055 KV Amsterdam, The Netherlands.

These authors advance the notion that striving for a "nursing" information system per se will not be sufficient to carry nurses into the 21st century. Indeed, we need to redefine nursing's informational requirements within the contexts of: future health care delivery, the notion of integrated systems, and innovative applications of available technologies. For the purposes of this paper, information technology refers to all manner of data and information management, manual and automated systems, and communication devices as used by nurses in the performance of their work.

2. Nurses and Information Technology

Information technology is being used daily by nurses working in diverse roles and settings. Nurse administrators use information technology to capture and measure nursing workload, to support the management of human and fiscal resources, and for the purposes of quality assurance monitoring. The specific tools employed range from a simple adaption of a spreadsheet application (e.g. LOTUS 1-2-3) to the purchase of a sophisticated standalone or integrated system application (e.g. unit-based nursing workload linked to staffing and patient costing).

Information technology has been incorporated into the provision of patient care through the automation of clinical activities including: order entry, nursing care planning, and documentation. Although such systems are increasingly desirable, a very small percentage of health care organizations in North America had implemented a clinical information repository system.

Additional benefits of information technology are being realized in meeting the learning needs of nurses and patients. Nursing research activities such as data retrieval and statistical analyses have also been expedited through the use of information technology.

Historically, a majority of hospitals made the decision to purchase and implement *clinical* information systems because of the need to improve the timeliness and accuracy of documentation and the efficiency of interdepartmental communication. It would appear that these goals have been achieved within most organizations that have implemented hospital-wide systems.

3. Outcomes Realized

Based upon interviews with nurse administrators ($n = 12$) from Canadian and U.S. hospitals, there are some common perceptions of the benefits derived from clinical information systems to date [7]. The most consistently cited outcomes include: (a) the standardization of practice by providing clear guidelines for documentation and an up-to-date policy and procedure reference, (b) more attention to accountability for practice, (c) increased precision of documentation, and most commonly, (d) decreased clerical tasks performed by nursing staff. Some administrators also reported a reduction in medication errors and a decrease in disputes between individuals (e.g. between nurses and physicians with regard to physician orders) and departments (e.g. the system provides confirmation of specimens being received in the labs).

Changes relevant to nursing administration were reported to include: (a) a decrease in costs related to overtime—because of less time being spent charting at the end of shifts, (b) the ability to assign cost of nursing services per case type, (c) the ability to satisfy accreditation requirements, and (d) improved legibility and completeness of patient records.

Several attitude changes were reported as a direct result of introducing a clinical information system. Nurses became more acutely aware of the need to preserve "hands on care"; the humanistic components of practice. Some staff became more acutely aware of confidentiality issues relevant to patient information. Whether fully computerized or not, most reported the development of a dependency on the system; this had become most evident during system downtime. For some administrators, this dependency translated into a need for staff education about the system's fallibility. Others reported that in some instances nurses were overly confident in the accuracy of system inputs and outputs (e.g. physician orders). In these situations, the need to scrutinize computerized data was stressed as being no different than in the world of manual systems. Despite these changes and improvements in the efficiency of information flow, administrators reported that nurses were experiencing information overload worse than in pre-system days. In many ways more documentation was being required, resulting in more paper and more information to process on a daily basis.

Disappointments with the limitations of existing systems and a demand for more technology and specific applications has begun to surface in institutions with a relatively long system history (greater than 10 years). The results reported by the administrators in these institutions suggests that the original purpose of systems dictated the outcomes. There were improvements in documentation and communication, and the processing of certain kinds of information had become more efficient. Enhancements to clinical practice and improved patient outcomes were not identified as part of the benefits realization.

Nurses have indicated that they want to see system developments which: (a) increase the focus on clinical practice, (b) increase the meaningfulness of clinical data, and (c) support clinical decision-making. Fully exploiting the possibilities of information technology for nursing, necessitates moving beyond the traditional conceptualizations of a nursing information system to that of an integrated clinical information system.

4. **Integrated Clinical Information System**

The term "nursing information system" is limiting in a hospital environment with a multi-disciplinary, multi-departmental patient care focus. A hospital information system in its entirety will be comprised of many inter- and intra-departmental applications designed to supply necessary patient-related information to serve corporate administrative and clinical patient-care functions. A clinical information system is integral to the overall hospital information system, has applications which are unique to nursing and others which derive data elements from complementary applications in other departments/disciplines.

The concept of "integrated systems" is becoming a familiar phrase in the health informatics literature [8,9]. Many existing hospital systems are comprised of several different systems supporting patient care and typically require several entries of the same data. The principle of integration implies that each patient data element is entered into a system with minimal replication and is accessible to all health care providers as necessary.

Ideally, nursing applications should be developed as components of an integrated clinical information system. Patient specific data are the focal point of integrated systems. Considering the multiple sources and users of patient data such a system would provide a common database accessible to all care providers. An integrated system would also support the recent trend of a case management approach to patient care. Clearly there is much patient data which is not exclusive to nursing. There is, however, a need to ascertain those components which are the exclusive responsibility of nursing. Such identification will expedite a more efficient and non-redundant collection of patient information. An integrated patient care system needs to accommodate various levels of users. Not only are the users of an integrated system professionally diverse, they may also be practicing at varying levels of expertise, from the in-house trained technician or aide to the clinical specialist in nursing, medicine, pharmacy, etc. Clinical information systems should: (a) make expert knowledge accessible to the practitioner, (b) provide cues to enhance practice and optimize patient care outcomes, and (c) assimilate practice and research findings to guide the nurse in day to day practice.

5. **Critical Issues for Informatization**

"Informatization" is the synergistic integration of computer, nursing, and information science which facilitates the generation of new knowledge for nursing practice [10]. Clinical information system developments should be driven by the ultimate goal of informatization: the management of outcomes. The successful attainment of informatization in clinical care delivery settings will be contingent upon an understanding of the informational requirements of care providers and the possibilities for meeting those needs given existing technology. Issues of an informational, technological, and organizational nature will need to be addressed in order to achieve such an understanding. The central leadership role of nursing in addressing these issues and the application of state of the art technology to clinical settings are identified as focal to realizing the epitome of an integrate clinical information system.

5.1 Informational

With increasing sophistication and insight, nurse researchers are attempting to disentangle and understand the complex processes of nurses' clinical decision-making [11,12]. Several nurses have addressed the relative value of computerized decision support tools for nursing practice [13,14,15,16]. Although there is a plethora of literature on decision-making, an understanding of the elements of information processing, clinical inference, and intuitive knowledge in nursing remains somewhat elusive. In the future, systems modelled on these processes will indeed simplify the tasks of organizing and interpreting clinical data, and hopefully result in more efficient and efficacious patient outcomes.

5.2 Technical

For many organizations, no matter which generation or configuration of information system was selected, the technology seemed to be outmoded within a few short months of implementation, if not purchase. The occurrence of premature obsolescence has been largely due to a propensity to under-resource these projects. Anticipating future technological advances and strategically designing a system infrastructure to allow for the integration of new technologies has been and continues to be a major challenge for information systems personnel and health care providers. The technical elements of data capture, processing, storage, and retrieval capacities will likely continue to evolve, becoming less costly with increased capabilities in multiple orders of magnitude. In the future, we can expect a clinical information system with the technical flexibility which allows for non-sequential/ multi-dimensional access to data.

Health care administrators are demanding increased system efficiency and immediate access to quality information. Care providers are seeking system support to ease the burden of increased clinical complexity in environments of declining human resources. Therefore, clinical information systems need to be designed such that meaningful information is accessible by whoever needs it, whenever they need it, and where ever they need it.

The key elements of clinical information for technical consideration are accessibility, portability, and user-defined data.

5.2.1 Accessibility

Evaluations of automated systems to support nursing information management have yet to provide a convincing argument for either central or bedside as a preferred location of access. We advance the notion of a compact, wholly portable device, with two-way communication for data entry, retrieval, and management. Moreover, as bio-technical research continues to develop improved, non-invasive, cost-effective patient monitoring/assist devices, increasing volumes of clinical data will be readily available to care providers.

5.2.2 Portability

System interaction should be possible from where ever the care provider legitimately requires access without impeding the delivery of patient care. The user interface should allow for multiple devices and modes of data entry, retrieval, and manipulation. The incorporation of multi-media capabilities (e.g. voice and image) and the accommodation of mouse, bar code, pen-based, and radio-frequency technologies will provide unprecedented opportunities in health care computing.

5.2.3 User Defined Data

A majority of clinical information systems have been designed on the basis of existing manual systems. Automating previous practice without evaluating re-engineering requirements adds limited value to the practice of care providers. Care providers must still sift through the volumes of data collected on individual patients and ensure that they have considered all data elements in the process of making a clinical judgement. However, if a system presented patient data and information to care providers in a manner not only unique to the scope of their practice, but also within the limits of their clinical expertise, the potential for added value would be tremendous.

5.3 Organizational

An organization's mission, philosophy, and goals should provide the foundation for the development of a philosophy of information management. Requisite to the operationalization an innovative information management philosophy is a clearly articulated strategic direction with unmitigated corporate support. A critical element of that support will be the acceptance and encouragement of process re-engineering to move the organization to successful informatization.

6. Directions for the Future

- Need for a corporate view to advance the development of wholly integrated clinical information systems.
- Need for a collaborative model between health professionals, information services, and vendors.
- Need for increased sophistication in the development of decision support tools for practice and administration. Systems should be designed to make decision support available to practitioners at all levels and incorporate current clinical data and research findings on a continuous basis.
- Need to apply new technology including multimedia and portable devices for the input, retrieval, monitoring and manipulation of data. The use of robotics should begin to provide more consistent data/information while assisting in the delivery of patient care and providing opportunities for improved process re-engineering.

References

[1] Saba V K and McCormick K A. *Essentials of Computers for Nurses*. Philadelphia: J.B. Lippincott, 1986.
[2] Gassert C A. Defining nursing information system requirements: A linked model. Proceedings: *The Thirteenth Annual Symposium on Computer Applications in Medical Care*. Washington, D.C.: IEEE Society Press, 1989:779–783.
[3] Graves J R and Corcoran S. Design of nursing information systems: Conceptual and practice elements. *J Prof Nurs* 1988, 4:168–177.
[4] Miller E. A conceptual model of the information requirements of nursing organizations. Proceedings: *The Thirteenth Annual Symposium on Computer Applications in Medical Care*. Washington, D.C.: IEEE Computer Society, 1989:784–788.
[5] Rieder K A and Norton D A. An integrated nursing information system—A planning model. *Comput Nurs* 1984, 2:73–79.
[6] Powell N. Designing and developing a computerized hospital information system. *Nursing Management* 1982, 13:40–45.
[7] Nagle L M. The impact of computerization on nurses' thinking. *Unpublished manuscript*, 1990.
[8] Ball M J and Douglas J V. Integration of systems for patient care. *Proceedings of Fourth International Conference on Nursing Use of Computers and Information Science*. New York: Springer-Verlag, 1991:110–114.
[9] Korpman R A. Integrated nursing systems: The future is now. Proceedings of Fourth International Conference on Nursing Use of Computers and Information Science. New York: Springer-Verlag, 1991: Addendum.
[10] Shamian J, Nagle L M, and Hannah K J. Optimizing outcomes of nursing informatization. In *MEDINFO 92* Lun K C, Degoulet P, Piemme T E, and Rienhoff O (eds.). Amsterdam: North Holland, 1992:976–980.
[11] Corcoran S, Narayan S, and Moreland H. "Thinking aloud" as a strategy to improve clinical decision making. *Heart Lung* 1988, 17:463–468.

[12] Thiele J E, Baldwin J H, Hyde R S, Sloan B, and Strandquist G A. An investigation of decision theory: What are the effects of teaching clue recognition? *J Nurs Educ* 1986, 25:319–324.

[13] Brennan P F and McHugh M J. Clinical decision-making and computer support. *App Nurs Res* 1988, 1:89–93.

[14] Cuddigan J E, Logan S, Evans S, Hoesing H. Evaluation of an artificial-intelligence-based nursing decision support system in a clinical setting. Proceedings: Third International Symposium on Nursing Use of Computers and Information Science. St. Louis: C.V. Mosby, 1988:629–636.

[15] Henry S B, LeBreck D B, and Holzemer W L. The use of computer simulations to measure clinical decision making in nursing. Proceedings: Third International Symposium on Nursing Use of Computers and Information Science. St. Louis: C.V. Mosby, 1988:485–491.

[16] Sinclair V G. Potential effects of decision support systems on the role of the nurse. *Comput Nurs* 1990, 8:60–65.

4
Toward a Uniform Language for Nursing in the US: Work of the American Nurses Association Steering Committee on Databases to Support Clinical Practice

RITA D. ZIELSTORFF, NORMA M. LANG, VIRGINIA K. SABA, KATHLEEN A. McCORMICK, and D. KATHY MILHOLLAND

1. Introduction

Unique representation of concepts is a prerequisite for computer-stored databases that are designed for retrieval, aggregation, and analysis of data. For many years, it has been the vision of the American Nurses Association (ANA) to achieve a uniform language for nursing practice, in order to be able to gather, store, retrieve, aggregate, and analyze data pertinent to the profession. Collaboration with inter- and intra-disciplinary groups is an essential prerequisite, as is integration with other health care data systems. In 1989, a charge was given to the ANA Cabinet on Nursing Practice to provide policy recommendations related to the development of database systems to describe and measure the quality and cost of nursing care. To carry out that charge, the Cabinet appointed a Steering Committee on Databases to Support Clinical Nursing Practice (hereafter referred to as the Steering Committee). This paper reports on the work accomplished by the Steering Committee to date and on its future plans.

2. Background

The Steering Committee consists of approximately nine individuals who represent a number of affiliations in the nursing community. There are

Reprinted with permission from *MEDINFO '95: Proceedings of the Eighth World Congress on Medical Informatics*; Greenes, R.A., Peterson, H.E. & Protti, D.J. (Eds.). 1995. Pp. 1362–1366. Edmonton, Alberta, Canada: Canadian Organization for the Advancement of Computers in Health (COACH).

academics, researchers, practitioners, administrators, educators, and policy makers in the group. The strength of the group is its diversity and its depth of expertise in a variety of areas. In addition, consultants from government and private organizations, as well as researchers in the field of language development in nursing, are frequently brought in to inform the Committee. The charge to the Steering Committee is to:

- Propose policy and program initiatives regarding nursing classification schemes, uniform nursing datasets, and the inclusion of nursing data elements in national databases.
- Build national datasets for clinical nursing practice based on elements contained in standards, criteria, and guidelines.
- Coordinate ANA's initiatives related to all public and private efforts regarding the development of databases and the relationship to the development and maintenance of standards of practice and guidelines and payment for the reform of nursing services [1].

The Steering Committee meets twice yearly to conduct its work and appoints task forces that meet as needed to complete their assignments.

3. Accomplishments to Date

3.1 Foundations

As a foundation for its work, the Steering Committee adopted some fundamental premises. It proposed definitions for terms that are commonly used in relation to classification work; it affirmed the tenets of the 1980 ANA *Social Policy Statement*, which advocated the Nursing Process as the framework for organizing nursing data (i.e., according to nursing assessment, nursing diagnosis, nursing interventions, and nursing-sensitive outcomes) [2]; and, it endorsed the Nursing Minimum Data Set (NMDS) as the essential set of data elements that must be included in any databases or record systems that describe nursing practice [3, 4].

3.2 Analysis of Federal Databases

The Steering Committee has examined several large federally held databases for the presence of nursing-related data elements. These include the Health Care Financing Administration claims database and the quality of care databases. The details of this analysis are provided elsewhere [1]. The summary is that while linkages to some elements of the NMDS are evident, all of the elements are not found in the existing claims and quality of care databases. In particular, even when elements can be found that relate to some nursing assessments, diagnoses, interventions, and outcomes, there is almost never a linkage with a nurse provider; so it is not possible to assess the quality of care in relation to nursing care provided. Including the missing elements and relating this data to nurse providers is essential if full evaluation of the quality of patient care is to be determined. The Steering Committee is working to rectify this situation, by making specific recommendations to the appropriate agencies as to the data elements that must be included.

3.3 Nursing Data Elements in Bibliographic and Other Index Databases

The National Library of Medicine (NLM) maintains several large data-bases that index bibliographic data, expert systems, practice guidelines, and other knowledge sources for the practice of health care. Two of these indexing schemes are MeSH (Medical Subject Headings), which is used to index a vast number of biomedical and health citations, and UMLS (Unified Medical Language System), which is being developed to transcend the differences in medical and health vocabularies currently used to code health-related data [5]. The Steering Committee is working closely with NLM staff to augment the representation of nursing terminology in these and other databases maintained at the Library [1, 6]. In particular, the NLM staff have agreed to add to the UMLS all nursing vocabularies endorsed by the ANA through the Steering Committee. This work is currently in progress.

3.4 Toward a Uniform Language for Nursing: A Phased Approach

The Steering Committee recognized very early that imposition of a monolithic nomenclature on the profession would be unlikely to succeed at this point in nursing's history. No nomenclature had yet been developed that claimed to codify all of nursing. And yet, the development of a single nomenclature is an important goal, for all of the reasons stated earlier. After extended discussion, it was decided by the group to take a phased approach. First, all of the existing work in nomenclature development in nursing would be examined; second, criteria would be developed for recognizing classifications and nomenclatures that would be eligible for inclusion in an endorsed set of nomenclatures—so that those who were developing databases could select from among these the one(s) that best suited their purposes; third, a method would be developed that would map the concepts among these classifications—so that databases coded in di-verse systems could be mapped to each other. This process would result in a Unified Nursing Language System, similar to the NLM's concept of a Unified Medical Language System, but representing only nursing practice terminologies. Finally, it was hoped that through the mapping process, a common set of concepts would lead to the "discovery" of a Uniform Language, one that could be accepted by all of the profession as representing the essential elements of nursing practice: assessments, diagnoses, interventions, and outcomes. This approach is shown schematically in Figure 1.

Criteria for Recognizing Nomenclatures

The Steering Committee adopted the following criteria for recognizing vocabularies and classifications for clinical practice. Vocabularies/classifications for clinical practice should:

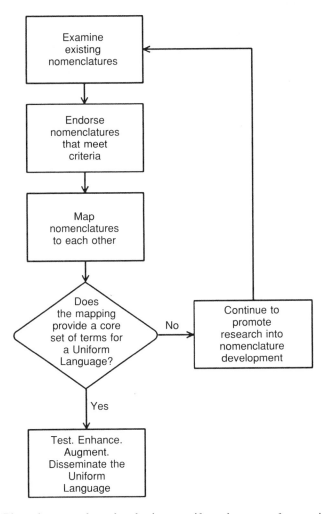

FIGURE 1. Phased approach to developing a uniform language for nursing practice

1. be clinically useful for making diagnostic, intervention, and outcome decisions;
2. be stated in clear and unambiguous terms, with terms defined precisely;
3. have been tested for the reliability of the vocabulary terms;
4. have been validated as useful for clinical purposes;
5. be accompanied by documentation of a systematic methodology for development;
6. be accompanied by evidence of a process for periodic review and provision for addition, revision, or deletion of terms;
7. have terms that are associated with a unique identifier or code.

Criteria for recognizing classification schemes used for nursing research or to classify nursing literature were also adopted. Terms should:

1. be stated in clear and unambiguous terms;
2. have been validated as useful for classifying its domain;
3. have a taxonomic structure that is conceptually coherent;
4. be accompanied by documentation of a systematic methodology for development;
5. be accompanied by evidence of a process for periodic review and a provision for addition, revision, or deletion of terms;
6. have terms that are associated with a unique identifier or code.

In the course of its review, the Steering Committee noted that there has been much commendable, scientifically grounded research in the development of nursing nomenclatures and taxonomies. The Committee has formally recognized the following:

• North American Nursing Diagnosis Association (NANDA) Approved List of Nursing Diagnoses [7]
• The Omaha System [8]
• Home Health Care Classification [9]
• Nursing Interventions Classification [10]

Several additional classifications are under consideration for formal ANA recognition. The Committee recognizes that, at this time, no one vocabulary is used consistently throughout the country, nor are the existing vocabularies fully established. Indeed, the use of multiple vocabularies and classifications for nursing's rich language is consistent with the diversity of purposes for which the schemes are used.

Mapping the Nomenclatures

Task forces have been developed to begin mapping the nomenclatures to each other. Expertise in nursing classification, nursing nomenclature, and the broader field of nosology is being applied. At this point, progress is very encouraging and confirms that: a) the task is possible, and b) the results are useful.

4. International Activities

In addition to the work described above, the Steering Committee has been active in promoting the inclusion of nursing-related data in international classification systems. The Steering Committee Chair (NL) is a consultant to the World Health Organization's Unit of Nursing and the International Council of Nurses to work jointly on the development of a classification of nursing that could be included in the WHO's Family of Disease and Health-Related Classifications. Subsequently, the ICN began work on an International Classification of Nursing Practice (ICNP).

5. Future Plans

The Steering Committee will be continuing the work on mapping nursing nomenclatures and, as that work progresses, will map the nursing nomenclatures to external classification systems such as ICD and CPT. This work will be coordinated with ongoing projects such as the UMLS and the work of the Computer-Based Record Institute Workgroup on Codes and Structures. Additional nursing nomenclatures will be considered by the Steering Committee as those products mature sufficiently for review. The work of the many informatics standards groups, such as Health Level Seven, CPRI, and ASTM, will be monitored to ensure that the structure and content of these standards includes nursing nomenclature and data elements.

6. Conclusion

The charge to the Steering Committee is very broad and will doubtless be ongoing. However, significant progress has been made to identify and target priority areas that will move forward nursing's agenda of having national databases that reflect nursing practice for the purposes of quality assessment and costing. With the support of the American Nurses Association, and with the cooperation of nurse researchers, practicing nurses, federal agencies, and policy-making bodies, the goal is within reach.

Acknowledgments. The following were members of the Steering Committee on Databases to Support Clinical Nursing Practice from 1989 through 1992: Norma M. Lang, PhD, RN, FAAN (Chair); Rita D. Zielstorff, MS, RN, FAAN (Vice-Chair); Carole Hudgings, PhD, RN; Ada Jacox, PhD, RN; Jane Lancour, MS, RN; Margaret L. McClure, EdD, RN, FAAN; Kathleen McCormick, PhD, RN; Virginia K. Saba, EdD, RN, FAAN; Thomas E. Stenvig, MS, MPH, RN, CNAA. Consultant and ANA staff to the Steering Committee during that period were: Patricia Prescott,

28   R.D. Zielstorff, et al.

PhD, RN, FAAN; D. Kathy Milholland, PhD, RN; Karen S. O'Connor, MS RN.

References

[1] Lang N. M., Hudgings C., Jacox A., Lancour J., McClure M., McCormick K., Saba V. K., Stenvig T. E., Zielstorff R. D., Prescott P., Milholland K., & O'Connor K. S. *Toward a National Data Base for Nursing Practice.* Washington, DC: American Nurses Association (In press).
[2] American Nurses Association. *Social Policy Statement.* Kansas City, Mo: Author (1980).
[3] Werley H. H. & Lang N. M. (eds). *Identification of the Nursing Minimum Data Set.* New York: Springer Publishing Co. (1988).
[4] Werley H., Devine E., Zorn C., Ryan P., & Westra B. "The Nursing Minimum Data Set: Abstraction Tool for Standardized, Comparable, Essential Data." *American Journal of Public Health* (1991) 81(4): 421–426.
[5] Humphreys B. L. & Lindberg D. A. B. "Building the Unified Medical Language System." In Kingsland L. C. III (ed). *Proceedings of the Thirteenth Annual Symposium on Computer applications in Medical Care.* Washington DC: IEEE Computer Society Press (1989): 475–480.
[6] McCormick K. A., Lang N., Zielstorff R., Milholland D. K., & Saba V. "Toward Standard Classification Schemes for Nursing Language—Recommendations of the American Nurses Association Steering Committee on Databases to Support Nursing Practice." *Journal of the American Medical Informatics Association.* (In press).
[7] North American Nursing Diagnosis Association. *Classification of Nursing Diagnoses: Proceedings of the Tenth Conference.* Carroll-Johnson R. M. (ed). Philadelphia: Lippincott (1994).
[8] Martin K. S. & Scheet N. J. *The Omaha System: Applications for Community Health Nursing.* Phila: WB Saunders (1992).
[9] Saba V. K. "The Classification of Home Health Care Nursing Diagnoses and Interventions." *Caring* (1992) 11(3): 50–57.
[10] Iowa Intervention Project. *Taxonomy of Nursing Interventions.* University of Iowa (1992).

5
A New Paradigm for Computer-Based Nursing Information Systems Twenty Care Components

Virginia K. Saba

1. Background

The Twenty Care Components provide a new paradigm for computer-based nursing information systems. They provide the structure for documenting the nursing process. They are used to assess, cost, evaluate, and statistically analyze as well as link the documenting of the nursing process phases. The Twenty Care Components were derived from empirical data from a recently completed home care classification study [2]. The purpose of the study was to develop a method to assess and classify home health Medicare patients to predict the resource requirements and determine their care needs for nursing and all other home care services; it also measured their outcomes of care [5].

A national stratified sample of 646 home health agencies (HHAs) collected retrospective data on 8,840 discharged cases. Data was abstracted on their entire episode of home health care (admission to discharge). The study data included 40,361 nursing diagnoses/patient problems and 73,529 patient services (skilled nursing services, treatments, activities, and/or interventions) provided during the episode of care. They were collected as narrative statements, which had to be coded for computer processing so that the study data could be statistically analyzed.

The coding strategy developed has since been called the *Saba Home Health Care Classifications (HHCC) of Nursing Diagnoses and Interventions*. The HHCCs consist of 145 nursing diagnoses with three expected outcomes and 160 nursing interventions with four type intervention actions. Each of the schemes is classified according to the Twenty Care Components [3, 4].

Reprinted with permission from *MEDINFO '95: Proceedings of the Eighth World Congress on Medical Informatics*; Greenes, R.A., Peterson, H.E. & Protti, D.J. (Eds.). 1995. Pp. 1404–1406. Edmonton, Alberta, Canada: Canadian Organization for the Advancement of Computers in Health (COACH).

2. Description of Care Components

A Care Component is defined as a cluster of elements that represent a behavioral, functional, psychological, and physiological care patterns. The Twenty Care Components were especially designed to code, classify, and statistically analyze the four taxonomies. They were developed for coding the four phases of the nursing process—nursing assessment, nursing diagnoses, nursing interventions, and care outcomes. They make it possible to link these four phases, resulting in a new paradigm designed to classify and statistically analyze nursing process. The care components provide a holistic approach toward assessing clinical nursing practice. They differ from the "body systems chapters" used to classify medical diseases and conditions as found in the International Classification of Diseases (ICD). They are defined in Table 1.

3. Uses of Care Components

The Twenty Care Components can be used to assess, document, cost, evaluate, and statistically classify as well as link the four nursing process phases. They offer a new paradigm for nursing and provide a holistic approach toward coding and statistically classifying clinical nursing practice. Because they can statistically link the four phases of the nursing process, clinical nursing practice can be tracked and audited; outcomes can also be evaluated. The linked phases will provide nursing care profiles to develop integrated care protocols and/or plans.

The use of the care components make it possible for computer-based nursing information systems to store, process, and statistically analyze the nursing care of patients. They can be used to predict resource use, determine care requirements, and develop clinical care paths for the electronic documenting of nursing care. Such systems will make it possible to provide nurses with the on-line interactive capability to assess, evaluate, and revise their care as needed. Such systems will enhance the decision-support systems and improve the decision-making of nurses.

A standardized classification of nursing practice can be integrated easily with other clinical data. They can be compared across health care settings and used for discharge planning and the continuity of care data sets. They can be used to determine the cost as well as the payment of nursing care.

4. Conclusions

This new paradigm for computer-based nursing information systems consists of Twenty Care Components that provide a means of coding, classifying, and statistically analyzing nursing taxonomies. They provide the

TABLE 1. Home health care classification—20 care components: alphabetical list with definitions

---

1. *Activity component*
   Cluster of elements that involve the use of energy in carrying out bodily actions.
2. *Bowel elimination component*
   Cluster of elements that involve the gastrointestinal system.
3. *Cardiac component*
   Cluster of elements that involve the heart, blood vessels, and circulatory system.
4. *Cognitive component*
   Cluster of elements involving the mental and cerebral processes.
5. *Coping component*
   Cluster of elements that involve the ability to deal with responsibilities, problems, or difficulties.
6. *Fluid volume component*
   Cluster of elements that involve liquid consumption.
7. *Health behavior component*
   Cluster of elements that involve actions to sustain, maintain, or regain health.
8. *Medication component*
   Cluster of elements that involve medicinal substances.
9. *Metabolic component*
   Cluster of elements that involve the endocrine and immunological processes.
10. *Nutritional component*
    Cluster of elements that involve the intake of food and nutrients.
11. *Physical regulation component*
    Cluster of elements that involve bodily processes.
12. *Respiratory component*
    Cluster of elements that involve breathing and the pulmonary system.
13. *Role relationship component*
    Cluster of elements involving interpersonal, work, social, and sexual interactions.
14. *Safety component*
    Cluster of elements that involve prevention of injury, danger, or loss.
15. *Self-care component*
    Cluster of elements that involve the ability to carry out activities to maintain oneself.
16. *Self-concept component*
    Cluster of elements that involve an individual's mental image of oneself.
17. *Sensory component*
    Cluster of elements that involve the senses.
18. *Skin integrity component*
    Cluster of elements that involve the mucous membrane, corneal, integumentary, or subcutaneous structures of the body.
19. *Tissue perfusion component*
    Cluster of elements that involve the oxygenation of tissues.
20. *Urinary elimination component*
    Cluster of elements that involve the genitourinary system.

---

structure for documenting the nursing process and link the phases using a holistic approach. The care components can be used to assess, document, cost, evaluate, as well as link the nursing process phases. They are classes that can be used to compare nursing care across health care settings, nationally and internationally. They can be used as the data standard for the different taxonomies being developed for nursing assessment, diagnoses, interventions, and outcomes.

The Twenty Care Components have been recognized by the American Nurses Association as the classes for the Saba HHCC; we now need to use them [1]. We need to statistically analyze nursing care across health care settings, nationally and internationally. We could compare nursing care on-line and interactively, making it possible for nurses around the world to communicate and compare their care paths and protocols.

References

[1] American Nurses Association. *Toward standardization of nursing practice.* Washington, DC: ANA (1992).
[2] Saba V. K. *Home health care classification project.* Washington: Georgetown University, (NTIS# PB92-177013/AS) (February, 1991).
[3] Saba V. K. "The classification of home health care nursing diagnoses and interventions." *Caring* (1992a) 10(3): 50–57.
[4] Saba V. K. "Home health care classification." *Caring* (May 1992b) 10(5): 58–60.
[5] Saba V. K. & Zuckerman A. E. "A new home health care classification method." *Caring* (October, 1992) 10(10): 27–34.

6
Nursing Intervention Lexicon and Taxonomy Preliminary Categorization

Susan J. Grobe

1.0 Significance

The nursing action (or intervention) and the individual's response to care represent a central phenomenon that is an essential component of the record of nursing care. The absence of a systematic and uniform way of referring to nursing care phenomena presents an important obstacle to the automation of nursing records. Even when automated systems are employed, the use of narrative, natural language to record nursing interventions usually precludes the retrieval of nursing interventions for abstraction and summarization. On the other hand, use of automated systems that demand rigidly controlled vocabulary and structured menu terminology choices inhibit practitioners from freely expressing their impressions in sufficiently individualized detail. Consequently, discovery of methods that allow nurse clinicians to describe their care without unduly restricting their choice of terminology represents an important area of investigation.

This study is important for three reasons: first, it focuses on nurses' natural language expressions of clinical care activities; second, it demonstrates that scientific methods can be used to build dictionaries and thesauri of nursing intervention clinical terms and indicates that these terms can be used for classification purposes; and third, it suggests that, once the dictionary or lexicon of clinical terms is available, it may be possible to design automated methods by which nurses' clinical terms can be effectively abstracted and classified.

Reprinted from *MEDINFO '92: Proceedings of the Seventh World Congress on Medical Informatics*, Lun, K.C., Degoulet, P., Piemme, T.E. & Rienhoff, O. (Eds.). 1992. Pp. 981–986, with kind permission from Elsevier Science—NL, Sara Burgerhartstraat 25, 1055 KV Amsterdam, The Netherlands.

In summary, the language methods used in this study are important because they demonstrate preliminary attempts by which nursing intervention terminology can be used for automated abstraction and classification. Once a local dictionary or thesaurus has been established and the language methods described, validated and confirmed, it is possible that data from electronic care records can be automatically abstracted and mapped to a "metathesaurus" of uniform nursing terms. As a result, data can be aggregated across settings and made accessible for retrieval for a variety of purposes.

2.0 Purpose

The purpose of this paper is to report on the language-based methods used for the preliminary categorization and classification of 1317 nursing intervention statements generated by masters' prepared practicing nurses ($N = 94$). The language paradigm was used for the study because of the relative instability of clinical language and the necessity to continually update automated systems' data dictionaries as well as respond to terminology changes that occur. Thus, language-based methods are useful both for the derivation of the classification system and for its continual updating. Furthermore, language-based methods can be used to deal with subtle variations in nursing terminology, synonyms and differences in the meaning of terms based on the context of their use. Language-based methods allow for terminology variation and may be useful for establishing a uniform terminology that can be used to bridge different vocabularies.

3.0 Review of Literature

Nursing actions have been classified in a variety of ways using four primary approaches. These approaches have ranged from categorizations derived by summarizing lists of nursing interventions to categorizations produced from systematic study and validation-based approaches. None of these approaches, however, has been developed using language methods. Furthermore, few classifications have been developed using a systematic research approach. Even fewer classifications have been validated through their use with automated clinical record systems. Only two classification systems could be found in which one or more of the following criteria were met: systematic development through the use of a research based approach, validation by an individual other than the developer, or, validation through use in an automated systems environment [1–3]. These classification systems are also similar in that they permit the categorization of nursing interventions from the context of community health nursing.

Several categorization schema, derived from summarizing lists of nursing interventions, have been proposed. One of the earliest of these proposals was developed by Campbell [4]. She proposed seven nursing intervention categories: assistive, hygienic, rehabilitative, supportive, preventive, observational, and educational, and has used four categories to present a revised list of interventions: nursing treatments, nursing observations, health teaching, and medical treatments performed by nurses [5]. Snyder proposed the following category scheme for the nursing interventions identified in her book: movement and proprioceptive strategies, cognitive strategies, sensory strategies, and other strategies [6]. Bulechek and McCloskey used four categories to group a list of nursing interventions: stress management, lifestyle alteration, acute care management, and communication [7]. Similarly, McFarland and McFarlane described two ways in which nursing interventions could be categorized: by the level of assistance represented by the intervention and by types of activities performed. They proposed ten categories of nursing interventions that include: ongoing assessment and monitoring, coordination of resources and health care services, emotional support or therapy, guidance or counseling, teaching, acting for or doing for the patient, collaborating with the patient, referring the patient to other health team members, monitoring the environment, and supporting and teaching the family [8]. Saba, O'Hare, Zuckerman, Boondas, Levine, & Oatway categorized nursing actions, in order to codify them, as: assess, direct care, teach, and manage [9]. Finally, the Sigma Theta Tau Directory of Nurse Researchers' categories, derived from researchers' reports of the topics of their research, includes only two intervention categories: physiological and psychosocial [10].

A second way nursing intervention category schemes have been derived is by describing nursing activities, actions, or functions. Hagen described the domain of nursing care activities as: nursing care plans; provision for safe and comfortable patient environment; meeting physical needs of patients; meeting physiological needs of patients; meeting psychological, social and religious needs of patients; implementing medical regimen for patients, teaching patients and/or family; keeping records of nursing care given to patients; and, evaluating the patient's responses to nursing interventions [11]. Both Barnard [12] and Joel [13] proposed a four category model of nursing intervention categories. That proposed by Barnard included monitoring, information giving, supporting, and therapy while that proposed by Joel included teaching, supporting, medical facilitation, and compensation for diminished functional status. Scholtfeldt [14] identified appraisal, compensatory, sustaining and supporting, guiding and teaching, stimulating and inspiring strategies as nursing action categories while Phillips [15] identified doing for, monitoring, arranging for, assessing, and socializing as primary nursing action categories. Kasch [16] described nursing as including information, influence, comforting, and relaxational and identity functions while Friss [17] described nursing actions as assisting, intervening, informing, and coordinating.

A third way that nursing intervention categories have developed has been from consensus activities. Resulting from a Nursing Minimum Data Set consensus conference, Werley and Lang initially proposed a 16 category classification system that was subsequently reduced to seven categories [18]. These categories included surveillance and/or observation, supportive measure, assistive measure, treatment and/or procedure, emotional support, teaching, and coordination. In a paper presented at a consensus conference, Corless and Riordan described the following categories of nursing care activities: personal support-coaching, advocacy, education, physical support-activities of daily living, therapeutics-for-healing, symptom control and cure or cure related acts, and, assessment-monitoring [19]. In a paper presented at a nursing diagnosis conference, Bulechek and McCloskey, described the following seven groups of nursing activities: assessment activities to make a nursing diagnosis, assessment activities to gather information for a physician to make a diagnosis, nurse-initiated treatments in response to nursing diagnoses, physician-initiated treatments in response to medical diagnoses, daily essential function activities, activities to evaluate the effects of nursing and medical treatments, and administrative and indirect care activities [20].

A fourth way that nursing intervention categories have developed has been through systematic nursing research. One of the earliest studies conducted to investigate the categorization of nursing actions was reported by Verhonick, Nicholas, Glor, & McCarthy [21]. These investigators identified the following categories of nursing action: therapeutic (prescribed by a physician), supportive (based on nursing judgment and independent of a physician's order), and four other categories consisting of different options about phoning the physician. Ciuca reviewed over 1100 nursing care plans and described seven groups comprised of a total of 56 possible nursing activities [22]. His groups (categories) were as follows: group 1 entries related to medications, treatments, monitoring of vital signs, intake and output and diagnostic studies; group II actions related to prevention of harmful sequelae; group III actions related to preservation of body defenses; group IV actions related to elimination; group V actions related to comfort measures; group VI actions related to emotional support; and group VII actions related to rehabilitation and discharge planning.

Kane, Kingsbury, Colton, & Estes analyzed 222 reported nursing activities and developed seventeen categories of patient needs clustered into three large categories: coordination of care, direct client care, and health promotion and client self-care [23]. This study was conducted to validate clinical nursing activities for the purpose of establishing content validity for the nursing performance examinations for the United States National Council of State Boards of Nursing. The first two categories of nursing activities grouped under coordination of care included: staff development and collaboration, and quality assurance and safety. The second group of eleven activity categories, grouped under direct client care, included: planning/managing client care; protecting client; meeting acute physical needs; preparing clients for procedures; monitoring clients at risk; assisting clients with mobility needs; controlling pain; meeting client needs related to parenting; performing routine nursing activities; and meeting acute emotional/behavioral needs. The third group of four activity categories grouped under health promotion and client self-care included: assisting clients with self-care; helping clients cope with stress; supporting client's family; and, immunizing/screening.

Two other studies have been conducted in which intervention classifications for community health nursing use have been proposed. The first one that resulted in a classification of nursing activities was the Taxonomy of Ambulatory Care developed by Verran [3] and later used by Cohen, Arnold, Brown, & Brooten [24] to validate nursing activities in neonatal transitional care follow up. The categories of nursing activities identified by Verran included: patient counseling, health care maintenance, primary care, patient education, therapeutic care, normative care and nonclient centered care [3]. Cohen et al [24] used Verran's taxonomy to determine if all the nursing interventions employed by the nurse specialist providing follow-up care for neonatal infants could be adequately captured thereby confirming the heuristic value of Verran's taxonomy. The second scheme for classifying nursing interventions, by Martin and Scheet of the Omaha Visiting Nurse Association, has four categories: health teaching; guidance and counseling; treatments and procedures; case management and, surveillance [1–2]. Under development and testing since 1975, this classification scheme is currently used in the automated system used by this Visiting Nurse Association to plan and record nursing care. It is also used for quality improvement efforts by the agency.

Thus, while several classifications of nursing activities or interventions have been proposed from a variety of perspectives, The Taxonomy of Ambulatory Care Nursing [3] and the Omaha Intervention Scheme [1–2] are the only two intervention classifications that have been validated either through use in an automated system or through an empirical investigation. Although both schemes have been developed using an empirically based inductive approach, neither has been developed nor validated using language methods as proposed in this study.

4.0 Study Purpose

The purpose of this phase of the study is to define the categories for nursing interventions, use the categories for classifying the lexicon of nursing intervention statements, and validate the adequacy of the classification using automated natural language methods.

4.1 Study Methods

In this study, a nursing intervention statement consists of a verb phrase and one or more noun phrases. In study phase I, subjects were instructed to enter "nursing intervention statements" into a Hypercard instrument that contained 12 case studies of community health clients. They were asked to begin each intervention statement with a verb and were also prompted to enter synonyms for each of the verbs used. The instrument has been described previously [25]. No other definition of a nursing intervention statement was given to the subjects. All intervention statements and verb synonyms that were entered by 94 masters prepared nurses were captured and used in this phase of the study. Thirteen hundred and seventeen intervention statements constitute part of the lexicon that served as the body of nursing intervention statements used.

4.2 Procedures

The general categories for nursing interventions were established through a variety of semantics-based approaches. Initially, similar verb terms were mapped (placed in clusters of verbs with similar meanings) and faceted (placed in larger maps to illustrate the broader than and narrower than relationships and the verb terms' equivalence) [25]. Using the knowledge gained from the mapping and faceting procedures, three different investigators used all subjects' interventions to propose categories and their definitions. This iterative process was repeated until consensus was reached on both a category definition and on the interventions that fit into the category.

The preliminary nursing intervention categories, their definitions and selected intervention examples follow. In this preliminary classification, no distinctions are made in terms of whether the interventions were considered dependent or independent, whether they represent direct or indirect care, or whether they were nurse initiated or physician initiated. All interventions entered by the subjects were used.

Based on the analysis of nursing intervention statements, the following categories of interventions were identified: care environment management (CEM), care need determination (CND), care information provision (CIP), care vigilance (CV), care vigilance-specific (CVS), therapeutic care-general (TCG), therapeutic care alternatives (TCA), therapeutic care-cognitive understanding and control (TCCU&C), therapeutic care-psychosocial (TCP), and therapeutic care-specific (TCS). Twelve hundred and forty nursing interventions were assigned to one of these ten categories with 100% agreement by the three independent investigators.

Care Environment Management (CEM)

The deliberative cognitive, physical, or verbal acts which influence the sum total of all the conditions, resources, and services that make up the care surroundings. (Care surroundings may include the immediate physical environs or extend to the family, neighborhood, or community.)

Examples: Arrange needed supplies close at hand for client, i.e., towels, etc. Refer to community self-help group for cardiac patients and families; Develop flash cards to decrease frustration.

Care Need Determination (CND)

The process of gathering information to reach a rational decision that reflects what is judged necessary for individuals who are the focus of care. This process may be either one time or at periodic intervals. (Individuals may be the client, family, significant other(s), or care giver.)

Examples: Assess patient's physical abilities and areas of difficulty; Ask patient to describe how he cares for his feet; Determine current mobility/immobility status from last nursing assessment.

Care Information Provision (CIP)

The communication of facts, thoughts or sentiments to individuals who are the focus of care. (Individuals may be the client, family, significant other(s), or care giver.)

Examples: Instruct family and patient on the care of incisional sites; Demonstrate with patient the mechanics of blood sugar testing; Explain to patient that she would breathe more easily if she cut down on smoking.

Care Vigilance (CV)

The ongoing process of observing and monitoring for maintaining an awareness of the general state or condition of individuals who are the focus of care. (Individuals may be client, family, significant other(s), or caregiver.)

Examples: Assess peripheral pulses; Monitor vital signs q4 hours; Weigh patient every visit.

Care Vigilance Specific (CVS)

The process of observing and monitoring to become alert to or to determine that a problem or potential condition exists that may require a nursing response.

Examples: Assess groshong catheter site for signs of infection; Note amount of blood in stools; Monitor degree of edema QID.

Therapeutic Care-General (TCG)

The deliberative cognitive, physical, or verbal patient-specific procedures, therapies, and medications directed toward the maintenance or improvement of physical health or status of individuals who are the focus of care. (Individuals may be the client, family, significant other(s), or caregiver.)

Examples: Apply lotion to body q8 hours; Keep in semi-Fowler's position; Elevate feet.

Therapeutic Care-Alternatives (TCA)
The deliberative cognitive or verbal activities directed toward offering alternatives for consideration by individuals who are the focus of care. (Individuals may be client, family, significant other(s), or caregiver.)
Examples: Explore options for alternative methods of providing comfort and pain relief; Investigate alternative actions to smoking cigarettes; Encourage patient with wife to examine other housing opportunities available to them.

Therapeutic Care-Cognitive Understanding & Control (TCCU & C)
The activities that support choices or decisions directed toward increasing the patient and family's understanding, promoting physical or psychological independence, or gaining control.
Examples: Reinforce husband's decision to provide care for client; Allow patient to be as independent as possible; Support client's decision to live alone while stressing caregiver desires to be of assistance.

Therapeutic Care-Psychosocial (TCP)
The deliberative cognitive, physical, or verbal activities directed toward support or improvement of psychological status of individuals who are the focus of care. (Individuals may be the client, family, significant other(s), or caregiver.)
Examples: Encourage husband and client to discuss feelings about her illness; Discuss her feelings about loss; Reassure patient regarding issue of addiction.

Therapeutic Care-Specific (TCS)
The deliberative cognitive, physical or verbal patient-specific goal-directed procedures, therapies, and medications directed toward the maintenance or improvement of physical health or status of individuals who are the focus of care. (Individuals may be the client, family, significant other(s), or caregiver.)
Examples: Encourage fluid intake to liquify secretions; Apply warm compress to back for pain relief; Position to avoid dependent edema.

5.0 Results

Using these category definitions, three nurse investigators independently placed the entire set of nursing intervention statements ($N = 1317$) into one of the ten categories. An overall agreement of 100% was achieved for 86.7% ($N = 1240$) of the interventions. An overall agreement of 66% or less was obtained for 77 of the 1317 interventions.

The 1240 interventions that had been independently categorized with total agreement by the three researchers were then subjected to categorization by a rule based expert system, Id-3. The overall percentage of correct judgments (using the investigators' categorizations as the criterion) achieved by Id-3 was 89.7%. Thus when 1240 interventions were assigned to categories by Id-3 using its system rules, 128 interventions were misjudged. The percent correct for each category is reflected in Table 1.

TABLE 1. Correct judgments by category by Id-3

Category	Interventions (N)	Percent correct by Id-3
CEM	394	0.96
CIP	299	0.91
CVS	81	0.95
TCG	158	0.89
TCS	29	0.86
CND	155	0.84
TCP	67	0.82
TCCU	11	0.81
TCA	10	0.80
CV	36	0.47

5.1 Discussion

Id-3's misjudgments ($N = 128$) are being examined using knowledge of their erroneous category placement in an attempt to determine the possible reasons for the misjudgments. Possible alternatives being examined include Id-3's rules, their application, or data dictionary improvements. Revision of these preliminary categories and perhaps the combination of some categories may be indicated when these analyses are complete. The revised category scheme with its new definitions will again be subjected to independent investigators' categorization to establish a criterion for comparison. Use of Id-3 and other linguistic methods will be attempted to achieve the most robust intervention category scheme possible for contrast with natural language analyses using different procedures.

References

[1] Martin K, Scheet N, Crews C, and Simmons D. *Client management information system for community health nursing agencies.* (NTIS Accession No. HRP-090723). Springfield, VA: National Technical Information Service, 1986.
[2] Martin K, and Scheet N. *The Omaha system: Applications for community health nursing.* Philadelphia: W.B. Saunders, 1992.
[3] Verran J. Patient classification research: new directions. *West J Nurs Res* 1983, 5: 91–93.
[4] Campbell C. *Nursing diagnosis and intervention in nursing practice.* New York: John Wiley and Sons, 1978.
[5] Campbell C. *Nursing diagnosis and intervention in nursing practice.* New York: John Wiley & Sons, 1984.
[6] Snyder M. *Independent nursing interventions.* New York: John Wiley & Sons, 1985.
[7] Bulechek G M, and McCloskey J C. *Nursing interventions: Treatments for nursing diagnoses.* Philadelphia: W.B. Saunders, 1985.
[8] McFarland G, and McFarlane E. *Nursing diagnosis and intervention: Planning for patient care.* St. Louis: C.V. Mosby, 1989.
[9] Saba V K, O'Hare P A, Zuckerman A E, Boondas J, Levine E, and Oatway

D M. A nursing intervention taxonomy for home health care. *Nurs Health Care* 1991, 12: 296–299.

[10] Hudgings C, Hogan R, and Stevenson J S (eds.). *Directory of nurse researchers* (3rd ed). Indianapolis: Sigma Theta Tau International, 1990.

[11] Hagen E. Conceptual issues in the appraisal of the quality of care. Paper prepared for the conference on Assessment of Nursing Services. Publ. No. (HRA) 75–40. Washington, DC: USDHEW, 1975: 133.

[12] Barnard K. *ANA social policy statement.* Paper presented to the University of Texas Student Nurses' Association, Austin, Texas, 1984.

[13] Joel L A. Preparing clinical specialists for prospective payment. In *Patterns in education: The unfolding of nursing.* New York: National League for Nursing, 1985.

[14] Schlotfeldt R. Vision for the future. *The Schlotfeldt Lecture.* (Available from The Frances Payne Bolton School of Nursing, Case Western Reserve University, Cleveland, Ohio), 1985.

[15] Phillips L R. Caring for the frail elderly at home. In L. R. Phillips (ed.), *A clinician's guide to the critique and utilization of nursing research.* Norwalk, CT.: Appleton–Century–Crofts, 1986: 130–160.

[16] Kasch C. Toward a theory of nursing action: Skills and competency in nurse-patient interaction. *Nurs Research* 1986, 35: 226–230.

[17] Friss L. What do nurses do? *J Nurs Adm*, 1977, 7: 24–28.

[18] Werley H H, and Lang N M. (eds). *Identification of the nursing minimum data set.* New York: Springer, 1988.

[19] Corless I B, and Riordan J J. Nursing care: A user-friendly approach—identifying the cutting edge questions. In J. Stevenson, and T. Tripp-Reimer (eds.), *Knowledge about care and caring: State of the Art and Future Developments.* Kansas: American Academy of Nursing, 1989: 53–64.

[20] Bulechek G M, and McCloskey J C. Nursing intervention taxonomy development. In JC McCloskey, and HK Grace (eds.), *Current issues in nursing* (3rd ed). St. Louis: C. V. Mosby, 1990: 23–28.

[21] Verhonick P, Nicholas G, Glor B, and McCarthy R. I came, I saw, I responded: nursing observation and action survey. *Nurs Res* 1968, 17: 38–44.

[22] Ciuca R L. Over the years with the nursing care plan. *Nurs Outlook* 1972, 20: 706–711.

[23] Kane M, Kingsbury C, Colton D, and Estes C. *A study of nursing practice and role delineation and job analysis of entry-level performance of registered nurses.* Chicago: National Council of State Boards of Nursing, Inc., 1986.

[24] Cohen S M, Arnold L, Brown L, and Brooten D. Taxonomic classification of transitional follow-up care nursing interventions with low birthweight infants. *Clin Nurs Spec* 1991, 5: 31–36.

[25] Grobe S J. Nursing intervention lexicon and taxonomy: Methodological aspects. In E J S Hovenga, K J Hannah, K A McCormick, and J S Ronald (eds.), *Nursing informatics '91: Proceedings of the fourth international conference on nursing use of computers and information science.* New York: springer-Verlag, 1991: 126–131.

[26] McCloskey J, Bulecheck G, Cohen M, Craft M, Crossley J, Denehy J, Glick O, Kruckeberg T, Mass M, Prophet C, and Tripp-Reimer T. Classification of nursing interventions. *J Prof Nurs* 1990, 6: 151–157.

7
An International Classification for Nursing Practice

JUNE CLARK

The particular contribution of this paper to the Workshop is to offer a global perspective on a shared problem. It is a cruel paradox that while we "know" that nursing is universal because the human needs that it exists to meet are universal, we have at present no empirical means of comparing nursing practice across countries, or even across clinical settings or client groups within a country. We do not yet have terms which are precisely defined or universally agreed in any one language, let alone across languages, in which to express what Florence Nightingale[1] once called "the elements of nursing": that is, what nurses do, in response to what sorts of problems, with what sorts of effects.

Communicating among ourselves about nursing is, and always has been, important, but communicating with other people about nursing has acquired a new urgency in all countries as we are forced to recognize that the value of nursing can no longer be considered self-evident, but has to be made visible in the information systems which all countries are developing as part of their efforts to manage health care.

The International Classification for Nursing Practice (ICNP) project is being undertaken by the International Council of Nurses—an organization made up of the National Nurses Associations (NNAs) of well over a hundred countries across the five continents of the world. Language in its everyday sense is a daily issue for such an organization: ICN has three "official" languages in which all its work is conducted (English, French, and Spanish), but its members practice their nursing in literally hundreds of different languages and dialects.

Reprinted with permission from *Informatics: The Infrastructure for Quality Assessment and Improvement in Nursing: Proceedings of the Fifth International Nursing Informatics Symposium Post Conference*, Henry, S.B., Holzemer, W.L., Tallberg, M. & Grobe, S.J. (Eds.). 1995. Pp. 24–31. San Francisco, CA: UC Nursing Press.

It is especially appropriate to reflect on such a problem at an international conference, and I am certainly not the first to do so. Almost a century ago a nurse who attended one of the earliest meetings of the International Council of Nurses wrote:[2]

> While attending a special meeting of the ICN in Paris, I was naturally at once struck by the fact . . . that the methods and the ways of regarding nursing problems were. . . . as foreign to the various delegations as were the actual languages, and the thought occurred to me that . . . sooner or later we must put ourselves upon a common basis and work out what may be termed a "nursing esperanto" which would, in the course of time, give us a universal nursing language. . . .

In the ninety years that have passed since then, nursing has developed enormously, but the gap which Hampton Robb identified has not yet been remedied.

Now, at last, we are taking up the challenge: developing a universal language and classification for nursing practice has been called by the International Council of Nurses "Nursing's Next Advance."

History and Context

I think it is important not only to explain a little of the history of the ICNP project but also to try to place it in the context of other similar work happening around the world.

First, we have to recognize that while nursing is a very ancient art, it is a young discipline which has only recently begun the scientific process that Harmer,[3] as long ago as 1926, commended to nursing as follows:

> It may be emphasized here that if nursing is ever to make even a remote claim to being a science, or even to being conducted on a scientific basis, it must be built up like all branches of science; that is, by the most careful, unbiased observation and recording of often seemingly trivial details from which—by organizing, classifying, analyzing, selecting, inferring, drawing and testing conclusions—a body of knowledge or principles are finally evolved.

Medicine was, of course, a little ahead of us. The International Classification of Diseases (ICD), which began more than a century ago, has now reached its Tenth Revision[4] and spawned a whole family of classifications, a point to which I will return later because one of the issues which has emerged in the ICNP work is the extent to which we should draw on these medical classifications and the extent to which we should invent our own.

In nursing, it was the USA which was first in the field. This audience will be familiar with Werley's work, from the late 1960s onward, on the Nursing Minimum Data Set,[5] the nursing diagnosis work led by the North American Nursing Diagnosis Association since the 1970s;[6] the classification systems developed by nurses such as Grobe,[7] Martin,[8] McCloskey and Bulechek,[9] and Saba,[10] and the efforts to support and coordinate this work made by the

American Nurses Association. The reasons why this development began first in the United States are probably to be found in the US systems of nursing education and of financing health care. It is significant but unsurprising that the resolution to the International Council of Nurses Council of National Representatives at Seoul in 1989 that led to the establishment of the ICNP project, was proposed by the US. But in particular, the identification by the American Nursing Association, as part of its work on standards of practice during the 1970s, of "assessment factors, nursing diagnoses, interventions and outcomes" as the elements for a nursing practice classification, has had a profound effect on the shaping of the ICNP concept.

Developments in countries outside the U.S. began later, but have accelerated rapidly during the 1990s. In 1991, when we undertook our initial literature review and our first survey among our (then) 105 member nursing associations and the (then) 21 WHO Collaborating Centers for Nursing,[11] we were able to identify some work in Australia and the beginnings of work in a few other countries, but not much, for example, in Europe. By 1994, classification activities were happening all over Europe, and in 1995 a new organization—the Association for Common European Nursing Diagnoses, Interventions and Outcomes (ACENDIO)—was launched. It is clear that the impetus for this development is coming from two sources: from the accelerating concern in all countries with cost containment and resource management in health care, and from the rapidly developing science and technology of informatics which is providing the systems necessary to support these activities.

The History of ICNP

The ICNP project is the result of a resolution of the ICN Council of National Representatives at its meeting in Seoul in 1989. Proposed and seconded by the American Nurses Association and the Canadian Nurses Association, the resolution asked that ICN encourage member NNAs to become involved in developing classification systems for nursing care, nursing information management systems and nursing data sets, to provide tools that nurses in all countries could use to identify nursing practice and describe nursing and its contributions to health.

The resolution was referred by the ICN Board of Directors to its Professional Services Committee (then chaired by Dr. Margretta Styles), which appointed consultants, first to study the feasibility of such a project and subsequently to take the work forward. The three consultants are Norma Lang (from the USA), Randi Mortensen (from Denmark), and myself.

Norma Lang and I began in 1990 (Randi Mortensen was appointed later) by setting out the vision in the form of a proposal to the ICN's Board of Directors.[12] A description of the proposal was published in the International Nursing Review in 1992.[13] In this document we set out the shape of the project, in particular its goals and its criteria, to which I will return in a minute.

We have no full time staff or research team, so sometimes I fret that progress has been slow. On the other hand, when I look back, I can see that what has been achieved has been considerable.

Since 1990, when we began work, this is what we have done:

1.   We undertook a preliminary literature search and we have done three small surveys of member associations to identify classification systems in use or being developed around the world.[11]

2.   We got together a Technical Advisory Group of nurses from six countries (Israel, Nepal, Chile, Kenya, Jamaica, and Japan) who met in Geneva to test the feasibility and applicability of the work to date at global level. This is very important because one of our key challenges is to ensure that any system avoids the trap of what I call "cultural imperialism" and is applicable in all countries.

3.   We made a first draft list, derived from the literature, of terms currently used to describe nursing diagnoses, interventions, and outcomes. This initial list is recognized to be highly selective and is biased by its overreliance on English language sources; and it is certainly not comprehensive. For example, the UK Nursing Terms Project alone has already generated some 20,000 terms currently used by UK nurses. The list does not yet incorporate any attempt at classification beyond alphabetical ordering under the three headings of diagnoses, interventions, and outcomes. The list, and the updating of the literature review, are being maintained by Dr. Madeline Wake at Marquette University, Wisconsin.

4.   We have invited our 114 member NNAs to submit new terms (labels) and have published guidelines to help people to do it.[14]

5.   As part of our commitment to collaborate with the WHO Department of Epidemiological and Health Statistical Services and the WHO Collaborating Centers for the Classification of Diseases, we have undertaken a review of ICD-10 and related classifications to identify labels which are relevant to nursing, and a preliminary report of this work is included in an ICN Working Paper published in 1993.[12]

6.   We made three presentations at the Quadrennial Congress of the ICN held in Madrid in June 1993—a plenary session, a special interest session, and a poster session. All three were extremely well attended, demonstrating a quite overwhelming interest and enthusiasm for ICNP by nurses from many countries.

7.   We help an Advisory Meeting on the Development of an Informational Tool to Support Community-Based and Primary Health Care Nursing Systems, which was generously funded by the W.K. Kellogg Foundation and held in Mexico in February 1994.[15] This meeting brought together nurses from selected countries in Africa and North and South America to

explore the potential of the ICNP for nursing in primary health care. This, too, is a major challenge because ICN is totally committed to the development of primary health care, and, unfortunately, most of the work and the systems developed to date are very oriented to acute care in hospitals. Another workshop is to be held in December 1995, in Taiwan.

8. Most recently, the consultants and technical advisers met in Geneva in June 1995, to work on developing the taxonomic structure—we call it the architecture—which will eventually enable the terms we have already collected, and the new terms emerging from the work of nurses in many countries, to be arranged in a logical system that everyone can share.

The Scope of ICNP

The challenge is enormous. But we do have a clear idea of what the task involves.

An International Classification for Nursing Practice involves:

naming, sorting and linking
phenomena which describe
what nurses do, for what human conditions
to produce what outcome

We know that this involves identifying and naming what Florence Nightingale[1] called the "elements of nursing."

*   nursing problems/diagnoses
*   nursing actions/interventions
*   nursing outcomes

We have modeled the structure of the task to show how each stage leads on to the next.

The diagram (Fig. 1) shows how the practicing nurse finds words (labels) for the elements of her/his practice. When standardized among nurses, these words become a nursing nomenclature and can be combined to form a language for nursing. This nomenclature can be sorted according to agreed-upon principles to form a classification.

The nomenclature can be used in a nursing minimum data set (NMDS), which is a minimum set of items with uniform definitions and categories concerning nursing. Many countries have already identified the need for collection, storage, and retrieval of nursing data, making it important to have a uniform nomenclature and classification of nursing practice so that meaningful and comparative data can be collected.

The data that are labeled according to a nursing nomenclature, structured into a nursing language and classified by means of common features (an ICNP), can be collated for inclusion in a nursing minimum data set, which in turn can be fed back into nursing practice at the center of the

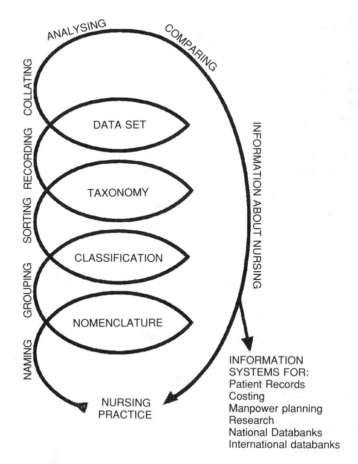

Figure 1. Development of nomenclature in nursing.

spiral. Thus the continuous process of development, refinement, and modification in response to external change.

As you can see, the title ICNP is a kind of shorthand. We could not resist using the initials ICN, but you can see that the process involves developing a language, a classification, and, eventually, a nursing minimum data set, which in turn can be incorporated into a country's larger information systems. But the most important thing to note is that the spiral begins and ends in nursing practice.

The Political Dimension

The creation of an ICNP involves not only the technical tasks inherent in any kind of classification or information system; it is a huge exercise in communication, politics, and diplomacy which sometimes makes me think that the UN Security Council has it easy! For example, here are the goals which we proposed in our Strategic Plan:[12]

Goal 1   To develop an ICNP with specified process and product components.

Goal 2   To achieve recognition by the national and international nursing communities.

Goal 3   To ensure that the ICNP is compatible with and complementary to the WHO Family of Classifications, and the work of other standardization groups such as the International Organization for Standardization (ISO) and its related groups, including the Comites European de Normalisation (CEN), and to secure inclusion of ICNP in relevant classifications.

Goal 4   To achieve utilization of ICNP by nurses at country level for the development of national databases.

Goal 5   To establish an international data set and a framework that incorporates the ICNP, the nursing minimum data set, a nursing resource data set, and regulatory data.

You can see immediately that these goals cannot be achieved by technical means alone, nor can they be achieved by the consultants or ICN alone. They require the collaboration and commitment of many people in many organizations and many countries. And achieving that is a mammoth political and diplomatic task.

The criteria we specified that ICNP must meet, demonstrate even more clearly the complexity of the task, and I will use these criteria also to identify some of the issues that have emerged during this developmental phase, to which I referred earlier. The criteria are:

1. Broad enough to serve the multiple purposes required by different countries and, as we now recognize, to serve the multiple purposes of information systems within countries;
2. Simple enough to be seen by the ordinary practitioner of nursing as a meaningful description of practice and a useful means of structuring practice;
3. Consistent with clearly defined conceptual frameworks but not dependent upon a particular theoretical framework or model of nursing;
4. Based on a central core to which additions can be made through a continuing process of development and refinement;
5. Sensitive to cultural variability;
6. Reflective of the common value system of nursing across the world as expressed in the ICN Code for Nurses;

7.   Usable in a complementary or integrated way with the family of disease and health-related classifications developed within WHO, the core of which is the International Classification of Diseases.

Each of these criteria raises issues that are political and philosophical as well as technical.

First, "Broad enough to serve multiple purposes. . . ." The issue here is not so much the variability among countries, as the particular perspectives and purposes that determine the collection and use of data within any one country.

We have found from our surveys and our consultative meetings that nurses in most countries collect and record data, including data about nursing, for epidemiological and management purposes. These data are often collected by nurses at the local level, and simply "passed up the line" to be aggregated at the hospital or national level, often with no feedback that might be used by nurses. The selection of what data are to be collected is not made by nurses and is not necessarily relevant to nursing purposes.

For example, we have found that many countries collect data about nursing activities, usually in the form of a tally list of things like numbers of immunizations given, or numbers of patients seen, per day or per month. But the selection of activities to be recorded, as the nurses from the countries of Africa and Latin America at our Mexico meeting told us, means that while about 20% of nursing activity is recorded, about 80% is not. Moreover, the 80% which is not recorded includes, in particular, activities such as teaching, corn-selling, and the "basic" or "activities of living" care which many of us would regard as the core of nursing.

Some countries, including the UK, have recognized the deficiencies of this approach, and are shifting the focus from a top-down, information technology-led statistical approach, to a bottom-up, clinically led approach, in which clinicians collect and record data for their own clinical purposes, and the necessary managerial and epidemiological data are extracted from this. This is certainly how we would like to see the ICNP used—hence its title: an International Classification for Nursing Practice. This is also what is referred to in our second criterion as being "seen by the ordinary practitioner of nursing as a meaningful description of practice and a useful means of structuring practice."

But before moving specifically to the second criterion, there are other issues in the words "broad enough." Most of the classification systems developed for nursing to date, reinforced by the fact that they have been developed in North America and tend to have been technology led, are about nursing in hospitals. We need systems which describe nursing in schools, in community settings, in rural primary health care clinics, indeed, in primary health care in all its forms. One of the outcomes of the Mexico meeting was to demonstrate the different kinds of problems and interventions that were the stock-in-trade of nurses working in primary health care settings, especially in rural areas and in less developed countries. We recognized too that we have to find ways of describing problems, diagnoses, and interventions that apply to groups (such as a whole community) as well as to individuals.

"Broad enough" also raises the issue of hierarchies or levels in classification. For an international system, how detailed should the categories be? In recording nursing activities, for example, would a broad division into five or six categories be more realistic than the very detailed systems already in use in some countries? I do not know, but I am convinced that a top priority must be to find some way of recording the 80% of nursing activity that is completely invisible and therefore unrecognized and undervalued.

These issues also relate to our second criterion, "Simple enough to be meaningful to the ordinary practitioner." Clearly, we need systems that do not depend on computers, simply because, in many settings, computers are not available. The ICNP has to be as usable by a primary health care nurse practicing from a mobile clinic or under a tree in rural Africa as by a nurse operating a battery of sophisticated equipment in an intensive care unit in New York.

The words "structuring practice" lead directly into our third criterion, "Consistent with a clearly defined conceptual framework . . ." Does nursing have clearly defined conceptual frameworks and, if so, which one should we choose? The use of nursing models in general is much less prevalent, and is considered much less important, in some countries than in the United States. The concept of nursing diagnosis, let alone the language of the nursing diagnosis literature, is unfamiliar in many countries and positively rejected in some.

It will not be easy to achieve a global consensus, but our surveys and consultative meetings to date have identified two concepts that appear to be universal or at least widespread, and that can therefore provide a starting point:

1. The use of the nursing process as a means of structuring nursing practice; and
2. A focus on the "basic needs" or "functional patterns" or "activities of living" derived from the work of Henderson which has already been translated into 24 languages, with several more translations into Eastern European languages in preparation.

The architecture of the ICNP is still being thought out, but the three consultants have agreed on the broad principles of a taxonomy. There is a lot more work to be done, and what we have done so far is not yet ready for publication. But I can tell you that, in line with the purposes for the ICNP which we set out in our original proposal, ICNP will provide a structure that will enable nursing interventions to be linked with nursing diagnoses and outcomes.

For nursing diagnoses, we have indeed included the concepts identified by Henderson, but we want also to make provision for diagnoses that apply to groups as well as to individuals—to families and whole communities. We know that this part of the system will be especially important for nurses working in primary health care, but we have found very little published work in this area, so we are looking to nurses currently working with families and communities in primary health care to send us terms and definitions, using those Guidelines to which I referred earlier.[14]

For nursing interventions, we have agreed to work on a system that explicitly identifies those activities such as teaching that are under-developed in most existing classifications and that enable them to be linked to our classification of nursing diagnoses.

Our work on outcomes is still at a very early stage, but we have agreed to use the term "nursing sensitive" outcomes, and again to link them with nursing diagnoses and nursing interventions.

Our fourth criterion specifies "a central core to which additions can be made." Any system must, of course, be dynamic and not static, and that is why the first of our goals specifies that ICNP must have "process and product components." ICNP must reflect and be responsive to the changes and developments in the nursing practice which it attempts to describe.

But this criterion also raises issues of compatibility with other systems, not only with the WHO systems, which I will return to in a moment, but with national level multidisciplinary health information systems which several countries, including the UK, are now developing. In no way could ICN impose, nor would it wish to impose, a new system on people's existing systems. We need a broad framework into which other systems can be crossmapped.

The fifth and sixth criteria raise issues about cultural variability across countries and sensitivity to the value base of nursing. I put these two together because, while most nurses will recognize and respect the reality of cultural differences among the people whom nursing serves in the different countries of the world, we often do not recognize the strength and variability of the culture of nursing itself. For example, we sometimes tend to assume that the values that underpin nursing in the Western world, which are in fact derived from the Greek/Judeo/Christian historical traditions of Western Europe,[17] are universal. But Eastern and non-Christian traditions and approaches may be very different. For example, Japanese people may not attribute the same value to the individual as does American or British nursing. In some cultures, "self-care" or "patient participation" may not be seen as desirable goals, and the harsh reality is that for nurses in some countries of Eastern Europe and the former Soviet Union, the concept of "care" is not a value, let alone the basis of a science.

The final criterion refers to "the family of disease and health-related classifications developed within WHO." This raises the fundamental issue, which I mentioned earlier, of the extent to which we can draw on existing classifications, which are primarily medical, and the extent to which we should invent our own. Opinions are sharply divided and strongly held. There is conflict between the ideal and the reality. For example, at the Mexico meeting, participants from all the African and Latin American countries complained of the inadequacy of the systems which they were using, but recognized that, whatever nursing might decide, the ICD and other similar systems would continue to be the main methods of data collection in their countries. Our present work plan still includes a commitment to the preparation of an "Application of ICD to Nursing" and an "International Classification of Procedures in Nursing," using the framework and format of the WHO family of classifications. But there is considerable debate about the wisdom of this course, lest it detract from the need to develop nursing's own systems based on nursing values and conceptual frameworks.

Strengths and Weaknesses, Limits and Opportunities

In discussing these criteria which we specified in our original proposal that the ICNP must meet, I have highlighted some, but by no means all, of the philosophical, conceptual, and political issues that have emerged during the developmental phases of the ICNP project. I think it is important also to recognize some of the limits.

First, the ICNP is not a panacea; it is merely a tool which nurses can use in whatever way they want and for whatever purposes. It will be of no use unless it is used and, as with any tool, we will have to learn how to use it well.

Second, it will only be as good a tool as we make it. For example, it will enable us to describe the full range of nursing practice only if it contains appropriate labels (terms) from all fields of nursing practice—so I repeat my plea for more work to be done on describing the nursing diagnoses and interventions used in community nursing and primary health care.

Third, if we do not value it, then nobody else will. There is a tendency, at least in the United Kingdom, to regard activities such as this as "mere theorizing," some kind of trivial intellectual game for academics which has no relevance to "real" nursing. I believe this attitude is dangerous because it ignores the importance that computerized information, and therefore information systems, are beginning to have on the determination of health care, especially health care resources, in all our countries. As Norma Lang has frequently pointed out: "*If you can't name it, you can't control it, finance it, research it, teach it, or put in into public policy.*"

But I do believe that "limits" are just things that you have to step over in order to see the beauty beyond. And I do believe that for the ICNP, the view beyond the limits is very beautiful indeed.

If an International Classification for Nursing Practice were adopted on a worldwide basis and used to summarize data that were routinely and continuously collected, the benefits for nursing would be immense: for nursing practice, nursing administration, nursing research, nursing education, nursing policy, and health care policy.

For Nursing Practice, an ICNP would:

- provide a framework and a structure for nursing documentation that would encourage more precise and consistent documentation of nursing care and provide data to be used as a basis for individual clinical decision-making;
- facilitate documentation (and therefore recognition) of those nursing actions (e.g. those concerned with health promotion, identifying and utilizing people's own strengths and capabilities, and coordinating care) that are not at present explicitly documented, recognized, or costed;
- improve continuity of nursing care for patients who are transferred across settings by improving the quality of information about their nursing needs and previous nursing care;
- facilitate the collection and use of data for measuring and monitoring quality of care and for development of nursing practice standards and guidelines and quality assurance.

For Nursing Administration/Management, an ICNP would:

- facilitate the measurement of clinical nursing care for evaluation and other purposes;
- refine nursing resource allocation methodologies and improve ability to estimate the need for nursing as a basis for planning, budgeting, and resource allocation;
- enable investigation of the cost-effectiveness of nursing by relating nursing interventions to outcomes;
- enable investigation of the effectiveness of differential staffing patterns relative to patient dependencies (acuity);
- enable comparison of clinical nursing data and human resources data across units, regions, and countries;
- enable description and analysis of trends based upon data about clinical nursing practice.

For Nursing Research, an ICNP would:

- facilitate descriptive research on the kinds of problems that are the focus of nursing, and on the types of intervention that nurses use to tackle them;
- stimulate and facilitate comparison of nursing diagnoses/problems across settings, locally, regionally, nationally, and internationally;
- facilitate studies of the effectiveness of nursing treatments by relating nursing diagnoses, actions, and outcomes;

- permit the creation of a national and international database for development of nursing science, knowledge, and theory building.

For Nursing Education, an ICNP would:

- provide a framework for curriculum planning and evaluation;
- provide a direct communication link between the curriculum and the practice arena;
- encourage research-based teaching by providing a similar communication link between curriculum and research data;
- encourage the integration of information management into basic, post-basic, and continuing education.

For Nursing Policy, an ICNP would:

- make visible the full range of nursing practice, including the nursing contribution to health promotion and prevention of illness;
- enable sound data instead of anecdotal information to serve as the basis for informed decision-making and policy formulation;
- facilitate the definition of the evolving scope of practice for regulatory purposes;
- facilitate the definition of nursing roles for socioeconomic purposes.

For Health Care Policy, an ICNP would:

- identify the role of nurses in the multidisciplinary team and the contribution of nursing to multidisciplinary health care, especially in primary health care;
- provide nursing data comparable with and complementary to existing health care data;
- propose additional elements for epidemiological study;
- enable the inclusion of nursing data in cost-benefit ratios and quality assurance;
- enable the inclusion of nursing data in measurements of universal health status.

The resolution of the issues which I have highlighted will not be quick or easy. But I am optimistic and eager to accept the challenge, and I know that there are many nurses around the world who share my aspirations.

In the UK we have a joke which seems particularly appropriate to this occasion:

Question: How do you eat an elephant?
Answer: One bite at a time.

The task is enormous, but it is fundamental to the continued development and recognition of nursing. It is the kind of project that never ends but for which there is a timely beginning: Now. With justification, it has been called "Nursing's Next Advance."

References

1. Nightingale F. Notes on Nursing. 1959.
2. Hampton Robb I. Report of the Third Regular Meeting of the International Council of Nurses. Geneva: ICN, 1909.
3. Harmer B. Methods and Principles of Teaching the Principles and Practice of Nursing. New York: Macmillan, 1926.
4. World Health Organization. International Statistical Classification of Disease and Related Health Problems: Tenth Revision. Geneva: WHO, 1992.
5. Werley HH, Lang N. Identification of the Nursing Minimum Data Set. New York: Springer Publishing, 1988.
6. North American Nursing Diagnosis Association. Nursing Diagnoses: Definitions and Classifications. Philadelphia: NANDA, 1994.
7. Grobe SJ. Nursing Lexicon and Taxonomy: Preliminary Categorization. In Lun KC, Degoulet P, Peimme TE, Rienhoff O, eds. MedInfo91. Geneva: North-Holland, 1992:981–86.
8. Martin KS, Scheet NJ. The Omaha System: Applications for Community Health Nursing. Philadelphia: Lippincott, 1992.
9. McCloskey JC, Bulechek GM, eds. Nursing Interventions Classification (NIC). St. Louis: Mosby, 1992.
10. Saba VK. The classification of home health care nursing: diagnoses and interventions. Caring Magazine. 1992;11:50–6.
11. Wake M, Murphy M, Affara F, Clark J, Mortensen R. Toward an International Classification for Nursing Practice: a pilot litenture review and survey. Int Nurs Rev. 1993;40:77–80.
12. International Council of Nurses. Nursing's Next Advance: Development of an International Classification for Nursing Practice: Final Proposal. Unpublished, 1991.
13. Clark J, Lang N. Nursing's next advance: an International Classification for Nursing Practice. Int Nurs Rev. 1992;38:109–112.
14. International Council of Nurses. Guidelines for Submitting Labels to the International Classification for Nursing Practice. Geneva: ICN, 1994.
15. International Council of Nurses. Report of an Advisory Meeting on the Development of an Information Tool to Support Community-Based and Primary Health Care Nursing Systems. Geneva: ICN, 1994.
16. Henderson V. Principles of Basic Nursing Care. Geneva: ICN, 1977.
17. Lanara VA. Heroism as a Nursing Value. Athens: Author, 1991.

8
Evaluating Information Support for Guideline Development

L. McQueen, Kathleen A. McCormick, and Carole Hudgings

1. Background

In November, 1989, Congress amended the Public Health Service Act to create the Agency for Health Care Policy and Research (AHCPR) in order to promote the quality, appropriateness and effectiveness of health care services and to improve access to these services. The strong emphasis on outcomes and effectiveness research led to the initiation of many creative new projects designed to promote the quality of health care in the United States. One of the most innovative ideas to reach fruition was the creation of a program to facilitate the public-private creation of clinical practice guidelines.

Within AHCPR, the Office of the Forum for Quality and Effectiveness in Health Care (the Forum) has primary responsibility for facilitating the development, periodic review, update and evaluation of guidelines and the medical review criteria, standards of quality and performance measures related to the guidelines. Guidelines are defined by the Institute of Medicine as, "systematically developed statements which assist practitioner and patient decisions about appropriate health care for specific conditions" (1990), and are based on the analysis of relevant published scientific data relevant to the topic. Current interest in guideline development has soared in recent years and more than 1500 guidelines are currently being produced or updated by professional associations or other groups in the United States. This trend is expected to continue as outcomes and health services research gain increasing attention in the health care reform agenda.

The Forum presently manages the development, review, update and evaluation of twenty-three guidelines by multidisciplinary panels of experts

Reprinted from *Nursing Informatics: An International Overview for Nursing in a Technological Era*, Grobe, S.J., Pluyter-Wenting, E.S.P. (Eds.). 1994. Pp. 705–709, with kind permission from Elsevier Science—NL, Sara Burgerhartstraat 25, 1055 KV Amsterdam, The Netherlands.

and health care consumers charged by Congress to review the scientific evidence related to their topic. Some AHCPR-supported panels are coordinated through contracts, while others are coordinated directly by AHCPR. Medical review criteria, standards of quality and performance measures for each guideline are also developed, updated and evaluated. The instigation and management of this ambitious program would be impossible except for appropriate uses of various technologies, including the personal computer. The importance of information planning and support has been recognized from the beginning, as technology is used to maximize the efficiency of guideline development and production.

Nurses play key leadership roles in all aspects of AHCPR-supported guideline development. Nurses serve as panel members or chairs on all AHCPR-supported guideline panels, and as projects officers, directing guideline development for AHCPR.

The complexity imposed by the AHCPR methodology require that all available supports be given to each panel and that efficiency be constantly monitored and promoted. In addition to the guideline itself, each panel produces four other documents, totaling more than 1200 pages, during the 12–18 months allotted for initial development. These five guideline products are developed after extensive literature searches are conducted and the scientific evidence is amassed from relevant published literature related to the topic. Each panel is also required to conduct an open meeting for the public, peer and pilot review the draft documents, and consider cost impact to their recommendations. The amount of data collected and the speed and sophistication required for complex analysis during the short development time demands that resources be planned and expended carefully.

Personal computers were implemented in ways which optimize both the quality of the final product and the management of the complex processes involved in guideline development. The Forum Director and the Senior Health Policy Analysts who manage the guideline panels recognized from the beginning that the ambitious schedule would be impossible unless every aspect of project management were made as efficient and effective as possible. Direction regarding the appropriate uses of technology is one of the many ways AHCPR supports the needs of each panel.

Management decisions made while planning the information support for the panels were influenced by the reports in the literature. Since there are no citations in the nursing literature directly related to computer applications for the management of guideline development, the international literature related to information systems and guideline development was generalized while planning the implementation of the information system support needed for guideline development. Publications related to clinical practice guidelines by Gardner[1] (1992), Musen[2] (1992) and others were considered, in addition to the nursing and other scientific literature related to decision-support and information system management (McCormick[3] 1991; Suwa[4] 1982; Petrucci[5] 1992; Bloom[6] 1987; Okada[7] 1988).

Based on these and other publications, the information support was planned to provide fast and effective technology, while planning resource expenditures carefully. The complexity of the guideline development process and the guideline documents themselves provided the incentive to simplify the requirements for the end-users, guard against any excess implementations, while providing the capability to generate all of the needed applications and communications. A management decision was also made to frequently evaluate the end-user satisfaction, and use the feedback to change and upgrade the system on a regular basis.

2. System Description

Hardware, software, and professional support is provided by AHCPR for each guideline panel. IBM compatible 486 computers are provided to the co-chairs of each panel, and are used by the methodologist, writer/editor and others developing each guideline. Although the 500 experts and consumers now serving as panel members and chairs have personal preference for the software needed, the Forum has found standardization of some of the software between panels to be essential, while allowing for flexibility and personal preference for other applications. The consistent use of some identical software between panels assures that all documents can readily be converted to electronic media for on-line dissemination and reduces the difficulties and delays associated with the preparation of manuscripts and camera-ready copy for each of the five guideline documents printed during the intense production phase. Wordperfect 5.1 is used for all content and the production of tables, and Harvard Graphics is used for all figures. Pro-Cite 3.5 is used to input, manage, organize and format the references and bibliographic information used in developing the guidelines products. The bibliographic information for each reference is entered as a record in the Pro-Cite database either by manual entries or importation from other on-line databases. Since each panel reviews up to 100,000 abstracts and 1000 full-text articles, the consistent maintenance of the Pro-Cite database is crucial to the management of the literature. The MacFlow program is used for algorithm development. Procomm Plus, Grateful Med, Lotus 123, and utilities packages are also provided. Although on-line support is included with several of the packages, the Forum provides additional user support as needed. The Forum provides the education necessary to assist all users and to update the systems to accommodate individual needs.

For some applications, the Forum has assisted users to design systems which not only include the standardized software, but also incorporate personal preference for other, additional programs. Several panels, for example, use different relational database, spreadsheet, and statistical analysis software packages. Whenever the use of a different software package promotes the efficiency of guideline development, efforts are made to accommodate these preferences.

AHCPR has balanced individual preferences with the need for all panels to use similar software which readily allows for the creation of products which meet specified formats. Panel chairs are frequently asked to provide feedback about the system and to communicate additional needs to the Forum. Verbal and written interviews directly related to use and satisfaction are routinely administered and discussions regarding computerization are included in management meetings. A database on a commercial relational software package is maintained at the Forum for this purpose. The feedback is used when planning how to best meet the on-going needs of the panels. The end-user satisfaction with the required software is of primary concern and on-going evaluations are made, particularly for Pro-Cite. Based on the feedback received, the system has evolved and improved over time. Additional software and hardware standards are added, after they are tested by individual panels. For example, the routine use of fax-modems is now being tested and may become a standard means of communication between the panel chairs, members, consultants, AHCPR and the methodologist. Two other panels are pilot testing the use of a network in which all panel members can more easily communicate and transfer information.

The Forum has created centralized computer systems to compliment the systems used by individual panels. Two large administrative databases allow the Forum to compare data related to the functions and management of the twenty-three panels now working to develop or update clinical practice guidelines. The information gained from these databases allows for the

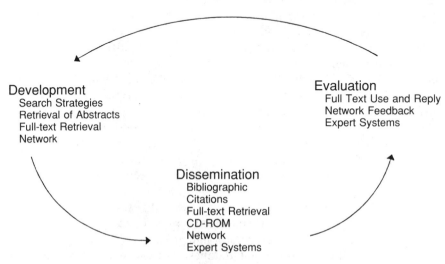

FIGURE 1. Feedback for guidelines.

evaluation of existing strategies and the analysis of costs, thereby promoting efficient guideline development.

The systems described above to support guideline development are one part of the overall plan created by the Forum for using personal computers as a workstation. Figure 1 shows the model of using computers during development, dissemination, and evaluation. This model illustrates how the computer output for bibliographic citations, full text retrieval, CD-Rom, networks, and expert systems during evaluation, eventually provides feedback for guidelines updated on a regular schedule after release.

3. Conclusions

Nurses at AHCPR have planned, implemented, managed, and evaluated the use of personal computers to facilitate the development and update of clinical practice guidelines. The scarcity of published nursing literature on computer applications associated with guidelines motivated these nurses to publish their findings. IBM compatible 486 personal computers equipped with WordPerfect 5.1, Harvard Graphics, Pro-Cite, Procomm Plus, Grateful Med and other software are supplied to each panel and user support is provided as necessary. This technology is used as each panel reviews extensive literature searches and produces five scientific documents in twelve to eighteen months. The appropriate use of technology for this project has occurred due to careful planning "efficient" and effective use of resources, provision of sufficient end-user support, evaluation of the system, and revision or expansion of the system over time. Communication and on-going adaptations to the needs of the users has resulted in the creation of a system which promotes the final goal of guideline development.

References

Book:
[1] Gardner E. (1992). *Putting guidelines into practice.* Modern Healthcare 1992, September: 24–26.

Book:
[2] Musen A, Tu S and Shahar Y. (1992). *A Problem-solving model for protocol-based care: from eoncocin to eon.* Proceedings of Medinfo 92, Amsterdam: Elsevier Publishing September: 6–9.

Book:
[3] McCormick KA. (1991). *Future data needs for quality of care monitoring, DRG considerations, reimbursement and outcome measurement.* IMAGE: The Journal of Scholarship, 23,4–7,1991.

Book:

[4] Suwa M, Scott AC, and Shortliffe EH. (1982). *An approach to verifying completeness and consistency in a rule-based expert sytem*; AI Magazine (US);3(4),16–21.

Book:

[5] Petrucci K, Jacox A, McCormick K, Parks P, Kjerulff K, Baldwin B, and Petrucci P. (1992). *Evaluating the appropriateness of a nurse expert system's patient assessment*; Computers in Nursing 10(6),243–249.

Book:

[6] Bloom C, and Salano F. (1987). *A nurse expert system to assign nursing diagnosis.* Computers in Nursing, 5(4),140–145.

[7] Okada J, and Okada O. (1988). *Prolog-based system for nursing staff schedule implemented on a personal computer*; Computers in Biomedical Research, 21(1),53–56.

Article:

Field MJ, and Lohr RN (editors) (1990). *Clinical Practice Guidelines: Directions for a New Program* Institute of Medicine Report, National Academy Press.

Article:

Hadorn DC, McCormick KA and Diokno A. (1992). *An annotated approach to clinical guideline development.* Journal of the American Medical Association, 267(24).

9
ComputerLink: An Innovation in Home Care Nursing

Patricia Flatley Brennan

1. Background and Research Objectives

Nurses of the late 20th century face many challenges as they diagnose and treat human responses. Some of these challenges arise from the complexities of life and disease processes which confront humans. Other challenges arise from the psychological, temporal, geographical, or physical barriers to reaching and intervening with persons in need. The purpose of this project was to determine the feasibility of using commonly available computer technology to circumvent barriers to the delivery of nursing care, and to deliver services in a timely and convenient manner.

Caregivers of persons with Alzheimer's Disease (AD Caregivers) were selected as an important target group in need of nursing care and for whom barriers arising from time constraints, shame, and distance presented formidable obstacles for obtaining necessary services [1]. Over five million family members and friends provide home care support for persons with AD. Most of these caregivers find meaning and fulfillment in the caregiver role; yet, due to the stress and demand of caregiving, many become vulnerable to physical health decline and psychological distress [2]. Thus, nursing care is needed to aid the AD caregiver in meeting the caregiving role expectations and to help this population avoid the negative consequences of caregiving.

The nursing care required by AD caregivers include social support, professional counselling, and assistance with the challenges of caregiving, such as gaining information about or confidence in the decisions they make for themselves and the person for whom they provide care [3]. Traditional methods of providing these types of service require face-to-face contact between the caregiver and nurse at meetings and counselling sessions. Notwithstanding the benefits of face-to-face encounters, many AD

Reprinted from *Nursing Informatics: An International Overview for Nursing in a Technological Era*, Grobe, S.J., Pluyter-Wenting, E.S.P. (Eds.). 1994. Pp. 407–413, with kind permission from Elsevier Science—NL, Sara Burgerhartstraat 25, 1055 KV Amsterdam, The Netherlands.

caregivers cannot avail themselves of these services because they lack the time or ability to travel to the meetings, or because the caregiver suffers from shame or embarrassment. Therefore, nursing care is needed, and nurses must examine and creatively employ technology to insure the delivery of the service. One technology with great potential for transcending physical, psychological, temporal or geographic barriers is computer networks.

Computer networks, electronic links between remote sites, provide a mechanism for nurses to reach AD caregivers in their homes in a manner that is timely and convenient. Computer networks support asychronous communication; that is, the sender and receiver need not be present simultaneously. This aspect permits a caregiver to leave a message for a nurse, and review the response, when it is convenient for the caregiver to do so. Conversely, the nurse need not wait for a mutually convenient time to respond to the caregiver's request for information; rather, he/she can respond as needed at a time convenient to the nurse. Additionally, computer networks allow caregivers to communicate with each other in the same timely and convenient fashion, thus mimicking many of the features of a support group without requiring the caregivers to leave home and come to a central site.

Computer networks also support a "broadcast" communication; messages relevant to many individuals can be posted once and delivered to all involved persons. Computer network also provide pathways into repositories of information, such as electronic data bases and encyclopedias. Nurses can prepare materials for caregiver education and teaching once, and then make these materials accessible to the caregivers as they need so. Computer networks provide portals into specialized programs that can guide the caregiver through complex decisions and analyses, thus facilitating nurse's use of adjuvants to individual counselling strategies.

A team of nurses and social scientists developed the ComputerLink, a specialized computer network having three functional components: a communications area, a decision support system, and an electronic encyclopedia. Built within an existing free, public-access computer network, the ComputerLink provided a pathway for nurses to reach individuals at home, in a timely and convenient manner. ComputerLink also provided a central repository for programs and information resources likely to be helpful to the person at home.

2. Presentation of Methods

2.1 The ComputerLink

The ComputerLink consists of hardware, phone lines, software and nursing interventions. The ComputerLink was designed to provide three major types of nursing services to AD caregivers: social support, clinical advise and information and decision support. Caregivers accessed these services through computer terminals placed in their homes. ComputerLink was available 24 hours a day for an 18 month period, and caregivers could access the system as often as they desired. One nurse served as nurse moderator; she logged onto the system daily, read and responded to caregiver comments as needed, and maintained the currency of the information available through the network.

Social support, defined as both peer and professional support, was available through the communications area. The Communication area permitted several options for public and private communication among caregivers and between caregivers and the nurse moderator. In an unrestricted bulletin board (The Forum) any user could read, post and respond to issues of concern and interest. Private electronic mail afforded one-to-one interaction away from the scrutiny of others. In a special feature combining private mail with The Forum, called Q & A, caregivers could send questions anonymously to the nurse moderator, who posted the answer to the question for all to read.

In addition to responding to specific requests for information through the communications areas, the nurse moderator also provided structured information through the Electronic Encyclopedia. The Electronic Encyclopedia included over 150 short articles designed to enhance self-care, understand issues about Alzheimer's Disease and about the experience of caregiving, and promote home-based management of the person with Alzheimer's Disease. Caregivers could browse through the Electronic Encyclopedia in a screen-by-screen manner, selecting topics from a key-word listing, or search using specific words and phrases for the information of their choice.

Supporting caregivers through complex decisions can occur through interpersonal interaction, either individually or in the open bulletin board discussions. In addition, in the decision support module, caregivers could work though a decision problem on their own. English-language questions guided users in an analysis of a self-defined decision problem. For some users, the decision problems focused on selecting living arrangements. For other users, intimate questions of relationships served as the focus of the analysis. The analysis strategy, decision modelling [4], helped the user focus on the values and trade-offs that occur during difficult choices. The decision support module permitted caregivers to explore their values, and to select choices that best meet their own stated values.

2.2 Research Design and Procedures

Subjects in the 18-month randomized field experiment included 98 individuals who considered themselves to be the primary caregiver of a person with AD, sixty-six females and 32 males. Caregivers were randomly assigned to a placebo or experimental (ComputerLink) conditions. Subjects also completed self-report inventories at the beginning and end of the

TABLE 1. Demographic summary of ComputerLink Caregivers

Age	60.8 years (s.d. 14.92)	**Caregiver relationship**	
		Spouse 26 (57%)	
Gender	Male 14 (33%)	Daughters or 11 daughters-in-law (24%)	
	Female 33 (66%)	Son 3 (6%)	
		Other 7 (13%)	
Race	Black 14 (33%)		
	White 33 (66%)		
Years of school	<12 years 14 (33%)		
	>12 years 33 (66%)		

study. Research nurses visited the homes of caregivers, installed the necessary equipment, and trained caregivers in the use of the ComputerLink. Caregivers accessed ComputerLink via Wyse 30 terminals placed in their homes. A 1200 baud modem provided the connection between the terminal and the standard telephone line. Caregivers entered the ComputerLink through the CWRU modem bank. Successful access occurred in over 95% of desired encounters.

Because the present report deals only with caregivers who used ComputerLink, Table 1 summarizes the profile for ComputerLink users. Care recipients were predominantly spouses (60%) and parents (31%), and required care for an average 34.5 months (s.d. 26.8). This sample is representative of other study samples of caregivers of elderly patients [5]. Thirty-two percent of the subjects stated that they care for someone in addition to person with AD. Twenty-six of the subjects (26%) in this sample placed their loved one in a nursing home made during the one-year period of involvement. This incidence represents substantial evidence that caregivers are making decisions about health service use, such as nursing home placement.

3. Results and Discussion

The ComputerLink was active for 540 days. Caregivers accessed the system on 3875 occasions (median 2.5 uses per week). All caregivers used the system on at least three occasions; one caregiver accessed ComputerLink on over 575 occasions. A typical encounter lasted 12 minutes, and included use of two or more functions. Table 2 summarizes the use of ComputerLink by feature.

The communications area was used most often; in this area caregivers could interact with each other in a public, "bulletin-board", a private mail service or through a nurse-advising service in which caregivers could post confidential questions. The Forum received the most attention from the

TABLE 2. ComputerLink feature uses (Note: Caregivers use one or more function of each access)

Feature	# of uses	Duration in minutes (SD)
Forum	3312	9.87 (12.15)
Private mail	2019	5.78 (09.34)
Q & A	878	3.14 (04.95)
Electronic Encyclopedia	541	9.34 (10.32)
Decision support	106	7.65 (07.92)

caregivers. The nurse entered the Forum daily and posted messages whenever necessitated by direct request or professional judgment that such comments would enhance peer support.

Caregivers sought direct contact with the nurse in several ways. First, they sent 27 private mail messages to the nurse, with topics ranging from requests for assistance with the computer system to questions about managing specific problems with the person with AD. Second, of the 749 messages posted in the Forum, 50 made a direct reference to the nurse moderator. The nurse moderator posted 88 messages in this area. Finally, caregivers asked thirty questions in the Q & A area. Interestingly, the caregivers accessed this section to read questions and responses 20 times more often than they did to ask questions.

The Electronic Encyclopedia and the decision support module received less attention by the caregivers than did the more interactive functions of the system. Within the Electronic Encyclopedia caregivers sought information on the care of the person with AD more often than any other topical area. The 106 uses of the decision support module included analysis of such decisions as placement of a mother in a nursing home or return to work.

3.1 Discussion

The evidence presented here demonstrates that ComputerLink provided a vehicle for nurses to reach and support AD caregivers. The system proved easy for caregivers to access and use. Communication services, moderated by the nurse, receive the most attention by the caregivers. The surprising pattern of caregiver use of the Q & A section suggested that in addition to using ComputerLink to reach peers, caregivers also employed it as a pathway to professional contact.

The disproportionate access to the Forum relative to the private mail section of the ComputerLink suggests that the most extensively valued nursing intervention was the provision of social support. While peer contact was available under both "public" (Forum) and "private" (private mail) conditions, the caregivers participating in this study sought the more public environment. Because support groups are a common, but under-used mechanism for facilitating peer support among AD caregivers [6] it is likely that these caregivers were seeking out similar types of experiences in the electronic media.

Caregivers made most use of those parts of the system supporting interaction among peers or between caregivers and the nurse. It is possible to consider such nursing strategies as providing information on request and facilitating social support as "active" interventions. In contrast, then, the construction of an information utility (Electronic Encyclopedia) or the provision of adjuvant programs (decision support) may be considered indirect nursing strategies (indirect because the nurse is instrumental in providing access, but not directly involved in implementing the nursing strategies than of the indirect nursing strategies available through ComputerLink).

Preliminary evidence indicates that ComputerLink enhances caregiver decision making confidence, and serves as a viable medium for nurses to provide social support, education, and clinical interventions to home-bound AD caregivers in a manner free of time and space boundaries. Caregivers are more likely to use the interactive rather than the broadcast features. ComputerLink represents an efficient use of technology to support a new approach to nursing care.

3.2 Generalizability of ComputerLink Nationally and Internationally

Certain features of the ComputerLink suggest that this intervention is likely to be successful in a variety of communities in the US and world-wide. First, although the participants in this project were AD caregivers, their performance suggests that ComputerLink may be desirable whenever nurses need to reach individuals in remote areas who face ongoing complex health management challenges. The success of ComputerLink with individuals of all age groups indicates that advancing age is not a barrier to successful use. The nature of the services provided here (information, decision assistance, social support) were tailored to the needs of this particular group; it is possible that other groups may require a different mix of services. While not all nursing interventions can be delivered in an electronic medium, many may be effectively delivered so. The challenge remains to nursing to evaluate the needs of the target population and determine how to best employ existing technologies to delivery nursing care.

Some aspects of the technology may preclude its use in certain developing countries. For example, a stable electrical supply and access to phone lines is required to implement a home-based electronic pathway for nursing care. Telephone service, whether satellite-mediated or not, is also necessary to make the link between the remote sites and a central site. Finally, the ability to insure privacy of telecommunication transmission is a necessary precursor to the effective use of technology in delivering nursing care to remote sites.

Acknowledgment. Supported by a grant from the National Institute on Aging, #AG8617, Patricia Flatley Brennan, PhD, RN, FAAN, Principal Investigator.

References

[1] U.S. Congress, Office of Technology Assessment. (1990). Confused minds, burdened families: finding help for people with Alzheimer's Disease & other dementias. (Report No. OTA-BA-403).

[2] Brody EM. Patient care as a normative family stress. *Gerontologist* 1978, 25:19–29.

[3] Haley WE, Brown SL and Levine EG. Experimental evaluation of the effectiveness of group intervention for dementia caregivers. *Gerontologist* 1987, 27:376–382.

[4] von Winterfeldt D and Edwards W. *Decision Analysis and Behavioral Research.* Cambridge: Cambridge University Press, 1986.

[5] Stone R, Cafferata GL and Sangl J. Caregivers of the frail elderly: a national profile. *Gerontologist.* 1987, 37:616–626.

[6] Noelker LS and Bass DM. Home care for elderly persons: Linkages between formal and informal caregivers. *J Geron: SocSci* 1989, 44:S63–70.

10
Combining Telecommunications and Interactive Multimedia Health Information on the Electronic Superhighway

Mary Anne Sweeney and Diane J. Skiba

1. Introduction

The multimedia health promotion programs of *The Healthy Touch® Series* from The University of Texas Medical Branch in Galveston (UTMB) have been incorporated into the health information section of the Denver Free-Net (DFN), located at the University of Colorado Health Science Center (UCHSC) in Denver. The multimedia programs are accessible in the OUTREACH Network sites located in rural Southwestern Colorado and Northwestern Colorado. The OUTREACH (On-Line Urban to Rural Education and Community Health) Network, whose goal is to "expand and augment rural health care services through a set of user-friendly community computing systems," is the link to the programs from each of the rural community locations.

The multimedia programs were added to with an established computer network to provide residents of the rural areas with two key enhancements to their computer information resources. The multimedia programs are multisensory and appeal to a wide variety of learners to capture their interest while obtaining health promotion information and parenting skills. The programs are helpful to people who are not in a position to rely on their reading skills. The Denver Free-Net currently provides only text-based materials in other sites, which must be read from the screen by learners. This requires a high level of literacy skills.

The second contribution of the multimedia programs is the availability of audio tracks in Spanish. The Denver Free-Net provides information exclusively in English.

Reprinted with permission from *MEDINFO '95: Proceedings of the Eighth World Congress on Medical Informatics*; Greenes, R.A., Peterson, H.E. & Protti, D.J. (Eds.). 1995. Pp. 1524–1527. Edmonton, Alberta, Canada: Canadian Organization for the Advancement of Computers in Health (COACH).

2. The Denver Free-Net

The Denver Free-Net's electronic network serves as the common thread across all specialties participating in the OUTREACH Network activities. The Denver Free-Net is an electronic community computing system that provides public access to community resources [1]. The system is an extension of the School of Nursing's original electronic bulletin board, NurseLink. Seed money for DFN was given by The Colorado Trust, a philanthropic foundation whose mission is to improve the health care of Colorado citizens, in March of 1992. The system opened in January 1993 and has over 24,000 registered users. The Professional Advisory Board, in operation since the summer of 1992, has a primary role to guide and govern the development of the Denver Free-Net and serve as an ambassador of the system by promoting the concept of community networks. The Board consists of health care professionals, librarians, information specialists, and telecommunication specialists.

3. The OUTREACH Network

The OUTREACH (On-Line Urban to Rural Education and Community Health) Network is an innovative project to support the elimination of barriers to care in rural areas by expanding telecommunications capacity and extending the use of community networks. The community networks discussed in this paper exist in a physical sense and are active stakeholders in building community capacity. But they also exist in "cyberspace," the electronic world of the information highway. In both senses, this project will increase the interactive capabilities of the rural health professional, provider, and consumer to access human, institutional, and knowledge based resources located within and outside of their geographic area.

The mission of the OUTREACH Network is to expand and augment rural health care services through a set of user-friendly community computing systems. The systems include a publicly accessible Internet resource, the Denver Free-Net, which specializes in health care issues. A second component is a public state-wide Internet library project called Access Colorado Library Information Network. The third component is a local community computing effort called the Yampa Valley Bulletin Board System (BBS). The last system is another local community computing effort called DAVID, Database and Vicinity Information Directory. The Yampa Valley BBS and DAVID serve two large rural areas in Colorado. The OUTREACH Network will provide these two rural regions in Colorado with access to the wealth of health care resources available at the University of Colorado Health Sciences Center and the University Hospital.

The two rural regions, selected because of their commitment to the community computing concept, rural health needs, and their positioning for telecommunications, are wired to the University of Colorado Health Science Center. Rural health care professionals and consumers have, over a three year period, electronic access to a variety of health care resources and communication services at a local, state, and national level. The project involves two rural areas, Southwestern and Northwestern Colorado, with "on-ramps" to the Information Highway. The project will specifically decrease professional isolation of rural health care providers, increase professionals access to knowledge resources, and increase access to numerous health care specialties such as Geriatric Care, Substance Abuse, Cancer, Women's and Men's Health, School Health, and Native Americans Mental Health issues.

The OUTREACH Network will also promote the goals of Healthy People 2000 and will be one of the few publicly available networks for consumers to access health care resources to encourage their active participation in health decisions. The rural communities and academic health center will partner with local Cooperative Extensions to facilitate their Decisions for Health Initiatives in the State of Colorado.

4. The UTMB Interactive Multimedia Intervention

Educators, researchers, and clinicians at The University of Texas Medical Branch in Galveston (UTMB) have developed an interactive educational intervention that can be individually tailored by learners to get the information they need [2]. The intervention is quite different from the more traditional fare of instructor-driven materials, such as the text in printed brochures, instructional videotapes, or even organized classes. The educational materials in the UTMB interactive multimedia programs appeal to a wide range of learners because there is variety and choice in both the way information is presented and the order in which it appears. According to Lubin [3], interactive multimedia programs empower individuals who have different learning styles, especially those who are just not good at traditional learning with texts. Interactive multimedia uses technology to bundle together multiple collections of information into a single program or application. The collections of information can be full motion video, computer data, animation, graphics, still-frame slides, and stereo audio [4].

The UTMB interactive educational intervention started out as a series of interrelated health promotion programs for new mothers to use in learning to care for their infants. The audience of learners soon broadened to include families and friends interested in these young infants as well as their older brothers and sisters. This is in concert with a move to expand the role of the patient as consumer to include family members [5]. The UTMB-produced *Healthy Touch*® *Series* now provides access to health education resources for families and other small groups of learners on topics ranging from nutrition and immunization to safety around the home [6]. It is a resource for a wide variety of learners who can make choices about the topic, the order of presentation, the language of presentation, and the pace of the instructional material.

Learners stay involved with the programs because their participation is required at multiple decision points all along the way. Complex and extensive information is broken down into manageable components. Patients "navigate" through the choices about the information, so attention and responses are required of them every few minutes throughout the program. This feature helps to keep learners engaged with the programs despite the distractions of busy, noisy clinics.

5. The Healthy Touch® Series

The Healthy Touch® Series consists of four programs that were developed to provide health promotion information to patients and families in maternal-infant settings. The following titles were produced: *Feeding Your Infant, Home "Safe" Home, Immunizations on Parade*, and *Having a Healthy Pregnancy*.

The multimedia programs were designed from the outset to provide a comfortable and non-threatening learning environment that would put learners at ease; that would provide an overall approach of enjoyment or fun so they would be motivated to continue to learn; and would present a style that would appear to be very non-technology-oriented. The program was also designed to accommodate bilingual patients with comparable versions available in Spanish and in English.

One section of the program, *Feeding Your Baby*, includes a visit to a computerized grocery store. Colorful foods are pictured on the shelves, and the learner can navigate in any direction around the 3-D grocery store. A discovery learning experience has been constructed in which the patient can: touch the sign above the food (to hear the label rather than read it); touch the food (to hear animated audio sounds such as sizzling bacon and get information on nutrient values or age-appropriateness of the foods); or touch the animated grocery cart and move to a new aisle.

Screens were created with PC Paintbrush, imported as DIB files directly into the authoring system, Authorware Professional 2.0, and combined with digital audio files to be delivered via Soundblaster Pro. The files were mastered on a CD-ROM disc because of the large file size of both the digitized graphics and bilingual audio files. (The version of the grocery store with the English version print and audio track was nearly 100MB alone.) Digital video technology was also used for teaching program content. Digital video was scaled in windows by using a video digitizer card and video compression technology [7].

A second example from the series shows how the flexibility in the design can accommodate varied learning needs and styles. In the safety program, entitled *Home "Safe" Home*, the learner is offered a choice of relational courseware formatting or linear formatting. The relational format is the best choice when learners are encouraged to explore all factors affecting the task or concept being taught [1].

In the "safety house," learners choose between a "browsing" mode and a "tour" mode. In the browsing mode, learners wander into the locations of their choice in the 3D house, garage, or yard and select any items they want to explore. For example, if they touch the medicine cabinet in the bathroom, the door opens to display medicines and many of the other usual items. When touched, each item in the cabinet responds with an animation and an audio file of information about the particular substance. On the other hand, the "tour" mode offers a selection of tours that have been developed in a linear format to assist in providing organization and structure for the new information. For instance, the Fire Safety tour visits only the locations in the house that contain items related to potential fire hazards or burns. The learner has the opportunity to touch the items to see the animation or hear the fire safety audio message that relates to it, but she cannot move to other non-fire-related items in the room if they are on the tour.

6. The Project Sites

The rural population served by this project consist of residents of southwestern and northwestern Colorado. The total square mileage (25,689) of the counties affected by the project is larger than ten states. All but two of the counties are classified as frontier counties. Two of the counties—LaPlata and Routt—are one step up from frontier counties and are classified as low density counties. Both of Colorado's Indian reservations—the Southern Ute and the Ute Mountain Ute—are located in the southwestern area.

Several workstations have been established in these rural communities for access to this "telemultimedia" resource. Once on the system, the learner "enters" this educational resource center by selecting the health information section of the Denver Free-Net. A brief explanation of *The Healthy Touch*® *Series* and its content ends with a menu of choices for accessing specific topics. As soon as the learner designates a choice, the specific CD-ROM title is "up and running," triggering a contact with the Texas portion of the network for activation of a tracking file for electronic record keeping, for data collection, and for storage of files if troubleshooting is required.

The workstations include the following hardware: a touch-sensitive monitor with SVGA capability, a quad speed CD player with 6 CD capacity, a soundcard, speakers, a modem, and a printer. The approximate cost of the workstation configuration is $6,000 each.

References

[1] Skiba D. & Mirque D. "The electronic community: An alternative Health Care Delivery System." In Grobe (ed). *Nursing Informatics: An International Overview for Nursing in a Technological Era.* Holland: Elsevier (1994).

[2] Sweeney M.A., Mercer Z., Oppermann C., McHugh D., & Murphy C. "Innovative designs in multimedia programs for clinical teaching." In *MEDINFO '92, Proceedings of the Seventh World Congress on Medical Informatics.* Amsterdam: North-Holland (1992).

[3] Lubin D. Making multimedia accessible. *Multimedia Monitor* (1993) 11:24–29.

[4] Anderson C. & Veljkow M. *Creating Interactive Multimedia.* Glenview, IL: Scott, Foresman and Company (1990).

[5] Gustafson D. "Expanding on the role of patient as consumer." *Quality Review Bulletin* (1991) 17(10):324–325.

[6] Sweeney M.A., Mercer Z., Lester J., & Oppermann C. "Multimedia interventions in maternal-infant community-based clinics." *Proceeding of Fifth International Conference on Nursing Use of Computers and Information Science* (1994—in press).

[7] Luther A. *Digital Video in the PC Environment.* New York: McGraw-Hill Book Company (1989).

11
The Electronic Community: An Alternative Health Care Approach

DIANE J. SKIBA and D.T. MIRQUE

1. Background

Health care expenditures in the United Sates have reached staggering proportions, 761 billion dollars in 1990 representing 12.2% of the gross national product (GNP) [1]. There is consensus among the health care professions that much of the injuries and illnesses contributing to this cost can be prevented through widespread adoption of improved safety practices and healthier lifestyles [2]. The promotion of health and prevention of disease are the basis of the health care reform movement and of the government initiative, Healthy People 2000. Health promotion and disease prevention are considered methods to: dramatically cut health care costs, prevent premature onset of disease and disability, and help all Americans achieve healthier and more productive lives [3]. The National Agenda for Health Care is based upon three assumptions: personal responsibility is a key to good health, health care should be accessible and available to every citizen, and that prevention is described in its broadest perspective [3]. In Colorado, these initiatives are examined by a governor-appointed task force, the Colorado Health Care Reform Initiative [4].

To achieve the health goals, individuals must understand the relationship between lifestyle behaviors and their medical consequences. Individuals must have readily accessible health care information to promote this understanding. Further, the broad definition of health must extend beyond the notion of absence of disease. The World Health Organization defines a

Reprinted from *Nursing Informatics: An International Overview for Nursing in a Technological Era*, Grobe, S.J., Pluyter-Wenting, E.S.P. (Eds.). 1994. Pp. 388–392, with kind permission from Elsevier Science—NL, Sara Burgerhartstraat 25, 1055 KV Amsterdam, The Netherlands.

76

healthy community as "one that includes a clean, safe, high quality physical environment and a sustainable ecosystem; provision of basic needs; an optimum level of appropriate, high quality, accessible public health and sick care services; and a diverse, vital and innovative economy" [5]. To date, most printed information as well as computerized information systems remain accessible to only health care professionals [2]. Many [6, 2, 7] believe that taking self-care and health promotion into the home is of critical value in resolving the health care crisis. According to McDonald and Blum's [8] report, 95% of all first-line health decisions are made at home or in the workplace by the person and family or friends. Additionally, most people (60%) wait too long to handle health care problems resulting in longer, more complex and costly care [8]. Certainly home health care and community based clinics are popular mechanisms advocating these notions of self-care and health promotion concepts [9].

An alternative for health care delivery advocates the use of computers and telecommunications. Information access and communication can be available on a 24 hour basis, 365 days a year. This approach is of particular importance for rural areas which traditionally have suffered from serious problems with health care access [10]. A recent report [8] states that a telecommunication infrastructure could provide health care to the neediest segments of our population. Health-oriented telecommunications "could save hundreds of billions of health care dollars over the next two decades" [8]. According to this report, this proposed interactive network could provide: access to patient electronic medical records, integration of clinical databases and preventive care, self-care medical advice and other health care information to consumers. The provision of distributed health information and health decision-making tools coupled with communication pathways to health care professionals will promote greater self-responsibility for one's health.

A review of the literature examining the use of electronic networks for the delivery of health care provided encouragement for the development of this project. The use of a computerized network to support persons living with AIDS/ARC [11] and support for caretakers of Alzheimer's patients [12] provided a solid foundation for the efficacy of health-oriented telecommunications. In both instances, patients and caretakers were receptive of the technology and used the network for information retrieval and communication. Hassett, Lowder and Rutan [13] studied the use of bulletin boards by the disabled population and found the technology could provide information, services and support for this population and their caretakers. Another study [14] also concurred that it is feasible to use interactive, computer-based systems to support people facing health-related crises such as breast cancer and AIDS/HIV infection. Brennan [11] summarized that a computer network provided the balance necessary to promote social support while providing information access and tools to foster self-care.

2. Denver Free-Net

2.1 Denver Free-Net Development

Since 1987, the School of Nursing at the University of Colorado Health Sciences Center has operated an electronic bulletin board called NurseLink. With initial funding from the regional telephone service entity (US WEST), NurseLink was designed as a communication vehicle to disseminate research findings to nurses in local clinical agencies. After an extensive evaluation [15], a decision was made to redesign NurseLink from an electronic bulletin board for health care professionals into a community computing system for consumer access to information and communication mechanisms. The evolution of NurseLink to the Denver Free-Net was facilitated by the receipt of a grant from The Colorado Trust, a philanthropic foundation dedicated to promoting the health and well-being of the citizens of Colorado.

The Denver Free-Net is modeled after the community computing system, the Cleveland Free-Net. Community computing, as described by the National Public Telecomputing Network (NPTN), establishes a community resource that is freely accessible by the citizens through a computerized network. By using a personal computer, telecommunications software and a modem, the community can access a Free-Net system on a 24 hour basis. The community itself defines the information resources and provides the necessary support to maintain the information resources as well as to sustain the concept of an electronic community. The Cleveland Free-Net originated at Case Western Reserve University in 1984. Presently, there are 10 free-net systems available worldwide and all are members of NPTN.

2.2 Denver Free-Net Description

The mission of the Denver Free-Net project is to promote the concept of community computing to citizens in the state of Colorado. Specific goals are: to provide citizens with free and open access to community information resources, particularly in health and human services and to foster the development of health-oriented telecommunications as a means of health care delivery within the state of Colorado. The Denver Free-Net system is available to anyone who has access to a computer, modem and telecommunication software. The system is available 24 hours per day and can be reached via six dial in phone lines (303-270.4936) or via Internet (telnet to 140.226.1.8). People may login as a guest or as a registered user. A guest can browse the system and register as a user via an online registration process. Register users have interactive privileges through electronic mail, chat functions and the ability to post questions, answers or messages. Presently, a total of 20 concurrent users are allowed online.

The Denver Free-Net is best conceptualized as an electronic city where a user enters buildings such as the Post Office, the School House and the Health Care Community Center. It is a menu-driven system that provides information in several formats: read only text information, databases, question and answer forums, and online conversation mode. The opening screen is the main menu and contains the numerous buildings a user can enter. As one can see, the buildings are similar to those in existence in many communities throughout the world.

2.2.1 Health Care Building

Let us take a tour of the Health Care Building and view a sample of the information and communication exchanges available. It is important to remember that the Denver Free-Net is a dynamic system in which new information can be added on a daily basis. The Health Care Building contains numerous menu selections categorized into several broad areas. One area focuses on health promotion and prevention materials categorized according to the Healthy People 2000 goals. For example, the Aurora Prevention Partnership, a federally funded resource center with educational materials, is listed under the goal—substance abuse. Another example is a list of "consumer tips" provided by sources such as University Hospital, Colorado Department of Health and the FDA. Also included in this broad category is the Consumer Health Question and Answer (Q & A) moderated by a consortium of medical librarians. The Q & A allows consumers to leave questions about health promotion and an experienced consumer health librarian provides an answer within a day or two. The Q & A sections are the most interactive component of the Free-Net system. The Q & A provides a comfortable, non-threatening environment for consumers to ask questions openly without fear of ignorance or embarrassment. This is a particular useful method for consumers to ask questions about sensitive topics. A similar Q & A is under construction for school health area. This Q & A is targeted for adolescents who will be able to leave anonymous questions to be answered by school nurses.

A special community area is the Support Group Center that houses a database of support groups available in the Denver metropolitan region. The Support Group Center, initiated by the Denver Free-Net staff, is continually updated by community information providers. The database contains over 600 support groups with specific information about the group, meeting times, address, phone numbers and contact person. All groups are classified by keywords to represent their focus areas such as grieving, cancer patients, eating disorders, etc. The database has simple searching capabilities. There are plans to develop the searching capabilities.

Another room focuses on AIDS/HIV and contains a variety of information: online publications, a database of support group and discussion groups. A highlight of this room is an AIDS discussion area that is part of a worldwide USENET newsgroup. This communication mechanism, delayed time discussion groups, allows users to participate in discussions with people from around the world.

Various organizations such as the Alzheimer's Group and the Parkinson's Disease Group maintain areas in the health care building. Information includes items such as support group listings, newsletters, position papers (i.e. Directions in Alzheimer's research), and Frequently Asked Questions (FAQ) section that contains answers to consumers' most commonly asked questions.

The University of Colorado Health Sciences Center maintains a building which contains separate areas for the schools of nursing, medicine, dentistry and pharmacy. A variety of information and Q & A's are housed in this area. For example, the School of Nursing lists its courses, academic schedule, student and school newsletters, faculty phone numbers, faculty research interests and research announcements. The Colorado Nursing Task Force maintains information about the differentiated practice models and articulation programs available in Colorado and operates a Q & A to guide nurses about educational and career opportunities available statewide. The Health Sciences Library also maintains a room with a current list of available journals, available library courses, announcements and a newsletter. There is also a gateway for a connection to the Colorado Alliance of Research Library (CARL) system. The gateway provides a connection to a remote computer (telnet capability) that houses the CARL system. Computer conferencing classes are being planned by the School of Nursing with its outreach students using the discussion/newsgroup format available on the Denver Free-Net.

Online publications for health care professionals are also available in the Health Care Building. For example, the Center for Disease Control's biweekly publication of Federal Drug announcements and Weekly Mortality and morbidity Reports are available via the *Health InfoComm Newsletter*. Health care professionals can read these documents within hours of their release rather than waiting for their arrival via the postal service.

These examples of the health care building are but a small fraction of what is available in this electronic city. The examples, though, represent a wide variety of information and communication formats. Information is available in various formats: text only (most of which can be downloaded) and searchable databases. Communication vehicles include Q & A formats, delayed time discussion and news groups, computer conferencing and the ability to connect to remote computers via the telnet function. Other capabilities of the Denver Free-Net system are described in the subsequent section.

2.2.2 Electronic Mail (email) and Chat

Registered users have two additional communication mechanisms available: email and chat. Each registered has full Internet mail access. In the

Post Office, a user can check their mail, send mail, create a signature file, and use the directory services to find a user login name. Electronic mail includes messaging and the attachment of files to messages. The Communications Center Building allows one to communicate with others online. The chat function allows both a one-on-one chat or a multi-user chat. The one-on-one chat allows you to talk in real time to another registered user who is currently on the system. A multi-user chat allows several users to talk in real time. Both functions are quite popular and many of our Internet users partake in this function. This function will be particularly useful for our outreach students who can chat with each other and the instructor.

2.2.3 Other Buildings

The Denver Free-Net boasts a wealth of consumer-based information in other buildings; the latest weather report for most North American cities can be found in the Science Building; the current performing arts schedules in the Arts Building; an electronic library in the Schoolhouse; the ability to explore other established Free-Nets in the Communications Building. As one can see a variety of essential consumer information exists to complement the Health Care Building and fosters the healthy community concept.

3. Current Usage

The Denver Free-Net officially opened to the public on January 12, 1993. At the time of this writing (September, 1993), there are over seven thousand registered users. Most users are from the Denver metropolitan area and represent age groups from teenagers to senior citizens. Uses from other Free-Nets throughout the United States and other Internet users in the United States and from various countries (France, England, China, Germany, Finland, Bulgaria and Italy) are also registered. Numerous health care projects have been initiated with the Denver Free-Net being used as a communication vehicle and as an information dissemination mechanism.

Besides the registered users, there are over 500 information providers who contribute information to the various buildings. In addition, a multitude of volunteers help to maintain the system by serving on committees, as technical back-up staff and moderators of special interest groups or discussion areas (Q & A's). Without the participation of the community, the Denver Free-Net would not exist.

Since the time period between the paper submission and presentation is lengthy, we know the health care applications of this system will increase dramatically over the next year. Therefore, the conference presentation will focus on the impact of this system as an alternative health care delivery system.

4. Summary

The Denver Free-Net project is achieving its mission to promote the concept of community computing in the state of Colorado. Health care and human services information is widely being distributed to all segments of the population. The uses of electronic community network is offering many opportunities as an alternative health care delivery system and is promoting the concepts of self-care, consumer-health care partnerships, and healthy communities. It is important to remember that "Telecommunications is not an end in itself but a means to an end which is to break down barriers . . . and . . . that the highway of the 21st Century will transmit information, not people" [10].

References

[1] Office of the Actuary, *Health Care Financing Administration*, Press Release, March, 1991.

[2] Melmed A and Fisher FD. *Towards a National Information Infrastructure: Implications for Selected Social Sectors and Education.* New York University, 1991.

[3] *Healthy People 2000: National Health Promotion and Disease Prevention Objectives.* Full report with commentary. Washington, D.C.: United States Department of Health and Human Services (PHS #91-50212).

[4] *Colorado's Health Care Action Plan: From Concept to Proposal to Solution.* Denver: Governor Roy Romer's Office, 1992.

[5] Colorado Trust Unveils Strategic Study. *The Colorado Trust Quarterly* 1992.

[6] Grundner TM and Garrett R. Interactive Medical Telecomputing: An alternative Approach to Community Health Education. *N Engl J Med* 1986, 15:982–985.

[7] Olson R, Jones MG and Bezold C. *21st Century Learning and Health Care in the Home: Creating a National Telecommunications Network.* Washington, D.C.: Institute for Alternative Futures and The Consumer Interest Research Institute, 1992.

[8] McDonald MD and Blum HL. *Health in the Information Age: The Emergence of Health Oriented Telecommunication Applications.* Berkeley, CA: University of California, 1992.

[9] Shugars D, O'Neil E and Bader J. *Health America: Practitioners for 2005, An Agenda for Action for U.S. Health Professional Schools.* Durham, NC: The Pew Health Profession Commission, 1991.

[10] Puskin D. Telecommunications in Rural America: Opportunities and Challenges for the Health Care System. *Ann N Y Acad Sci* 1992, 670:67–75.

[11] Brennan P, Ripich S and Moore S. The Use of Home-Based Computers to Support Persons Living with AIDS/ARC. *J Community Health Nurs* 1991, 8:3–14.

[12] Brennan P, Moore S and Smyth K. ComputerLink: Electronic Support for the Home Giver. *ANS* 1991, 13:14–27.

[13] Hassett M, Lowder C and Rutan D. Use of computer network bulletin board systems by disabled persons. In: SCAMC '92. Frisse M (ed). New York: McGraw-Hill, 1992: 151–155.

[14] Gustafson D, Bosworth K, Hawkins R, Boberg E and Bricker E. CHESS: A computer-based system for providing information, referrals, decision support and social support to people facing medical and other health-related crisis. In: SCAMC '92. Frisse M. (ed). New York: McGraw-Hill, 1992: 161–165.

[15] Skiba D and Warren C. The impact of an electronic bulletin board to disseminate educational and research information to nursing colleagues. In: Nursing Informatics '91. Hovenga E, Hannah K, McCormick K and Ronald J (eds). Berlin: Springer-Verlag, 1991: 704–709.

12
Nursing Collaboratory Development via the Internet

Linda K. Woolery and J. Yensen

1. Definition of an International Nursing Collaboratory

The Nursing Collaboratory is based on concepts described by Wulf [1] and consists of researchers who participate in research laboratories and nursing research projects through Internet communication and collaboration. The Nursing Collaboratory is affiliated with the Virtual Nursing College (VNC) that was developed to provide distance education delivery through intelligent use of technology, where distance could be two blocks from the computing center or two continents away.

One of the evolutionary trends required for a virtual nursing college is that of ease of access. Hardware solutions are dipping in price and rapidly increasing in availability. It is feasible and now do-able to have glass connectivity and hence very high optical transfer rates. It is likely that, in the near future, houses and buildings will have built-in wide band width plug-in ports for cable, glass, and satellite transmitted data. Data storage will be in the form of distributed storage site hubs, similar to airport hubs. This is starting to occur now and the time frame for super-connectivity is within 5–7 years.

Perhaps of more interest in the VNC domain is the problem of data management. On the Internet, there are already the beginnings of knowbots (software whose entire function is to wander the Net and look for specific violations of HTML in HTML document depositories and report back to the owner) and global area menu harvesting (ALIWEB) to keep WWW servers current. Future local knowbots will spend their time roaming through our own data files looking for associations and connectivities, only some of which have been established by the user. Knowbot software will learn about the activities and interests of the owner by monitoring

Reprinted with permission from *MEDINFO '95: Proceedings of the Eighth World Congress on Medical Informatics*; Greenes, R.A., Peterson, H.E. & Protti, D.J. (Eds.). 1995. Pp. 1349–1352. Edmonton, Alberta, Canada: Canadian Organization for the Advancement of Computers in Health (COACH).

computer activity and data transmissions. The knowbot software develops a dynamic profile of its owner and then intelligently scans all of Internet, plus 650 TV channels etc. and establishes IURLs (Intelligent User Resource Links) on a daily basis. The software assembles the IURLs into menus and presents them to the owner at pre-established intervals. You, the owner, can then choose to follow any or all of the menu options as you wish. Pursuit of a link that yields poor returns (however defined) may be handled by assigning a priority rank or probability to the link. The next time you see the menu, this priority will be reflected in menu ordering. This allows the user to constantly redefine what is currently important. The software will also contain propositional intelligence (i.e., when queried it can support how and why it established the link).

2. Nursing Collaboratory Model and Components (Figure 1)

Distributed Systems Technology

The Nursing Collaboratory functions in a distributed systems technology environment that includes the wide area network of planet earth. Information overload will be managed through personal "knowbots" that are programmed to search the Internet as both data producing filters and information producing filters for the researcher's specified domain of inquiry. Knowbot software is intelligently constructed and does not limit its owner to the knowbot profile (i.e., if you accidentally stumble on control tower tapes and find it important, you hot-key the "serendipity" flag of knowbot and it stores your find and offers you an optional profile amendment quiz). The quiz is a database front-end that is intended to take care of new owner interests that may occur outside of computer activities and TV channel monitoring—such things have been known to happen! Knowbot does not prevent you from random or erratic searches. If you are engaged in such an activity, knowbot asks politely if you want this material indexed and added to your profile; it is possible to turn on or off certain kinds of

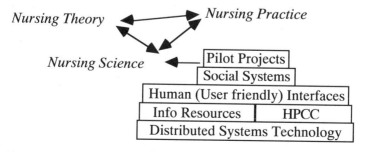

FIGURE 1. Nursing collaboratory model and components.

activity monitoring so that knowbot is not confused. Your questions about the human propensity to be curious etc. are not defeated by knowbot, but rather enhanced. Thus, from a research laboratory or office anywhere in the world, a researcher can acquire raw data, library resources, and other information from anywhere on the planetary Internet web. While there are many issues that relate to client-server and distributed systems technology, it is important to understand that the technology exists now, and the Nursing Collaboratory research environment is developing because it is currently possible, from a technological standpoint.

Information Resources

The "information age" provides nurses with vastly expanded information resources; traditional journals and textbooks become too rapidly outdated and replaced with online, up-to-date digital libraries around the world. Again, personal knowbots manage information by filtering the Internet's vast resources for search strings that are specified (or programmed) by the researcher to compile relevant resources at the local level for the researcher's analysis and review.

HPCC = High Performance Computing and Communications

The technology to support a global distributed systems environment and planetary information resources is foundational for Nursing Collaboratory development. Communication can take many forms (e-mail, listserv, snailmail, fax, voice telephone, and future videoconferencing). But, high performance communication implies Internet transmission of all types of data/information using voice, technology, and video conferencing from small pocket-sized computers with wireless infrared transmission as these technologies are further developed. Traditional forms of communication have already given way to e-mail and listserv discussions among Nursing Collaboratory researchers.

Human (User Friendly) Interfaces

Mosaic (http://www.ncsa.uiuc.edu/SDG/Software/Mosaic/NCSAMosaic-Home.html [as of 6/94]) and Cello (http://www.law.cornell.educello/

Research Project Management	Research Development Resources
Budget	Funding
Data Management	Collaborating/Consulting
Data Analysis	Data Acquisition
Human Resources	Literature
Task Lists	Proposal Development Tools
Results Reporting	
Publishing Resources	

FIGURE 2. Screen design for the Nursing Collaboratory.

cellotop.html las of 6/94]) are just two examples of already developed friendly human interfaces used to access the Internet. In addition, user friendly knowbot packages are at various stages of development and testing (as well as various stages of user friendliness). The following functionality is planned for Nursing Collaboratory screen design, with prototype development beginning at multiple sites around the world (Figure 2).

Social Systems

Technology does not operate in a vacuum and often succeeds or fails based upon the social systems into which it is introduced. The Nursing Collaboratory development teams understand this phenomenon and work closely with current and potential Nursing Collaboratory researchers to develop and sustain social systems that support and promote the goals and objectives of individual researchers as well as the Nursing Collaboratory at large. Strategies to develop Nursing Collaboratory research teams include front-loading teams with knowledgeable, talkative, and diverse personalities that can stimulate scholarly discussion of ideas and sustain the teams through periods of disagreement and conflict. The Nursing Collaboratory teams are addressing social systems by front-loading teams with already active Internet users who are "talkative," diverse, and tolerant while generating provocative discussions. There is a developing sense of community and "belonging" that will be important to sustain as further social systems develop within the Nursing Collaboratory.

Pilot Projects

Pilot work involves iterative development, prototyping, and research elements that help define and refine the work of collaboratory researchers. Shared proposal development, shared data, shared analyses and interpretations, and shared manuscript development are ongoing activities for Nursing Collaboratory researchers. On-line Internet consultation saves travel time and money and permits expert consultation even on limited research budgets. Pilot projects must fit within a nursing research-theory-practice paradigm to advance the profession's body of knowledge.

3. Opportunities

The Nursing Collaboratory provides opportunities for nurse researchers to be more productive through cooperation and collaboration. Research is strengthened through multi-site replication. One principle that guides Nursing Collaboratory development is that things need to change; another is that the rate of change is itself accelerating; yet another is that current rule sets are inadequate to apply to future possibilities. Whether we like it or not, practice-driven disciplines require causative logic at most levels i.e., we need to be able to substantiate or support why we "do" certain things in order to influence certain desirable changes of state (outcomes). A corollary of this is that nursing research may reduce the need for peer evaluation/peer review through the more appropriate strategy of small scale multi-site replication. As an example, if you develop a strategy for effective enhancement of adaptation in women recently diagnosed with breast cancer and do a reasonable well designed study, you may end up with insufficient power or failure to reject a key hypothesis. (As you know, a lot of research ends up in this state!). Now, through VNC and all its sites and resources, several practitioners working with such women may say that the acid test is it if it works for them. This is external validity proceeding without experimental grounds. But, if you reconceptualize the whole thing, trying out your strategies is no longer a replication, but rather an extension of your work at another site. If several of us try out your approaches at different sites, we overcome the obstacles. In this way, the discipline advances much more effectively and in fact all research (and practice) becomes collaborative.

Expanded social systems networking creates a community of researchers that exchange ideas and provides professional and personal support for individual researchers. Improved communication and collaboration minimize duplication and redundancy such that knowledge development in an individual researcher's work builds on an already publicized domain (where one exists), or communicates to the Nursing Collaboratory teams that a new domain of knowledge building is now in progress. Knowledge domains are mapped, and links are identified and described to help articulate a coherent body of nursing knowledge. Incremental and supplemental knowledge building that is scrutinized by international Nursing Collaboratory researchers (in the spirit of cooperation and collaboration) will help define and advance the science (and maybe the art) of Nursing.

4. Issues

Various issues arise when new modes of communicating and collaborating are made available through the Nursing Collaboratory. Hardware and software reliability issues are crucial to Nursing Collaboratory research, since nurses cannot communicate and collaborate when Internet links and transmissions fail. Also, it is important to verify, or authenticate, the expertise of a potential research collaborator. It is equally important to verify the reliability and accuracy of data sources. Security and confidentiality issues related to patient data exist as in all research modes. But security and confidentiality of methodologies and tools that secure competitive funding will also arise. An issue of "ownership" (both of data and research strategies) must be dealt with. The people issues (i.e., (un)willingness to share and collaborate) involve monumental tasks in nursing that will be difficult to resolve in some situations. Awareness of these issues is an important place to begin, and researchers will acknowledge that these issues exist outside the Nursing Collaboratory. Answers and solutions are works-in-progress.

5. Current State of Nursing Collaboratory Development

Activities (as of July 1994)

The VNC team developed the Nursing Collaboratory idea, initial goals, initial issues list, and first research team meeting. A group of nursing informatics researchers gathered in San Antonio, TX (USA) in June 1994 to form a Nursing Collaboratory team that would focus on the research and development of expert systems and decision support for nurses. This group shared ideas and updates on their current research projects and debated many of the issues involved in their research domain. The group is in the formative stage and communication and collaboration has just begun. While the first meeting was held in person (part of the social systems of current paradigms), ongoing "meetings" and continued work are conducted over the Internet. A collaborative project is under development, and preliminary work on Internet tools has begun.

Nursing Collaboratory Goals (as of July 1994)

1. To build an international community of researchers in nursing domains.
2. To support scholarly research that defines and refines nursing knowledge.
3. To support Nursing Collaboratory researchers both personally and professionally.
4. To promote communication, cooperation, and collaboration that enhances research efforts and avoids redundancy and duplication of research efforts.
5. To sponsor multi-site replication that provides for highly cost-effective research extending into high statistical power and rapid implementation of findings.
6. To identify and resolve issues that arise in Nursing Collaboratory research efforts.
7. To promote health and well-being for citizens of planet Earth.

Nursing Collaboratory Development Team (as of July 1994)

Jack Yensen (Langara College—Vancouver, British Columbia, Canada)
Linda Woolery (University of Missouri—Columbia, Missouri, USA)
Linda Thede (Kent State University—Kent, Ohio, USA)
Members of the Expert Systems and Decision Support Research Team

Reference

[1] Wulf W.A. "The collaboratory opportunity." *SCIENCE* (1993) 261(5123):854–855.

13
Data Protection and Nursing; A Technical and Organizational Challenge

A.R. Bakker and Maureen Scholes

Introduction

The application of computers in health care and in particular in nursing offers new possibilities for improved communication and coordination. These possibilities look very attractive and already now we see a rapidly increasing use of computer facilities throughout the whole health care system. We should realize however that application of computers also has its disadvantages. The flexible communication facilities introduce an increased risk for unauthorized access to data that might harm the privacy of the patient. Storing data in a computer memory and processing it automatically is quite attractive from different points of view (direct support of the patient care process, management support, quality assurance, etc.), however we should realize that computers might fail either because of problems in the hardware, the software or the operations. Such failures might lead to loss or modification of data. When computers are used intensively in the health care process, we become quite dependent on their facilities. Failures in the information system can lead to interruptions in the service. In those situations the essential data might be unavailable and we should think on beforehand what to do in such situations.

In this paper the various aspects of data protection are discussed first. Next it is indicated which types of measures might be taken to reduce the risks involved. The increasing use of information systems in health care should go hand in hand with increased awareness of the data protection aspects. Also the impact of changing technology will be considered in this paper. At the end it is suggested that nurses be aware of these risks and play an active part in setting-up a data protection policy.

The authors strongly believe that information processing will be of tre-

Reprinted with permission from *Proceedings of Nursing and Computers: the Third International Symposium on Nursing Use of Computers and Information Science*; Pp. 94–102. Daly, N. & Hannah, K.J. (Eds.). 1988. St. Louis: The C.V. Mosby Company.

mendous importance for both the quality and the efficiency of our health care system in general and nursing in particular. However we should not introduce these new technologies thoughtlessly. It is our responsibility to find a balance between improved services and increased risks.

Data Protection: Its Three Components

The terminology in the data protection field is often confusing. The terms: privacy, security, safety, confidentiality are being used, without clear definition. In this paper we will follow the terminology used by working group 4 of International Medical Informatics Association (IMIA) (Griesser et al 1980). We distinguish three components:

Usage integrity
Data/program integrity
Availability

Usage Integrity

The storage and communication facilities of computerized health information systems do not only supply valuable functions for authorized health care professionals, they also lead to an increased risk that unauthorized users get access to sentive data either directly via terminals, or by means of database query facilities. Also linking of computer systems may increase the risks. We should be aware of the fact that access to data that are essential for the health care process may lead to an intrusion of the patient privacy. For instance the fact that somebody has been admitted to the hospital, with a certain diagnosis or treatment may effect his social functioning. Many patients will not appreciate if data about their behaviour in the hospital would be made available to unauthorized people.

Data/Program Integrity

Maintenance of data integrity means that the quality, availability and accuracy of computerized data and programs remains the same as the source documents and it has not been exposed to accidental or malicious alteration, loss or destruction. In the health care system we are primarily concerned about accidental loss or destruction. Nevertheless there are some examples of malicious alteration. Loss of data might occur because of hardware failures, software failures or human errors in the operations. A major risk is the "improvement" of programs, sometimes leading to serious errors.

Availability

Protection of the availability of data and resources includes all measures which are required to preserve the availability of the health information system in total or of any part or service related to it.

The information system is meant to support the health care process and to replace (at least in part) the manual recording and communication system. Also the organization of the institution will be adapted to take full advantage of the health information system. One should realize, however, that the availability of the system will never be 100%, although measures can be taken to approach this ideal situation. One should define on beforehand what has to be done in case of nonavailability of the system or specific data. One of the problems is that patients will be present in the hospital 24 hours/day and will need care. In practice an availability of over 99.5% can be realized (at considerable costs) but even then one should be organized for a situation where the system would not function for one day in a period of three years.

Professional Responsibilities

It is remarkable that the concern about data protection often comes rather from data processing professionals than from endusers. In our era the trust in technology is so large that we are hardly inclined to think about its weaknesses. An adequate approach towards data protection needs awareness of the user community. This paper is to some extent an alarm message. On the other hand it gives indications about the solutions that will be available if we are prepared to pay attention to this aspect in a multi disciplinary approach.

Data Protection Tools and Measures

Many measures and tools are available to support an adequate data protection policy around health information systems. Measures can belong to the categories hardware, software and organizational. In this section only a global indication will be given of available measures. For details reference is made to the literature [E.J.O. Velders, A.R. Bakker 1987, G. Griesser et al. 1980].

First of all there are measures to support user identification. Based on this user identification within the software authorization checks can be implemented that take care of hiding data that should not be accessible to the specific user involved. User identification usually is achieved by a personal password system sometimes supported by magnetic batch reading facilities. User identification is mainly implemented to achieve adequate usage integrity. In addition to it procedures are necessary for handling of output and data carriers.

In the area of data integrity the following common measures can be listed:

Checks on validity and consistency of input data.
Periodic checks on the contents of the database combined with statistical
    checks.

Periodic copying of the database combined with logging of all mutations
in the system. Based on these safecopies and the logging files recovering
software opens the opportunity to reconstruct the database in case it
might be corrupted (by hardware, software or organizational reasons).
Procedure for the handling of safecopies.
Access control to the computer facilities.

To obtain adequate program integrity the following measures can be
considered:

No program development tools in the production environment (preventing
the carelessly "improvement" of production programs)
Inspection of all new programs offered for production
Acceptance testing of new versions using copies of the production files.

To obtain a high availability amongst others the following measures are
proposed

Back-up equipment; even full duplication is often applied
Automatic fire extinguishing
Access control to the computer facilities
On call maintenance and support

Outside the health care field cryptography is sometimes applied for
messages transmitted in the network. For the time being this measure in
general seems overdone in health information systems. The only place
where cryptography is often applied is in the storage of passwords within
the information system. In that case often an irreversible scrambling is used.

A good regulation for the information system is important to get a clear
insight for both users and patients about the aims and main structure of the
information system. Moreover the right of the patients as to information,
inspection, correction, deletion, refusal, should be described. For users the
regulation should make clear what their rights and responsibilities are. The
regulation should clearly describe how complaints should be handled.
Moreover the procedures around the supply of data should be stated
clearly.

Data protection is becoming a key issue in health information systems. The next section will make clear that we are only in initial phase
and that the role of information systems in the health care will increase
rapidly in the years to come. New technologies will on one hand help us
to extend the benefits of such systems. On the other hand these new technologies will have an increasing effect on the risks. Instruction and training
of users seems indispensable to arrive at an atmosphere where adequate
data protection is recognized as a common interest of both users and
patients.

The set of measures chosen in a specific situation should be geared to the
estimated risks that do exist. In literature methods are suggested to come to
an adequate set of data protection measures.

Present Trends and Developments

The data protection challenge in health information systems is not static. The use of computers in health care is spreading rapidly; this leads to:

More functions within the information system, supporting gradually more vital activities in the institution. Amongst these functions one can think of not only direct communication functions (like order entry and reporting) but also of functions with a direct effect on patient care like drug supply and medication schemes. Sometimes direct control of processes is supported by computer systems.

More users, each with their specific need for data; almost all disciplines will be involved as users of an integrated health information system.

More terminals/workstations to supply access facilities for these users. In nursing a terminal at the bedside is advocated these days.

More types of data in a coherent database; leading to more possibilities to combine data. As facility attractive for research support but a risk for the privacy.

Besides the extended use of computers one should notice that technology is developing rapidly. The new technology has a lot of attractive aspects for the information systems. In this paper it is emphasized that there are not only advantages and benefits but also risks that should be taken seriously.

The Application of Personal Computers

PC's can be used either as stand-alone facility or as intelligent workstations of a health information system. Often data protection aspects around stand-alone PC's are neglected with as argument that those systems have only a limited capacity and scope. To some extent this will be true, however the capacity of present PC's is comparable with that of "large computers" some 15 years ago. Pretty large databanks can be organized in PC's and when these databases contain medical data all usual data protection questions are applicable. These questions do not only relate to usage integrity but also to data/program integrity. The professional climate that in general exists around "large" health information systems is often missing when PC's are applied. So procedures about safecopying and checks on consistency of the database are often not reliable. The procedures about modifications in the software are often sloppy which may lead to serious errors. Also in a PC environment quality assurance on programs is a must.

When PC's are used as workstations of a health information system often the facility exists to derive data from the central database and store it in the PC for local processing. In such a set-up it is difficult to keep control over the data that might be stored on floppy disks and can easily be transported to other computers leading to breaches of privacy. Another risk is if the data are down-loaded but not kept up-to-date which might lead to errors in appreciation of medical situations. This might harm the patient directly.

Another risk of intelligent workstations is the possibility that repeated access attempts are generated from a PC with the risk that the access control system is violated. As a special measure to reduce this risk significantly a gradually increasing waiting-time can be implemented after failing access attempts.

Data Communication

The fast developments in data communication hardware and networking software facilitate the easy exchange of data between different computers. There is a clear tendency to construct links not only within the hospital but also across its borders. It is becoming more and more clear that we need more thinking and study about the rules for exchange of medical data within the hospital and even more across its borders. Although there are some technological challenges here the major problem in our feeling is the lack of a well-accepted code of conduct in this area. This holds true for both the exchange of data within the health care process as around medical research. As long as such rules are missing it might be used by technicians as an excuse for not implementing appropriate measures. The medical and dataprocessing profession should not wait for each other but cooperate to come to acceptable solutions.

Smart Cards

Smart Cards or chip cards create the possibility to supply patients with a machine readable medium that they carry themselves. On such a card a variety of health care data can be stored.

When thinking about a possible widespread use of this medium the following data protection issues come to mind:
What are the risks for privacy if the card is lost or stolen.

In certain situations the fact that a person has a smart-card holding at least part of this medical data might lead to pressure on him to reveal those data (e.g., in application procedures).
Since the medium would be carried by the patient himself a wide variety of health professionals might get access to the data. The risk exists that the data will be used outside the context and mis-interpretation might occur.
Standardization in both hardware, data structure, and data description is a need to make the smart-card a useful tool in the health care field.

Terminals at the Bed-Side

Wide-scale use of terminals at the bedside would imply a complete change of the information processing scenario in a hospital. Although terminals are being used already on a large scale (e.g., in Leiden University Hospital the number of terminals amounts to 800 now), they are situated in more or less specific working locations like reception desks, laboratories, radiology departments, ward stations, personnel department, pharmacy, etc.

The use of the terminals at the bedside would be different from the average present use in the following respects:

Use of the same terminal by a variety of disciplines: almost all people directly involved in patient care (mainly nurses and physicians) but also the patients themselves.

The terminals will in general be used very often for retrieval and input of limited amounts of data. This means that the "sessions" will be short. Sophisticated log-on procedures would be a burden.

Most hospital information systems are nowadays built on the principle that all functions a user is authorized for can be carried out from any terminal throughout the institution. For bed-side terminals there should be additional restrictions. It is suggested that from a bed-side terminal only data of the specific patient in that bed can be accessed easily and that access to data from other patients is only possible after additional checks on user of authorization. The following suggestions are made:

At the bed-side terminal only a limited subset of the functions of the health care system would be made available.

User identification is necessary to avoid the risks that patients destruct data recorded about them in the database.

The use of identity cards might help to simplify the log-on procedure.

One even could think of a situation where the patient himself could have access to his own data and some general hospital data without explicit log-on.

One should make special provisions to avoid the risks that visitors of the patients get access to the data either by operating the terminal or by viewing data that are on the screen.

The Role of the Nurse and Her Responsibility

Respecting a patient's privacy, not talking about him or her outside the hospital, weighing one's works carefully, keeping the nursing record accurately and safely: all such things nurses have been taught since the time of Florence Nightingale. Additionally, nurses have watched over the doctors' case notes and prescription charts, keeping them carefully and converting his works as required into actions.

Furthermore, national or local rules are usually formulated to accompany the prescription chart and ensure the safe administration of medicines.

At first sight the new rules for Data Protection, although entirely sensible, seem to add little to the good practice concerning information that has been, and still is, the consistent aim of the nursing profession. Why then should nurses need new guidelines for data protection?

There are, I would suggest, four main reasons for considerations.

The Effect of Increased Volume of Data and Need for Control

Computers and associated information technology can bring so much more information to the nurse, and to the bedside of a patient. Large volumes of information can subsequently be stored—much more than previously possible in hand-written report books or kardex. The computer stored data can easily be linked with or transferred to other systems within or outside the patient/client setting. Whereas, even if using photocopying machines it is time consuming, and requires a conscious decision to link and transfer data from manual reports.

Thus, it is timely to issue the Data Protection rules which, put simply, requires us to know from where we obtain data about patients, think why we need it, use it for that purpose alone, not disclose or transfer it to others without permission from the patient, keep it accurately, up-to-date, and store it for no longer than is necessary.

The Effect of Increased Use of Computer Held Information on Patient Privacy—And Need for a Balance

Previous and indeed most current manual systems are certainly not watertight in keeping confidentiality. Nevertheless the report book of kardex was often jealously guarded by Sister, kept away from prying eyes and certainly away from the patient himself or his family. Similarly a computer system has to balance privacy against the considered proper use of information.

Thus, it is timely to issue Data Protection rules that require us to state who has access to the computer stored information, who has the right to change it, and who to disclose it and to whom. This requires us to rethink about the roles of the extended team of health professionals caring for a patient or client:

Was the information or data collected for them?
Have they a need for it rather than a right to have it? Does the team vary over the 24 hours and does the use then differ?

The Effect of the Changing Attitudes of Society to Information—Rights, Responsibilities, and Litigation

"Ownership" of manual data was, and until recently, seldom spelled out but generally understood—the "Doctors" case notes, the "Sisters" kardex, for example. It was also generally understood that the Administrators stored these securely and retrieved them as required.

The patient was never supposed to see his record, although his lawyer occasionally sought access to it. Attitudes are changing rapidly, particularly about ones personal information about which it is felt one should have access and the right to change it, if wrong.

The changes are embodied in the Data Protection legislation, giving the patient access to his data, except rarely if thought to cause him serious harm.

Thus it is timely to issue guidelines about computer held information which state who owns the data, who has a right to the information and what are the responsibilities for its handling.

"Weighing the words carefully" has never been so important as now. If the patient considers his care was inadequate or harmful resulting from some inaccurate, incomplete or out-of-date computer held information, he has a legal right to seek compensation for this.

Similarly, if information is disclosed to an unauthorized person and if this harms the patient in some way—perhaps affecting career or family—he has a right to seek redress.

"Talking on the bus" needs an up-dating but is still a high profile topic for nurse education.

The Effect of Other Professionals Data on Nursing—A Need for Clarity

Nurses collect data for other members of the health team and also carry out treatment using their verbal or written orders. Manual systems have often been ambiguous, or not up-to-date and in need of changing. Hence the rules for example of prescribing and administration of drugs referred to earlier. Computer held systems offer direct links between professionals highlighting their interdependence. The highly complex relationships between one professionals decisions, automated equipment and another professional's actions can at best contribute greatly to a patient's care and at worst cause serious harm.

Challenging the system on behalf of the patient will be increasingly necessary, and observations as important as ever they were in Nightingale's time.

References

G.G. Griesser et al. (1980) Data Protection in Health Information Systems—Consideration and Guidelines. North Holland, Amsterdam.

E.O.J. Velders, A.R. Bakker, E.L.A. Flikkenschild, Method for selection of data protection measures. Proceedings MIE '87, of the seventh International Congress, Medical Informatics Europe Conference, A. Serio et al eds. (1987) Vol. 1, pp. 46–52.

14
Structuring Nursing Data for the Computer-Based Patient Record (CPR)

Mary L. McHugh

1. Components of Successful Design

Properly designed, the Computer-based Patient Record (CPR) has great potential. It can be used to facilitate continual improvement of quality patient care. At the same time, it can help with cost control. The CPR can produce these advantages by improving accessibility and utility of data related to patient care. Ultimately, it should enable clinicians to better understand the effects of clinical decisions on patient care outcomes. Clinicians can use that new knowledge to change practice in a way that improves the success of clinical protocols. The key to achievement of these benefits lies in the design of the system. The purpose of this paper is to describe one facet of the design of the CPR; design of the structure for the clinical content of the CPR.

Design of the CPR has four main components. They are, design of the hardware configuration, database management system (DBMS) design, applications software design, and design of the structure of the content data to be placed in the CPR. Details of the hardware design are usually a function of the requirements of the software. Users specify the requisite functionality of the applications software. Vendors design the internal structure of their software packages to meet the customer's requirements. Sometimes, customers and their consultants collaborate with vendors on software design. When the system involves a database, the specific DBMS software must be purchased or developed. Once the DBMS is selected, the file structures and the internal linkages among the various databases, files and tables or records must be addressed. These layers provide the foundation for a powerful computer based clinical record. With a clinical database, an additional layer of structure needs to be developed. That layer consists of the structure of the clinical information that is to be placed in the

Reprinted from *Nursing Informatics: An International Overview for Nursing in a Technological Era*, Grobe, S.J., Pluyter-Wenting, E.S.P. (Eds.). 1994. Pp. 302–307, with kind permission from Elsevier Science—NL, Sara Burgerhartstraat 25, 1055 KV Amsterdam, The Netherlands.

CPR. Structuring of the content data to be accessed and stored by the system is as important to the success of a CPR as is the computer-based medium itself.

History has demonstrated the problems with simply "computerizing" existing paper systems. The benefits of the CPR were not achieved when vendors transferred existing documentation models designed for paper record systems to a computer record system. The primary problems with that approach were inefficiency and the inability of users to aggregate data across groups of patients for the purposes of analysis of clinical and financial performance. If the promise of the CPR is to be realized, a paradigm shift in the structuring of patient care documentation is required. Data selection, mapping, coding schemes, data item interrelationships, and data retrieval and analysis processes and technology must be changed so that they provide a better fit with a computer information system paradigm [2].

At St. Francis Regional Medical Center in Wichita, Kansas, the theory and practice of clinical documentation is being shifted from a paper-based standard to an electronic record paradigm. The old charting paradigm focused on documenting patient assessments and clinicians' actions. It was organized around clinical services. It promoted department specific forms, which were unstructured or minimally structured. Narrative descriptions were common, as was a weak focus on outcomes. Data retrieval was often difficult and time consuming. The new paradigm focuses on the patient's problems and care requirements, and changes in health and functional status as the focus of the documentation system. It employs highly structured forms composed almost entirely of coded data elements. Many of the concepts and ideas used in this redesign were derived from the writings of Dr. Lawrence L. Weed. Further clarification was obtained when Dr. Weed came to St. Francis in 1991 to discuss his ideas with members of the hospital staff involved in documentation system redesign.

2. System Functionality and Design Processes

As suggested by Weed [1], the new system has been designed to *guide* as well as document care. Design focused on ways to reduce the incidence of clinical errors, to streamline documentation, and to improve the quality of information in the chart. Thus, the entire system is designed to support care quality. It guides practice by using flow sheets rather than narrative charting formats. Flow sheets list as many of the clinical assessment, intervention and evaluation activities performed by nurses as possible. Clinical errors of omission are reduced by a format that inherently reminds the nurse of care that needs to be performed. The new format is expected to facilitate quality improvement efforts by making available in a timely manner, data required to track care processes, and to monitor and evaluate the outcomes of patient care. It is also expected to help support many of the financial analysis, clinical, research, and education needs that are now so poorly supported by the manual systems.

The St. Francis task force began by identifying the purposes to be served by the new system. The task force recognized that the first and most important purpose for the patient record was communication of clinical events. The patient record or "chart" is to be used to help the care givers to record their observations and their actions. These recordings are used by all care givers involved with the patient to communicate care directions, patient health and knowledge deficits, and other information that will help to ensure that optimal care is delivered by all staff who come into contact with the patient. In addition to clinical communication, the chart needs to be used by utilization review personnel, by representatives of third party payers who check for correct billing and quality of care provided. The chart is also the legal record of care and must sometimes be made available to attorneys and to the patients. Regulatory agencies, such as public health departments, nuclear regulatory agencies, and environmental protection agencies, among others, may require certain patient records to evaluate compliance with various regulations. Finally, it was recognized that a tool that made explicit the logic of clinical decision processes [3] would serve our mission as a teaching hospital better than the existing model.

The Task Force recommended a charting methodology focused on the patient rather than the caregiver, with location of care or procedures as the center of the documentation effort. That is, the clinical record would be designed around the need to identify patient problems, record clinical actions taken to deal with those problems, and document the effects on patient health status or functional status of those clinical services. (It is understood that a "problem" may be either an actual or potential problem.) Intrinsically, the new approach will meet Joint Commission on Accreditation of Health Care Organizations requirement that the linkage between caregiver actions and patient problems be explicit. It will also enable clinical managers to begin the process of linking costs of care to patient outcomes.

3. Documentation System Redesign Principles

There are two basic drivers for the new system. The first driver is focused on diagnoses. The diagnoses made by each of the clinical subspecialty practitioners are logged onto the *Patient Problem List*. The Patient Problem List is envisioned as becoming the "driving force" for clinical action planning. All other documents are being designed to support problem identification, to document plans and interventions designed to resolve or ameliorate those problems, or to document outcomes of care. In this way, the system will make clear the thinking of clinicians, and the logic of clinical decisions. The system is designed to replace the nursing care plan and other clinical care planning documents. An important goal of the new system will be parsimony. That is, the least amount of paper (or file space) needed will be used to capture the maximum amount of clinical information.

The nurses on the task force identified an issue important to nurses that was not addressed by our consultants or by the POMR literature. Nurses must repeatedly document some of the same assessment/monitoring and care items over the length of stay. Some of these items are not associated with a problem but rather with unit routines and basic hygienic care. The system had to support documentation of *both* problem-derived and other nursing care documentation needs. This was accomplished with the second type of forms. The second driver of the system is the set of *Flow Sheets*, composed of highly structured screens or paper forms. The flow sheets are used to document assessment data, interventions and patient outcomes in the form of changes in functional or health status. These structured forms are similar to the flow sheets that have long been in use in most critical care units. The entire documentation system is being redesigned around these two drivers. Once the drivers were selected, design principles were elaborated to guide the redesign process.

The principles of chart redesign are:

1. The organization of the chart forms and data elements selected for inclusion are designed to represent the structure of care.

2. All possible information is recorded coded data elements rather than a narrative format.

3. The documentation format is designed with as many items of assessment, diagnosis, interventions, and patient care outcomes specifically named in lists. The clinician chooses words from the list to enter into the clinical record. The choice made by the clinician is represented by a code in the computer's memory.

4. The record is integrated around patient problems, rather than fragmented into forms that reflect the hospital's departmental and service structure. Thus, the patient problem list becomes the organizing focus of clinical documentation.

5. The structure of the flow sheets is specifically designed to help maintain minimum standards of care. This principle is actualized through flow sheets that guide assessment and care. The words used in the flow sheets, and the sequencing of the interrogatory structure of assessment and care documentation are designed to prevent errors of omission by supporting memory and clinical pattern recognition.

4. Goals and Anticipated Outcomes of the Redesigned Documentation System

Use of these principles produces a document that offers many memory supports to the nurse. Blanks in a document serve to remind the nurse to perform an assessment, or to provide a treatment. The Medication Administration Record (MAR) in use by most hospitals is a document that exemplifies many of the desired characteristics. Each of the patient's ordered medications is listed, along with the correct dose, time of administration, route, and if appropriate, concentration in admixture. These items serve to help nurses maintain a high degree of accuracy in medication administration. The new forms are designed to garner these benefits for the majority of patient care work of the nurse.

The main objective of the redesign is to develop a more effective and efficient clinical documentation system. The system will be used for the following purposes: improve quality of care through improved clinical communication, maximize reimbursement, support accreditation of the medical center and service units within the center, meet the requirements of regulatory agencies, and when necessary, provide legal evidence of care.

The anticipated outcomes of the redesigned documentation system are:

1. The system will increase overall efficiency by reducing the amount of time and effort staff spend entering or retrieving data from the clinical record.
2. The system will make recording and retrieving clinical information substantially easier for physicians.
3. The redesigned documentation system will facilitate and document care integration across and among the departments.
4. The system will lower clinical errors of omission as well as errors related to incomplete or missing documentation.
5. The system will improve clinical communication by increasing the ease with which important information can be retrieved as well as by decreasing problems of incomplete or missing documentation, and by increasing the legibility of the record.
6. The system will make clear the linkages among patient problems, care delivered and the effect of that care on patients outcomes.
7. The system will reduce the volume of the clinical record.

5. Goals of the Redesign Process

The task force also delineated a variety of goals for the documentation system redesign process itself. It was recognized that a healthy, inclusive process would increase the probability that the main objectives would be achieved. The process goals were:

1. Representatives of all patient record user groups would be included in the redesign effort. Where feasible, legitimate external users were to be consulted about redesign concepts or products.
2. To the extent possible, the system would encourage house-wide, common forms rather than area or specialty specific forms.

3. To the extent possible, the system is to avoid the use of narrative notes. This is to be accomplished through the use of codifiable data formats, such as numeric entry, checklists, graphic representations of information, etc.

4. The system was to be designed to serve as a memory support system for clinicians.

5. Data entry simplification was to be an important goal for both the manual and computer-based implementations of the new documentation system.

6. The system was to be designed to provide a method by which the outcomes of patient care could be clearly and concisely documented.

7. The system design process was to focus on ways to reduce data redundancy in the clinical record.

6. General Approach to Documentation and Rationale

The new documentation system is a Patient-Centered, Problem-Oriented charting system. The patient-centered chart will be achieved through a focus on the list of patient problems. (Depending upon the preference of each hospital's medical staff, the list of medical diagnoses may head up the problem list, or physician documentation may be kept entirely separate.) Nursing at St. Francis uses the NANDA words and coding scheme for nursing diagnoses in the design of the nursing component of the documentation system. Other nomenclatures and coding schemes such as those developed at Iowa [4] are under review.

The new documentation system is designed to be parsimonious. That is, it must be concise, yet extremely complete. The quality of succinctness will be achieved by limiting redundancy and the amount of narrative charting as much as possible. Forms and procedures are being redesigned to avoid repetitive entry of the same data. For example, if nursing has recorded information about the patient's family and living situation, social service will need only to ask information that is not already collected. The patient's age and gender are standard items stamped or printed onto every form. The nursing assessment has this information. There is no reason for any other form to have a place for the clinician to re-enter the patient's age and gender. Parsimony is also encouraged through checklists, numeric representations of information, and other forms of entry that can be coded. Narrative charting is not parsimonious.

Reduction of narrative charting carries a variety of benefits to the institution. First, it takes more time to write a paragraph than to make two or three check marks on a list. Second, personal script is often illegible. Numeric or check list formats are far more likely to be understandable to the user. Third, this approach helps to reduce the amount of extraneous and unnecessary notation often found in narrative notes. Superfluous items increase the volume of the chart without a concurrent increase in communication. Even more serious, such notations may be prejudicial to the hospital, its staff, or physicians in litigation. Fourth, narrative charting makes the job of those who must perform quality studies, abstract the chart, or otherwise search out and summarize information across multiple patients, very time consuming and difficult. Fifth, the design of flow sheets (which is the basis of the codifiable charting format) intrinsically serves to support the memory of the caregiver. Sixth, narrative charting formats offer no supports to the memories of clinicians. Seventh, the specific structure chosen by St. Francis uses the initial nursing assessment to lead directly into identification of the nursing diagnoses, which then—along with the medical diagnoses—form the patient problem list. Thus, the system serves to focus and guide care as well as to document care.

The St. Francis clinical record system is being reengineered to provide many memory supports in aid of complete documentation. Common care-related items are listed for check-off to help remind staff of important items that are easily forgotten. Insofar as possible, care information was represented numerically, or through checklists and codifiable formats. The new Nursing Admission Assessment is designed to guide the nurse through a complete assessment, and to extract information from that assessment to use in building the problem list. The reason for these new approaches is futuristic, and at the same time pragmatically focused on the current need for efficiency and a very high degree of completeness (effectiveness) in the St. Francis clinical documentation system. Existing research demonstrates that a minimum of 35% to 40% of nursing time is spent handling information. Given the cost and cyclical scarcity of nursing resources in the United States, and the very high complexity of St. Francis patients, the need to achieve the most efficient use of nursing staff time is critical.

Incomplete or inaccurate charting is most serious. It is ineffective for the purpose of clinical communication. It can therefore have deleterious effects on the quality of patient care. Insufficient documentation can have very serious financial and perhaps even public image consequences for the institution. HCFA publishes information about mortality rates in hospitals, and has a stringent quality review system that can provide very severe punishments for quality problems in hospitals. Since those quality reviews are based on review of the clinical record, a complete, concise clinical record is an important tool for demonstrating quality care to third party payers and other reviewers.

The proposed system will eliminate the Nursing Care Plan (NCP). Information in the NCP should be in the clinical record. Nurses complain the NCPs are very difficult and time consuming to generate, yet have contributed little to quality patient care. Using a Problem-Centered system creates a mindset in which actions are deliberate, and explicitly related to recognized patient problems and needs. The NCP was a device to encourage such deliberate action. The new system is focused on impelling the caregiver to consciously act in an organized manner that is directed toward solution of the patient's problems and needs that the NCP becomes unnecessary as a separate document. With a more structured format, the work of coders, abstracters and reviewers should be greatly streamlined. A variety of approaches could be used. Many of the items these staff need could be easily located on the problem or intervention lists, or placed on a flowsheet type of form. In an automated system, these items could be retrieved with the help of a code. Third, the volume of the chart may be reduced, thus saving costs associated with paper purchases, record storage costs and people time in searching form information on the chart.

7. Conclusion

The proposed changes are a significant departure from typical paper-based, manual documentation systems. The paper systems can best be described as care giver, service center or department focused or procedure focus. The new paradigm is focused on the patient and his/her problems and needs. It also is designed to take account of the need to provide a system to support human memory in a complex, rapidly changing work environment. The paper-based model depended far too much on human short and long term memory. As a result, human limitations too often resulted in clinical errors. The redesign of the structure of the documentation system will serve as a support system as well as a documentation system to clinicians. As a result, patients will receive better care; and the best justification for an automated system is that it improves patient care.

References

[1] Weed LL. *Medical Records, Medical Education, and Patient Care: The Problem-Oriented Record as a Basic Tool.* Cleveland: Press of Case Western Reserve University, 1969.
[2] McHugh ML. Increasing Productivity Through Computer Communications. *Dim Critical Care Nsg* 1986 5(5):294–302.
[3] Weed LL, and Zimny NJ. The Problem-Oriented System, Problem-Knowledge Coupling and Clinical Decision Making, *Phys Ther* 1989, Jul;69(7):565–8.
[4] Bulecheck GM and McCloskey JC. Nursing Intervention Taxonomy Development. In: *Current Issues in Nursing* 3rd ed. McCloskey JC, Grace HK (eds). St. Louis: CV Mosby Company, 1990.

15
Educating Nurses to Maintain Patient Confidentiality on Automated Information Systems

T. Hebda, L. Sakerka, and P. Czar

1. Privacy and Confidentiality

Privacy and confidentiality are concerns in health care. Once access to the patient's record was limited by its location and physical form. Now 75 or more persons have access to a patient record. [1] And, computerized information systems (IS) permit decentralized access. This reduces wait time for record access, but it increases opportunities for unauthorized access.[2,3] This paper defines confidentiality, discusses legal safeguards, reviews related literature, and outlines measures at two institutions to protect confidentiality.

While the terms privacy and confidentiality are used interchangeably, they are different. Privacy is defined as a state of mind, a specific place, freedom from intrusion, or control over the exposure of self or personal information.[4,5] Information privacy refers to the individual's ability to choose the extent to which, and the time and circumstances under which his attitudes, behavior, and beliefs will be shared with others. Information privacy includes the right to insure accuracy of records, and the right to confidentiality of information that has been collected by an organization.[6]

Confidentiality connotes a relationship in which information is disclosed.[7] It is dependent upon the loss of privacy. Unlike privacy, which is controlled by individual choice to reveal information, confidentiality is controlled by the person(s) to whom information is disclosed. Confidential information can be sensitive if disclosed to inappropriate persons. Inappropriate disclosure of confidential information may result in harm to employment, reputation, or personal relationships, and possible exploitation.[5] In the case of medical records, health care professionals are morally obligated

Reprinted from *Nursing Informatics: An International Overview for Nursing in a Technological Era*, Grobe, S.J., Pluyter-Wenting, E.S.P. (Eds.). 1994. Pp. 635–638, with kind permission from Elsevier Science—NL, Sara Burgerhartstraat 25, 1055 KV Amsterdam, The Netherlands.

by their professional code of ethics to maintain confidentiality of information as there can be no privacy of medical records without confidentiality.[8] Some states have regulations, statutes, and case law recognizing the confidentiality of medical records and limiting their access. A breach of confidence may lead to disciplinary action inclusive of revocation of license.[9] Such disciplinary measures generally apply only to physicians.[10] Confidentiality is essential to the relationship between health care provider and recipient. Anything that threatens confidentiality may keep people from seeking care or making disclosures required for treatment.[11]

2. Legal Protection in the U.S.

Laws to protect automated records cannot keep pace with technology.[12] Legal literature reveals an increased awareness of threats to medical record privacy but limited protection. In 1980 proposed federal legislation called for a time limit on consent to release information, standardized procedures for record access, a log of all parties accessing any medical record, and stiff penalties for obtaining records under false pretenses. Unfortunately the Privacy of Medical Information Act bill was defeated.[13]

Protection of medical records varies from state to state. Only some states have privacy laws which include private record keepers such as insurance companies and hospitals.[10] Some states provide criminal sanctions for the violation of confidentiality statutes and have monitoring agencies in place. But even with criminal sanctions and monitoring agencies, enforcement is generally up to the patient whose privacy was violated. Quantifying damage is difficult. Specific security measures for the possessors of confidential health care information are not required in all states.[5] Ohio case law has found unauthorized disclosure of medical information by anyone in a confidential relationship with the patient an actionable tort.[9]

3. Review of the Literature

Given the limited legal protection for patient records, the health care institution and professional must maintain patient confidentiality.[1] Unfortunately, weak data protection policies encourage information abuse. Any, and all elements of the IS can threaten its security including all levels of nursing personnel. Nonprofessionals are not bound by a professional code of ethics. But, even many RN's revealed that they had accessed information on patients not under their care.[14–17] This has implications for the structure of IS and treatment of personnel.

Data protection must be built into the system. Institutions need clearly stated security policies that are enforced.[7,18–20] Everyone with IS access should sign a statement that pledges to uphold patient confidentiality and acknowledges the consequences for failure to do so. Data protection can also be achieved through limited access to hardware and software. Access to software can be achieved through user specific sign on codes that are changed frequently, eliminated upon employee departure from a unit or the institution, and limit access to a need to know basis. Codes should not be borrowed or exchanged. Unattended terminals should have an automatic sign off feature. And, tracking user access and changes must be possible. But perhaps the best way to safeguard patient information is through the creation of a structure that supports privacy and confidentiality. Users tend to ignore access rules and ignore possible ethical and legal implications. Personnel need periodic reminders of what constitutes professional, legal, and ethical practice and behavior, and their responsibility to safeguard patient confidentiality.[2,7,14,15,17,21,22]

4. A Tale of Two Institutions

St. Francis Medical Center is a Technicon Data System (TDS) hospital in Pittsburgh, Pennsylvania. St. Francis emphasizes the importance of patient confidentiality in several ways. First, all staff sign a form upon issue of their access code. This document states that violation of patient confidentiality constitutes grounds for dismissal. Staff are told that their access code is their legal signature and that it should be treated accordingly. Codes are distributed in sealed envelopes. Many staff keep their codes with them until transcription area.

Automated information systems also provide the technology to easily violate patient confidentiality. In recognition of this fact, the basic concepts of patient privacy and confidentiality must be even more heavily emphasized in the basic education of nurses and training of ancillary personnel. Continuous reinforcement of these concepts must be an integral part of IS training. Periodic reminders about patient confidentiality must also be a part of ongoing education for all employees. IS professionals must still recognize that humans will be curious. The successful IS strategy must address ways to maximize utilization of computer technology while planning ways to promote patient confidentiality. Steps to reduce temptation to inappropriately access records must be addressed through institutional policy and IS structures.

References

[1] Calfee, B. Confidentiality and Disclosure of Medical Information. *Nurs Manage* 1989, 20 (12):20–23.
[2] Eleazor, PY. Risks Associated with Clinical Databases. *Top Health Rec Manage* 1991, 12 (2):49–58.

[3] Haddad, A. The Dilemma of Keeping Confidences. *AORN* 1989, 50 (1):161–164.

[4] Kmentt, KA. Private Medical Records: Are They Public Property? *Medical Trial Technique Quarterly* Winter 1987, 33:274–307.

[5] Winslade, WJ. Confidentiality of Medical Records: An Overview of Concepts and Legal Policies. *Journal of Legal Medicine* 1982, 3 (4):497–533.

[6] Murdock, LE. The Use and Abuse of Computerized Information: Striking a Balance Between Personal Privacy Interests and Organizational Information Needs. *Albany Law Review* 1980, 44 (3):589–619.

[7] Romano, C. Privacy, Confidentiality, and Security of Computerized Systems: The Nursing Responsibility. *Comput Nurs* 1987, 5 (3):99–104.

[8] Maciorowski, L. The Enduring Concerns of Privacy and Confidentiality. *Holist Nurs Pract* 1991, 5 (3):51–56.

[9] Johnston, CE. Breach of Medical Confidence in Ohio. *Akron Law Review* Winter 1986, 19:373–393.

[10] Miller, M. Computers, Medical Records, and the Right to Privacy. *J Health Polit Policy Law* 1981, 6:463–488.

[11] Fry, S. Confidentiality in Health Care: A Decrepit Concept? *Nurs Econ* 1984, 2 (6):413–418.

[12] Nasri, W. Legal issues of computers in healthcare: liabilities of the healthcare provider. Paper presented to the Tri-State Nursing Computer Network Pittsburgh, Pennsylvania. March 19, 1992.

[13] Morihara, J. Computers, the Disclosure of Medical Information, and the Fair Credit Reporting Act. *Computer/Law Journal* Summer 1982, 3:619–639.

[14] Curran, M and Curran, K. The Ethics of Information. *JONA* 1991, 21 (1):47–49.

[15] Regan, BG. Computerized Information Exchange in Health Care. *Med J Aust* 1991, 154 (2):140–144.

[16] Solomon, T. Personal Privacy and the "1984" Syndrome. *Western New England Law Review* Winter 1985, 7:753–780.

[17] Wogan, MJ. New Technologies Raise Concerns about Protecting Patient Confidentiality. *Hosp Patient Relat Rep* 1991, 6 (2):1–2.

[18] Barber, B. Guardians or Gizmos. *Health Serv J* 1991, 101 (5262):33–34.

[19] Lochner, MA. Legal issues pertaining to clinical record systems. Paper Presented at the Medical Information Systems Association, Incorporated Spring 1991 Meeting: Achieving the Competitive Edge. April 24, 1991.

[20] Williams, FG. Implementing Computer Information Systems for Hospital Based Case Management. *Hosp Health Serv Adm* 36 (4):559–570.

[21] Grady, C, Jacob, J and Romano, C. Confidentiality: A Survey in a Research Hospital. *J Clin Ethics* 1991, 2 (1):25–30.

[22] Powell, D. Plugging the Leaks in Data Networks. *Networking Management* 1992, 10 (6):29–32.

16
Data Bank—A Model System for Assuring the Public's Health, Safety, and Welfare

Marsha Kelly

Introduction

In September of 1980, the National Council of State Boards of Nursing (NCSBN) established a national disciplinary data bank for nurses. The Nursing Disciplinary Data Bank was established to provide a mechanism for Boards of Nursing, as members of NCSBN, to report disciplinary action against RNs and PNs to be central source for distribution to all Boards of Nursing, on a monthly basis. Such sharing of disciplinary actions was viewed as a mechanism for safeguarding the public's health, safety, and welfare. With each Board of Nursing having access to information about nurses reported to the Data Bank, the endorsement process for granting a Registered Nurse (RN) or Practical Nurse (PN) license became a system better able to assure the public that its safety and welfare were being protected.

Board participation in the established Nursing Disciplinary Data Bank System was not universal in the beginning. As the System gained usefulness for the Boards, especially in the endorsement process for granting a RN or PN license, most Member Boards joined the System and have continued to participate by submitting reports on actions taken against RNs and PNs in their respective jurisdictions.

System Evolution

The Nursing Disciplinary Data Bank System was operated as a manual system from its initiation in 1980 through 1985. In January 1984, the process of converting the manual system of compiling a monthly report

Reprinted with permission from *Proceedings of Nursing and Computers: The Third International Symposium on Nursing Use of Computers and Information Science*; pp. 549–559. Daly, N. & Hannah, K.J. (Eds.). 1988. St. Louis: The C.V. Mosby Company.

of all actions against RNs and PNs to a computer system was begun with completion in January 1985. The conversion required coding over 6000 individual records into computer receivable codes and entering those records into a central data file system. This initial conversion provided the capability for aggregate statistical information, relative to the type of disciplinary cases and the resultant actions, to be produced. These monthly statistical reports have been revised and updated over time and are now routinely circulated with the monthly reports. In addition, an annual summary of all data reported in a calendar year is produced.

Files and File Structures

The current hardware system that accommodates the storage, retrieval, and report functions for the Disciplinary Data Bank is a DEC Microvax II. It has a 456 Megabyte disk with nine million bytes of memory. Software for the hardware system is the Unix Operating System and the Unify Relational Data Base System. The following data file categories exist within the Disciplinary Data Bank Program:

Biographical file
Aliases (aka) file
Licenses file
Case header file
Actions file
Violations file
Comments file

The data contents in each of these files are set forth in the Record Layout presented in Table 1.

For each report received four types of records are added: the case header record, the action detail record(s), the violations detail record(s) and the comments record(s). The case header record is linked to the biographical record by having the nurse ID number as one of its data fields. The violations, actions, and comments records for a case are keyed to each other and the case header record by having the case number as one of the data fields in each of these records.

Report Process

Entry into the Disciplinary Data Bank begins with the receipt of a report on an individual RN or PN from one of our 61 Member Boards. Each Member Board uses a universal form to report actions taken against licensees. The form consist of four sections as follows:

TABLE 1. Record layout

Biographical file
    Nurse ID Number
    Name (first, middle, last, maiden)
    Highest nursing degree held
    Birthday
    Social security number
    Jurisdiction of original license
    Original license type
    Original License Number
Aliases
    Nurse ID number
    Alias (AKA)
Licenses
    Nurse ID number
    Licensing jurisdiction
    License type
    License number
Case header
    Case number
    Nurse ID number
    Address (at time of hearing)
    Month and year reported
    Jurisdiction reporting
    Date of action
    License type being disciplined
    License number being disciplined
Action detail
    Case number
    Action ID number
    Was action stayed? (Y or N)
    From-to dates (when applicable)
Violation detail
    Case number
    Violation ID number
Comments record
    Case number
    Comment

Section A—Biographical and unique identifier information
Section B—Action taken and duration of action listing nine common actions as well as an "other" category
Section C—Case description listing five categories with specific actions under each category
Section D—Final disposition actions with an authorizing signature

Additionally the form provides space for comments or further data pertinent to the case reported on the reverse side of the form. The form goes through periodic review and update, but the essential data elements listed above are viewed as the necessary inclusions in any form used for reporting individual disciplinary cases.

When the National Council receives a disciplinary report from a Member Board, a search of the component file to see if previous reports have been processed for that nurse is completed. It follows from the above that the search procedure should allow the operator to search on each of the data elements in the master (biographical) record. To make these searches efficient, the program has built B-trees (special fast-access tables) for each of the data elements. The average access time to search all the current records in the system for a match on a field is 2 to 7 seconds.

If the nurse is identified in the search the original National Council identification number is assigned to the current report. If the nurse is not found in the system, an original number in sequence is given. The data from each report is entered and on the last day of each month, a monthly report of all records entered from the first working day of the month to the last working day of the month is produced.

This monthly report and aggregate statistical data for the month is circulated to the National Council Member Boards. The aggregate data is tabulated by nurse category, type of action, case description, and total number of reports for each Member Board. Subsequent to each monthly report an aggregate statistical report for a calendar year is prepared and circulated in January following the end of the previous calendar year.

Disciplinary Data Band Aggregate Data

In 1984, NCSBN commissioned Ruth Elliott and Margaret Heins of the Tennessee Board of Nursing to conduct a longitudinal study of the Nursing Disciplinary Data Bank to ascertain the characteristics of the disciplinary actions taken by state boards of nursing. The study further included the development of a computer program and report form that would provide more differentiated data about the types of case descriptions for which action was being taken by boards of nursing. The final report of the Elliott and Heins Study entitled *Disciplinary Data Bank: A Longitudinal Study* was distributed July 1987. Data related to the type of disciplinary actions and case descriptions reported from that study and the data reported from the 1987 Calendar Summary Data are presented in Tables 2–5.

As Tables 2 and 4 indicate, probation, suspension, and revocation are the most common types of action taken when RNs and PNs are disciplined for violations of Nursing Practice Acts by Boards of Nursing. The Tables further reveal the increase of use of Boards of Nursing of the actions of summary suspension, voluntary surrender, limitation of the license, and the use of fines when disciplining a nurse.

Tables 3 and 5 reveal that action involving drugs and the administration of drugs are the most frequent description given in discipline cases of RNs and PNs by Boards of Nursing. The Tables further reveal an increase of

TABLE 2. Summary of disciplinary actions registered nurses and licensed practical nurses, 1980–1986

Action	RN		LPN	
	Cases	Percent	Cases	Percent
License denial	240	2	80	2
Limitation	298	2	35	1
Probation	3,164	25	1,074	23
Reinstatement	860	7	321	7
Revocation	2,942	23	1,057	23
Summary suspension	85	1	36	1
Suspension	2,556	20	1,017	22
Voluntary surrender	573	5	253	5
Letter of reprimand	88	1	51	1
Action cleared	476	4	186	4
Reinstatement denied	96	1	82	2
Other	1,400	11	453	10
Total	12,778	102	5,995	101

discipline cases against RNs and PNs related to misconduct in nursing practice.

System Success

The Nursing Disciplinary Data Bank and its statistical profile of disciplinary actions against RNs and PNs has gained national prominence. In 1986 and 1987 respectively the Veterans' Administration (VA) and the United States Public Health Service (USPHS) used the Nursing Disciplinary Data

TABLE 3. Summary of case descriptions registered nurses and practical nurses, 1980–1986

Case descriptions	RN		LPN	
	Cases	Percent	Cases	Percent
Action involving drugs	4,319	45	1,811	36
Inconsistent nursing practice	1,158	12	649	13
Misconduct in nursing practice	489	5	441	9
Administration of medicine	1,039	11	621	12
Crime convictions	486	5	543	11
Action in another jurisdiction	847	9	266	5
Failure to meet previous terms	25	0	13	0
Action cleared	489	5	240	5
False application	737	8	436	9
Total	9,589	100	5,020	100

TABLE 4. Summary of disciplinary actions registered nurse and licensed practical nurses, 1987

Action	RN		LPN	
	Cases	Percent	Cases	Percent
License denial	29	1	12	0.8
Limitation	74	2.5	11	0.8
Probation	827	28.3	378	26.6
Reinstatement	187	6.4	70	4.9
Revocation	367	12.6	184	12.9
Summary suspension	25	0.9	9	0.6
Suspension	548	18.8	323	22.7
Voluntary surrender	145	5	83	5.8
Reprimand	194	6.6	95	6.7
Action cleared	174	6.0	71	5.0
Reinstatement denied	18	0.6	10	0.7
Fine	109	3.7	63	4.4
Other	223	76	112	7.9
Total	2,919	100	1,421	100.0

Bank in a merge with their personnel records to purge any nurses working in their system with license that were suspended, revoked, or probated with conditions. The VA purge identified 18 RN and 13 PN personnel working in their system with encumbered licenses. The Public Health Service purge identified 13 RN and 5 PN personnel working in their system with encumbered licenses. As of April 1988, the USPHS will further use the Disciplinary Data Bank to screen applicants seeking RN or PN positions in their service.

In addition, the three branches of the military services have routinely been reporting cases of military disciplinary action since 1984. In 1984, the American Association of Nurse Anesthetists (AANA) sought permission to receive the Disciplinary Data Bank for the purpose of using the data to check against their file of certified nurse anesthetists. The Member Boards in July of 1984 granted that permission, and for a nominal fee, the AANA now receives the monthly report and have reported changing certification statuses of nurse anesthetists with disciplinary action resulting in suspended or revoked licenses.

The primary success of the system has been its provision of a mechanism for identifying nurses in the U.S.A., among a mobile nursing population, who are a potential risk to a public's health, safety, and welfare and who often seek a geographical cure to disciplinary action.

Unify Relational Data Base System

The Unify Relational Data Base System is particularly suited for systems where it is efficient and wise to have only one identifying master record for each entity (person) with a variable number of record types for

TABLE 5. Summary of disciplinary actions registered nurse and licensed practical nurses, 1987

Case description	RN		LPN	
	Cases	Percent	Cases	Percent
Action involving drugs				
Abuse	574	28.3	186	26.3
Diversion	597	29.4	212	29.9
Self-administration	419	20.7	125	17.7
Use on duty	165	8.2	58	8.2
Writing prescriptions	49	2.4	34	4.8
Other	224	11.0	93	13.1
Total	2,028	100.0	708	100.0
Inconsistent nursing practice				
Leaving duty station	15	3.8	21	8.3
Not maintaining minimal standards	164	41.0	110	43.5
Incompetent practice	97	24.2	45	17.8
Other	124	31.0	77	30.4
Total	400	100.0	253	100.0
Administration of medications				
Charting errors	142	27.6	82	28.7
Failure to follow orders	79	15.4	45	15.7
Failure to have stage witnessed	70	13.6	25	8.7
Failure to document administration	114	22.2	58	20.3
Other	109	21.2	76	26.6
Total	514	100.0	286	100.0
Misconduct relating to nursing practice				
Misconduct/other	280	80.7	13	16.6
Practicing beyond scope	24	6.9	23	11.7
Fraudulent practice	43	12.4	160	81.6
Total	347	100.0	196	100.0
Convictions				
Felony	68	21.7	79	38.0
Misdemeanor	35	11.1	62	29.8
Offense in other jurisdiction	209	66.6	67	32.2
Other offense	2	.6	0	0
Total	314	100.0	208	100.0

each data related to that entity (person), like the Disciplinary Data Bank.

Within this system the master record must contain data elements that are unique. Non-unique data elements must reside in sub-records. To illustrate: A nurse may have more than one married name over the course of her life. The system accommodates the need to have a married name and a maiden name in the master (biographical) record by saying that the biographical record contains the current married name and that any previous married names are in the alias file. Similarly, if a nurse had her name legally changed other than by marriage, the biographical file would contain the current legal name and the alias file would contain the previous legal name.

Maiden name within the Disciplinary Data Bank means not the last married name but the surname on a birth certificate. The program allows for a person to have one birthday and one "maiden" name in a lifetime and further allows for a person to have only one social security number in a lifetime since the law stipulates that, if a person gets assigned more than one in error, only one is valid. Thus, the requirements of a relational data base system are met by saying the data elements in the master (biographical) record are each unique; they are the only first, middle, last, and maiden name the people currently have and they are the only social security number, birthdate, and NCSBN nurses ID numbers they have. If we inadvertently assign a second NCSBN nurse ID number to a person, we take the same approach that the Social Security Administration takes; that is, the assignment of the second number is an administrative error and second ID number will be voided on discovery.

The operation of the system is easy to understand if you understand how the relational data base system cross-references the records that pertain to a nurse and/or a case. The alias records are keyed to the biographical file by the nurse ID number as each alias record has the same nurse ID number as her biographical record. Similar, the file containing data on other licenses held by the nurse are linked to the biographical file by having the nurse ID number in each license file record.

With the advent of statistical profile data, it also serves as a national mirror for the disciplinary problems faced by Boards of Nursing in carrying out their function as regulators of nursing practice. It additionally serves as the most comprehensive data source for monitoring specific types of disciplinary problems, in particular cases related to substance abuse, at a national level.

System Weakness

Though the Nursing Disciplinary Data Bank has been extremely successful as a tool for identifying nurses as risks to the public's health, safety, and welfare, and as a national statistical source for profiling types of disciplinary concerns in the nursing population at a national level, the System is not as complete, and therefore not as thoroughly reliable as NCSBN would like. Originally, only one Board of Nursing (Georgia PN) philosophically stated its inability to share data with the National Council, based on the belief that data are public information for the state of Georgia only; however, it and approximately seven other Member Boards have shared data sporadically or in some years not at all. Four of those Boards are territories and have alluded to the fact that discipline procedures have been poorly developed and staff support has not been available to pursue the disciplinary function of the Boards. The other three are small volume licensee jurisdictions.

One very large Member Board, in terms of number of licensees, the California RN Board of Nursing, did not begin sharing data until mid-year 1985. The California LVN Board, another large volume PN board, began sharing data only since becoming a member in July 1986.

With 100% participation, the system would become 100% reliable in fulfilling the two very distinct and important functions it presently serves. NCSBN will continue to monitor Member Board participation in an effort to encourage full participation and to eliminate this weakness of the System.

Another weakness in the present Nursing Disciplinary Data Bank System is the timeliness of the data. The National Council processes data within the month it is received. A monthly report is constituted of those reports, either RN or PN, that come in from the first working day to the last working day of a given month. That process is as timely as is manageable for a monthly report.

When the National Council receives data from Member Boards, however, the data being reported are on the average, four months old. Data are frequently a year to 18 months after an actual action has been taken. Though Member Boards have informally told us that some reports are held pending a challenge to the action taken by the Board, the delays are often due to slow processing procedures in sending reports to the National Council. Delays in reporting by Member Boards to the National Council with the automatic NCSBN internal delay of one month processing time, results in a five month lag time from case action to case reporting. NCSBN is concerned about this delay and will be investigating ways of decreasing the delay time in the future. Five months as an average length of time from case action to case reporting is a major weakness of a system that is based on providing data to protect the public's health, safety, and welfare, when nurses facing disciplinary action often seek a geographic cure for their discipline problems.

Future System Implications

Full report and inquiry access for Member Boards to the Disciplinary Data Bank are presently being investigated. Such ability would allow Member Boards to directly query the system to identify if a nurse applying for licensure appears in the system. It would also allow the members to report directly to the system on a computer version of the report form instead of requiring hand generated forms filled out and mailed to the National Council office. Since the DEC Microvax II system will accommodate such access, the logistical problems of individual state ability to access the National Council computer system and quality assurance mechanisms for ensuring the integrity of the data, with such widespread access, are the only hindrances from current full implementation of report and inquiry access. Those hindrances are being addressed and such capability is expected by the end of 1988.

Overall System Evaluation

The System is providing a unique service to NCSBN's Member Boards, to the general nursing population and to the public at large. Even with its identified weaknesses, it has considerable strength for a system that has been in existence for only seven years and that has grown from a manually operated system in 1980 to a sophisticated computer-based system in 1988.

Its primary purpose is to serve as an identified base for a Member Board to reference before granting a license to an applicant for licensure in individual states. The mechanism serves to protect the public in a mobile society such as exist in the U.S.A. The data field established by the system serves as a prototype system whether its application is at a state, national or international level.

References

Elliott, Ruth L. and Heins, Margaret. *Disciplinary Data Bank: A Longitudinal Study*—A Monograph Presented to the National Council State Boards of Nursing, Inc., 1987.
National Council State Boards of Nursing, Inc., *Disciplinary Data Bank 1987 Calendar Year Summary Data*, 1987.

17
A Conceptual Model of the Information Requirements of Nursing Organizations

Emmy Miller

Nursing has been described in a variety of ways. By and large these definitions have focused on observable activities that nurses perform to help individuals and groups cope with conditions affecting their health. In an alternative to traditional task-based descriptions, nursing has been defined as "the diagnosis and treatment of human responses to actual or potential health problems" [1]. The diagnosis and treatment of human responses consists of information processing activities and the execution of nursing treatments. It is the information processing component that determines which nursing treatments will be offered; therefore, the activities, or work, of nurses can be viewed as information processing.

Nurses in clinical and administrative practice process data into useful information. In the clinical setting, the nurse obtains data about the patient and then processes these data into nursing diagnoses and associated nursing interventions, as well as recognizing and responding to significant medical symptoms and other disease-related findings. In administrative nursing practice, the nurse manager processes data from nursing unit activities into information for managing unit operations and for strategic planning for the nursing organization.

Data collection, storage, and processing are critical aspects of nursing practice. However, nurses have not yet assimilated the language or concepts of computerization on a wide scale. Indeed, a recent study of inpatient health care agencies showed that only 7 percent of those health care agencies with automated systems used these systems for nursing care planning, while only 4 percent documented nursing care in their information system [2].

Three related issues play a role in the identification of the information needs of nursing organizations. These issues are the current state of com-

Reprinted with permission from *Proceedings: Thirteenth Annual Symposium on Computer Applications in Medical Care*, Kingsland, L.C. (Ed.). 1989. Pp. 784–788.
© 1989, American Medical Informatics Association (formerly SCAMC): Bethesda, MD.

puter systems in health care organizations, the lack of a well-defined data set for nursing, and the absence of models representing data and information relevant to clinical and administrative nursing practice that can be used to guide the design of automated nursing systems. This paper will examine current methods of data collection, processing, and storage in clinical and administrative nursing practice for the purpose of identifying the information requirements of nursing organizations. A conceptual model of the types of data necessary to produce the desired information will be presented and the relationships among data will be delineated.

Nursing Information: Current Issues and Strategies

Data from nursing practice and information about nursing services are important. Nurses deliver 90% of the care received by hospitalized patients [3]. Nursing personnel make up roughly one half of the personnel employed by a typical hospital, and salary expense for this group may approach 30% of total hospital expenditures [4]. Yet, nursing information is one of the least defined areas in terms of computerized health care applications [5].

Today, there are a variety of manual and automated systems to record or produce nursing information. Most were originally administrative support systems that were adapted for hospital or nursing use. In this adaptation, nursing information requirements were often determined by technical experts rather than nursing experts, resulting in a design that has restricted the nursing information system to performing as a recording system with limited capacity to provide nurses with information [6]. Another problem is that many of the commercially available computerized systems for health care organizations are single purpose stand-alone systems, such as patient classification systems, nurse scheduling systems, and documentation systems [7].

Health care organizations often have several single purpose systems in operation. Multiple systems can be quite useful for specific operational problems; however, it is difficult, if not impossible, to network these various products into a unified information system [8]. This "multi-system syndrome" results in untold hours of time spent attempting to relate clinical, census, payroll, and financial data with limited success as each system generally has unique reporting capabilities and uses different time-frames [9]. Yet, there are existing data in these computerized systems that could be used for clinical and administrative decision making, but the time and cost of retrieving, aggregating and analyzing these data are prohibitive.

The second issue in defining the information requirements of nursing organizations is the lack of a well-defined and agreed upon data set for nursing; however, progress is being made in this area. The Study Group on Nursing Information Systems identified six functional areas where nursing information is needed: patient care, resource allocation, personnel management, education, planning and policymaking, and investigation or research

[10]. As an outgrowth of this work, a Nursing Minimum Data Set (NMDS) has been proposed. Elements of the proposed NMDS cover three broad categories: nursing care elements, patient demographic elements, and service elements.

In the 16 data elements of the NMDS, there are four nursing care elements: nursing diagnosis, nursing intervention, nursing outcome, and intensity of nursing care. Demographic elements consist of a personal identification element, date of birth, sex, ethnicity, and residence. Service elements include the unique facility or service agency number, the unique health record number of the patient, the unique number of the principle registered nurse provider, the episode admission or encounter date, the discharge or transfer date, the disposition of the patient, and the expected payer of the bill [11].

The nursing care elements of the NMDS are based on the recognized thinking model of nursing, the nursing process; the key element is the nursing diagnosis, which names the patient's condition requiring nursing care, directs nursing intervention, and establishes parameters for outcome measures. A measure of the intensity of nursing care and designation of a unique RN provider also reflect concerns of professional nursing about nursing care needs of patients, allocation of nursing resources, and nursing accountability.

The third issue in regard to the information needs of nursing organizations is the lack of a model of nursing information that could guide the design of nursing information systems. A useful model of nursing information must reflect the conceptual foundations of nursing, contain the data to produce the desired nursing information, and promote the efficient collection, storage, and retrieval of information that can inform decision-making in clinical and administrative nursing practice. In addition, such a model can be used to design database structures that meet these requirements and assist nursing organizations in dealing with their information needs.

The Database Approach and Nursing Information

The database approach offers a number of ways for nurses in clinical and administrative practice to address the three issues discussed here. In order to benefit from the advantages of database technology, however, nurses must identify and define their information needs. These information requirements must then be transformed into data elements and structures that can be used in the design of a computerized database.

The database approach is especially useful in those situations where there is a need for interactive inquiry and update capability, an anticipated growth in data volumes, or an expected expansion in the range of decision making which must be supported by information systems [12]. As such, it is ideally suited to nurses who collect and record tremendous amounts of data about the health status of their patients and the nursing care services they provide. Flexibility, enhanced data integrity, and ease of information retrieval are database characteristics that make the adoption of database technology an important step for nursing organizations. Another important feature of database technology is the ability to aggregate nursing data for a variety of purposes. For example, the ability to retrieve and compare clinical data about nursing diagnoses with nursing hours projected by a patient classification system and with actual nursing hours provided for a nursing unit offers a more complete picture of nursing care that either set of data alone.

Two problems in database design have been identified by Blum [13]: what data should be included in the database and how these data should be organized within the database. The first problem is addressed through data modeling, while the second is dealt with by analysis. Data modeling is the representation of some real world object designed to convey some information about the object; a data model for a nursing organization would depict the necessary data elements to convey information about that organization. Relationships among the data are determined by analysis of the data elements in order to identify the ways that the data elements are used in the real world.

Database design is concerned with the identification of logical relationships among entities. An entity is an object, concrete or abstract, about which data are collected; the specific properties of an entity are its attributes. Attributes may be assigned values that are facts [14]. Logical relationships describe association or commonalities that exist between entities. For example, nursing diagnosis is an entity in the NMDS having the attributes of problem statement, etiology, and defining characteristics. The values of these attributes might consist of the nursing diagnostic labels, etiology statements, and defining characteristics found in the *Pocket Guide to Nursing Diagnosis* [15]. The entity, nursing diagnosis, has logical relationships with two additional entities, patient assessment and nursing interventions. These logical relationships are presented in Figure 1.

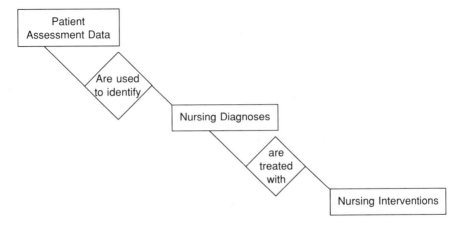

FIGURE 1. Logical relationships among three entities.

The database approach offers an important strategy for nursing organizations to deal with their information needs. In order to take advantage of the unique characteristics of database technology, nurses must delineate the essential data to be included in a nursing database and the desired nursing information output. The model of nursing information presented in the next section will describe broad information areas and the major categories of nursing data that should be included in a nursing database.

Overview of the Model

The model of nursing information presented here is a conceptual model; it offers a representation of the "real world" of clinical and administrative nursing practice. This real world is reflected in the definition of nursing as "the diagnosis and treatment of human responses to actual or potential health problems" [16], as well as the use of the nursing process as an organizing framework. The nursing process is the best known and most widely used scheme for organizing the collection, use, and storage of nursing data [17]. The model also reflects the elements of the NMDS.

In the model, data and information required for nursing practice have been conceptualized in three broad areas: Patient Care, Unit Operations, and Strategic Planning (See Figure 2). While a similar model was presented by Rieder and Norton [18], their focus was defining information requirements in ten functional modules for an automated nursing system, using a

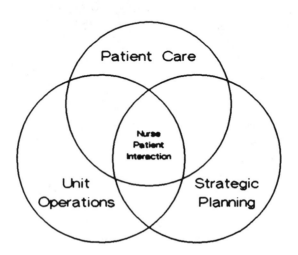

FIGURE 2. Information model for nursing organizations.

Table 1. Information requirements of nursing organizations major content areas and categories

Patient care		Unit operations		Strategic planning	
I.	Information about Human responses (Nursing diagnoses)	I.	Nursing unit activity	I.	Indicators of organizational performance
II.	Information about disease-related conditions	II.	Patient characteristics	II.	Organizational characteristics
III.	Additional information	III.	Nursing personnel	III.	Information about health care environment
		IV.	Actual nursing resource consumption		

systems analysis framework. In contrast, the model presented here is concerned with delineating the essential data and information for nursing organizations and representing that knowledge in a way that can be used for database design.

Each of the three broad areas in the proposed model—Patient Care, Unit Operations, and Strategic Planning—represents a set of data elements and their relationships (See Table 1). There is also substantial overlap between areas, which means data elements that produce meaningful information in one area may also produce meaningful information in another. For example, data about census and patient acuity for a particular nursing unit are helpful in constructing information for managing nursing unit operations and for strategic planning.

Data in the first category, Patient Care, are obtained through individual nurse-patient interactions, then processed into information about nursing care for an individual patient. When these data are aggregated to provide information for managing unit operations, they enter the second category of information for the nursing organization, Unit Operations. An analysis of data for the projection of trends in the needs for nursing care and the required nursing resources for Strategic Planning represents the third major information category. The information in these three categories can be considered to have a common foundation: the nurse-patient interaction. While information about nurse-patient interactions is a major component of Patient Care, it also contributes to information necessary for nursing unit operations and long range planning for the organization. Data from Patient Care must be aggregated to meet short- and long-term planning needs, and other types of data will be included in this analysis.

Patient Care

This category consists of the data and information necessary for nurses to provide care to individual patients. Three subcategories of information are found within this category: information about human responses, disease related information, and additional information that is not directly related to the patient's nursing or medical condition.

The first subcategory, information about human responses, is composed of pertinent assessment data and the nursing diagnoses, as well as the implementation and evaluation of the nursing treatment plan. The nursing diagnosis is the foundation of this category of information for nursing documentation, because nursing diagnoses describe human responses to actual or potential health problems nurses treat. In addition, nursing diagnoses within the context of the nursing process provide a framework for conceptualizing nursing practice, which is essential for efficient and effective processing of information.

A nursing diagnosis framework does not address the delegated medical responsibilities of nursing associated with the patient's disease or medical condition. The practice of nursing includes both of these areas, and any approach to processing nursing data must also include both. The second subcategory of information required for Patient Care describes disease related information, including signs and symptoms of diseases and medical conditions, the effects of medical therapeutics, and the execution of medical orders. Information in this category should be described using medical terminology, and does not usually fit into the nursing process framework.

Additional information is a subcategory of data that are not directly linked to either the patient's disease condition or human responses. The demographic and service elements of the NMDS fit in this subcategory. This category often reflects information necessary to meet legal, regulatory, or organizational requirements. An example would be that all patients have a notation in their record indicating that side rails are elevated and the bed is in low position, irrespective of any medical or nursing condition that might warrant the use of side rails. The impetus for recording much of the data in this subcategory is found in risk-management and legal concerns, rather than clinical considerations.

Unit Operations

Managing the operations of a nursing unit requires a related, but somewhat different set of data. While information from the Patient Care category comprises an important part of this information, it is generally necessary to convert these data into other forms. For example, a nurse may identify several nursing diagnoses for a particular patient; using this information in conjunction with demographic data and disease-related data, a nursing care plan is formulated, executed, and evaluated. For the nurse manager, this patient and nurse specific information must be transformed into aggregate data that can influence decisions about groups of patients' requirements for nursing care, the nursing personnel necessary to meet the requirements, and compliance of nursing care with quality indicators.

Information necessary for unit operations can be examined in four subcategories. The first is nursing unit activity, including data about unit census, occupancy rate, patient days, unit length of stay, and the number of admissions and discharges. Relevant patient characteristics are the second subcategory, and these data are provided to some degree by aggregate information about nursing diagnoses and disease-related conditions; however, this is usually augmented with patient classification or acuity measures in order to describe patients' requirements for nursing services.

The third subcategory of Unit Operations contains data about the nursing personnel assigned to the unit. Basic personnel data such as social security number, position number, address, educational preparation, licensure data, certifications, and continuing education activities are basic information needed by the nurse manager. Position control is another area where personnel data are required, including approved positions by category of personnel, salary rates, full-time equivalents, and filled/unfilled positions.

Data about actual nursing service resource consumption are the fourth subcategory of Unit Operations. Nursing diagnoses, nursing interventions offered, and their effectiveness in achieving patient outcomes provide important data about nursing services. Unfortunately, these data are often difficult to obtain, resulting in an absence of this type of information in determinations of nursing resource requirements and costs of nursing services [19].

Some types of data about nursing service resource consumption are available. Data about hours of nursing care provided, as well as nonproductive time, such as holiday and educational leave, are available and frequently used as indicators of nursing service delivery. Information in this area is often comparative in nature; for example, required nursing hours are calculated based on a patient classification system and nurse staffing levels are projected on that basis. A comparison of actual hours of nursing care and required hours is a recognized productivity measure [20]. The intensity of required nursing services is another comparative measure used to analyze nursing service consumption. A useful model of nursing information for managing nursing unit operations should include data about actual nursing conditions, or nursing diagnoses, and nursing interventions as well as data about required nursing hours and hours worked.

Another example of comparative information is seen in quality assurance monitoring. Documentation of nursing care is examined to establish compliance with recognized standards of care. Information about the actual services that nurses provide and comparison of those services with quality standards represents a critical area of information for managing nursing unit operations.

Strategic Planning

While operational planning is the setting of short-term goals, strategic planning is a long-range planning process. It is concerned with the formulation and implementation of strategies to accomplish specific organizational goals that extends from 3 to 5 years into the furture [21]. Information used in strategic planning addresses organizational performance as well as environmental influences on the organization.

The information required for the strategic planning will come from existing information in the first two areas: information for caring for individual patients and information for managing nursing unit operations. While the information used to manage nursing operations will play a role in the strategic planning process, this information must be organized to analyze historical trends in indicators of nursing service requirements and consumption, as well as indicators of goal attainment. This information can be used to identify problem areas and to forecast future demand for nursing services. In addition to this type of information, an environmental assessment is done to identify past, current, and future data that could affect the organization.

Conclusion

Nursing practice requires that data are processed into meaningful information for the nursing organization. This information exists in three major areas: providing care for individual patients, managing nursing unit operations, and strategic planning for the nursing organization. Many, if not all of the data elements identified in this model exist in health care organizations, either in manual form in the patient record or in automated form in single purpose systems; however, these data are often unavailable in their present form. Effective mechanisms for collecting, recording, storing, aggregating, and analyzing nursing data are required. Computerization and database technology have the potential to provide many useful strategies to accomplish this.

A nursing database, designed using the model presented here, would provide easy and efficient retrieval of nursing data; furthermore, the internal data structures of such a system would be organized in a manner consistent with the conceptual framework of nursing practice, the nursing process and reflect the proposed NMDS. To satisfy the information requirements of nurses in clinical and administrative practice, a model for database design is needed that reflects the data that are produced and used by nurses in their practice. In order to design and develop databases for nursing information that meet these requirements, a conceptual model of nursing information is required. The conceptual model of the information requirements of nursing organizations presented here is a step toward the design and use of such database systems.

References

[1] American Nurses Association (1980). *Nursing: A Social Policy Statement*. Kansas City, Mo.: The American Nurses Association.

[2] Ratliff, C., Summers, S., Resler, M., & Becker, A. (1988, March). *Computerized Nursing Diagnosis and Documentation of Nursing Care in Inpatient Health Care Agencies*. Paper presented at the meeting of the North American Nursing Diagnosis Association, St. Louis, Mo.

[3] American Hospital Association. Public Information Announcement, Prime Time, ABC, NBC, CBS, first six months of 1982.

[4] Levine, T. and Phillip, P. (1975). *Factors Affecting Staffing Levels and Patterns of Nursing Personnel*. Washington, D.C.: U.S. Department of Health, Education, and Welfare.

[5] Rieder, K.A. & Norton, D.A. (1984). An Integrated Nursing Information System—A Planning Model. *Computers in Nursing*, 2(3), 73–79.

[6] Graves, J. and Corcoran, S. (1988). Design of Nursing Information Systems: Conceptual and Practice Elements. *Journal of Professional Nursing*, 4(3), 168–177.

[7] Saba, V.K. & McCormick, K.A. (1986). *Essentials of Computers for Nurses*. Philadelphia: J.B. Lippincott Company.

[8] McHugh, M.L. (1986). Information Access: A Basis for Strategic Planning and Control of Operations. *Nursing Administration Quarterly*, 10(2), 10–20.

[9] Pinkley, C.L. and Sommer, P.K. (1988). An Integrated Nursing Management Information System: From Concept to Reality. In R. A. Greenes (Ed.), *Proceedings of the Twelth Annual Symposium on Computer Applications in Medical Care* (pp. 790–795). Los Angeles, Ca.: IEEE Computer Society Press.

[10] Study Group on Nursing Information Systems (1983). Computerized Nursing Information Systems: An Urgent Need. *Research in Nursing and Health*, 6, 101–105.

[11] Werley, H.H. (1987). Nursing Diagnosis and the Minimum Data Set. In A.M. McLane (Ed.), *Classification of Nursing Diagnoses: Proceedings of the Seventh National Conference* (pp. 21–36). St. Louis, Mo.: The C.V. Mosby Company.

[12] Loomis, M.E.S. (1987). *The Database Book*. New York: Macmillan Publishing Company.

[13] Blum, B.I. (1986). *Clinical Information Systems*. New York: Springer-Verlag.

[14] Loomis, M.E.S. (1987). *The Database Book*. New York: Macmillan Publishing Company.

[15] Kim, M.J., McFarland, G.K., & McLane, A.M. (1986). *Pocket Guide to Nursing Diagnosis*. St. Louis, Mo.: The C.V. Mosby Company.

[16] American Nurses Association (1980). *Nursing: A Social Policy Statement*. Kansas City, Mo.: The American Nurses Association.

[17] Grier, M.R. (1984). Information Processing in Nursing Practice. In H.H. Werley & J.J. Fitzpatrick (Eds.), *Annual Review of Nursing Research* (Vol. 2, pp. 265–287). New York: Springer Publishing Company.

[18] Rieder, K.A. & Norton, D.A. (1984). An Integrated Nursing Information System—A Planning Model. *Computers in Nursing*, 2(3), 73–79.

[19] Prescott, P.A. (1986). DRG Prospective Reimbursement: The Nursing Intensity Factor. *Nursing Management*, 17(1), 43–46.

[20] Spitzer, R. (1986), *Nursing Productivity: The Hospital's Key to Survival and Profit*. Chicago, Il.: S-N Publications.
[21] Strasen, L. (1987). *Key Business Skills for Nurse Managers*. Philadelphia: J.B. Lippincot Company.

18
Utilizing Computer Integration to Assist Nursing

Marianne Hujcs

Introduction

The ability of a hospital information system to integrate data from various programs provides users many opportunities to tailor the computer to meet their individual needs. Specifically, nurses utilizing computers at the bedside have often perceived the computer as another task to be learned rather than a benefit to their practice. However, the capability of integration of the HELP system at LDS Hospital in Salt Lake City, Utah, has provided staff nurses the opportunity to design specific reports and utilize computer generated alerts which are perceived as helpful tools that save time and assist in patient care delivery. In addition, integration has also raised some challenges for nursing to determine the scope of documentation and how best to utilize the computer. The purpose of this paper is to discuss the development of one example of a tool, the Charge Nurse Report, how this report and computer generated alerts are utilized, and the impact on nursing.

Integration of a Hospital Information System

Demands for large amounts of information from various sources, especially in critical care, have encouraged the development of ways to process this information for the user [1,2,7]. Gardner et al. has identified four functions of the computer in the critical care setting [1]:

(1). physiologic monitoring containing microcomputers that acquire, process, store, and display data and can sound alarms when variables become life threatening. (2). computers to facilitate timely and accurate communication of data to and from multiple sources (laboratory, blood bank, surgery, and radiology) within the

Reprinted with permission from *Proceedings: Fourteenth Annual Symposium on Computer Applications in Medical Care*, Miller, R.A. (Ed.). 1990. Pp. 894–897. © 1990, American Medical Informatics Association: Bethesda, MD.

hospital, making patient information more readily available for use in patient care. (3). medical record-keeping, which enables consistent patient care. (4). expert computer systems used to make nursing and medical decisions and augment the capabilities of those staff caring for critically ill patients.

The ability to process this information from various sources is the result of integration. Having a hospital information system to collect data from physiologic monitors and hospital departments physically separated from each other and communicate that information to multiple health care providers, is a great asset in patient care. Integration not only allows this enhanced communication but also relieves the task of collecting that information from staff nurses. Blaufuss [2] stated that "the information system must be interactive. If it is set up as a separate computer system, nurses may still be forced into the same role as in a manual system—pulling all of the information areas together and trying to make them relate to each other" [2].

Integration allows a centralized patient data base to be generated. Having a centralized data base allows individualization of the patient record and individualization of any reports generated from that record.

Since the installation of the HELP system, on-going development has focused on utilizing integration. As a result of this development, several reports which collect information for the care-giver have been created. The intensive care unit (ICU) shift report and ICU rounds report are two examples of daily reports used in the ICU setting. The ICU shift report displays patient data such as vital signs, intake and output, medications administered, and current lab results. The rounds report, used most consistently by physicians, collects a 24 hour summary of lab results, vital signs, medications, and nutritional data. Contributions from staff nurses led to the development of a charge nurse report to assist nurses in communicating patient status at the end of a shift. The charge nurse report also utilizes integration.

Computer generated alerts, another example of integration, have always been a facet of the HELP system. These alerts assist the user in identifying data that falls outside of pre-programmed normal ranges. Alerts are also generated in the pharmacy program when a medication is scheduled if that medication has a contraindication with previously scheduled medications or a known hypersensitivity exists. Development of computer generated alerts to assist nurses in documenting standards of care is in progress.

Identifying Tools to Assist Users

Development of new programs or tools to assist staff requires the contribution of those personnel. At LDS Hospital, various Users Groups for physicians and nurses exist in order to provide a forum for communication of ideas, problems, or needs pertinent to computer utilization. For example, the ICU User Group consists of two staff nurses from each of the intensive care units; the group is purposely kept small to allow adequate communication and discussion. Often, the staff nurses identify their own needs through quality assurance monitors or daily practice issues. The User Group determines the feasibility or practical application of the tool and recommends whether to pursue further development.

Once a need is identified, suggestions are taken to the Nursing Information System Committee and the Medical Informatics Department. Programmers are then assigned to the task of developing the tool. After a test program is developed, the User Group tests the tool for any obvious problems. After testing is completed, the program is installed on the nursing divisions. The User Group trains their own staff to use the program and follows up with communication for revisions or further suggestions.

Similar input is solicited when computer generated alerts are developed. Staff nurses and physicians assist in determining normal ranges and how an alert should be displayed [3]. Staff nurses also contribute to the on-going development of alerts in the nurse charting program.

Utilizing a Charge Nurse Report in the ICU

The purpose of the charge nurse report is to decrease the amount of time needed by the charge nurse collecting information on patients at the end of the shift and reporting that information to the next shift. The goal of the ICU User Group developing this report was to decrease the amount of overtime due to the nurse to nurse report at the end of a shift. This report is generated by the charge nurse; it contains patient specific data stored in various programs. After the printout is obtained, the charge nurse collects information on general problems regarding the patients that may impact staff assignments (i.e. hemodynamic instability, transporting to x-ray or surgery).

The charge nurse report consists of a current patient list, room number, patient identification number, diagnosis and attending physician, information collected from the admit/discharge/transfer (ADT) program. The report also lists current infusions and rates including TPN, vasopressors, and maintenance solutions, data which is stored in the medication program and medical information bus (MIB). Current arterial blood gases, ventilator settings, and FIO_2 (fraction of oxygen therapy) are included; this data is collected from the laboratory and respiratory therapy charting programs. Finally, the report also generates information from the nurse charting program: Glasgow Coma Score and level of consciousness.

The uniqueness of the HELP System allows this report to be tailored to each specific ICU; it is possible to program this report for each unit with unit specific information. For example, in the Shock-Trauma ICU, monitoring of patient coma score is deemed important by the charge nurses since head-injury patients are frequently admitted there. However, in the Thoracic ICU where post-operative open heart surgery patients are admitted, coma score has little significance; the charge nurses prefer to report the ECG results. The charge nurse report can be programmed differently to provide individualization.

Since the implementation of this report in all ICU's, the charge nurses have found that general charge nurse report time has decreased allowing more time for bedside report and thus decreasing overtime. Also, the charge nurses have felt a more thorough report is given to the on-coming shift since some of the information can be lost in a completely verbal report. Finally, the charge nurse report is seen as a benefit of computerization and has changed some staff nurse perceptions.

Computer Generated Alerts in the ICU

The HELP System utilizes alerts in many programs. The goal of alerting is to assist users to identify life-threatening conditions promptly [3,4].

One such example is the arterial blood gas interpretation. The interpretation consists of a range of possibilities including hypoxemia and acid-base alerts. Presently, in the ICUs, bedside terminals exist in all patient rooms allowing rapid and frequent examination of results. The alerts are reported with the specimen lab values. As expected, the significance of the computer-generated alert is different among the experience level of the nurse. For example, experienced ICU nurses state that they rapidly recognize any abnormal result without prompting from the computer; however, less experienced nurses state that the alert assists them with interpretation, especially if the alert is reporting an acid-base abnormality. Nurses also state that the computer alert can not be interpreted without a clinical exam of the patient. The computer alert is more significant on the acute care units where bedside terminals do not exist in all patient rooms. The lab result automatically prints out at a central nursing station; the report is collected by a unit secretary. If an alert is generated, the unit secretary promptly notifies the nurse caring for the patient to examine the report.

Laboratory alerting capabilities were expanded in 1987 with the installation of the Computerized Laboratory Alerting System (CLAS) [3]. This system was designed to improve reporting of life-threatening conditions via the lab results review program. A previous study conducted after the implementation of CLAS showed that staff nurses identified alerts 54% of the time in the ICUs and 52% on the acute care divisions [3]. In contrast, the studies identified that physicians identified 32% of the alerts in the ICUs and 26% of the alerts on acute care divisions [3]. In addition, the study indicated an increase in physician response to alerts and a decrease in length of stay after implementation [3].

Another example of computer generated alerts is in the pharmacy program. Currently, when a nurse schedules a medication, an alert will be generated if there is a contraindication with a previously scheduled medication or a known hypersensitivity to that drug. Nurses state that the physician directing the patient's care is notified of the alert and changes are made appropriately. Often, the alert recommends monitoring of plasma drug levels, as is the case with aminoglycosides; this alert is also discussed with the physician and usually results in such monitoring. In fact, a study conducted at LDS Hospital by Gardner et al. identified physician response and attitudes with the pharmacy alerting system and determined that in 1989, physician compliance with "action-oriented" alerts was 100% [4]. Often, these alerts were relayed to the physicians by nurses, especially in the ICU.

Eventually, computer generated alerts will assist the nurse in documenting standards of care. Presently, nurses have identified deficiencies in documentation through quality assurance monitors. These items have been added to the nursing data base in order to improve documentation of the standard of care; development of alerts for nurses to chart these items is in progress.

Challenges for Nursing

The ability to generate specific reports and alerts raises several challenges for the nursing profession. Among the first issues to be addressed is the establishment of standards for documentation and acceptable response time to meet these standards. For example, the computerized nursing care plan currently in place within the HELP system allows standards of care to be programmed [5]; computer generated alerts can notify staff to provide adequate documentation. The challenge for nursing is to determine what time-frame is acceptable and reasonable for adequate documentation in addition to what information is to be stored in the patient record. The question is then raised, should alerts be generated every two hours; or, perhaps, if the patient condition is stable, every eight hours would be adequate. Parameters determining patient normals could be developed identifying which patients would need more frequent monitoring.

A second issue for nursing which follows the question of adequate documentation is quality assurance. Computerization of the nursing process allows concurrent review of the patient record and identification of problems as they occur [5]. Quality assurance issues, then, can be immediately addressed. Therefore, the challenge to nursing is to establish what should be monitored. Nursing can utilize the computer to collect data for quality assurance and decrease individual chart reviews in an effort to make the process more efficient. At LDS Hospital, staff nurses complete quality assurance monitors on a monthly basis; much of the data they collect is in the computerized patient data file.

Utilizing the computer prospectively leads to yet another challenge for nursing. Computer generated alerts and reports can be developed to identify patient needs on admission so that planning can begin to assist that patient. In a time when health care is facing its own challenge to provide the maximum amount of care in a minimum amount of time, the need for discharge planning to begin immediately and for identifying factors which decrease length of stay are essential. As a result, alerts determining discharge needs can be developed. In addition, nursing can identify those factors that prolong length of stay and use the computer in alerting staff to the problem. For example, the admission of a head-injury patient to the ICU can be tracked by a nursing case manager. The computerized nursing history can alert staff to potential needs for physical and occupational therapy and eventual placement in a rehabilitation unit. Currently, at LDS Hospital, development of a falls alert is in progress. The purpose of this tool is to alert staff to those patients most at risk to fall out of bed, etc. and to implement safety measures as needed [6]. In addition, development of a wound/skin assessment tool is also in progress. Eventually, this tool will collect data from the nurse charting program and identify those patients at risk for decubitus ulcers and alert the skin care team for intervention.

Finally, the challenge of nursing research needs to be addressed. Studies on the efficacy of computers in nursing need to be conducted. For example, how frequently do computer generated alerts alter nursing practice and how does this change affect patient outcomes or length of stay? Some studies have been conducted in this area [3,4]; however, as more alerts are being developed, they, too, should be studied. In addition, cost comparisons on using the computer to improve patient care should be performed. These studies would justify nursing time in projects such as discharge planning and encourage budgeting for further studies. Research on the type of nursing diagnoses generated could also be conducted. For example, identifying the most frequently utilized nursing diagnosis within a certain patient population could lead to the development of alerts to assist staff in planning patient care.

Utilizing computers within nursing is increasing greatly. The opportunity for developing computers to assist nurses is a priority. Integration within a hospital information system allows such development. Nurses have the challenge to integrate computers into their practice and have an impact on patient care as well.

References

1. Gardner RM, Bradshaw KE, Hollingsworth KW. Computerizing the intensive care unit: Current status and future opportunities. *J Cardiovasc Nurs* 1989;4:69–78.
2. Blaufuss JA. Computer technology. In Spicer JG, Robinson MA (eds). *Managing the environment in critical care nursing*. Baltimore, MA: Williams & Wilkins, 1990: pp 93–104.

3. Bradshaw KE, Gardner RM, Pryor TA. Development of a computerized laboratory alert system. *Computers and Biomedical Research* 1989;22:575–587.
4. Gardner RM, Hulse RK, Larsen KG. Assessing the effectiveness of a computerized alert system. (To be presented: Symposium on Computer Applications in Medical Care 1990).
5. Blaufuss JA. Promoting the nursing process through computerization. In Salamon R, Blum B, Jorgensen M (eds). MEDINFO 86 BV North-Holland: Elsevier Science, 1986: pp 585–586.
6. Blaufuss JA, Tinker A. Computerized falls alert—a new solution to an old problem. Proceedings of Twelfth Annual SCAMC Conference. Silver Spring: IEEE Computer Society Press, 1988: pp 69–71.
7. Gardner RM, Shabot MM. Computerized ICU data management: pitfalls and promises. *Int J of Clin Mon and Comp* 1990;7:99–105.

19
Role of the Nurse in Implementing Nursing Information Systems

Rita Axford

Introduction

New roles and responsibilities are emerging in nursing as we become aware of the profession's information systems and the benefits of the computer as a tool to manage them more effectively. This new technology challenges us to do more than learn to operate new machinery. The complexity and cost of different computer systems and rapid changes in hospital computer technology require nursing leaders to have an understanding of many key issues. Only a sound knowledge of hospital information systems and a keen understanding of nursing practice and the information systems which support it will enable us to obtain computer tools useful to the profession. This paper will overview the general structures and functions of hospital information systems, describe common nursing information systems, detail the nurse decision-makers' role in system implementation, and finally, share principles for computer user training derived from a review of the literature and from the author's professional experiences as a nursing systems analyst/computer trainer.

Hospital Information Systems (HIS): An Overview

The specific set of elements of a hospital information system will be unique to each institution depending upon the structure, size, philosophy, clientele, and resources of the organization. Computer systems may be described in terms of machinery in their hardware. While knowing the difference between a mainframe and a personal computer, between a "dumb terminal" and a local area network are useful, it is the understanding of the

Reprinted with permission from *Nursing Informatics '91: Pre-Conference Proceedings*; Turley, J.P. & Newbold, S.K. (Eds.). 1991. Pp. 35–42. Heidelberg-Berlin, Germany: Springer-Verlag.

structure and functions of the information component the computer manipulates which enables the nurse decision-maker to conceptualize and communicate nursing's information processing needs.

The structures of HIS vary. Some are wholly integrated. That is, each operation of the system has equal access to data; data are entered only once and at their source. Some systems interrelate less cohesively, sharing data on a limited basis, i.e. interfacing systems. A person may be used at intervals to interpret and verify selected data (a "human interface"). And some systems stand alone. This is the least efficient structure as redundant entry of data is generally necessary, delays are created, and there is increased opportunity for error.

An HIS model may be useful for understanding common terminology, interrelationships, and purposes of the health care industry's information base. Hospital computer systems can be described in terms of three non-discrete categories. Financial/Administrative systems automate such activities as cost accounting, receivables, payables, the general ledger, payroll, and property management. Decision-support systems assist management in the analysis of data produced by other (generally computerized) systems. Examples include case-mix and diagnostic related groups (DRG) analysis, medical records abstracting systems, incident reporting, workload management, and rostering systems. Clinical/departmental systems are designed to assist a clinical department such as pathology, pharmacy, or nursing, with its information management and may serve any or all of the following functions for the specific department: planning, scheduling and documentation of services, quality monitoring, and cost analysis.

Office automation functions do not fit neatly into this model, but are a key part of an HIS. These functions include word processing of supporting documents like policies and procedures, electronic scheduling, diaries, and electronic mail. The rapid expansion of microcomputer applications in the workplace during the 1980s redirected many hospital computer implementation plans as managers saw the immediate value of inexpensive and accessible word processing, database management, spreadsheet and graphic applications.

Nursing Information Systems (NIS): Key Elements

Nursing may use each of the systems just described. NIS include the financial, decision-support and office automation functions. Nursing also has unique departmental/clinical information systems needs. These clinical systems can be seen to mirror nursing's professionally dependent and independent functions within hospitals: managing the patient environment and providing direct nursing care. The two clinical information systems fundamental to an efficient nursing department are its order communications and nursing clinical record-keeping systems.

Order communications systems (also called order entry, order management, or patient information systems) track patient data from admission through discharge automating information collection at every phase of the patient's stay. While specifics may vary, the prime thrust of this system is to communicate data between nursing care areas and the ancillary or support areas. Patient supplies can be ordered electronically and ancillary departments provided with computerized requests for services, clinical reports, and costing data. Electronic communication of patient orders for diagnostic and therapeutic services can provide nursing with a log of services and with outcomes or results reporting. Patient scheduling can be accomplished both for the service departments and for the individual patient. This system provides nurses, physicians, and other health professionals with information which aids patient care delivery while simultaneously providing data for effective resource management.

An order communications system is a most complex system in terms of the scope of interdepartmental interactions and the number of people using the system. Development and installation of the order communication system, by whatever nomenclature, is complicated and fraught with difficulties. The number of departments involved, their respective political and power relationships within the organization, and the amount and level of compatibility of computer systems with each department, all impact on its complexity. This is often the most expensive system a hospital ever invests in, and while it is an interdepartmental information system, nursing is, by virtue of the number of users, the amount of time on the system, and the number of entry and retrieval interactions, its primary user. Nursing must therefore, have high level involvement in system design and implementation. We must understand, explain, and assert our requisites for patient information management.

Nursing clinical record-keeping systems automate the documentation tools used in nursing: care plans, flowsheets, progress notes, and graphics. These systems are relatively new to the marketplace and vary in complexity, flexibility and cost. The most sophisticated of these automate aspects of the clinical decision-making process and may be called "expert systems." Simpler systems automate the documentation process by storage of protocols and standard care plans for retrieval by the nurse for specific individualization. Flowsheets for continued documentation of patient responses to nursing care may be constructed on the computer from the patient's care plan. Costing for nursing care services can be an important by-product of this system.

Decision support systems that serve the nursing department include resource management and quality monitoring systems. A number of software vendors provide rostering and dependency systems of varying degrees of sophistication. Programs that assist the budgetary process are available in the form of general-purpose spreadsheets and as specific budget packages tailored to an institution's own budgetary protocols. Employee record-keeping functions are often similar for the nursing department, personnel, employee health, and staff development, and may be part of an integrated system or a separate system with a shared data base.

Quality assurance information comes in a variety of forms depending on the questions being asked, the data being examined, and the methodology for analysis and reporting selected. Likewise, the computer tools vary. A quality monitoring system can be purchased as a stand-alone system with its own vehicle for data collection, input, and analysis or may be an integral part of a clinical system. Alternatively, inexpensive and capable systems have been developed from generic spreadsheet, statistics, and graphics packages.

Guidelines for Decision-Makers

Instrumental decision-makers enact a variety of roles in the hospital hierarchy and include charge nurses, middle managers, and directors of nursing. Armed with a global understanding of the kinds of computer systems we need, nurse decision-makers are prepared to participate with their management colleagues in the cost-benefit analyses needed for effective computerization decisions. Identification of all costs and benefits is difficult as many outcomes are obscure and far reaching. The following may each be useful to evaluate:

BENEFITS
    Time savings through
        Reduced duplication in charting and retrieving clinical data
        Less time communicating relevant patient data
        Less time developing patient care plans
    Money savings through
        Decreased use of professionals in clerical activities
        Better compliance with patient care plans
        Better risk management due to fewer charting omissions
        Fewer forms
        Reduced overhead in managing resources
    Improved human satisfaction through
        Better interpartmental communications
        Improved patient and family outcomes
        Increased professional autonomy by access to critical information

COSTS
    Time expended on
        Planning and developing systems
        Implementing large scale change and educational processes
        Installing the system and initial data base

Money expended on
   Purchasing and maintaining machinery and materials
   Personnel cost outcomes such as attrition or sabotage
Human dissatisfaction related to
   Industrial issues through changing work requisites
   Role ambiguity
   Computer anxiety
   Perceived depersonalization

A critical question remains: In light of current resources and overall department goals and priorities, what is the cost of implementing versus NOT IMPLEMENTING a given computer system, relative to the expected benefits as we know them now? The rapid change in the capabilities and the costs of computer technology makes answering this question difficult as well as tentative. Today's answer requires frequent re-examination.

In addition to cost-benefit analysis, other strategies useful in the computerization process include mobilizing key people to explore the critical issues collectively. This role ensures liaison between nursing, data processing, and other computerization decision-making sub-groups. Information processing decisions are often political and require collaboration and compromise. Adequate nursing resources including people, time, and expertise must be allocated for successful planning, selection, education, and implementation. Appropriate staff involvement helps guarantee success of an effective system.

Often organizations purchase computer systems from companies specializing in these products. When dealing with vendors it is important to ask if your organization has worked satisfactorily with this supplier before, and if possible, to find other hospitals who have also dealt with them. Careful deliberation and questioning can ensure a satisfactory purchase. You need guarantees about the specific applications and the hardware requirements to support them. Determine the true status of each application. Has the vendor actually installed each feature or are applications being developed specifically for you. Find out about the skill level and experience of their installation team: what is required of hospital resources including personnel, space, and money. Other questions to consider include:

How does the product protect the confidentiality of information about your patients?
What provisions have been made for upgrading the software as needed?
How much flexibility is allowed in the design and content of the various screens?
What are the noise levels and space requirements of terminals and printers?
How much scheduled downtime is required for maintenance?
What back-up systems are planned?

Good equipment and well-designed software are two of the essential ingredients of successful system implementation. System user training is the third. Plan it in detail: who will do the instruction and the evaluation; what teaching methodology will be used; what resource materials will be needed; who will prepare them; and what is the expected implementation schedule and time commitment?

Computer Training: Principles and Experiences

The structure of a training program provides the foundation for user success. Established learning principles are as applicable to computer training as to any other teaching-learning environment. Specifically, effective computer training needs organizational support. It should accommodate individual variations in learning styles, address cognitive, affective, and psychomotor aspects learning and, embrace adult learning principles.

Learners vary in their response to written, oral, or graphic presentation of information. Information can be presented verbally and a written syllabus provided with instructions and pictoral representation of information. Audio-visual adjuncts and a healthy dose of humor aid a didactic presentation. Some learners perform better when working in groups; some when solo. While there is an inherent efficiency in group learning, individual or paired practice at computer terminals is most effective. Since group size must be limited because of the need for immediate feedback during interactive learning activities, experienced trainers recommend a group size limited to ten learners for one trainer and only one or two learners per terminal. Attention span for learning activities is enhanced if breaks in learning tasks are provided at hourly intervals. Reduce competing demands for learner attention through legitimized training sessions in off-duty time.

Computer training encompasses all the domains of learning: cognitive, affective, and psychomotor. Nurses are skillful at recalling new information, and more important, are great problem-solvers when given appropriate tools. Instructing users about system structure and about additional "help" resources is invaluable. It is worth noting that the initial start-up steps of using a computer system usually involve specific commands for which no amount of problem-solving capability will help. A clear, comprehensive, and available user manual is essential as nurses begin to use a system. This document contains information different from the sequenced learning activities of the computer training syllabus. User manuals require highly specific system instructions with detailed indexing for easy reference. Identification of experienced resource people on the wards can also help reinforce learning and keep frustration at a minimum.

There is an unmistakable affective component to learning about computers. Computer-phobia is a real phenomenon and may be manifested in resistant behaviors. Computers commonly threaten the status quo, thus creating many real or imaginary fears. At the very least, many nurses must return to the role of novice learner and begin the often uncomfortable process of mastering new and unfamiliar skills. Computers also threaten to change decision control and social norms within an organization. Nursing unit managers may resist computerization of rostering if these decisions have offered them significant influence and control over their staff. Barriers to computerization may emerge if nurses feel that computers deprive patients of professional contacts or invade their privacy. A pro-active stance is needed to reduce apprehension and resistance about a new computer installation. Assess the pre-implementation environment, identify expected changes and threats, mobilize resources for planned change, market the computerization effort, and involve users in the design, implementation, and evaluation of the system.

The psychomotor component of the computer learning also must be acknowledged. Generally rudimentary keyboarding skills are sufficient to operate a well-designed, "menu driven" system (one in which the user selects an option from a pre-determined list of choices). While penlights, touch-screens, and bar codes have limitations, they may be useful alternatives if user keyboarding skills are known to be limited.

Principles of adult learning have application to all adult learning activities. Examples of the application of these principles to computer training include:

Adults Learn Best when it is in response to a felt need.

Staff nurses often feel they are "drowning in documentation." When instituting a nursing care planning documentation system, emphasis on the benefits to patient care through rapid, legible, and retrievable documentation can serve to capitalize upon this learning principle. Similarly, computer applications for nurse executives are best taught by learning activities dealing with the analysis of common management problems.

Adults respond best to immediate applications of new knowledge.

Application, practice, and hands-on experience are essential to effective computer training. Because of their interactive nature, computers are very effective teaching devices for self-paced and experiential learning. Transfer of learning can be maximized by using training exercises that are as close to real applications as possible.

Adults mobilize their experience repertoires.

The majority of nurses have used computers—perhaps only their automatic bank teller card. Comparing the steps of "logging on" a computer to bank card access is one of the many analogies that can be used successfully.

And finally, adults want to be treated as such.

A collaborative relationship where there is mutual diagnosis and shared goal setting is more likely to succeed. Computer training lends itself to mastery-oriented learning with clear, predefined expectations and goals.

Summary

Nursing leaders are currently faced with complex and costly decisions about how to computerize nursing department information systems. The unique configuration of the computer systems in a hospital and the goals and priorities of the nursing department influence the outcomes of these decisions. Being informed about the many options for computerization, facilitating communications between nursing, other clinical departments, and the system provider, and ensuring effective computer training are powerful determinants of successful role implementation for NIS developers.

References

Axford R: Implementation of nursing computer systems: A new challenge for staff development departments. *Journal of Nursing Staff Development* 1988; 4:125–130.

Flaugher P: Computer training for nursing personnel: Suggestions for training sessions. *Computers in Nursing* 1986; 4:105–108.

Gibson S, Rose M: Managing computer resistance. *Computers in Nursing* 1986; 4:201–204.

Ginsberg D, Browning S: Selecting automated patient care systems. *Journal of Nursing Administration.* 1985; 15:11–21.

Knowles M: *The Adult Learner: A Neglected Species (3rd ed.).* Houston: Gulf Publishing, 1984.

Simpson R: Technology: Nursing the system. *Nursing Management* 1990; 21:46.

20
An Integrated Nursing Management Information System: From Concept to Reality

CONNIE L. PINKLEY and PATRICIA K. SOMMER

Introduction

The healthcare environment today is radically different from that of the near past. In this era of cost constraint, information to guide decisions is a prime commodity. The lack of such essential information is insupportable. U.S. Navy Admiral Grace Hopper [1], an early pioneer in information system development, points out that the cost of not having information is usually overlooked when calculating the cost of producing information. One does not have to look far to demonstrate the substantial costs incurred by inappropriate, incomplete, or inaccurate data.

Davis [2] differentiates "information" from "data" based on the recipient's perception of relevance in making decisions. The ease and efficiency the user experiences in interpreting computer outputs as information must play a formative role in computer system design. Specifications for new systems often emphasize computer process, rather than user product criteria.

Historical and emerging influences shaping the development of information systems used by nurses are presented. Broad system objectives and assessment factors are proposed to guide the definition and design of a Nursing Information System (NIS). The University Hospitals of Cleveland Nursing Management Information System (NMIS) illustrates the emphasis on user products in the system design process. The challenge is to blend capabilities and constraints existing within a particular institution with the needs of nurses for information products supporting and enhancing their decisions.

Reprinted with permission from *Proceedings: Twelfth Annual Symposium on Computer Applications in Medical Care*, Greenes, R.A. (Ed.). 1988. Pp. 790–795. © 1987, American Medical Informatics Association (formerly SCAMC): Bethesda, MD.

Developmental Issues in Information Systems for Nurses

Historical Influences and Their Impact

An overview of the traditional situation of the nurse reveals systems have often been designed without appreciation of the type and presentation of data required to support nursing decisions. Existing information has often been structured and prioritized to meet the needs of others within, or outside, the hospital system.

Process Driven Design

General systems theory concepts of input, throughput, and output are frequently used to model information system design. These terms provide an organizational scheme for information system components and processes. The terms fail to define the ultimate information product. Nurses passively receiving data from the system are likely to find themselves immersed in outputs with little information value. They then attempt to approximate desired information products by reformatting and revising available data.

Multi-System Syndrome

Systems usually develop along functional and departmental organizational lines. Financial systems are usually the first to be computerized. As other systems are added, each with unique reporting functions and capabilities, they seldom communicate. Discrepant timeframes are often used, creating an interpretive dilemma. Untold hours are spent attempting to relate clinical, census, payroll, and fiscal data.

Regulatory Requirements

Governmental and other regulatory agencies have significantly influenced hospital information system development. The precedence of external requirements is easily discerned when viewing the particular elements being collected, counted, and reported in a given year. If reimbursement is tied to an element, it most assuredly drives the report system.

Data necessary for external accounting of hospital services cannot be assumed to also meet the need of the nurse clinician, manager, or the profession as a whole. The lack of systematic collection of nursing data nationally represents a vacuum in which health care policy is defined. The absence of information is as powerful as its presence might be in determining policy for, and practice of, professional nursing.

Organizational Structure

Hierarchical management structures promote downward accountability and flow of information. Standardization of administrative and managerial reports usually occurs. Reports do not differentiate the type and/or specificity of data required to support decisions at various levels in the organization.

Rarely can standardized reports and data from which they are constructed address the complexity of nursing management decisions. This results in a lack of relevant information products. For example, productivity measurements based only on patient data/FTE comparisons do not discriminate the critical role of nurse experience. In addition, standardized reporting systems are slow to adapt to dynamic information needs. Midnight census, though a deteriorating indicator of patient throughput, continues as the measure of unit activity.

Emerging Influences and Their Implications

We are in a health care future shock mode. Adequate decision support is crucial if nurse managers/administrators are to meet the needs:

To be competitive
To conserve resources
To anticipate and plan for change
To remain flexible, and
To design creative alternatives.

Organizational Change

Drucker [3] characterizes the information-based organization as one that directs the flow of information and accountability for decisions to those closest to the point of product production, or delivery. Accelerated change in health care has compressed time in which decisions are effected. Decentralized organizational structures have broadened the control and responsibility for clinical and operational decisions at the unit level. The Head Nurse Manager needs specific information to effectively respond.

As reimbursement systems have changed, the necessity to define, quantify, cost, and develop quality measures for nursing products is inescapable. Nursing product data are needed to explain resource utilization patterns, length of stay, and to devise alternative patient care delivery models in product-line management systems. These data facilitate strategic planning, marketing, and resource projection. Classification systems based on time/task measures, converted to resource allocation numbers, are not useful in tracing or evaluating the qualitative impact of nurse service over time, and are impotent to stimulate change.

Professional Practice Models

The role of the professional nurse in patient care management is increasingly clear. Nosek [4] demonstrated the high explanatory power of patients' nursing diagnoses in evaluating length of stay. Determining the patient's need for nursing, the optimal environment of care, the expertise and resource allocation of the nurse, and evaluating the clinical outcomes of patient care management strategies are of prime importance for quality and cost management.

Nursing databases must meet the demands experienced by practitioners. Included are 1) enhanced communication across settings; 2) identification of existing relationships among clinical data, nurse provider data, and operational data; and 3) assessment of cost, quality, and appropriateness of patient care management. Systems must facilitate identification of patients at risk, selection of management strategies, measurement of patient care outcomes, and generation knowledge through research.

Definition of Nursing Data

In addition to the need for clinical and operational data to support nursing decisions within institutions, the broader needs for nursing data are gaining recognition. Information system development can be guided and expanded from elements identified in the Nursing Minimum Data Set, Werley, Lang, & Westlake [5]. As uniform nursing data become available they can be used in research, policy development, and reimbursement at a national level, Jencks & Dobson [6]; Halloran & Kiley [7].

Participation in System Design

Nurses are gaining in awareness. They are developing knowledge, discrimination, and expectations for quality information products. Increasing numbers of jobs hybridize professional nursing and informatics expertise. This creates an opportunity to design data output that is efficiently translated to information by the user. Practitioners have an opportunity to utilize data for decision-making previously unattainable.

Garnering resource commitments to the development of information systems result from conscious prioritization over other competing goals. Nurses must articulate the relationship between information and effective care. Nurses must be intimately involved in strategic planning, system evaluation, and cost/benefit analyses.

Defining and Designing Nursing Information Systems

Computers are purchased to extend our capabilities, increase our efficiency, and broaden the domain of data to which we can effectively respond. Are the expectations inappropriate and unachievable, or have we simply failed to define the task sufficiently? The challenge is to develop systems that emulate, facilitate, and/or stimulate nurses' thought processes. These are best articulated by nurses who understand nursing decision processes and appreciate computer capabilities.

Information systems necessitate a wide range of data access to service clinicians, managers, and administrators. Identification of data types, sources, and interfaces is fundamental to constructing a usable system. The flexibility and capability for data manipulation, immediacy and style of presentation, must be defined and synchronized with the institution's capability to support the volume and types of usage desired.

Institutional size and resources are major determinants in system design. Similar objectives may be achieved by various system configurations. Having identified the information products desired, analysis of existing and desired input, throughput, and output processing configurations can begin.

Input

Information goals must be reduced to discrete data elements serving as precursors to information products. In addition to data generated by the nurse through documentation or classification systems, relevant data can be procured through integration with the Hospital Information System (HIS) databases. Traditional database management fostered independent definition, creation, and maintenance of HIS components along departmental lines. The orchestration of database management, providing shared access, avoiding redundancy, and storing data in formats that promote flexible use, while protecting data integrity and security, is paramount.

Failure to integrate nursing data with the broader HIS severely limits the scope of information products. Often, nurses are forced to chose between the limitations of independent nursing data collection and processing systems, or create a more extensive system by initiating redundant data entry. Neither option is desirable, or necessary, in the current technological environment. Systems can be networked and data shared, or transferred. The higher initial costs and complexity of design outweigh the limitations and/or data maintenance requirements of independent systems.

Table 1, though not exhaustive, describes types of data desired to produce NMIS information products. Figure 1 illustrates data input sources in the integrated NMIS.

Input Objectives

1. Minimize interference with patient care, while capturing summarized clinical data;
2. Avoid re-entry of data entered at other points in the HIS;
3. Store data sufficiently detailed for multiple information products;
4. Ensure adequate data representation, accuracy, and durability for shared data;

TABLE 1. Data requirements of an NMIS

Data type	Sample data elements
Patient specific data	* Hospital service data: admission, discharge, Los, care locations, referral source, discharge destination, disposition
	* Social/demographic data: age, sex, race, zip, guarantor
	* Medical ICD-9 codes, DRGs
	* Nursing diagnoses, goals
	* Primary Nurse, care providers
Professional provider data	* UHC Employment/experience role progression, service location(s), status, tenure
	* Professional experience education, prior experience, certification
Operational data	* Patient movement patterns: admission, discharge, transfer; census, patient care days,
	* Nursing hours data by type: staffing patterns, educational hours, administrative hours
	* Nurse work pattern data
Fiscal data	* Personnel cost by type of hours paid
	* Supply/equipment expense
	* Budget data and variance

5. Employ standards for parallel and compatible coding schemes to relate diverse data sources.

Input Assessment Areas

1. Corporate philosophy and data access policy emphasizing institutional, rather than departmental, data ownership;
2. Established system for assuring data security and the integrity of shared data;

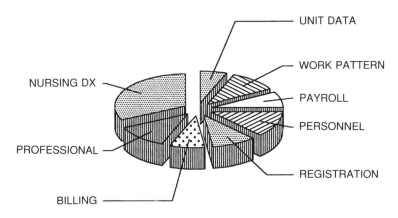

FIGURE 1. Nursing Information System Data Sources.

3. Information Services Department able to create software and data access links between systems;
4. Strategic plan for information system development;
5. Determination of the suitability and cost of data input methods for nursing data.

Throughput

The complexity of decisions often necessitates flexible analysis of the same data set, focused on differing dimensions. The user's ability to interact with information products through immediate reorganization and multiple presentation methods supports creative exploration complex analysis, and problem-solving. Data base management, statistical analysis, and graphic software create open-ended opportunities. However, speed and ease of retrieval are often sacrificed as flexibility increases. Specialized applications may be required when these qualities are important.

Throughput Objectives

1. Establish requirements for security and availability of data, systems, and equipment;
2. Utilize standardized database software when possible to reduce cost, and increase flexibility, retrievability, and usability;
3. Provide multiple levels of data manipulation using compatible database management, statistical analyses, and graphic software;
4. Develop application software when specialized needs exist.

Throughput Assessment Areas

1. Database and analysis, graphic software present or planned;
2. Degree of flexibility, modularity, and integrative potential of vendor solutions;
3. Programming capability to address required modification of system software as needed and to pursue internal application development;
4. Characteristics of desired information products: frequency, flexibility, immediacy required;
5. Online support capacity, i.e. access, response time, terminal availability, and utilization patterns;
6. Degree of user skills and independence desired and supported.

Output

The attempt to structure information outputs supporting and emulating user thinking processes requires assessment and participation of the user. Inattention to the system output/user interface can result in a communication mismatch; data that are not perceived as information.

Various strategies for presentation can be applied in designing information products. Frequently, the primary goal of the user is to identify exception, or deviation from the norm. When presented in this format, the user no longer has to sort through the data to identify relevant material. Trending, and presentation of multiple related factors with possible correlation, promotes identification of patterns of interest. Graphic illustration expedites the interpretive process. Progressive levels of summarization are often desired in report design.

Output Objectives

1. Select, merge, calculate, summarize, and display data according to user needs;
2. Present information that enhances a reliable and valid interpretation by users;
3. Achieve and maintain data accuracy;
4. Provide timely, flexible access to information products.

Output Assessment Areas

1. User ability to articulate information needs and characteristics;
2. User patterns for data organization and interpretation;
3. User sophistication, interest, and independence in data management;
4. Frequency, specificity, complexity of data required;
5. Flexibility and interactive requirement in data use;
6. Options promoted or limited in the computer environment.

NMIS Development at University Hospitals of Cleveland

The core nursing data element in the University Hospitals of Cleveland Nursing Management Information System was established in 1985 with the implementation of the Nurse Patient Summary classification system using nursing diagnosis [8]. This represents a philosophical commitment to describing the patient's need for nursing, determined through professional judgement of the nurse, as the cornerstone for nursing decisions. (Halloran & Kiley [9]; Halloran, Patterson, and Kiley [10]).

Data entry is accomplished through barcode scanning into hand-held terminals. These data are transmitted to the mainframe daily. This provided an efficient data collection method minimizing disruption to patient care. Data collection programs are being expanded to: 1) identify other care providers, 2) communicate Nurse Alert messages, 3) track professional development activities, 4) provide report request capabilities, and 5) enable generic, user defined data collection.

The volume and demand for flexible manipulation, presentation, and turnaround times could not be addressed through a system limited to batch processing of standardized reports. A twofold development strategy emerged to supplement periodic reporting: 1) rapid, online data retrieval facilitating clinical care, and 2) database management capabilities for unique and complex information needs.

The HIS development strategy in the U.H.C. environment nurtures the concept of an integrated data system through the formulation of a data access policy and through the installation of data management, statistical analysis, and graphics software systems. Not all software bridges desired are in place, but they are on the horizon.

Obstacles encountered most frequently resulted from data deficiencies. Unilateral decisions in data management will continue to occur and impede HIS integrated use until much more formalized communication is established in the context of a strategic information plan. Parallel coding schemes have not been integrated or standardized in systems posing challenges to integrated reporting. Increased interdepartmental communication, and synchronization is desirable. The roles for information management and support are dynamic. The strategic planning process provides opportunities and challenges as the merit of each system proposal is weighed.

Conclusion

The achievement of an integrated information system requires active administrative support and resource commitment over an extended developmental phase. The impact of the institution's strategic plan, existing hardware and software capability, and support for internal development are decisive factors in the feasibility and staging of system pursuit.

This paper highlights the importance of a clear understanding of the information product to be operationalized in computer processing systems. Prioritization of the product over the process design that results in information, rather than data output. Objectives and assessment considerations for each phase in the input, throughput, and output process have been presented.

"Man's mind, once stretched by a new idea, never regains it original dimensions" (Oliver Wendell Holmes). Access to a broad database, designed to address the information needs of nurses potentiates an exploratory and explanatory power often unimagined. While the ease and cost of obtaining stand-alone nursing information systems is attractive, the capabilities of an integrated NMIS are incomparable.

References

[1] Hopper G. (1986). Keynote address, Digital Equipment Corporation User Symposium. Dallas, Texas, May 1986.

[2] Davis, G.B. (1974). *Management Information Systems: Conceptual Foundations, Structure and Development* (p. 123). New York: MacGraw-Hill Book Company.

[3] Drucker, P.F. (1988). The coming of the new organization. *Harvard Business Review,* 66 (1) 45–53.

[4] Nosek, L.J. (1986). Explanation of hospital stay by nursing diagnoses, medical diagnoses, and social position. *Dissertation Abstracts International, 47,* (7), 2840-B. (University Microfilms No. DA8622844).

[5] Werley, H.H., Lang, N.M., & Westlake, S.K. (1986). Brief summary of the Nursing Minimum Data Set Conference. *Nursing Management,* 17 (7) 42–45.

[6] Jencks, S. & Dobson, A. (1987). Refining case-mix adjustment: the research evidence. *New England Journal of Medicine,* 317 (11) 679–686.

[7] Halloran, E.J., & Kiley, M.L. (1988). The complexities of case-mix adjustment. *New England Journal of Medicine,* 318 (8) 520–521.

[8] Halloran, E.J. (1983). Staffing assignment: by task or by patient? *Nursing Management,* 15 (2) 39–45.

[9] Halloran, E.J., & Kiley, M.L., (1984). Case-mix management. *Nursing Management,* 15 (20) 39–45.

[10] Halloran, E.J., Patterson, C., & Kiley, M.L. (1987). Case-mix: matching patient need with nursing resource. *Nursing Management,* 18 (3) 27–42.

21
Knowledge and Knowledge Acquisition for the Development of Expert Systems for Nursing

CAMILLE GROSSO

Residing within the field of Artificial Intelligence, knowledge acquisition is the process of locating, collecting, and refining knowledge for the development of knowledge based systems (Harmon & King, 1985). It is the transfer of expertise from a person to the system. Knowledge is an integrated collection of facts and relationships basic to competent performance (Harmon & King, 1985). Townsend and Feucht (1986) extend the definition to include heuristics that can be used to solve problems. A common dictionary definition is that knowledge is an acquaintance with facts, truth, or principles as from study or investigation.

Knowledge acquisition can be a manual process or automated. In the manual process, the knowledge transfer is accomplished through a knowledge engineer; that is, an individual skilled in assessing problems and building knowledge systems (Townsend & Feucht, 1986). When the knowledge sought is from an expert, the resulting knowledge systems are expert systems.

A nurse's knowledge is an integrated collection of facts, experience, and relationships basic to competent practice. This knowledge is acquired through formal and informal experience, discovery, learning, insight, or investigation. There is a need to understand what rules of thumb, intuition, and judgment are present in expert nursing practice. Expert computer systems developed for nursing will harness this expertise for problem solving in specific patient care areas.

This paper will explore expertise, knowledge, and the knowledge acquisition process.

Reprinted with permission from *Proceedings of Nursing and Computers: The Third International Symposium on Nursing Use of Computers and Information Science*; pp. 422–430. Daly, N. & Hannah, K.J. (Eds.). 1988. St. Louis: The C.V. Mosby Company.

Expertise

The Relevance of the Mental Model

It is evident in the Artificial Intelligence literature that the nature of expertise and the mental model of human information processing have played a large role in the development of expert systems. The underlying assumption appears to be that understanding the mental activities associated with problem solving is the way to proceed to expert system development.

In fact, in the merging of cognitive psychology and computer science has come understanding of the human expert and machine learning. This point is well made by Pylyshyn (1984) and Selfridge, Dickerson, and Biggs (1987) who say the next generation of expert systems will be termed cognitive expert systems. They propose that future systems will need to be modeled on expert human reasoning and learning in order to demonstrate performance, robustness, and flexibility. Cognitive expert systems will have the following characteristics: qualitative causal models and large-scale, event-based memory structures; the ability to learn through real world natural language interaction; and the ability to request information that has not been provided. Work in the mental model and by extension the knowledge acquisition process with a knowledge engineer makes sense in this light.

Expert Tasks

The consumer or user of expert services can expect certain generic tasks to be within the realm of the expert (Hayes-Roth, Waterman, & Lenat, 1983). The expert interprets data to determine meaning. The interpretation must be rigorously complete in spite of noisy and errorful data. This means dealing with partial information, hypothesizing between contradictory data, identifying when information is uncertain, and being able to support conclusions reached with evidence.

The expert also diagnoses or fault finds, based on interpretations of data. The expert diagnostician must understand the system; know that faults can be masked or intermittent; know that there may be faulty sensors; know that some data may be inaccessible or dangerous to get; and understand the need to combine partial models or understanding.

Another task is monitoring, which means interpreting signals from the environment and sounding alarms. False alarms must be avoided for the expert to maintain credibility.

Prediction is forecasting the future from models of the past and present. This process requires the expert to reason about time-related events. The expert works with incomplete data, multiple possible futures, diverse data found in unlikely places, and with outcomes viewed as contingent.

Planning is also an expert task. Planning is devising a way to achieve goals by establishing priorities and through actions. Since the consequences of a plan are never fully known, a plan must be tentative and focus on the important considerations. The planner must be comfortable operating in the face of uncertainty, and possible goal interactions, and be ready to deal with contingencies.

Hawkins (1983) would add other expectations of an expert. Experts must learn and interact in the language of the user. This allows the expert to understand the user's meaning even when the meaning is implicit. Further, an expert acts as a knowledge broker between specialists. This intermediary role allows a clearer picture of predictions and plans, and the consequences of both. This role allows for conflict resolution when conflicts arise, by identifying alternative approaches.

Finally, the expert is able, when called upon, to justify his actions and recommendations.

The Expert Nurse

Benner (1984) defines expertise in nursing as hybrid of practical and theoretical knowledge that develops when a clinician tests and refines his or her knowledge in actual clinical situations. The skills of the expert are those rules of thumb, hunches, intuition, and facile judgment that develop over time and with experience (Michie & Johnson, 1985). The expert nurse has personal experience of problems solved, personal expertise or methods for solving problems, and a personal rationale for choosing a method (Weiss & Kulikowski, 1984).

The expert is one who is widely recognized as being able to solve problems in a particular clinical area (domain). Expertness is related to specialization and high-quality performance. Decision-making is rapid and accurate. The knowledge is highly aggregated, abstracted, and condensed which allows the expert nurse to make inferential leaps to conclusions (Hayes, Waterman, & Lenat, 1983). What distinguishes the expert from the non-expert is the ability to recognize large-scale patterns and quickly form reasonable hypotheses relying on short cuts or heuristic (Abraham, 1986). Heuristics are mental strategies used to manage knowledge and inferential tasks operating, in this case, in the clinical domain. Heuristics provide the basis for quick, coherent, but occasionally erroneous interpretations of new experience (Nisbett & Ross, 1987).

Some common heuristics employed by nurses in clinical situations can be briefly described:

Availability in memory. The accessibility of events in memory can aid in judgmental tasks.

Representativeness. In making a judgment, the degree to which the salient features of the object are representative of, or similar to, the features presumed to be characteristic of the category, is assessed.

Relief in the "Law of Small Numbers." The law posits that people in general and nurses specifically will readily draw inferences from limited amounts of information.

Unusualness. One of the features of the clinical event was rare or unusual.

Ambivalence. One of the features of the clinical event to be used in problem solving were inconsistent with each other leading to checking for adverse interactions.

Inconsistency. Two or more of the features of the clinical event to be used in problem solving were inconsistent also leading to checking for adverse interactions.

Faultiness. A particular feature had caused trouble before so it seems a likely source of new troubles.

The implications for clinical inference and whether or not these heuristics lead to faulty decisions will not be discussed here. The reader is referred to the work of Abraham (1986), Abraham and Krowchuk (1987), and Krowchuk (1987).

Experts develop first by acquiring knowledge and general principles regarded as basic to their discipline. With practice, and frequently under the tutelage of a mentor, the expert gains experience and recompiles what he knows. At this stage of development, the process is one of moving from a descriptive to a procedural view; what Benner notes as progression from use of abstract principles as a basis for judgment to the use of concrete experiences. As the experienced nurse becomes expert, knowledge is clumped into heuristics and domain specific theories, and held in long term memory. Benner would say that it is at this stage that the clinician perceives the patient in "wholes," in which only selected bits are relevant. The heuristics are considered shallow knowledge that suffices until the expert is faced with a really difficult problem. At this time the deep knowledge of first principles and general theories is called upon for problem solving (Harmon & King, 1985).

Expert nurses are not necessarily adroit at communicating the hows of their knowledge, which contributes to the knowledge acquisition complexity. Generally, however, they are known to their colleagues and coworkers and are trusted, respected, and believed in through their reputation and standing (Hart, 1986).

In the United Stated, the profession of nursing recognizes expertise in two widely known ways. The first is certification through the American Nurses' Association and through specialty practice organizations; the second is through the clinical ladder programs operating in hospitals and other health care organizations. Clinical ladders formalize criteria for recognition of different levels of expertise. Clinicians seeking recognition are evaluated by committees of their peers. Selection denotes a certain level of accomplishment and practice. Recognition of expertise carries with it the responsibility for clinical leadership.

Knowledge

Knowledge Structures

A person's understanding of the world around him is made up of general knowledge of objects, people, events, and their characteristic relationships. The knowledge may be held as beliefs of theories; or in more schematic ways as frames, scripts, or prototypes.

Nursing Knowledge

Nursing has reached agreement that nurses as clinicians and scientists deal with the central concepts of persons, health, and the environment (Fawcett, 1983; Flaskerud & Halloran, 1980; Fitzpatrick & Whall, 1982; Gortner, 1984; Meleis, 1985). Distinctions can be drawn between knowledge development as it relates to the content of nursing, i.e. the person, health and environment and how these interact and influence the other; and clinical inference as the process of nursing, i.e. how nursing decisions are determined and the outcomes of those decisions on patients.

Meleis (1987) calls for knowledge development as it relates to the content of nursing. Knowledge development must focus on the substance of nursing which is the phenomena and the theoretical propositions that evolve from practice. It is through the integration of theory, research, and practice that meaningful theories will emerge. The focus must be on domain concepts and questions. Nursing phenomena are the human phenomena of the health and well-being of individuals in exacting with their environment. The trend in development of the content of nursing is away from medical cure, illness, and prescribed tasks towards care environment, and the perception and meaning of the situation for all individuals (Meleis, 1986).

Clinical inference is a cognitive process by which data about a patient is interpreted and processed by a clinician in order to produce a nursing diagnosis (Abraham, 1986; Abraham & Krowchuk, 1987). Clinical inferences are related to the processing of multiple sets of observations, facts, and other information sources (Fitzpatrick, 1987). Four patterns of knowing or knowledge have been identified by Carper (1978) and extended by Chinn and Jacobs (1987). Each of these patterns is interrelated and knowing arises from the whole of nursing experience. The four patterns are: (1) ethics, the component of moral knowledge in nursing; (2) esthetics, the art of nursing; (3) the component of personal knowledge in nursing; and (4) empirics, the science of nursing. The purpose of knowing is choice so as to act in the best interest of the patient.

How the patterns of knowing can be emulated in expert systems for nursing has been discussed by Abraham and Fitzpatrick (1987). Ethical knowledge to the extent that codes of conduct have been defined can be emulated. What poses difficulty is that part of ethical knowledge that is grounded in intuition and emotion. Personal knowledge because of its idiosyncratic nature would be most difficult to include in an expert system. Esthetic knowledge is that which involves the perception of meaning derived from the context of a unique situational experience (Shuster, Mills, Davidson, Ransom, & Ross, 1987) so would be difficult to emulate. Empirics as that that describes, explains, or predicts phenomena is most amenable to emulation in expert systems. It perhaps can be argued that in the patterns of knowing that are not solely cognitive, i.e. ethical, personal, and esthetic, as the thinking processes of nurses are more clearly understood and as the number of nurses so studied increases in number, further insights into the dimensions of the patterns of knowing may be gleaned.

Knowledge Acquisition

Perspective

Knowledge acquisition according to Hayes-Roth, Waterman, and Lenat (1983) is the extraction and formulation of knowledge derived from extant sources, especially from experts. It must be discussed within the context of knowledge engineering since knowledge engineering is the discipline that deals with the development of expert systems. The knowledge engineer is an individual whose specialty is assessing problems, acquiring knowledge, and building expert systems. This person usually has training in cognitive science, computer science, and artificial intelligence.

Knowledge Engineering

It is the knowledge engineer who creates means for people in the marketplace to capture, store, distribute, and apply knowledge electronically. The knowledge engineer "engineers" knowledge, that is, converts it to applicable forms (Hayes-Roth, 1984). The knowledge engineer defines the domain, defines the representational theory, and acquires the knowledge.

The knowledge acquisition process is a bottleneck in the development of expert systems because of the small numbers of knowledge engineers available. Research is focusing on machine learning to streamline the process. The need remains, however, for basic research on human information processing since until expert systems deal with reasoning and knowledge at a semantic or conceptual level their application will remain at a superficial level (Hoffman, 1987).

It is forecast that there will soon be an explosion of expert system development in the marketplace. That problems remain does not seem to be an impediment. Uses are prophesied for all aspects of business and the professions. Harmon and King (1985) state that this is because there is a need for new approaches to business organization and productivity, a need for expertise, a need for knowledge, a need for competence, and finally a need for smart automated equipment.

The Knowledge Acquisition Process

Knowledge acquisition has been already defined as the transfer and transformation of problem-solving expertise from some knowledge source to a program. The source can be human experts, textbooks, databases, and one's own experiences (Hayes-Roth, Waterman, & Lenat, 1983). To acquire the knowledge, the knowledge engineer listens to the domain expert for certain broad kinds of knowledge such as classification schemes. He also listens for basic strategies in performance. Finally, he listens for justifications of the associations and methods used for problem-solving.

Stages of Knowledge Acquisition

Hayes-Roth, Waterman, and Lenat (1983) discuss five stages of knowledge acquisition. The first stage is identification of the problem to be solved. The problem has to be characterized with terms and key concepts clarified. The domain expert gives descriptions and explanations of problem-solving along with the related reasoning. This process is recycled until a refined statement of the problem is achieved. A goal should be mutually arrived at and a commitment of resources made.

The conceptualization stage follows. Key concepts and relationships are made explicit. Answers are sought to questions concerning the types of data available, the names of sub-tasks and strategies. An effort is made to draw and label hierarchal and causal relationships. Representational theories can help to direct the conceptualization, but a hard and fast choice of representation should not occur at this point (Cooke & McDonald, 1986).

The formalization stage involves mapping the key concepts, subproblems, and information flow into more formal representations. The concepts provide clues as to the nature of the hypothesis space. The result of this stage is a partial specification for building a prototype.

The implementation phase follows closely in that it maps the formalized knowledge into the representational framework. The domain knowledge made explicit during the formalization stage specifies the data structures, the inference rules, and the control strategies.

The final stage is that of testing and evaluation. The prototype may fail at this stage because of errors in any part of the prototype. Errors need to be found so that the system may be revised.

Knowledge Acquisition Difficulties

The knowledge acquisition process is an art since there are no known formal methods. Usual practice is to interview experts and analyze recorded verbal protocols. This is less than ideal since it involves introspection on the part of the expert, interpretation on the part of the knowledge engineer, and considerable communication between the two. The potential for errorful conclusions is great. Additionally it may be difficult for the expert to express knowledge in ways that are concise and complete.

Another problem is that of a representation mismatch. This is likely to happen since the traditional methods of acquiring knowledge are representationally driven. A method that is knowledge driven would minimize this problem (Cooke & McDonald, 1986).

Machine Learning

As noted earlier, research effort is being directed at machine learning to open the bottleneck and diminish the problems discussed. Teiresias (Davis, 1979) is a program designed to provide interactive transfer of knowledge from the expert to a system in a high level dialogue conducted in natural language. This is considered learning by being told or advice taking. This program offers the expert a framework for the explication of new domain specific knowledge. It encourages the formalization of implicit knowledge. This system also has a model of its own knowledge so is able to determine if a piece of new knowledge fits.

As Hayes-Roth, Waterman, & Lenat (1983) note, automated knowledge acquisition is still very much in the experimental stage, but work is progressing. Possible benefits these authors identify are the possibility that automated methods might prove more competent than humans for acquiring and fine-tuning certain knowledge and they may significantly reduce the high cost of knowledge engineering.

As developments in machine learning and parallel processing come to fruition, then the promise of expert systems will be realized.

Summary

This paper explored the knowledge acquisition process. It was noted that in order to understand the process, it was necessary to first look at the nature of expertise and knowledge. Those concepts laid the foundation for the discussion of knowledge engineering in general and knowledge acquisition in particular. Machine learning and automated knowledge was noted as one possible way to open the bottleneck and resolve some of the difficulties experienced in knowledge acquisition. The interest in expert systems for nursing is high; research efforts are being reported widely. If there are to be computational models of nursing practice, they must arise out of a synergy of nursing science and artificial intelligence. Nursing must be comfortable with concepts of knowledge engineering. The resulting systems will disseminate knowledge and expertise consistent with nursing's 24-hour presence with the patient.

References

Abraham, I. L. (1986). Diagnostic discrepancy and clinical inference: A social-cognitive analysis. *Genetic, Social, and General Psychology Monographs, 112,* 41–102.

Abraham, I. L. & Fitzpatrick, J. J. (1987). Knowing for nursing practice: Patterns of knowing and their emulation in expert systems. In W. W. Stead (Ed.). *Proceedings: The Eleventh Annual Symposium on Computer Applications in Medical Care.* Washington, DC: The Computer Society Press.

Abraham, I. L. & Krowchuk, H. (1987). *Heuristic aspects of clinical inference in nursing.* Manuscript submitted for publication.

Benner, P. (1984). *From novice to expert: Excellence and power in clinical nursing practice.* Menlo Park, CA: Addison-Wesley.

Carper, B. A. (1978). Fundamental patterns of knowing in nursing. *Advances in Nursing Science, 1*(1), 13–23.

Chinn, P. L. & Jacobs, M. K. (1987). *Theory and nursing: A systematic approach* (2nd ed.). St. Louis: The C. V. Mosby Co.

Cooke, N. M. & McDonald, J. E. (1986). A formal methodology for acquiring and representing expert knowledge. *Proceedings of the IEEE, 74,* 10, 1422–1430.

Davis, R. (1979). Interactive transfer of expertise: Acquisition of new inference rules. *Artificial Intelligence, 12,* 10–157.

Fawcett, J. (1983). Hallmarks of success in nursing theory development. In P. L. Chinn (Ed.). *Advances in nursing theory development* (pp. 3–17). Rockville, MD: Aspen.

Fitzpatrick, J. J. (1987). Etiology: Conceptual concerns. In A. M. McLane, (Ed.). *Classification of nursing diagnosis.* St. Louis: C. V. Mosby Co.

Fitzpatrick, J. J. & Whall, A. (1983). *Conceptual models of nursing:* Analysis and application. Bowie, MD: Brady Co.

Flaskerud, J. H. & Halloran, E. J. (1980). Areas of agreement in nursing theory development. *Advances in Nursing Science, 3*(1), 1–7.

Gortner, S. R. (1987). To build the science. In S. R. Gortner (Ed.) *Nursing science methods: A reader.* San Francisco: University of California.

Harmon, P. & King, D. (1985). *Expert systems.* New York: John Wiley & Sons, Inc.

Hart, A. (1986). *Knowledge acquisition for expert systems.* New York: McGraw-Hill.

Hawkins, D. (1983). An analysis of expert thinking. *Int. J. Man-Machine Studies, 18,* 1–47.

Hayes-Roth, F. (1984). The knowledge-based expert system: A tutorial. *Computer,* September, 11–28.

Hayes-Roth, F., Waterman, D., & Lenat, D. (Eds.) (1983). *Building expert systems.* Reading, MA: Addison Wesley.

Hoffman, R. R. (1987). The problem of extracting the knowledge of experts. *AI Magazine, 8*(2), 53–67.

Krowchuk, H. (1987). *The effects of stereotypes and diagnostic labels on the clinical inference of nurses.* Unpublished doctoral dissertation, Case Western Reserve University.

Meleis, A. (1986). Theory development and domain concepts. In P. Moccia (Ed.). *New approaches to theory development* (pp. 3–21). New York: National League for Nursing. (Pub. No. 15–1992).

Meleis, A. (1987). Revisions in knowledge development: A passion for substance. *Scholarly Inquiry for Nursing Practice, 1*(1), 5–19.

Michie, D. & Johnson, R. (1985). *The knowledge machines: Artificial intelligence and the future of man.* New York: William Morrow and Company, Inc.

Pan, J. Y-C. & Tenenbaum, J. M. (1986). PIES: An engineer's do-it-yourself knowledge system for interpretation. *AI Magazine, 7,* 4 (Fall) 62–69.

Pylyshin, Z. (1984). *Computation and cognition.* Cambridge, MA: The MIT Press.

Shuster, P., Mills, E., Davidson, L., Ransom, J. & Ross, D. (1987). *How do you know? A description and analysis of four ways of knowing in nursing.* Manuscript submitted for publication.

Selfridge, M., Dickerson, D. J., & Biggs, S. F. (1987). Cognitive expert systems and machine learning: Artificial intelligence research at the University of Connecticut. *AI Magazine, 8,* 1, 75–79.

Townsend, C. & Feucht, D. (1986). *Designing and programming personal expert systems.* Blue Ridge Summit, PA: Tab Books, Inc.

Weiss, S. M. & Kulikowski, C. A. (1984). *A practical guide to designing expert systems.* Totowa, NJ: Rowman & Allanheld.

22
A New Nursing Vision

VIRGINIA K. SABA

The electronic information highway is our new vision for nursing in the 21st century. Nursing must travel on this invisible highway to ensure the visibility and viability of the profession. Currently, nursing is involved in two developments concerning this highway. The first is becoming a partner in the National Information Infrastructure (NII), which will improve the quality and efficacy of patient care to support tomorrow's health care delivery system. The second is the development and utilization of nursing information resources and services available on the information highway.

Background

In the late 1960s, the information highway emerged as a new computing technology called an electronic network. It was designed by the Department of Defense (DoD) to transmit digital data from one computer to another. The new initial electronic network was called the Advanced Research Projects Agency Network (ARPANET). It was designed to link the major research centers conducting military research that required the high-speed computing power of supercomputers to the DoD. In the 1970s and early 1980s, several other large regional networks were developed for educational institutions so that researchers could link and access the computing power of supercomputers. In the late 1980s, ARPANET was replaced by the National Science Foundation Network called NSFNET (Figure 1). It initially consisted of five supercomputers connected via NSFNET to each other. As a result a nationwide system of linked supercomputers was created. This led to the concept of a network of networks called Internet (Glowniak & Bushway, 1994).

Reprinted with permission from *Nursing Leadership Forum, 1(2)*; Saba, V.K. 1995. Pp. 44–51. New York, NY: The Springer Publishing Company, Inc.

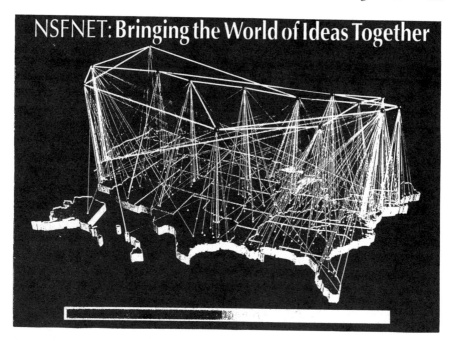

NSFNET: Bringing the World of Ideas Together

FIGURE 1. *Source*: Cox, Donna; Patterson, Robert; NCSA/University of Illinois at Urbana-Champaign. Used with permission.

The Internet

Internet is the world's largest collection of computer networks, linking millions of local networks together. It is the electronic information highway used to communicate, transmit, and retrieve digital computer data via fiberoptic lines. It is similar, but different, from telephone networks which use on-line analog (sound wave signals) communication. The internet is, in essence, a "free" worldwide electronic communication network that is not controlled by any single organization or country, even though several commercial "outernets" charge for incoming and outgoing services (Falk, 1994).

The internet not only provides different services and resources, but also offers different tools and protocols, "roadmaps" to connect with other local networks anywhere in the world. A user needs a computer with a communication software program to connect directly to a local network "node" which, in turn, facilitates the interaction between the user's computer and another local network on the internet highway. The local network "node" is not only used to access resources via the highway, but it can also act as "host" server for a resource that it may develop and offer to others on the highway.

National Information Infrastructure

Our first involvement with the information highway is in the development of the National Information Infrastructure (NII). The concept of the NII emerged from a Forum convened in 1991 by the Secretary of the Department of Health and Human Services (HHS). The Forum envisioned that an NII should be developed to support health and health care in the United States. The NII is proposed as an interconnected communication wide-area network that would link computer systems in health care facilities in and across different settings. The NII is considered to be the key technological network that supports another federal program's mission for health care, the High Performance Computing and Communication (HPCC) Program, a multiagency effort designed to develop and apply high-performance computers to help solve the nation's problems, including health. This program, initiated to implement the High Performance Computer Act of 1991, authorized the construction of a new high-speed computer communication network to connect governmental agencies, educational institutions, and scientific organizations. The HPCCP Program is viewed as providing the technological foundation for the NII (Fitzmaurice, 1994; Office of Science and Technology Policy, 1993; Work Group on Computerization of Patient Records, 1993).

The Secretary's Forum envisioned the NII as the technology that should be used to implement the Agenda for Health Care Reform by helping to reduce administrative costs while improving the quality of care for the health care delivery system. The Forum recommended that the NII should be used, not only to transmit electronic claims data and payment transfers, but also to link and share health care information of a computer-based patient record (CPR) among health care facilities, administrators, payers, providers, and consumers.

The Forum also identified the limitations of today's computer-based health information systems as often fragmented, duplicative, and only partly computerized. As a result the Forum determined that to implement the NII, national data standards not only need to be developed, but also the content and the structure of the electronic patient record, newly named the computer-based patient record (CPR). Together they should provide for the electronic interchange of the CPR, and the transmission of the data from one computer system to another in different health care facilities and settings, while ensuring security and preserving privacy and confidentiality. The Forum created several workgroups including the Workgroup for Electronic Data Interchange (WEDI), an industry-led task force, mandated to streamline health care administration through standardized electronic communication (WEDI, 1993).

National Data Standards

National data standards for the content and structure of CPR are being developed by several organizations including nursing. Data standards are characterized as rules and definitions that permit two or more disassociated computer systems to share common data elements. They are needed for several different types of CPR databases. The greatest need is for the "primary" CPR databases in all systems within individual health care facilities that are used to collect, document, process, and integrate patient care data. Data standards are also needed for "secondary" databases that are transmitted from one facility to other facilities in different settings over time. Still other data standards are needed for the design and transmission of "aggregated" databases for varying purposes such as federal funding, research, and/or Longitudinal Health (Life-Long) Records. Additionally, others are needed for the digital interchange of a variety of data forms: namely, text, images, video, and sound. Finally, standards are needed to access and retrieve data from bibliographic retrieval systems, electronic texts, and knowledge-based databases that use different vocabularies (Hammond, 1994).

Nursing Practice Standards

The vision for nursing to become a partner in the NII is critical to ensure our visibility in our nation's health care delivery system. We need not only to become an equal partner in the clinical care of patients and be reimbursed for our services, but we must also translate our clinical practice standards to electronic data standards. Nursing practice standards, as recommended by the American Nurses Association (ANA), provide the framework and content for documenting patient care using the nursing process. However, the electronic data standards for the content and structure of the six steps of the nursing process are not standardized. Therefore, we need to develop standards for coding and classifying clinical nursing practice so that the nursing process can become an integral part of the CPR and ultimately the NII. Once thy are developed, we can incorporate them in our nursing information systems (NISs) and integrate nursing data into the clinical patient record.

ANA Standards for Clinical Nursing Practice

For many years, the ANA has been involved in the development of Standards for Clinical Nursing Practice (1991). As early as 1973, the ANA introduced the first set of nursing practice standards that focused on the nursing process. In 1980, the Social Policy Statement endorsed the nursing process as the organizing framework for clinical nursing practice. The ANA continued to identify and classify the phenomena of nursing practice. In 1988, efforts were initiated to develop an international classification of nursing practice by submitting the International Classification of Nursing Diagnoses to the World Health Organization (WHO) for consideration for The Tenth Revision of the International Statistical Classification of Diseases and Related Health Problems (ICD-10) (Fitzpatrick et al., 1989).

In 1990, the ANA House of Delegates recognized the Nursing Minimum Data Set (NMDS) as the essential set of data elements that should be included in any database or electronic patient record. In 1991, ANA published its revised standards of care for clinical nursing practice that encompass all significant actions taken by nurses in providing nursing care. The nursing process was expanded to include six nursing care steps: assessment, diagnoses, outcome identification, planning, implementation, and evaluation.

ANA Database Steering Committee

In 1989 the ANA Cabinet of Nursing Practice appointed a Steering Committee on Databases to Support Clinical Nursing Practice. The committee was mandated to:

- Propose policy and program initiatives regarding nursing classification schemes, uniform nursing data sets, and the inclusion of nursing data elements in national databases;
- Build national data sets for clinical nursing practice based on elements contained in standards, criteria, and guidelines;
- Coordinate ANA's initiatives related to all public and private efforts regarding development of databases and the relationship to the development and maintenance of standards of practice and guidelines and payment for reform for nursing services (Lang, et al., in press).

The ANA Database Steering Committee took several steps toward developing computer-based data standards for clinical nursing practice. Even though the committee recognized the need for a standardized nursing classification to document the nursing process, they noted that there was no one accepted standardized nursing vocabulary, classification, or taxonomy currently used to document and code the different steps of the nursing process. To date, the ANA Database Steering Committee has endorsed not only the NMDS, but also formally "recognized" four nursing vocabularies and/or taxonomies as possible data standards for documenting nursing practice:

- NANDA Taxonomy I—Revised
- Saba Home Health Care Classification (HHCC)

- The Omaha System
- Nursing Intervention Classification (NIC).

Nursing Minimum Data Set

The Nursing Minimum Data Set (NMDS) advocates a common core of data with uniform standardized definitions and terminology. The purposes of the NMDS are "to establish comparability of nursing data across clinical populations, settings, geographic areas, and time, through identification of data categories, variables, or elements; and uniform definitions of these for use in nursing's clinical practice and administrative, research, and educational endeavors" (Werley & Lang, 1988, p. 7). The NMDS includes 16 data elements categorized in three broad categories: (a) four nursing care elements, (b) five patient/client demographic elements, and (c) seven service elements.

NANDA Taxonomy I—Revised

NANDA Taxonomy I—Revised, developed by the North American Nursing Diagnosis Association (NANDA), provides a classification scheme to classify and categorize nursing diagnostic labels, or conditions that necessitate nursing care. Each nursing diagnosis is delineated by defining characteristics, related factors, and/or risk factors that describe a condition that can be observed or inferred in client interactions (NANDA, 1991). Taxonomy I was also coded according to the structure of ICD-10 and categorized according to nine human response patterns.

Saba Home Health Care Classification

The Home Health Care Classification (HHCC) of Nursing Diagnoses and Interventions was developed by Saba and colleagues to classify, code for computer processing, and analyze the study data for the Georgetown University Home Care Classification Project. The HHCC is used to assess, document, code, and classify nursing diagnoses, their expected outcomes, nursing interventions, and their types of nursing intervention actions. They can also be used to track critical paths, determine costs, and measure outcomes of home health care (Saba, 1992).

The Saba HHCC consists of 20 components of home health care used to classify and code: (a) 145 nursing diagnoses (50 two-digit major categories and 95 three-digit subcategories); (b) a nursing diagnosis modifier (three possible expected outcomes: *improved, stabilized*, or *deteriorated*); (c) 160 unique nursing interventions (60 two-digit major categories and 100 three-digit subcategories); and (d) a nursing intervention modifier (four possible types of nursing actions: *access*, *direct care*, *teach*, or *manage*).

The Omaha System

The Omaha System is a client-focused taxonomy of nursing problems, nursing diagnoses, and health-related concerns. Developed by the Omaha Visiting Nurse Association (Omaha, Nebraska), this system provides a structure that can be used to document community health nursing. It consists of three main areas: (a) a problem classification scheme consisting of four domains encompassing 40 problems, 5 problem modifiers, and clusters of problem-specific signs and symptoms; (b) a problem rating scale for outcomes consisting of three 5-point Likert-type subscales; and (c) an intervention scheme, a taxonomy of nursing actions with three distinct hierarchical levels (Martin & Scheet, 1992).

Nursing Intervention Classification

The Nursing Intervention Classification (NIC) was developed by McClosky and Bulechek (1992) as part of the Iowa Intervention Project. NIC is a standardized list of direct care treatments designed for practitioners to document their care and assess their impact on patient outcomes. The basic scheme consists of 336 intervention labels, each with a definition and a set of nursing activities. It is hierarchical, with three levels that can be coded (McClosky & Bulechek, 1992).

International Classification of Nursing Practice

In 1988, when ANA submitted the NANDA Taxonomy I to the WHO for inclusion in the ICD-10, action was deferred until the taxonomy had international acceptance. As a result, in 1989, the International Council of Nursing (ICN) (114 member countries) passed a resolution initiating a project to devise an International Classification of Nursing Practice (ICNP) (ICN, 1993). The goal was to develop an international classification of nursing practice that, when accepted internationally, could be submitted to the WHO for inclusion in the Family of Diseases and Health-Related Classifications.

The ANA Database Steering Committee has been involved in this process since the four taxonomies and nomenclatures "recognized" by the committee have been included in the first phase of the project. At this time. ICNP consists of several possible classifications, three of which are alphabetized lists of all the terms used to describe nursing diagnoses, nursing interventions, and nursing outcomes. The ICN Committee hope that the ICNP will be used by nurses around the world so that they could participate in health-related information systems within and across settings and countries.

Uniform Nursing Language System

The ANA Database Steering Committee is also working toward developing a Uniform Nursing Language System (UNLS). The committee has taken a three-phased approach: (a) examine existing taxonomies and nomenclatures; (b) recognize and endorse a set of nomenclatures (four have been recognized); and (c) map concepts among the taxonomies so that they can be coded in diverse systems (Lang et al., in press).

The UNLS will be processed similar to the Uniform Medical Language System (UMLS) developed by the National Library of Medicine (NLM), initiated in 1986. The UMLS facilitates the computer mapping and retrieval of multiple machine-readable biomedical information resources including linking Medical Subject Headings (MeSH) with the clinical data classification systems such as the International Classification of Diseases (ICD) and Current Procedure Terminology (CPT) and other medical knowledge-based coding systems. Such linkages can also be used to facilitate the integration of databases in the CPR (Humphreys & Lindberg, 1989).

At this time, the four ANA "recognized" nursing vocabularies have been entered into the UMLS and will be linked to each other using the UMLS method of computer mapping concepts. All taxonomies will remain distinct and will be able to travel on the information highway. However, through the mapping process, it is envisioned that common nursing practice concepts could emerge that may lead to a unique UNLS that the entire profession could accept as representing clinical nursing practice using the nursing process (McCormick, Lang, Zielstorff, Milholland, & Saba, in press).

Data Standards Organizations

The ANA Database Steering Committee has also become actively involved in several organizations that are coordinating and developing other national data standards for CPR to ensure that nursing data are considered for inclusion in the CPR. This is critical, since most of the existing patient care data standards do not include nursing terms but rather primarily use medical coding and classification schemes that the federal government accepts for reimbursement and payment purposes.

The two major medical classification schemes used as the basis for data standards include the International Classification of Diseases: Clinical Modification (ICD-9 CM) and Current Procedural Terminology (CPT) codes. The ICD-9 CM is used for reporting and coding of payment of medical services in hospitals, whereas the CPT codes are used for reporting and coding medical services and procedures performed by physicians and/ or other eligible providers in out-of-hospital settings. However, neither of these schemes codes specify nursing services. It is of interest that some advanced practice nurses are using these codes for reporting diagnostic conditions they treat and/or procedures they perform for reimbursement in their respective settings. (Several states allow payment for services provided by nonphysician providers.)

The organizations that have been involved in developing data standards have included ANA nursing representatives in their deliberations. However, agreement on the nursing data that should be included in the new emerging data standards has not been reached, and must be if nursing is to become visible in tomorrow's health care delivery system. This initiative will also influence and impact on our nursing vision. The major organizations involved in the development of national data standards include the following.

CPRI

The Computer-Based Patient Record Institute (CPRI) was established in 1991 as a result of an Institute of Medicine (IOM) study of CPR (Dick & Steen, 1991). The study report recommended that a private-nonprofit organization be formed for the primary purpose of coordinating all private and governmental initiatives and to take the lead role in accelerating standard activities to enable the routine use of the CPR. CPRI currently is focusing its efforts on the electronic structure for three major types of CPR health-related information: (a) common coding strategies, (b) content and structure of the CPR, (c) structure of the message exchange (CPRI, 1993). These types of information are critical to the new nursing vision and are the ones we need to address.

The Common Coding Strategy initiative refers to the utilization of standard patient, provider, and site of care identifiers. Identifiers for patients and facilities are essential for sharing data across settings and caregivers. Additionally, there is no universally adopted system for a patient identifier, place of care identifier, or type of provider. The standardization of these data elements needs to be resolved, and must include nursing as a type of provider (Hammond, 1994). At this time, professional nurses do not have a standardized identification number which is essential if we are to be identified as a patient care provider in the CPR.

The work group that is addressing the content and structure of the CPR uses the classification and coding schemes accepted by the federal organizations. The goal is to determine an acceptable coding system for each kind of data for the CPR. The need for a common language that combines data structures and grammar for clinical care is being identified so that meaning-ful coded messages can be used and transmitted between CPRSs. The major domains identified, thus far, as needing a common language are drugs, diagnoses, symptoms and findings, anatomic sites, microbes and etiologic agents, clinical observations, patient outcomes, medical devices, units of measure, diagnosis study results, and procedures. It should be noted that, to date, nursing data are proposed but not identified in the common language.

The third initiative addresses the message standards for communication and electronic interchange of data from one organization to another, which also differ according to subject matter and kind of communication. There are several other organizations involved in electronic data transmission and communication standards, each focusing on different data interchange mes-sage standards.

HL7

Health Level Seven (HL7) standards organization is a standards group that grew out of efforts to design a "distributed open" hospital information system involving multiple vendors. HL7 protocols focus on standards for the electronic transmission of clinical data between multiple systems within institution transmission of medical orders; clinical observations, clinical data, and test results; admission, discharge, and transfer (ADT); and charge and billing data. HL7 has a subcommittee which is addressing the electronic data exchange of health care data dealing with patient care including nurs-ing care (CPRI, 1993; Milholland, 1994).

ASTM

The American Society for Testing and Materials (ASTM) is the oldest of the standards organizations developing heath care data interchange stan-dards. The major ASTM Committee on Computerized Systems is respon-sible for the development of patient care information standards. This committee has several subcommittees, each focusing on a different aspect of the content and structure of clinical data for all types of health care facilities and settings.

ANSI/HISPP

ANSI (American National Standards Institute's Healthcare Informatics Standards Planning Panel) is a private nonprofit organization that coordi-nates and approves standards efforts for the U.S.A. HISPP (Health Information Standards Planning Panel) is a another organization created in response to a request by a European standards organization to have a single U.S.A. organization to represent the U.S.A. standards effort. In 1992, ANSI HISPP was created to coordinate the development of health informatics standards as well as become the approving organization for the data standards organizations in the U.S.A.

ISO and CEN

There are other organizations involved in developing similar data standards in Europe and other areas around the world. Two important ones include the International Standards Organization (ISO) and the European Committee for Standardization (CEN). CEN Technical Committee on Medical Informatics has been established to develop standards for transmitting and communicating data among independent medical information systems. This group have also defined several nursing data elements for their standards.

National Nursing Networks

The second nursing involvement that impacts on our vision of the information highway is for nurses to become not only proficient users, but also developers of resources and services for the communication networks. This means developing local nursing networks that offer resources and services as well as using Internet to access a variety of nursing networks via the electronic information highway. Even though the network services and resources vary, they are being offered either as on-line data via telephone communication or digital data via Internet. Individual nurse researchers are also using Internet to share and communicate their research data. The major ones that highlight nursing's involvement in the information highway include the following:

Bibliographic Databases

There are the two traditional bibliographic databases that contain citations to the nursing literature—MEDLINE and CINAHL—both of which can be accessed on-line. Even though these have been available to nursing for several years, a major weakness is the lack of a common nursing language needed to link the nursing literature to nursing practice and be integrated into the CPR.

MEDLINE

MEDLINE is the on-line Medical Bibliographic database in the National Library of Medicine's (NLM) MEDLARS databases, which contains the world's largest collection of health-related bibliographic databases. It is indexed using a vocabulary called MeSH (Medical Subject Headings), which primarily contains biomedical and health-related terms, but it also has limited nursing labels for indexing the nursing literature (Saba, Oatway, & Rieder, 1989).

Grateful Med is the user-friendly on-line program available for accessing MEDLINE and other databases at the NLM. With Grateful Med, users can access, search, and retrieve bibliographic citations using a microcomputer that is connected to the NLM databases via a communication program, modem, and telephone lines.

CINAHL

The Cumulative Index for Nursing and Allied Health Literature (CINAHL) is the other on-line bibliographic database. It contains the largest list of nursing subject headings used to access its database that is similar but not identical to MEDLINE. The CINAHL vocabulary incorporates the MeSH subject heading for diseases, drug names, and anatomical/physiological concepts. It supplements these terms with over 2,000 unique headings designed specifically for nursing and allied health professionals. It is offered through several on-line communication services, including DIALOG, a commercial service.

Nursing Resources and Services

The Virginia Henderson International Nursing Library of Sigma Theta Tau International Nursing Library is now using the information highway for its Electronic Library. The Electronic Library can be accessed on-line or through Internet. It supports the mission of Sigma Theta Tau International and offers knowledge resources and library services, as well as disseminating nursing information and knowledge to its members.

The Electronic Library offers, at this time, two types of information. The first is the dissemination of databases from the Registry of Nursing Knowledge, which include Directory of Nurse Researchers, Research Conference Abstracts, Sigma Theta Tau Grant Recipients, Projects, and other similar databases. The second provides access to the on-line Journal of Knowledge Synthesis for Nursing, which is offering a full-text electronic version of its journal.

AJN Network

American Journal of Nursing Company (AJN) is developing a new national computer network, an on-line service called AJN Network. This network will be offered on Internet and become an HPCC initiative for implementing the NII. It will provide information to nurses in medically underserved communities. It will offer the following services: (a) a nurse consultant service for nurses to post questions; (b) a bulletin board for nurses to post problems for discussion; (c) computer-assisted instruction (CAI) programs that can be used for the continuing education (CE) credit; (d) patient information on various topics; (e) nursing-related national and international news; and (f) other resource databases of nursing interest.

ANA*NET

The ANA is developing ANA*NET, a combination of public and private databases compiled to assist and support ANA staff and State Nursing Associations by offering instant access for their information needs. ANA*NET not only provides essential national policy information to the state organizations, but also offers numerous nursing and health care databases, resources, and services including bibliographic, nursing practice, economic, and general welfare databases, e.g., Grateful Med and CINAHL (AJN, 1993).

NLN Electronic Accreditation

The National League for Nursing (NLN) is developing electronic software for a nationwide database that will be available on-line via Internet. Through a grant entitled "Gateway NLN: A Nationwide Information Link," NLN is developing a system and the resources that will address nursing educational issues in the nursing community. It is envisioned that the NLN Information Link will be primarily used for transmitting data to/from schools of nursing for the NLN accreditation process (NLN, 1993).

E.T. Net

The Educational Technology Network (E.T. Net) is an on-line computer conference network offered by NLM. E.T. Net is designed to link developers and users of interactive technology in health care education. It is a bulletin board system that electronically links developers and users of interactive educational materials. E.T. Net provides the opportunity via Internet for the users and developers to share reviews, as well as view new applications of interactive hardware and/or software (Sparks, 1993).

NCLEX-RN

NCLEX-RN is the computer-based testing for the Registered Nurse Examination which is now on-line. Students take the on-line examination at selected locations around the country via the information highway. On completion of the examination, the students could be informed of their grades but are not until a later date.

Several on-line bulletin boards have been developed for communication within the nursing community. FITNET ON-LINE is an electronic bulletin board that provides valuable information on software, hardware, interactive video, CAI, and other materials requested by users. The Nursing Informatics Working Group of the American Medical Informatics Association is offering its members information about Internet and on-line resources in health care. Nursing Informatics Associations are communicating with their members by transmitting their newsletters and other information on-line. Still many other services are being developed as nurses become more knowledgeable about using and traveling on the electronic information highway.

Summary

The new vision for nursing—to travel on the information highway—is another challenge for nursing's role in the 21st century. Nursing is becoming involved in the development of the National Information Infrastructure (NII) and the High Performance Computing and Communication (HCPP) Program, which has significant implications for the nursing profession and the role we will play in the Agenda for Health Care Reform and the visibility of nursing. Such involvement will enable nurses to access clinical information about their patients, their care, and their patients' particular health conditions from the literature, and predict outcomes from knowledge-based databases at the point of service.

This new nursing vision can improve the quality and efficiency of patient care, improve the nations health status, and reduce health care costs. The NII should support, transmit, and communicate health information systems, CPR systems, and more specifically, the nursing process within and across health care facilities and settings.

The development of nursing resources and services for travel using the on-line communication networks including Internet also demonstrates another nursing involvement for our vision, one that will use the electronic information highway. The most significant nursing databases, resources, services, and networks are described.

Questions for the Nursing Profession

Listed below are questions for consideration by the American Academy of Nursing. We need to discuss and make recommendations for the nursing profession. They include:

- Should we develop a formal strategic plan for how the nursing profession should use the information highway?
- What can be done to initiate reimbursement for nursing care and thus be included on the Medicare/Medicaid claims forms?
- What clinical nursing practice data should be included in the implementation of the CPR databases so we can be visible in the NII?
- Will nursing professionals—clinical practitioners, administrators, educators, and researchers—support a UNLS, a common nursing language, for documenting, coding, and classifying the nursing process, nursing practice, and nursing literature?

Acknowledgment. This article was presented as a briefing paper for the American Academy of Nursing, 1994 Annual Meeting and Conference, Phoenix, Arizona on October 22, 1994.

References

American Journal of Nursing (1993). Nursing education computer network to be developed. New York: AJN Press Release.

American Nurses Association. (1980). *Social policy statement.* Kansas City, MO: Author.

American Nurses Association. (1991). *Standards of clinical nursing practice.* Kansas City, MO: Author.

Computer-Based Patient Record Institute, Inc. (1993, April 30). *Position paper: Computer-based patient record standards.* Chicago: Author.

Dick, R. S., & Steen, E.B. (Eds.). (1991). *The computer-based patient record: An essential technology for health care.* Washington, DC: Institute of Medicine, National Academy.

Falk, B. (1994). *The Internet roadmap.* Alameda, CA: SYBEX.

Fitzmaurice, J. M. (1994, June). *Putting the information infrastructure to work: Health care in the NII.* Rockville, MD: Agency for Health Care Policy and Research, PHS, U.S. DHHS.

Fitzpatrick, J. J., Kerr, M. E., Saba, V. K., Hoskins, L. M., Hurley, M. E., Mills, W. C., Rottkamp, B. C., Warren, J. J., & Carpenito, L. J. (1989, April). Translating nursing diagnosis into ICD code. *American Journal of Nursing, 89,* 493–495.

Glowniak, J. V., & Bushway, M. K. (1994). Computer networks as a medical resource. *JAMA, 271,* 1934–1939.

Graves, J. R. (1994, Fall). Updates; Virginia Henderson International Nursing Library. *Reflections, 20*(3), 39.

Hammond, W. E. (1994) The role of standards in creating a health information infrastructure. *International Journal of Bio-Medical Computing,* (34), 29–44.

Humphreys, B. L., & Lindberg, D. A. B. (1989). Building the unified medical language system. In L. C. Kingsland, III (Ed.). *Proceedings of the Thirteenth Annual Symposium on Computer Applications in Medical Care* (pp. 475–480). Washington, DC: IEEE Society Press.

International Council of Nursing. (1993). *International classification of clinical nursing practice.* Geneva, Switzerland: Author.

Lang, N. M., Hudgings, C., Jacox, A., Lancour, J., McClure, M., McCormick, K. A., Saba, V. K., Stenvig, T. E., Zielstorff, R. D., Prescott, P., Milholland, K., & O'Connor, K. S. (in press). *Toward a national data base for nursing practice.* Washington, DC: ANA.

Martin, K. S., & Scheet, N. J. (1992). *The Omaha System.* Philadelphia, PA: W.B. Saunders.

McClosky, J., & Bulechek, G. (1992). *Taxonomy of nursing interventions.* Iowa City, IA: University of Iowa.

McCormick, K. A., Lang, N., Zielstorff, R., Milholland, D. L., Saba, V. K., & Jacox, A. (in press). Toward standard classification schemes for nursing language: Recommendations of the American Nurses Association Steering Committee on Databases to Support Clinical Nursing Practice. *Journal of the American Medical Informatics Association.*

Milholland, D.K. (1994, May/June). Health level seven. *Computers in Nursing, 12,* 138–139.

NLN. (1993, Fall). NLN recipient of Internet grant. *Connections,* p. 3.

North American Nursing Diagnosis Association. (1991). *Taxonomy, I. Revised-1990.* St Louis, MO: NANDA.

Office of Science and Technology Policy (1993). Grand challenges 1993: *High performance computing and communications.* Washington, DC: Federal Coordinating Council for Science, Engineering, and Technology.

Saba, V. K. (1992, March). The classification of home health nursing diagnoses and interventions. *Caring, 11*(3), 50–57.

Saba, V. K., Oatway, D. M., & Rieder, K. M. (July/August). How to use nursing information sources. *Nursing Outlook, 37*(4), 189–195.

Sparks, S. M. (1993, Spring). National Library of Medicine offers nursing resources. *Reflections, 19*(1), 7.

WEDI (1993, October). *WEDI: Workgroup for electronic data interchange.* Washington, DC: Author.

Werley, H.H., & Lang, N.M. (Eds.). (1988). *Identification of the nursing minimum data set.* New York: Springer Publishing Company.

Work Group on Computerization of Patient Records (1993, April). *Toward a national health information infrastructure: Report of the Work Group on Computerization of Patient Records: To the Secretary of the U.S.* Department of Health and Human Services. Washington, DC: Author.

Part II
Clinical Practice

The first article on computer technology in the clinical environment to appear in a nursing journal was published in 1961. This article, entitled "Patient Monitoring Is More Than Just a Dream," authored by Rita Chow (1961), dealt with patient monitoring and was the forerunner of the articles in this section of the anthology. This section addresses the clinical component of nursing and demonstrates the quantum leap from 1961, when Chow described a physiological monitor that had no memory and was not able to interpret the parameters that were displayed.

The first group of articles could be classified as generic, because they take a broad view of computers in the clinical environment and provide the basis for the more specific articles that follow. McDermott provides the reader with an excellent introduction for examining "seamless" database management information systems that can provide optimal access to patient information systems and decision support. She utilized the Veterans Affairs Medical Center system as her example. Palmer describes the approach nurses need to take to adequately utilize information technology to benefit patient care. She clearly and concisely presents the nursing role in system analysis, questions to ask and answer, and benefits to expect. Zielstorff points out barriers in capturing and recording data that are related to clinical outcomes and then focuses on information requirements to capture, store, and utilize clinical outcome data. She provides an in-depth look at nursing-sensitive clinical outcomes presented in the literature and then describes how each observation has implications for system design. King discusses the computer-based collection of basic data by nursing providers of preventive services in the United Kingdom. King cautions against taking an "ad-hoc and piecemeal approach to system development and implementation." This caution should be heeded by all developers of computer technology. The last "generic" article by Yoder "delineates some of the benefits for nursing, along with possible dangers related to the development of computerized nursing information systems." This is an excellent comprehensive article that provides readers with a foundation on which to base their evaluations of present and future nursing information systems.

The remaining articles in this section have been grouped into the following three categories: nursing documentation, the critical/acute care environment, and expert systems. Nursing documentation is one of the areas that was most eagerly awaited by nurse providers when computer technology was first introduced into the clinical environment of health care facilities. The articles in this category provide a varied perspective of progress in this area of automation.

Grewal et al. provide a succinct look at the design and development of an automated nursing note and focus on standardization of nursing vocabulary and implementation of nursing assessment functionality. Prophet discusses the development and implementation of the Information Network for Online Retrieval and Medical Management (INFORMM) Nursing Information System (NIS) at the University of Iowa Hospitals and Clinics (UIHC). She describes the development of two computer-generated charts, namely the patient problem/nursing diagnosis form and the patient discharge referral form. Included is the justification for/and savings from such a system. Stoupa et al. focus on the implementation of information management in the ambulatory care setting. They describe the use of COSTAR V at the University of Nebraska Medical Center and demonstrate "how nursing information management has changed using a variety of computer record tools, including features of exam room data entry, specialized nursing displays, and problems based patient summaries."

The following articles on documentation offer a slightly different perspective. Lange and Rossi provide the reader with a description of work completed as of the publication of a long-term research program—namely, the development of a data model for integrated rapid care planning (IRCP). The result is an information management tool that could support nursing activities for multiple-assigned patients, with a nurses' shift worksheet. The importance of their research is that, with another step forward, their data model could be incorporated into an automated management tool for the nurse. This demonstrates the vision of our nurse researchers as they continue to focus on the future. In the second article, Lange presents another aspect of her larger study that was described in an article written with Rossi—that is, a study of the information needs sought by nurses at the beginning of a work shift, patterns of information seeking behavior, and time requirements. It is easy to conclude that the results of her study could certainly contribute to the design of future clinical nursing information systems.

Meehan offers a different concept—the use of bedside terminals by the patient rather than the nurse. Her topics include the role of the nurse in designing and defining the patient-oriented interface terminal, the interface, and the patient's utilization/interaction with the computer. She concludes that "the type and quality of (patient) interaction is the responsibility of nursing."

The last two articles in this "documentation" category appropriately address evaluation/benefits. Hovenga warns that "the use of bedside terminals alone does not determine . . . benefits . . . ; the effectiveness of the system plus the organizational climate within which it is used, determine this." This article includes an excellent summary of selected articles by authors who present the results of their studies on the benefits of computer usage. Shamian et al. begin with the premise that the more the nurse can close the gap between the source of information and the place to store it, the more effectively and efficiently the provider can work. This is a thoughtful article describing the seven factors that need to "be considered prior to commitment to point of care technology."

Critical/acute care settings have usually been the first clinical areas to receive computer technology support. This is understandable when one considers that, with the exception of finance/management systems, physiological monitoring has been the initial focus of most computer vendors servicing the clinical environment of health care facilities. So it is not uncommon to see numerous articles addressing automation in critical/acute care environments. Nurses have been most active with computer technology in this environment as researchers and clinical users. Milholland's article provides the results of her research on developing and testing a generic evaluation tool to measure the effectiveness of patient data management systems (PDMS) in critical care settings. Grewal et al. describe the design considerations of a bedside computer system in an intensive care environment. They take the reader step by step through the process of design application, revision, solutions, and implementation problems, with nursing assessment as the main focus. A benefit of this article is the continuous evaluation regarding benefits.

Wykpisz et al. take a different perspective on automation in the acute care environment by describing how a nurse researcher used the wrist actigraph to provide continuous noninvasive objective clinical measurement of patient activity-rest. This is significant, because the author illustrates how "new technology, along with computer hardware and software described, stretches our capability and can enhance knowledge of activity-rest patterns disrupted by illness and treatment, resulting in improvements in the patients' activity and rest leading to enhanced recovery and well-being."

The last category of articles moves the reader into the realm of artificial intelligence by discussing the exciting potential for expert nursing systems. Warnock–Matheron provides the nurse who lacks an understanding of expert systems with a concise, all-encompassing look at expert systems and their relation to clinical nursing practice. Cuddigan et al. help the reader move from the philosophical/theoretical to the actual example of an expert system. The authors discuss COMMES (Creighton Online Multiple Modular Expert System), which is a group of artificial intelligence-based expert systems designed to manage stores of professional knowledge required to make intelligent decisions about patient care. They restricted their discussion to the Generalist Nursing Knowledge base and the Nursing Protocol Consultant, which provide the nurse with the professional knowledge necessary to support clinical decisions and ultimately improve the quality of patient care. Portus's article on clinical path analysis is a fitting final article in this category, as it provides the reader with a basic and broad overview of a system and tool that must be understood if expert nursing systems are to be developed that ensure continuity of care with predictive outcomes.

All of the articles in this section focus on the clinical environment. They have provided readers with a wide perspective, from philosophical/theoretical discussions to specific and unique uses of computer technology to support patient care to the futuristic view of the potential of artificial intelligence for the enhancement of quality care by nurse providers. There is no limit as to what computer technology can do to improve the clinical environment for the patient—only our lack of vision as guardians of this environment is an obstacle.

23
Interfacing and Linking Nursing Information Systems to Optimize Patient Care

Susan McDermott

1. Introduction

Nurses spend a great deal of time gathering and assimilating information to provide patient care. Lange [1] notes that nurses spend the first part of their shift in information seeking behavior related to planning interventions and other patient activities. In addition, Lange notes that medication schedules and other information related to medications are the most frequently sought type of information yet assessments and nursing summaries require more time for retrieval. With computerized nursing documentation systems interfaced to other hospital systems more information would be available for nursing computer displays and reports. Many hospitals have or plan NIS based entirely upon a network of microcomputers not interfaced to HIS. Local area networks (LANS) are increasingly being utilized in hospitals because personal computers are becoming more powerful and capable of handling textual and graphic information which is a major requirement of nursing information systems.[2]

HIS and ancillary department systems, e.g. nursing, laboratory, radiology, and pharmacy, may run on different computers. Stand-alone systems or LAN based systems are often more advanced and provide more detailed information than HIS however both departmental and HIS applications need to share data.[3] HIS developers have a significant task to try and keep every application current whereas the specialized systems may more effectively create and update applications for a specific group of users, i.e., nurses. HIS vendors may purchase and interface nursing and ancillary department systems and market the entire package as an HIS.

Reprinted from *Nursing Informatics: An International Overview for Nursing in a Technological Era*, Grobe, S.J., Pluyter-Wenting, E.S.P. (Eds.). 1994. Pp. 197–201, with kind permission from Elsevier Science—NL, Sara Burgerhartstraat 25, 1055 KV Amsterdam, The Netherlands.

Significant benefits exist from integrating healthcare data collected by all of the computerized information systems in the hospital setting.[3] Valuable nursing outputs in the form of computer displays and reports should save nurses some of the data collection time. Transformation of data to information is also possible with computerized information systems. Patient assignment reports or intervention lists for an individual or groups of patients can put individual patient information in the nurses hand without copying the kardex and making notes from other documentation. With these tools, nursing care should be more organized, efficient, and effectively provided.

Change of shift reports may include the following data: medications, critical lab results, nursing interventions/orders, physician orders, e.g. IVs, catheters, previous V.S. and amount left hanging in Ivs, patients' schedules for PT, OT, radiology, and surgery. Integrated clinical databases can bring nursing, lab, radiology, pharmacy, medicine, surgery, dietetics, and other information together for informed clinical decision making. Nursing data is more useful when entered real time at the point of care and made immediately available to all of the patients' healthcare providers throughout the hospital.

2. Current Trends

The value of computerized information systems for nursing and hospitals is widely accepted therefore many institutions are hastening to purchase systems to meet information needs. Nursing and other hospital departments may purchase systems as an answer to their current local information needs without considering the long-term need to share clinical data across departments. Currently, networks and interfaces are employed to transmit data between systems and applications.[4] Many computer interfaces are one-of-a-kind which make them costly to build and maintain therefore minimal essential data is transmitted between systems. With stand-alone departmental systems the clinical data base is usually not completely interfaced with the HIS. For systems not interfaced, two terminals may exist in clinical areas, e.g., a HIS terminal and a lab terminal with their databases remaining separate and distinct. Linking systems for terminal emulation using windows provides a view onto one system from another system without data transmission between the systems. Interfaces actually transmit data between systems.

Data base management systems and telecommunications are two building blocks for trends in developing information systems. Databases make data integration possible and telecommunications brings information closer to the end users.[4] A hospital database consists of the collection of data within the hospital and its departments. If there are stand-alone departmental systems, the data may not be transmitted across systems unless data requirements have been well defined and appropriate programs have been implemented. An interface capable of transparently passing any requested set of data from one system to the second system is necessary to support integrating processes.[3] Local area networks allow the sharing of programs, data and peripherals by providing common access to local and remote resources. There is immense pressure to link resources to increase productivity. Technological innovation and commercial offerings for LANs is increasing because of users' demand for greater data transmission speed and capacity.[5]

Telecommunications and network terminology is quite complex to the nontechnical consumer and includes but is not limited to the following components. Several common types of networks are star, ring, and bus/tree connections. Types of LAN servers include file, mail, print, and gateway servers. To select a LAN one must understand its growth limits, available number of nodes, and data rate limits. The media used to connect LANs may be shielded and unshielded twisted pair, coaxial cable, or fiberoptic cable. Each of these have performance, cost, and installation issues. Hardware components include transceivers, multi-station access units, repeaters, and network interface cards. To interconnect LANs one must understand the physical layer relays, e.g., repeaters, amplifiers, and token ring stations as well as the logical link layer bridges, e.g. source routing bridges, transparent bridges, inter-operability, filter rate, and copy rate.[4]

Interface software may be written for one-way communication of data, e.g., lab data transmitted to a nursing information system, or bidirectional, e.g., NIS sending data to and receiving data from the HIS. Technical knowledge and experience is needed to understand what a computer department is recommending or a particular vendor is offering when a LAN is being discussed. Since telecommunications is a rapidly evolving field, the hospital computer department may not have the technical expertise needed for decision making, or to create and troubleshoot networks and interfaces. Vendors and consultants often offer services to install and maintain networks and interfaces. Although network terminology may be foreign to nurses, a diagram that labels each device in the LAN by function may assist in understanding networks. Technical advice is recommended before contract negotiations begin involving networks or interfaces.

"When a network is considered, the nursing informatician and nurse administrator may want to consider these types of questions. How many workstations may be added to the network? How many days of an active patient record can be maintained on-line? Are patients records archived or purged after x number of days? How much time will it take nurses to log onto the NIS? What is the average response time for other users who have the same or similar network?, How reliable will the link or interface to other systems be, i.e. percentage of time available? What, if any, data will be transmitted to and from the HIS? Interfaces may add costs to an already itemized bill. Are the data stored in a data base and can ad hoc reports be generated? Are the system and reports site configurable by non-programming staff? The answers to these questions are important in assuring desired benefits are realized from a NIS.

Networking to hospital information systems is becoming easier with interface standards development. Use of standards will facilitate technical progress toward the "plug and play" environment where all types of computers will easily and transparently transmit data between each other. Interface standards make it possible to build complex systems from simple standard parts.[5] Standards committees for facilitating patient data exchange include ASTM (American Society for Testing and Materials), HL7 (Health Level 7), MIB (Medical Information Bus), and MEDIX. HL7 does not require special software or specific network protocols. MEDIX is an application level protocol and is built on the IOS (International Organization for Standardization) protocol. The MIB committee has developed interchange standards for critical care devices such as physiologic monitors, automatic intravenous infusion pumps, etc.[5] ASTM standards deal mainly with the exchange of laboratory data. All three specify messages, record types and data elements. The focus has been on transfer of coded data, which provides definite advantages for database retrieval and decision making.[6]

3. Data Capture and Output

Completely stand-alone networks without an interface to a HIS eliminate benefits from the automated NIS data. Data on integrated systems may be readily accessed and utilized from a cathode ray tube (CRT) without combing through a chart that is usually less meticulously organized and complete. Various input screens and devices can be utilized to capture data for different disciplines. Similarly separate outputs can be designed for nurses, physicians, and the different clinical departments without duplication of data on separate information systems. Nursing, like other disciplines, utilizes specialized knowledge and skills throughout the nursing process therefore the information desired and how to display it on screens and reports may be unique.

4. The Decentralized Hospital Computer Program (DHCP)

The Decentralized Hospital Computer Program (DHCP) consists of approximately 20 separate clinical and administrative software applications that reside on a dual VAX mainframe system at the Washington, D.C.

Veterans Affairs Medical Center (VAMC). Applications include: admission, discharge, and transfer; medical record tracking; lab; radiology; nursing; allergies; vital signs; medicine; surgery; pharmacy; order entry; health summaries; dietetics; oncology; progress notes; consults; mental health; social work; and, quality management. The data entered through these multiple applications reside in an integrated data base. All programs and data may be accessed from every hospital CRT. With access to these databases, data from multiple applications may be displayed or generate a report. The data may also be sorted and manipulated from the database.

The recent implementation of physician order entry utilizing the DHCP applications at the Washington, D.C. VAMC allows physicians to enter all orders on patients. The orders are entered through the "Order Entry/ Result Retrieval" application. The orders are transmitted to the ancillary services applications, e.g. lab, radiology, and pharmacy. The nurses and physicians utilize the orders data base to review current orders on patients without searching through order sheets on the chart. Orders for a specific department may be displayed, e.g., all active pharmacy orders or all orders including discontinued and expired orders. All orders for all services may also be displayed in reverse chronological order.

From pharmacy orders nurses print automated medication administration records and pharmacy prints profiles without transcribing orders or later recopying the record. Nurses can also print current physician or nursing orders and utilize these as kardexes. Included in the nursing orders printout are the responsible physician(s), diagnosis, condition, V.S. frequency, activity level, I&O, etc. With an integrated database many providers can utilize the same information in a context most meaningful to their discipline.

In another application physicians, nurses, pharmacists, radiologists, and dietitians can enter and display allergies, i.e., in an allergies application, which then print on nurses' medication administration records, display on the CRT when physicians enter orders, and display and print on pharmacists' and dietitians' profiles. All of this occurs with the simple entry of allergies by any user.

The "Health Summaries" application retrieves information from all clinical applications mentioned previously plus a clinic scheduler. A health summary displays real-time data and may be interacted with on-line or printed. Specific data may be displayed or printed as requested, e.g., the amount of data may be altered or the format of the data may be changed. Health summaries have been created for the diabetic nurse practitioner, cardiac rehabilitation nurses, nursing home clinicians, pharmacists review of antibiotics and microbiology reports, dietetic profiles, cardiac clinic, inpatient medicine, surgery, et al. Each user may create a health summary to meet their needs. Without an integrated database, this type of data retrieval and output would not be available.

5. The Future

Open Systems Interconnection (OSI) represents the goal of the "seamless" DBMS, in which all data is available across platforms and applications. OSI is an architectural framework defining standards for linking heterogeneous computer networks. The term "open" denotes the ability of a computer of one design to connect with any other computer conforming to a reference model and the associated standard protocols. The goal is to have applications on one computer communicate with applications on another computer through the OSI environment.[4] This "plug and play" environment would eliminate the need for programming interfaces to exchange data between systems and applications. MEDIX is the standard intended to bring all clinical data interchanges within the ISO scope.

Two technology centers for healthcare information systems that now exist are the Hospital of the Future for Andersen Consulting is in Dallas and the Healthcare Information Technology Center for Coopers & Lybrand is in Parsippany, N.J. New technologies that enable disparate systems to communicate and share information are demonstrated.[7]

Although decision support and expert systems technologies are relatively rare in healthcare institutions today, they will clearly be a standard in future systems. Integrated clinical DBMS are the foundation of these advanced tools. Automation of simple alerts are among the first application of expert systems in hospitals. Many current systems provide clinical alerts. In DHCP, alerts are generated for duplicate orders, critical lab results, abnormal radiology reports, unsigned orders, and for order clarification.

6. Benefits to Patients

With the DHCP order entry/result retrieval system, orders are entered through one application and received instantaneously in all ancillary services. Patients' receive and are started on medications sooner, are having laboratory tests and radiology exams completed more quickly, and diagnostic results available sooner. Duplicate order checking also avoids the inconvenience of duplicate testing of the patient and its associated costs. To the patient these may mean earlier effective treatment and a shorter length of stay.

One of the challenges to each department is the implementation of effective quality improvement programs. Measuring and attempting to improve the quality of healthcare are becoming increasingly important and expensive. Outcomes from nursing interventions and their impact on the patients' outcomes and course of illness may be more easily tracked in an automated nursing data base. Nursing quality improvement (QI) and research are facilitated by information systems that are designed to meet these needs. QI and clinical nursing research provide objective feedback about the quality of clinical practices which should lead to better patient care.

7. Summary

Nurses' needs for information processing are in the early stages of identification and development. Who was it that said, "how do you know what to ask for unless you know (or can dream) of what's possible." NIS can so clearly assist in processing the volume of data in patient care, education, administration, and research. Increased attention must be paid to providing universal access to the clinical content of each department's data base.[3] Networking and integration strategy should build upon the existing technology base.[9] Ideally all information in the future will be available in an apparently "seamless" DBMS so that relevant data may be accessed for clinical decision support. Clinical warning or alert systems are available to bring prompt attention to critical clinical events. Nurses participating in system selections and strategic information system planning may benefit from understanding the value of linking and interfacing NIS and HIS using the current telecommunications standards as a method of achieving the "seamless" clinical DBMS and "plug compatible programming."

Connectivity of future NIS and HIS should be evaluated during selection processes to achieve the greatest access to clinical data for nurses. Hardware and software contracts must include the cost and time frame for systems integration. Standards utilized for systems must also be considered. Design, implementation, and evaluation proceed more readily when hardware and software integration is planned. Also, current and future software functionality are understood. When comprehensive nursing computer applications are accessible at the bedside including documentation, retrieving previous multi-disciplinary documentation, all clinical results, entering and retrieving orders, obtaining operating room and on-call schedules, using electronic mail, and accessing staffing schedules, nurses remain at the patient's bedside rather than calling for results, signing on to different terminals, or walking up the hall looking for patients charts and other information.

References

[1] Lange L. Information Seeking by Nurses During Beginning-of-Shift Activities. *Proceedings Sixteenth Annual Symposium on Computer Applications in Medical Care.* Frisse ME (ed). McGraw-Hill, 1993, 317–321.
[2] Poggio F. Little Packages with big power. A Micro-Network to Meet Nursing Information Needs. *Comput Nurs.* 1990, 8(6), 256–260.

[3] Haug P, Pryor T and Frederick P. Integrating Radiology and Hospital Information Systems: the Advantage of Shared Data. *Proceedings Sixteenth Annual Symposium on Computer Applications in Medical Care.* Frisse ME (ed). McGraw-Hill, 1993, 187–191.

[4] Held G and Sarch R. *Data Communications: A Comprehensive Approach* Edition II. New York: McGraw-Hill, 1989, 396–426 and 495–500.

[5] Ahituv N and Neuman S. *Principles of Information Systems for Management* Third Edition. Dubuque: William C. Brown, 1990, 587–622.

[6] McDonald C. Standards for the Electronic Transfer of Clinical Data: Progress, Promises, and the Conductor's Wand. *Fourteenth Annual Symposium on Computer Applications in Medical Care: Standards in Medical Informatics.* Miller R(ed). Los Alamitos: IEEE Computer Society Press, 1990, 9–14.

[7] Sideli R, Johnson S et al. Adopting HL7 as a Standard for the Exchange of Clinical Test Reports. *Proceedings Fourteenth Annual Symposium on Computer Applications in Medical Care: Standards in Medical Informatics.* Miller R (ed). Los Alamitos: IEEE Society Press, 1990, 226–229.

[8] Dunbar C. Technology Centers Showcase. *Comput Nurs.* 1991, 12(1), 24–25.

[9] Panko W and Wilson M. A Path to Integration in an Academic Health Science Center. *Proceedings Sixteenth Annual Symposium on Computer Application in Medical Care.* Frisse ME (ed). McGraw-Hill, 1993, 278–282.

[10] Greenes R. Promoting Productivity by Propagating the Practice of "Plug-Compatible" Programming. *Proceedings Fourteenth Annual Symposium on Computer Applications in Medical Care: Standards in Medical Informatics.* Miller R (ed). Los Alamitos: IEEE Computer Society Press, 1990, 22–26.

24
How to Harness the Power of Information Technology to Benefit Patient Care

BARBARA PALMER

Introduction

Today's nurses must not only apply a plaster but must also charge for it, chart the procedure, direct others to do the task and evaluate the outcome. In addition, they must manage their own budget, workload, activities of health and other personnel and still spend 40% of their time with patients. The profession is turning to Information Technology (IT) to assist.

If IT is to be a help, the nurses must use the information to question and improve nursing to maximise the use of nursing resources and to understand the effect of other professionals on the requirement for nursing resources (Figure 1).

The resulting benefits to patient care combined with the up-to-date information, will leave nursing in a politically powerful position to control its own future.

Learning from Experience

Because of the pace of technological change, the changing organizational requirements and the evolving capacities of hard and software, it is extremely difficult to plan for the new technology in a coherent way. There is high risk. The results are all too often a disappointment, in that the system usually does less than planned and the implementation almost always takes longer than estimated. However, many of the pitfalls can be avoided by taking a step at a time.

Nursing is ideally placed for this approach, however seldom have computing systems proved as useful to nurses as they have a right to expect. What went wrong? How can we learn from the experience? What has not

Reprinted with permission from *Nursing Informatics '91: Pre-Conference Proceedings*; Turley, J.P. & Newbold, S.K. (Eds.). 1991. Pp. 145–150. Heidelberg-Berlin, Germany: Springer-Verlag.

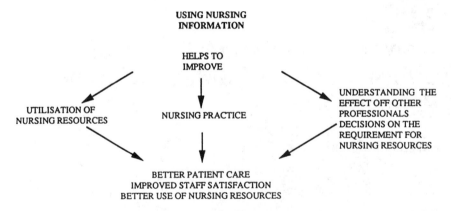

FIGURE 1. Using Nursing Information.

been given sufficient attention is the linking of the units' stated mission—objectives to the daily tasks performed by nurses in their unit. If IT is to be of help the nurses must be crystal clear about their purpose of the job and the key roles, skills and competences they need to achieve it (Figure 2).

In most instances, nursing information requirements were badly analysed and the human implications to patient care were ignored. The overworked

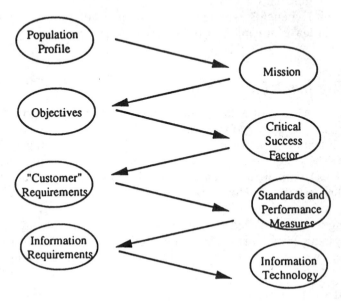

FIGURE 2. How Information Technology Supports Performance Measures and Improvement.

- Care planning
- Patient dependency/workload analysis
- Rostering
- Personnel

FIGURE 3. Nursing Information Systems.

nurse spends all her time on the day-to-day issues of caring for more dependent patients with less resources and assistance. And the stressed manager spends all her time in further stretching the ever decreasing resources and patching the subsequent holes. Neither had time or energy to see that computers could be the very professional tool to assist them in providing, planning and costing a quality service which answered the patients requirements.

To enable nurses to function most effectively, they must become more involved in business issues and work with the General Managers. Nurses cannot work in isolation. They must understand where to obtain the data, with whom to share it and how to use it. Nurses must set up the necessary information systems to monitor, cost, prioritize and evaluate their service. These systems should enable the nurse to seek and share information on the patients' behalf, and should provide the Ward Managers with the necessary information to assist decision making and to plan quality health care.

- Care planning
- Patient dependency/workload analysis
- Rostering
- Personnel

To obtain maximum benefit for nurses at all levels, these systems must be seen as part of a hospital or community information system (Figure 3).

Nurses in Systems Analysis

The first task of all nurses involved in systems analysis is to state clearly their information requirements. But this is not as easy as it sounds. Computerizing information in nursing does not mean, for example, that the inefficient, administrative, archaic paper recording systems should be simply transferred to a computer.

New systems need to be developed, and this means going back to basics: the patient. When the person is taken ill, each "episode of care" consists of a progression of events (Figure 4). The patient is assessed, his care planned, the treatment implemented and the outcome evaluated and costed.

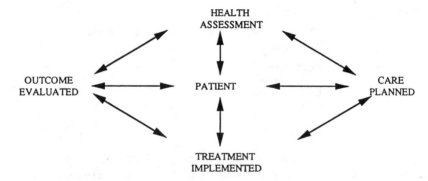

FIGURE 4. Episode of Care.

All of these procedures will generate information of different sorts to which other professions require access. Ward Managers are in a unique position to collect this type of information and to contribute to the wider aspects of health planning. Nurses are the originators of patient information, however, such information must be appropriate, accurate and accessible. This means that the technology used must allow information to be gathered where is originates—with the patient, not in the office or at the workstation, and this has implications to nursing practise.

The Implications of Computers on Nursing

To obtain the right nursing information which supports purpose and objectives, nurses must be open to question the assumptions concerning what is expected of them and whether expectations are being met. If we do not know what is expected of us or how effective we are we cannot plan and therefore cannot manage ourselves or others. It leads to loss of confidence and interest and so we take refuge in traditional safe tasks.

There are three main areas in nursing which computers will affect. These are:

How do we collect information? (source data capture)—technology must allow information to be gathered where it originates, alongside the patient (not in the office or at the workstation). The computer must be discreet and data input quick and easy, in a method suitable to the bedside which does not influence patient care.

What's the minimum information we can collect? (nursing minimum data set)—nurses should gather only information which is essential for patient care. Nurses currently spend a great deal of time and energy gathering data either for someone else or ostensibly for themselves which is never looked at (such as voluminous nursing histories). Nurses must become discerning users and collectors of information.

Which decisions need assistance? (decision support)—these systems must support rational decision making about individual patient care (not provide standard answers, for the nonexistent standard patient). The systems must support primary nursing and the nursing process and allow nurses to develop an individual care plan using an appropriate nursing model which indicates patient dependency and workload.

When nurses decide what information they need, they should take as their guide those things they use on a daily basis. These are broadly of two sorts: hard and soft. The hard information relates to performance measures, standards, rosters, patient throughput, etc. The soft sources of information—comments, hearsay, opinions, patients' appearance or written notes or comments. Both sorts must be easily understood and interpreted by the ward staff and by management.

Once the information has been accurately recorded at patient level, each ward/unit of care can then determine the best way to collate the information for its own purpose, to enable the most efficient and effective allocation of resources to maximize patient care.

Benefits to Patient Care

When nurses have a clear idea about the information they need, they will be able to judge what type of software system they need. It is vital for nurses to help choose the software system they will be working with to ensure that the system installed is one they own and are happy with and will not dictate or detract from patient care.

An integrated patient centered information system (of which the nursing systems are part) should provide benefits to the nurse and the patient from the time they enter hospital. If the system has been designed correctly all patient details will only have to be recorded once. It is not unknown at present for a hospital to hold this information in 20 different places—a waste of resources taking time away from direct care. The patient has often answered the same questions 4 times before treatment has even started!

Because information is held centrally, the potential for mistakes that result from the use of date information is reduced. As electronic communication is faster, ward orders and results can be sent and received more quickly; nurses do not have to waste valuable time chasing information.

The sharing of certain items of clinical data electronically makes the patient stay in hospital more comfortable. For example, when visiting other departments information badly written on scrappy pieces of paper does not have to be checked for accuracy, or result in repeating the procedure—a waste of resources and an increase in stress for the patient and nurse.

Workload measurements and flexible rostering also reduce wastage of resources. Staff is costed accurately and allocated to areas of greatest need—not to whoever complains the most. In the UK the average time spent on direct patient care is 55%. If this could be increased by even 5%, the implications for nursing budgets are enormous.

This increase in accurate communication need not be restricted to the hospital. With terminals in health centers community staff can both send and receive information enabling care to be planned and executed more cost efficiently and effectively. The ward is also a more pleasant place as it is quieter, with fewer frantic telephones. It can also be used for health education.

An often forgotten benefit to patients is that they can have their own daily agenda which allows them not only to take part in their care, but to plan in free time, trips to the hairdressers, chiropodists, etc. All those benefits mean that patients are happier, more satisfied and recover more quickly and therefore cost less. To obtain these benefits, nurses must be open to changes in practice (Figure 5).

Conclusion—Critical Evaluation

I hope I have shown that computerization can lead to new and improved ways of working with potential benefits to patient care, providing IT is seen as supporting rather than dictating the business.

However it will also lead to new kinds of organization. It will dramatically change nursing managers, who will have to become problem solvers rather than two way information relay links.

Ward Managers must also develop new attitudes to change. They must create an ethos which encourages nurses to take advantage of the opportunities new technology brings to improve their work and patient care. Indeed the full effect of computerized nursing systems can be realized only if nurses are prepared to use the information to change the nature of their work as they find smarter ways of doing things to benefit patient care.

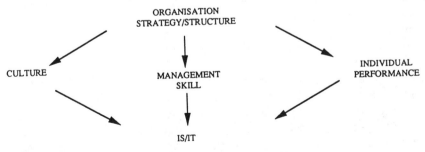

FIGURE 5. IT: The Catalyst for Change.

Then nursing will be politically powerful and will be making the invaluable contribution to the future of the country's health it always should.

References

- Caring for the 1990s, HMSO.
- Gareth Morgan, Riding the waves of change.
- B. Palmer (1989), The implications to clinical care of computerized nursing care plans.
- R. Hoy, IT injects new life into the nursing profession.
- B. Palmer (Feb. 1990), A smarter way of nursing. *Nursing Times*.

25
Capturing and Using Clinical Outcome Data: Implications for Information Systems Design

RITA D. ZIELSTORFF

The need for capturing measures of client outcomes has been recognized for decades by researchers, policy makers, administrators, payors, and practitioners. A variety of forces have made this need more urgent than ever. From a political perspective, policy- and law-making bodies are responding to consumers' demands for accountability from health care professionals for the results of their treatment plans.[1,2] Health care professionals themselves, through their professional organizations, have spent a great deal of energy developing guidelines that incorporate outcome standards.[3-5] The U.S. Joint Commission on Accreditation of Healthcare Organizations (JCAHO) has made outcome measurement a central focus of its "Agenda for Change."[6,7] Economic forces around the world are forcing the health care industry to move from its quality-at-any-cost paradigm to models that provide acceptable outcomes within limited costs.[8,9]

The demand for data to support examination of outcomes of health care has far exceeded our current capacity to respond.[10] The range of problems includes lack of agreement on conceptualization of the term "outcome"[11]; inadequate measures of outcomes[12]; and inadequate information systems to capture and manipulate data that would reflect outcomes.[13] This article focuses on one of those problems: inadequate information systems to capture and manipulate data that reflect clinical outcomes. In so doing, it will work within the current state of the art of outcome measurement. That is, while acknowledging that many conceptual and methodologi-

Reprinted with permission from *Informatics: The Infrastructure for Quality Assessment and Improvement in Nursing: Proceedings of the Fifth International Nursing Informatics Symposium Post Conference*, Henry, S.B., Holzemer, W.L., Tallberg, M. & Grobe, S.J. (Eds.). 1995. Pp. 87–91. Bethesda, MD: American Medical Informatics Association.

cal issues do exist, it also recognizes that acceptable, valid, reliable measures of *some* clinical outcomes are currently available, and that more will be developed. Furthermore, it asserts that linkages among outcome indicators and other essential related data (such as patient sociodemographic data, patient clinical data, and provider and site information) are required elements.

Background: Clinical Outcomes in Nursing

Because of the forces described earlier, a great deal has been written recently about nursing-sensitive clinical outcomes. Lang and Marek have provided comprehensive reviews of the literature related to outcomes of nursing care, which amount to a summary of the state of the art.[14–17] Hinshaw,[18] Strickland,[12] Hegyvary,[19] Ozbolt,[20] Higgins et al.,[21] Johnson and Mass,[22] as well as others have provided analyses of conceptual and methodologic issues related to outcome measurement in nursing. On a more concrete level, there are many examples of clinical articles that report upon specific interventions and their effects on patient outcomes.[23,24] After surveying this literature, one is struck by a few overarching observations.

The first is that there appear to be at least two very broad classes of outcomes: those that could be considered *generic*, i.e., pertinent to all consumers of health care services, and those that could be considered *condition related*, i.e., pertinent to subpopulations of patients who have specific diagnoses or procedures. For example, outcomes related to general physical functioning, such as mobility, may be considered generic outcomes, applicable to all clients. But an outcome such as reduced dyspnea following administration of oxygen in patients who have pneumonia is more pertinent to that subpopulation.

The second observation is that there appears to be a time dimension that must be taken into account in measuring and evaluating clinical outcomes. For example, degree of pain is an outcome that can often be influenced in minutes with appropriate intervention; however, degree of mobility may take days or weeks or months to reach desired levels, depending on the patient's clinical condition, procedures, therapies, etc. Therefore repeated measures over time may be required, and expectations of results will be different depending on the point in time at which the outcome is measured.

The third observation is that outcome-related data can come from several sources: from the patient, from biomedical instruments, from families and caregivers, and from health care professionals. Many outcomes are best judged by the patients themselves: degree of pain, ability to carry out daily activities of living, mood, satisfaction with care, quality of life.[25] Some outcome measures, such as vital signs and other physiological parameters, can be obtained from biomedical instruments attached to the patient or from instruments that analyze blood and other biologic products. Some outcome measures, such as affect, behavior, condition of the skin, social functioning can be observed by families and lay caregivers. Some outcomes, such as wound healing, respiratory status, family dynamics, are observed by the patient's health care providers.

The fourth observation is one that has probably occurred to the reader from the examples listed in the previous paragraphs: The single term outcome can be used at widely varying levels of abstraction, from very broad outcomes such as "health status" or "quality of life" to very specific outcomes such as "blood glucose" or "ability to bathe self." From an informatics perspective, this has implications for linkage and computation. For example, the dimensions of health status are often listed as physical, psychological, emotional and social functioning.[12] But are these *measures* of health status? Each of these dimensions has subdimensions. One aspect of physical function is the ability to perform activities of daily living. In turn, the subdimension "activities of daily living" is made up of its own set of sub-subdimensions, including eating, walking, bathing, dressing, etc. Each of these subsubdimensions can be measured on a scale that ranges, for example, from "independent" to "unable." Thus the atomic-level data element is "ability to bathe self" with a value such as "requires assistance." Ability to bathe self is but one of many measures that can be computed for a total score that reflects the broad outcome "health status." Ware and Sherbourne[26] have developed highly structured health status surveys as part of the work of the Medical Outcomes Study.

Of course, it is possible to simply ask patients whether they think their overall health status is "good," "fair," or "poor." However, the crudeness of the measure, the meaning and reliability of the information, and the questionable comparability among large populations of patients would seriously hamper any effort at relating outcomes to practice.

Implications for Systems Design

Each of these observations about outcomes has implications for systems design:

Generic vs. Condition-Specific

Automated documentation systems can cue the clinician to make pertinent observations related to outcomes. Logic must be specified so that cues for generic outcomes are provided for all patients, and cues for condition-specific outcomes are provided depending on the patient's diagnosis or procedure. Whenever possible, responses to the cues should be structured, with definitions early available to promote maximum objectivity and reliability.

Time Dimension

Immediate outcomes, such as pain relief after administration of analgesic, should be documented immediately, and appropriate technology should be provided to support that. Otherwise, the information becomes "old news," and may never be recorded, or may not be recorded in time to influence further decision making. If a specific medication in a specific dose is not providing pain relief, then that information must be recorded and acted upon before the time that the next dose is due. For maximum efficiency, this requires point-of care technology. In some cases, computer-generated alerts may be appropriate when recorded outcomes fall outside the range of the expected or desired.

In contrast, it is probably acceptable for visiting nurses to record functional assessments for their patients through the course of the day, and to hold transmission of this data to the central system until it is convenient, up to several hours later.

For outcomes that are measured repeatedly over time, the system should provide the ability to trend outcome data to support decision making. When patients are seen by multiple providers over extended periods of time, trended data can contribute to continuity of care and improved decision making. Another major implication of recording outcome measures over time is the necessity for a longitudinal record, one that begins with the patient's entry into the health system and continues throughout the entire health care episode, or more preferably, for life. Appropriate portions of the record must be made available to all authorized provident of care over time, no matter where they are, or where the data originated.

Multiple Sources of Outcome Data

Outcome measures should be captured as close to the time and source of their creation as possible. This follows a basic principle of information science that maintains that the less distance there is between the source of a signal and its receiving point, the less interference there will be with the signal, and the less distortion there will be in the information provided. This means that for outcomes that are best reported by the patient, the patient should have access to technologies that allow him or her to report these outcomes directly. In some instances, e.g., reporting functional status, this may be as simple as giving the patient a mark-sense form to complete that is subsequently fed into a mark-sense reader for automatic interpretation and storage. Summaries could then be generated automatically for the clinician to review, and to follow up on points that require further clarification. In other instances this may be as sophisticated as a patient's using a computer terminal directly to record his latest blood sugar, or perhaps using an automated telephone assistant to record his blood pressure,[27] or even perhaps wearing a monitor that transmits its measurements directly to a central receiving computer that interprets and stores the data for clinician review.[28]

When laypeople are expected to provide information related to outcome measures, it may be necessary to provide for their special needs in order to get the most reliable information. For example, native language, cultural background amount of education, and deficits in hearing, vision, or cognition all require special consideration in developing instruments and tools that elicit outcome-related data from patients and/or their families and lay caregivers. These factors are sources of "interference" that can distort the true outcome data, unless they are appropriately managed.

New technologies are on the horizon that will greatly assist with direct communication between the patient at home and the provider in a remote location. For example, home-based camcorders with links to the "information highway" could permit video-conferencing between patients and their health care providers and could allow observation of patients without the necessity for the patient to leave home. The patient's family could use the camcorder to record the patient's walking, or exercising, or could take pictures of the patient's wound. They could then transmit this information to the health center, where it could be viewed directly by providers, or analyzed automatically and summarized for the provider and the patient's record. Multimedia patient records that incorporate video and audio clips are already being described in the literature.[29] Telemedicine is an infant technology, with many hurdles yet to be overcome.[30] But it holds great promise for following patients directly through-out the course of care, and for directly capturing outcome data without the distortions of memory and perception. Perhaps in the future, "tele-healthcare" will be a routine aspect of follow-up care of patients.

Multiple Levels of Abstraction in Outcomes

For maximum utility, each outcome must be reduced to its atomic-level indicators, and each indicator must have a quantifying measure. Figure 1 illustrates the levels of abstraction that can occur, starting with the very high level "health status," down to an atomic-level indicator "bathing," with its measures. Not all outcomes will have as many levels of abstraction. Johnson and Maas, in their research at University of Iowa on classification of nursing-sensitive outcomes, have specified three levels: outcomes (the conceptual level), outcome indicators (the measurable concepts), and outcome measures (quantification of specific indicators).[22] To the extent that the measures are reliable and valid and can be treated as interval data, or at the very least as ordinal data, they will be more useful for aggregation and statistical manipulation.

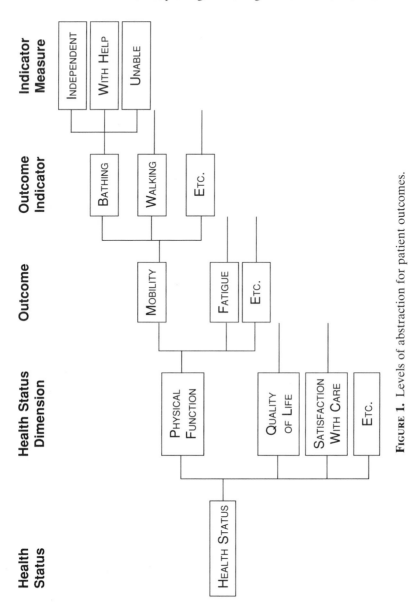

FIGURE 1. Levels of abstraction for patient outcomes.

Using Clinical Outcome Data

The previous paragraphs have focused on *capturing* clinical outcome data. However sophisticated the means of capturing data and however reliable and valid the measures are, this will not be sufficient unless systems are designed to allow maximum use of the data. There are at least five critical requirements related to this:

1.   The data must be stored in retrievable format, i.e., not embedded in the programs that capture the data, but in multipurpose databases.[31,32,33]

2.   The data must be stored according to standards that allow for data sharing across multiple hardware and software platforms.[34]

3.   There must be a way to link the outcome data to all of the factors that might influence outcomes: morbidities, comorbidities, procedures, treatments, interventions, patient sociodemographic data, provider-characteristics, organizational characteristics at site of care, etc.[11] Since it is unlikely that any one information system will contain all this information, the ability to retrieve pertinent information from different systems is a necessity.

4.   There must be some way to allow querying of the data, either directly or by downloading to standard data analysis packages.[31,33]

5.   There must be mechanisms in place to protect patient privacy and confidentiality.[10,35] For individual longitudinal records, data should only be provided to those who have authorized access. For pooled data, individual patient identifiers should either be stripped or encrypted.

If these requirements were met, computer-stored clinical records would be not just a passive record of events and observations, but a vital resource for managing individual clients, for evaluating quality and costs of care, for research, and for policy making.[13,20,33,34]

Conclusion

Most U.S. information systems of the past few decades have not been designed with a clinical focus. However, this picture is changing rapidly. Capture and utilization of clinical data are currently very "hot" items in clinical system development, as market forces demand an ability to assess both quality and costs of care. The advent of clinical pathways,[36] with their multidisciplinary focus on day-to-day accounting of de-signated tasks and expected patient outcomes, and the necessity to be able to analyze "variances" from the expected pathway, are creating a demand for systems that handle data in a highly structured way. These forces are mandating new system designs that rely heavily on structured, retriev-able databases. If care were taken to structuring these databases according to accepted standards, this development could well lead to the ability to create large pools of patient data that could be used for many purposes. Although many conceptual and methodological issues must be resolved with respect to outcome measurement and evaluation, the technology for capturing, storing, retrieving and analyzing outcome data is well within reach.

References

1. Agency for Health Care Policy and Research. Report to Congress: Progress of Research on Outcomes of Health Care Services and Procedures. Rockville, MD: U.S. DHHS, 1991. Publication no. 91-0004.
2. Roper WL, Winkenwerder W, Hackbarth GM, Krakauer H. Effectiveness in health care: An initiative to evaluate and improve medical practice. New Engl J Med. 1988;319:1197–1202.
3. American Association of Critical Care Nurses. Laguna Niguel, CA. Outcome Standards for Nursing Care of the Critically Ill. 1990. Available from the author.
4. American Medical Association. Chicago, IL. Directory of Practice Parameters. 1994. Available from the author.
5. American Nurses Association. Kansas City, MO. Outcome Standards for Rheumatology Nursing Practice. 1994. Available from the author.
6. McCormick B. Outcomes in action: the JCAHO's clinical indicators. Hospitals. 1990;64(19):34.
7. Nadzam DM. Infection control indicators in critical care settings. Heart Lung. 1992;21:477–81.
8. Relman AS. Assessment and accountability: The third revolution in medical care. N Engl J Med. 1988;319:1220–2.
9. Wennberg JE. Outcomes research, cost containment, and the fear of health care rationing. N Engl J Med. 1990;323:1202–04.
10. Agency for Health Care Policy and Research. Report to Congress: The Feasibility of Linking Research-Related Data Bases to Federal and Non-Federal Medical Administrative Data Bases. Rockville, MD: U.S. DHHS, 1991. Publication no. 91-0003.
11. Crane SC. A research agenda for outcomes research. In: Patient Outcomes Research: Examining the Effectiveness of Nursing Practice; Proceedings of the State of the Science Conference. Bethesda, MD: U.S. DHHS, 1992:54–62. Publication no. 93-3411.
12. Strickland OL. Measures and instruments. In: Patient Outcomes Research: Examining the Effectiveness of Nursing Practice; Proceedings of the State of the Science Conference. Bethesda, MD: U.S. DHHS. 1992:145–153. Publication no. 93-3411.
13. Stevic MO. Patient-linked data bases: implications for a nursing outcomes research agenda. In: Patient Outcomes Research. Examining the Effectiveness of Nursing Practice; Proceedings of the State of the Science Conference. Bethesda, MD: U.S. DHHS. 1992;198–202. Publication no. 93-3411.
14. Lang NM, Marek KD. The classification of patient outcomes. J Prof Nurs. 1990;6:158–63.
15. Lang NM, Marek KD. Outcomes that reflect clinical practice. In: Patient Outcomes Research: Examining the Effectiveness of Nursing Practice. Proceedings

of the State of the Science Conference. Bethesda, MD: U.S. DHHS. 1992:27–38. Publication no. 93-3411.

16. Marek KD. Outcome measurement in nursing. J Nurs Qual Assurance. 1989;4:1–9.

17. Marek KD, Lang NM. Nursing sensitive outcomes. In: Papers from the Nursing Minimum Data Set Conference. Ottawa, Ontario: Canadian Nurses Association. 1993:100–26.

18. Hinshaw AS. Welcome patient outcomes research conference. In: Patient Outcomes Research: Examining the Effectiveness of Nursing Practice. Proceedings of the State of the Science Conference. Bethesda, MD: U.S. DHHS. 1992:9–10. Publication no. 93-3411.

19. Hegyvary ST. Issues in outcomes research. J Nurs Qual Assurance. 1991;5(2): 1–6.

20. Ozbolt JG. Strategies for building nursing data bases for effectiveness research. In: Patient Outcomes Research: Examining the Effectiveness of Nursing Practice. Proceedings of the State of the Science Conference. Bethesda, MD: U.S. DHHS. 1992:210–18. Publication no. 93-3411.

21. Higgins M, McCaughan D, Griffiths M, Carr-Hill R. Assessing the outcomes of nursing care. J Adv Nurs. 1992;17:561–568.

22. Johnson M, Maas M. Classification of nursing sensitive patient outcomes. Presented at the meeting of the American Nurses Association Steering Committee on Databases to Support Clinical Nursing Practice, Washington DC, 1993.

23. Beal JA, Betz CL. Intervention studies in pediatric nursing research: a decade of review. Pediatr Nurs. 1992;18:586–90.

24. Bulecheck GM, McCloskey JC, eds. Nursing Interventions. Nurs Clin North Am. 1992;27(2).

25. Reiser SJ. The era of the patient: using the experience of illness in shaping the missions of health care. JAMA. 1993;269:1012–7.

26. Ware JE, Sherbourne CD. The MOS 36-Item Short-Form Health Survey (SF-36). Med Care. 1992;30:473–83.

27. Patel UH, Babbs C. A computer-based, automated, telephonic system to monitor patient progress in the home setting. J Med Syst. 1992;16:101–2.

28. Mou SM, Sunderji SG, Gall S, et al. Multicenter randomized clinical trial of home uterine activity monitoring for detection of preterm labor. Am J Obstet Gynecol. 1991;165:858–66.

29. Beck JR, Buffone GJ. A virtual chart and client management system. In: Proceedings of the 1994 Annual HIMSS Conference. Chicago, IL: Healthcare Information and Management Systems Society. 1994:95–107.

30. Denton I. Telemedicine: The new paradigm. Healthc Inform. 1993;10(11):44–50.

31. Grady ML, Schwartz HA. Automated Data Sources for Ambulatory Care Effectiveness Research. Rockville, MD: AHCPR, PHS, U.S. DHHS, 1993. Publication no. 93-0042.

32. McCormick KA. Nursing effectiveness research using existing data bases. In: Patient Outcomes Research: Examining the Effectiveness of Nursing Practice. Proceedings of the State of the Science Conference. Bethesda, MD: U.S. DHHS. 1992:203–9. Publication no. 93-3411.

33. Zielstorff RD, Hudgings CI, Grobe SJ. Next-Generation Nursing Information Systems: Essential Characteristics for Professional Practice. Washington, DC: American Nurses Assciation. 1993. Publication no. NP-83.
34. Dick RS, Steen EB. The Computer-Based Patient Record: An Essential Technology for Health Care. Washington, DC: National Academy Press. 1991.
35. Koska MT. Outcomes research: hospitals face confidentiality concerns. Hospital. 1992;66:32–4.
36. Lumsdon K, Hagland M. Mapping care. Hospital Health Netw. 1993;67(20): 34–40.

26
Information Technology and the Management of Preventive Services

Wendy King

Introduction

Medical care costs. Medical care is labour intensive, uses increasingly so-phisticated techniques and equipment and is subject to seemingly insatiable demand from raised expectations of consumers and from demographic changes. As medical science progresses, new techniques and possibilities are developed which creates tension between what is technically possible and what resources can sustain. This tension is further exacerbated by moral change: for example, recognition of the need to improve care for those with a mental handicap.

Prevention in Health Care

Prevention is widely acknowledged as a solution to the ever increasing cost of curing. It is considered to be better than cure and is regarded as the key to healthier living and a higher quality of life. Increasing attention is there-fore being paid to prevention in all health care settings and the preventive approach now permeates and informs all aspects of the health services. But while prevention is considered eminently desirable, is it affordable? Pres-sures on resources of money and manpower in the health services limits opportunities for new developments making it all the more essential that available resources are used to best effect.

Not all preventive measures necessarily require additional or massive resources. Much can be done by more effective deployment of existing staff and facilities and much will depend on encouraging members of the public to make better use of the preventive services already available. However,

Reprinted with permission from *Nursing Informatics '91: Proceedings of the Post Conference on Health Care Information Technology: Implications for Change*; Marr, P.B., Axford, R.L. & Newbold, S.K. (Eds.). 1991. Pp. 120–124. Heidelberg-Berlin, Germany: Springer-Verlag.

the redeployment of existing health care resources and the allocation of new resources requires appropriate planning and management. This requires health service managers to display a ready assessment of the effectiveness with which the service is meeting the needs and expectations of the people it serves. Specifically, they must develop real output measurement, against clearly stated management objectives.

In the last decade, changes to the way in which health services are managed in the United Kingdom (U.K.) have provided an improved administrative framework. It is now possible to look at priorities more comprehensively and to plan the allocation of resources more effectively. The main task of those who guide and manage the provision of health care is to ensure quality, contain costs and secure access to those who need it. This entails the making of choices.

Decision Making and Choice

Standard theories of choice view decision making as intentional, consequential action based on four issues:

- a knowledge of alternatives for action defined by the situation
- a knowledge of consequences of alternative actions
- a consistent preference ordering
- a decision rule by which to select a single alternative of action on the basis of its consequences for the preferences.

The Steering Group on Health Services Information (DHSS, 1984) said that, "Such choices and the decisions flowing from them are likely to be more consistent and more rational if they are taken in the light of correct and relevant statistical information. They will also be more easily explicable to the public, to professionals and others affected by them and thus often easier to implement. The result should be the provision of a good service for as many people as need it at least cost."

Information Systems

Harnessing the benefits of information technology to support the delivery of health care services was an obvious and evolutionary process for service managers. Not only would the capture of data enable them to define precisely what preventive services were, it would also enable them to monitor service delivery. Resource use could be assessed both in terms of efficiency, how well resources have been utilized irrespective of the purpose for which they were deployed, and effectiveness, whether the resources have been deployed in the best possible way.

In the U.K., the nursing providers of preventive services collect basic data to meet minimum national requirements and in the majority of cases, data collection is computer based.

The core of these information systems is activity data. Staff record details of the tasks that they have carried out including face-to-face client activity such as health promotion and screening, and client-related activity such as preparation for health teaching. This is supplemented by staff details and basic client biographical data. The aim is to produce output reports which can be used to inform decision-making and improve the management of services. The reality is a paper mountain of unused reports which are out-of-data, over-long or irrelevant to day-to-day management.

In the words of March (1982), "Decision makers and organisations gather information and do not use it; make decisions first, and look for the relevant information afterwards. In fact, organisations seem to gather a great deal of information that has little or no relevance to decisions." Further, Coddington and Moore (1987) observe that, "In general, the data available to health care managers are far more detailed and plentiful than those available in other industries. Nevertheless, there is a continuing obsession with getting still more data, and with deferring action until they are available."

Health providers have been seduced by the decreasing cost and increasing availability and flexibility of information technology, but are not necessarily reaping the rewards. As unsophisticated users of information systems, they have failed to avoid a major hazard in designing information systems described by Kast and Rosenzweig (1985), ". . . that of attempting to develop as much data as possible for use in the system. Voluminous data of many types might be collected and stored in case they are needed at some point in time. It is easy to see that massive amounts of useless data might result." They recommend that management information-decision systems should be evaluated on the basis of a cost-benefit analysis maintaining a balance between the cost of the system and the value of the information generated.

Tricker (1982) has noted that the demand for management information continues to grow as organizations become more complex, as the environment becomes more uncertain and as the rate of change of key business influences, including technology itself, accelerates. However, the value of an information source depends upon three factors: the decisions to be made, the precision and reliability of the information and the availability of alternative sources. The allocation of resources to information technology should therefore depend on a clear idea of how potential information might affect decisions. For example, if activity data predominates, pressure will inevitably be brought to bear upon staff to increase activity levels and thus efficiency. But if staff are delivering inefficient services, doing more of the same will conversely increase inefficiency.

Information Strategy

In their rush to implement information technology, health care providers have taken an ad-hoc and piecemeal approach to systems development and implementation. They have failed to appreciate the major impact that information technology will have on their organization because they lack an information strategy, a long-term, directional plan which will determine what information is to be gathered and how it will flow within an organization. It has two major aspects: the requirements of each function and the installation and use of Information Technology.

Developing an information strategy requires a change in thinking and needs to be undertaken within the context of the way in which the environment influences the basic functions of the organization. For each major area of service provision and related support services, service objectives and information flows around the business priorities and organization must be analyzed. Information requirements relating to service objectives can then be established including the identification of information flows which will relate care activity to targets, outcomes and resource utilization.

The result will be useful output reports. Activity is still likely to feature as an information requirement for preventive services, but in a much more limited way. For example, activity data is useful for services such as immunization programs, in which numbers of completed courses need to be counted for comparison against a target population, but this is less appropriate for a domiciliary visit.

Current information systems fail to recognize that each domiciliary visit has an overhead which is a cost to every visit regardless of the complexity of tasks carried out. Traveling to a home, gaining entry and conversing with the client and their family is a fixed cost. Individual activities are a variable cost which may accrue concurrently, or consecutively. For example, health education may occur during, or following a screening procedure. Separating those activities and managing them is impossible for both nurse and manager. Of much greater relevance is the reason for the visit or service target, and the outcome of that visit.

Service Objectives

The answer to effective and efficient management of preventive services therefore lies in detailing what it is the organization is trying to achieve. In other words, by setting objectives at every level of preventive services. "The introduction of information technology . . . does not challenge the . . . fundamental professional practice of the individual. The setting of workload objectives, however, does" (King, 1990).

For preventive services, objectives may be related to areas, target populations or programs of care. The crucial factor is that each objective must be capable of monitoring and managing by staff and that information systems collect appropriate data to support this process. Thus appropriate systems will only be procured with an information strategy built upon measurable service objectives.

Conclusion

In summary, it can be seen that despite the proliferation of information technology within the health care services, the failure of organizations to develop appropriate information strategies has diminished the potential return in terms of better client care.

Computers are about forty years old, information technology is much younger and the notion that information technology is strategic is newer still. Preventive services, more than any other health care area have emphasized the requirement for a comprehensive information strategy.

Preventive services are not delivered between the clearly defined parameters of hospital walls where patients in beds can be counted and diagnostic related groups identified. Preventive services are often opportunistic, less structured and less easy to define, a fact which has been highlighted by attempts to harness the benefits of information technology.

It is inconceivable that a nurse would deliver care to a patient without an assessment of their needs, a set of care objectives and a plan of care. Yet despite the pressure on health care resources we fail to adopt this simple process approach to considerable financial investments in information technology. While the move to preventive services has highlighted this deficiency, the lessons are applicable to all health care organizations. Treat information like a patient and the whole service will be healthier.

References

Coddington, D. C., & Moore K. D. (1987). *Market-driven strategies in health care.* Jossey-Bass.

DHSS. (1984). *Steering group on health devices information.* First Report: HMSO.

Kast, F. E., & Rosenzweig, J. E. (1985). *Organization and management.* McGraw Hill.

King, W. (Ed.). (1990). *Managing resources in community health*: Mercia Publications.

March, J. G. (1982). Theories of choice and making decisions. *Social Science and Modern Society, 20* (1).

Tricker, R. I. (1982). *Effective information management.* Oxford: Beaumont Executive Press.

27
Computerized Nursing Information Systems: Benefits, Pitfalls, and Solutions

Marianne E. Yoder

Naisbett (1982) has identified a "high tech/high touch" future, proposing that for every technological advance (high tech) that is introduced, a counterbalancing human response (high touch) must occur. Nursing has traditionally been an art of high touch. With the introduction of computerized patient information systems, nursing must counterbalance the dehumanizing effects of computerization with the humanizing effects of nursing. Hospitals have lagged considerably behind other businesses in integrating computers (Aiken & Mullinix, 1987). But as more and more hospitals incorporate computerized patient information systems, nursing will become highly dependent upon computer technology (Bongartz, 1988), much as our society is now highly dependent upon electricity. Computerization has the potential to greatly benefit patients and nurses alike. On the other hand, computerization has potentially detrimental effects. Nurses need to recognize some of these pitfalls and then prevent them through appropriate planning.

This chapter will delineate some of the benefits for nursing, along with possible dangers related to the development of computerized nursing information systems. Also, solutions to these dangers will be proposed. Each of these factors will be examined in terms of the effect on patient care, nursing research, nursing management, and quality assurance.

Patient Care

The advantages of computerized information systems for patient care are many. Health care from many different providers can become coordinated; pertinent information about past history and allergies is readily available;

Reprinted with permission from *Computer Applications in Nursing and Practice*; Arnold, J. & Pearson G. (Eds.). 1992. Pp. 138–144. New York, NY: National League for Nursing.

and scanning patient files to select those susceptible to an illness is easily possible with such systems (Creighton, 1978; Happ, 1983; Hiller & Beyda, 1981; Norris & Szabo, 1981; Snyder & Galante, 1984).

Computerized information systems also have the capability of extending nursing patient care through enhancing nursing efficiency and increasing productivity (Edmunds, 1984; Jenkins, 1988). Increased accessibility to patient data, automated ordering methods, along with computerized entry of progress notes, care planning, vital signs, medication administration, and online medication, dietary, or clinical reference libraries are but a few of the possibilities of such systems (Edmunds, 1984; Johnson, 1987).

Research has shown that computerized information systems decrease the amount of time nurses spend on the performance of clerical and communication activities, such as time spent communicating with other departments, telephoning, and searching for test results and laboratory reports (Hendrickson & Kovner, 1990; Staggers, 1988). Mowry and Korpman (1987) have estimated that $1^{1}/_{2}$ hours per nursing service employee per shift could be saved by using appropriate information technology. Although such systems have not decreased the amount of time nurses spend documenting care, research has supported the findings that computerized systems improve the quality and accuracy of patient record documentation by improving the completeness, legibility, and quality and number of nursing observations (Hendrickson & Kovner, 1990; Staggers, 1988).

The computerization of patient information, however, magnifies an age-old dilemma: the professional need for information versus the patient's right to privacy and confidentiality. The potential diminution of patients' rights brought by such systems has long been recognized. In the 1970s, the Department of Commerce's National Bureau of Standards appointed Alan F. Westin, professor of law and government at Columbia University, to study the effects of computerization on confidentiality of patient records. In the 381-page report, Westin concluded that the computerized health data systems were being created without (1) advance consideration for patients' rights, (2) sufficient consideration to what kinds of data were really necessary, and (3) sufficient control of confidentiality (National Bureau of Standards, 1976).

Hiller & Beyda (1981) echo Westin's concerns about what they describe as a universal unease asbout which patient information is "being tabulated and used, the extent of its accuracy, the necessity to control its dissemination, and the extent to which patients may have access to, and the opportunity to verify and correct, their personal medical records." No patient information system, whether manual or automated is 100 percent invulnerable to access by unauthorized personnel. The amassing of large amounts of data in a centralized location poses a greater threat to patient privacy than written information that is scattered geographically and is often disjointed. Without safeguards in place, anyone having access to the computer can have unlimited access to the data collected about patients. Levine (1980) cautions that the task of protecting patients' confidentiality remains an integral part of the relationship nurses share with patients.

Another hidden danger for nursing is the provision of patient care with limited access to the computerized patient information. If nurses are to adequately care for their patients, nurses must have the same access as physicians to the patients' data. Yet equal access to patient information is not seen as a universal right for nursing. Some would propose a hierarchy of information access with physicians having access to nurses' notes, but without nurses having access to physicians' notes (Dawson, 1983). One computerized system known to this author, used at a large teaching hospital in the southwest, allowed physicians and medical students access to laboratory reports, but denied access to nursing personnel.

The solution, then, is for nurses to have an active role in deciding what data should be collected, ensuring that the data is accurate, and determining who should have access to what data for what purposes. Strategies to prevent the identified pitfalls include surveillance, patient advocacy, and decision-making participation.

Nurses can help limit unauthorized use by seeking and supporting surveillance procedures such as user logs. Access to patient information should be attainable only through passwords or other levels of security (Romano, 1987). Nurses should not let others use their passwords and should not leave an active terminal running unattended. A solution could be terminals that have an automatic sign-off if left unattended for a set minimal time (Romano, 1987).

By far the most important way nurses can protect patients is through patient advocacy. Nurses as patient advocates must ensure that the patients' rights to privacy and confidentiality are not compromised during the creation and use of automated computerized information systems. Patient advocacy also includes offering explanations to patients about the collection and uses of data (Romano, 1987) and promoting patients' prerogative for access and verification of accuracy of the data collected.

Nurses should serve on the committees which decide what types of data are to be included in the information systems. Criteria for inclusion of particular data include not only relevancy and legality, but also consideration of the potential of patient harm in the event that information became accessible to an inappropriate source. Data should therefore be classified according to sensitivity (Romano, 1987). Not only will these criteria help protect patients, but they will also increase the relevancy of the data nurses will be entering into the system (Johnson, 1987).

Finally, nurses must take an active role in establishing who should have access to what patient information, and ensure that nurses attain and retain access to the patient data necessary for care. One solution is to have nurses serving on the information system committees in order to claim equal access to patient information.

Research

The development of large banks of computerized patient information offers the promise of new directions for nursing research. Although current information systems have not been designed to allow for easy retrieval of research data, the data will become available in a more organized form as these systems are further developed. The automated patient information system can be a valuable tool for research, possessing the capacity to save time and money (Kovner, 1989), especially in some types of research such as time series, retrospective, and secondary or meta-analysis. Such large data banks even provide the possibility of new types of research yet to be conceived.

Pitfalls exist in accessing the computerized information for research whether anonymity can or cannot be maintained. If anonymity cannot be maintained, then the problems of conducting research with computerized information is the same as with any research study, automated or not. However, when the data are so masked as to provide anonymity, guidelines are less clear. The assurance of anonymity does not necessarily guarantee the ethical use of the data. Demographic data can be analyzed (either accurately or inaccurately) to support conclusions about particular groups of patients which can lead to their stigmatization. The data are neither inherently good nor evil—only the uses determine the social significance.

The issue, therefore, is how to protect patients without stifling the advancement of nursing knowledge. Davis (1984) acknowledges that researchers accessing computerized information can invade patients' privacy. However, she also points out that a case can be made for the need of researchers to have access to the data for the advancement of knowledge. If nursing is to be research based, then the nurse–researcher must have access to available data. Strategies to prevent these problems involve the protection of human rights.

Whether using anonymous or known subjects, the procedures already in place to protect human subjects should be retained. Human subjects committees should screen all requests for access to the data for research purposes and weigh any possible risk against the possible benefits. Subjects must continue to give informed consent in those studies where anonymity cannot be maintained. In studies with anonymity preserved, the human subjects committee members must still consider the possible ramifications that any of the proposed variables may have, and the researcher must provide evidence of protection of patients' rights. Overall, research committees must discuss and establish ethical standards for conducting research using computerized data. Simultaneously, the issues of authority for access and assurance of scientific merit must be addressed, including what groups should have access to what information. The possibility of researchers' unethical utilization of data is no reason to prevent any utilization of the data for research purposes.

Management

The development of computerized patient information systems also provides the promise of many benefits to nurse managers. Automated systems can improve nurse–managers' efficiency and effectiveness by the way important information such as staffing patterns, nursing staff characteristics, nursing care efficiency, and client care costs are stored, organized, and retrieved (Kline, 1986). These systems decrease the time lapse between collecting data and making it available to the nurse-manager (Romano, 1990), thereby improving organizational problem solving, institutional planning, budgetary patterns, and needs projections (Kline, 1986). In addition, the information systems will make it easier to calculate a fee for nursing service (Johnson, 1987), and accurately assess the acuity level of patients' and thereby the staff's needs. Various staffing and scheduling programs that allow matching of patient acuity with staffing needs are already in place (Batchelor, 1985). Courtemanche (1986) reported that the installation of an automated nurse staffing schedule reduced the time managers spent on staffing from two days per month to two hours per month.

The programs in use, however, are prescriptive and not predictive. The staffing is therefore based upon the acuity levels measured daily, rather than upon the predicted acuity the patient will have. With the development of more extensive information systems, management will have a capability for even more precise staffing and scheduling. Such capabilities present a hidden source of harm for nursing service. Will the promised efficiency of such systems compromise the effectiveness of nursing care? Reliance on such scientifically precise data available through computerized scheduling has the potential to increasingly fragment patient care if, for example, staff nurses would continuously be "floated" to meet the designated "best" staffing/patient ratio to help contain costs.

The dilemma, then, is how to prevent fragmentation of nursing care through exclusive examination of the "bottom-line" when staffing. Such fragmentation of nursing care can lead to the depersonalization of the nurse and the patient, and can lead to a decrease in the effectiveness of nursing care given. Strategies to prevent this outcome entail better predictive scheduling.

The development of computerized patient information systems allows nurse-managers to uncover the relationship between patients' medical and nursing diagnoses and patient acuity, leading to better forecasting of staffing needs. For example, a patient with a particular medical diagnosis and particular nursing diagnoses predictably would need a certain amount of nursing care the first two days, a certain amount the next three days, and so forth. With the development of better forecasting, staff scheduling will become predictive, rather than reactive. Reliable forecasting can lead to more even workloads for units and provide a more rational basis for a patient admission to the skilled care of a particular cadre of unit-based primary care nurses. Fragmentation of nursing care will be prevented, while containing staffing costs.

Quality Assurance

Existing computerized information systems can be used for quality assurance. An automated patient information system has the ability to provide for evaluation and substantiation of the accountability of nurses and their practice. Such ability can be either enriching or detrimental for nursing, depending upon the purposes of the evaluation. The information system can contribute to the scientific base of nursing by providing a richness in description of what goes on between a nurse and a patient and by providing solid documentation of nursing outcomes. Also, manual data collection techniques for quality assurance is time consuming and expensive, but using information already contained in the automated systems can decrease collection time and expense (Kovner, 1989).

The major pitfall facing nurses is the misuse of the data in ways that can lead to the dehumanization of nursing and the possibility of an uncaring, mechanized state. Nurses have been taught to use the nursing process to solve problems and provide autonomous, theory-based or traditionally grounded care. Nursing has progressed beyond the rote learning of nursing techniques. Instead the teaching of scientific concepts and reasons behind the techniques associated with them enables a nurse to be flexible and adaptable in a variety of situations. However, computerization of patient information provides easily accessible data for which the productivity of individual nurses could readily be monitored and evaluated. Standards of care can be quantified and each nurse's performance "objectively" evaluated only "by the numbers."

Unfortunately, poorly thought out "objective" methods of evaluation can have potentially adverse effects on nursing because they threaten to stifle flexibility and adaptability. Nursing care would likely become increasingly standardized, rather than individualized. If employee productivity is closely monitored by management, will quota setting be far behind? Too frequently physicians and nurse practitioners in Health Maintenance Organizations already are expected to see a set number of patients in a set amount of time. Will bedside nursing become a set number of baths, dressing changes, and vital signs per unit of time? If so, then misuse of computer data will cause further depersonalization of the patient and dehumanization of nursing care. Nursing care will become task-"quota"-centered and not patient-centered.

The dilemma for nursing, therefore, is to find methods of evaluating and improving patient care without impacting negatively on patient-centered nursing. As Zielstorff (1983, p. 573) has stated, "the more humanistic [nurses] remain, and the deeper [their] skills in empathetic understanding and support, the less likely [nurses] are to be supplanted by computers." Strategies for preventing dehumanization of nursing consist of emphasizing patient outcomes, rather than nursing tasks.

Evaluation of nursing care should be based upon observable, measurable patient outcomes, and not upon quota-setting for nursing tasks. Patient outcomes must be established by a committee composed of patient-care nurses, nurse-managers, physicians, administrators, and consumers. Data management technology is not limited to numbers, so the outcomes established can include qualitative measures coupled with quantitative measures to further document the richness of nursing care.

Summary

Computerized patient information systems are two-edged swords. They hold considerable potential advantage to nursing, but they also have potential disadvantages that can be detrimental to nursing. Computerization holds many benefits for patient care, research, management, and quality assurance. Some of these benefits include a decrease in the amount of time spent on paperwork, along with assistance in planning nursing care. Further, computerization promises to offer vast patient databases from which researchers can design multivariate investigations involving large numbers of patients. Automated information systems also have the potential for improving forecasting and report generation and assisting in decision-making while decreasing time spent on tasks. Finally, patient databases can facilitate evaluation and substantiate accountability of nursing practice.

Computerized information systems, however, bring potential pitfalls such as invasion of patient privacy, unethical conduct of research, fragmentation and dehumanization of nursing care, and quota-setting based upon nursing techniques, which must be recognized and planned for. Although there are specific strategies for dealing with the individual dangers, nurses can help surmount any pitfall arising from computerization by taking an active role, rather than allowing others to set the agenda for nursing. Measures, such as educating themselves to some of the potentially detrimental effects and then preventing them through appropriate planning, will help prevent the dangers computerization can bring. Only by becoming actively involved in the planning and implementation of computer systems affecting their patients can nurses ensure that computerization will benefit nursing care.

References

Aiken, L., & Mullinix, C. (1987). The nurse shortage: Myth or reality? *New England Journal of Medicine, 317* (10), 641–45.
Batchelor, G. J. (1985). Computerized nursing systems: A look at the marketplace. *Computers in Healthcare, 6,* 55–56, 58.

Bongartz, C. (1988). Computer-oriented patient care. *Computers in Nursing, 6*, 204–210.

Courtemanche, J. B. (1986). "Gearing-up" for an automated nurse scheduling system in a decentralized setting. *Computers in Nursing, 4*, 59–67.

Creighton, H. (1978). The diminishing right of privacy: Computerized medical records. *Supervisor Nurse, 9* (Feb), 58–61.

Dawson, J. (1983). Can computers replace doctors? *Private Practice* (June), 68–71.

Davis, A. J. (1984). Ethical issues in nursing research. *Western Journal of Nursing Research, 6*, 351–353.

Edmunds, L. (1984). Computers for inpatient nursing care: What can be accomplished. *Computers in Nursing, 2*, 102–108.

Happ, B. (1983). Should computers be used in the nursing care of patients? *Nursing Management, 14* (7), 31–35.

Hendrickson, G., & Kovner, C. T. (1990). Effects of computers on nursing resource use: Do computers save nurses time? *Computers in Nursing, 8*, 16–21.

Hiller, M. D., & Beyda, V. (1981). Computers medical records, and the right to privacy. *Journal of Health Politics, Policy and Law, 6*, 463–487.

Jenkins, C. (1988). Automation improves nursing productivity. *Computers in Health-care, 9*, 40–41.

Johnson, D. (1987). Decisions and dilemmas in the development of a nursing information system. *Computers in Nursing, 5*, 94–98.

Kline, N. W. (1986). Principles of computerized database management: Considerations for the nurse administrator. *Computers in Nursing, 4*, 73–81.

Kovner, C. (1989). Using computerized databases for nursing research and quality assurance. *Computers in Nursing, 7*, 228–231.

Levine, M. E. (1980). The ethics of computer technology in health care. *Nursing Forum, 19*, 193–198.

Mowry, M., & Korpman, R. (1987). Evaluating automated information systems. *Nursing Economics, 5*, 7–12.

Naisbett, J. (1982). *Megatrends*. NY: Warner Communications.

National Bureau of Standards. (1976). *Computers, health records and citizen rights* (SD CAT C. No.: C13.44:157). Washington, DC: U.S. Government Printing Office.

Norris, J., & Szabo, D. (1981). Removing some impediments to development of America's third- and fourth-generation health care delivery systems: Legal aspects of computer medicine. *American Journal of Law & Medicine, 7*, iii–viii.

Romano, C. A. (1987). Privacy, confidentiality and security of computerized systems: The nursing responsibility. *Computers in Nursing, 5*, 99–104.

Romano, C. A. (1990). Innovation: The promise and the perils for nursing and information technology. *Computers in Nursing, 8*, 99–104.

Snyder, K. M., & Galante, M. M. (1984). Medically intelligent computer systems—a nurse's view. *Journal of Clinical Computing, 12* (6), 185–192.

Staggers, N. (1988). Using computers in nursing: Documented benefits and needed studies. *Computers in Nursing, 6*, 164–170.

Zielstorff, R. D. (1983). Microtechnology and the future of nursing, in R. E. Dayhoff (Ed.). *Proceedings of the Seventh Annual Symposium on Computer Applications in Medical Care* (pp. 572–577). Silver Spring MD: IEEE Computer Society Press.

28
Design and Development of an Automated Nursing Note

Ruby Grewal, Joyce Arcus, Johnetta Bowen, Kevin Fitzpatrick, William E. Hammond, and Liza Hickey

1. History

In the mid 1980s the Surgical Intensive Care Unit (SICU) staff began searching for a bedside computer system. Their goal was to find a system that would create a computerized medical record, reduce the clerical burden on the staff, and provide the necessary data for patient care and research in a unique and meaningful fashion. In the fall of 1987 the SICU staff approached the TMR staff with a proposal to develop a bedside computer system using TMR as the platform. TMR [1] is a comprehensive computer-based medical record system developed at the Duke University Medical Center (DUMC) in an evolutionary fashion over the past twenty years.

2. Introduction

It was decided that if the system was to succeed it must first be useful to the nursing staff. To be useful the system had to reduce the transcription burden on the nurses and better organize the large volume of data that they were collecting. The elements of the nursing process include: Assessment, Planing, Implementation, and Evaluation [2]. We choose the assessment portion of the nursing process as the first task to be developed in the system. It was chosen because of its potential impact on the nursing staff and because it caused the least amount of disruption to the existing paper documentation system. A computer committee consisting of nursing representatives, TMR representatives, and Duke Hospital Information System (DHIS) representatives was organized to begin the design of the automated nursing note. The goal was to create a menu driven data entry system based

Reprinted from *MEDINFO '92: Proceedings of the Seventh World Congress on Medical Informatics*, Lun, K.C., Degoulet, P., Piemme, T.E. & Rienhoff, O. (Eds.). 1992. Pp. 1054–1085, with kind permission from Elsevier Science—NL, Sara Burgerhartstraat 25, 1055 KV Amsterdam, The Netherlands.

on a standardized vocabulary that would allow the nurse to systematically document a patient's condition.

3. Standardized Vocabulary

The development of the automated nursing note began with the creation of a standardized vocabulary. The nursing committee met weekly for over a year to develop this vocabulary. The vocabulary includes items such as body locations or sites, descriptors, and quantifiers. The SICU nurses were accustomed to writing a patient assessment by reviewing the patient's condition organized by body system. The committee analyzed the content of each body system assessment, such as neurological, cardiovascular, and respiratory, and determined the evaluations that were made about each body system. Once an outline for a system was developed, the potential responses for each evaluation were determined. New evaluations and responses are continually being added to the dictionary. Currently there are over 750 evaluations that can be made and over 1200 standardized responses in the vocabulary. Figure 1 shows the primary neurological data entry menu. If item 1, behavioral appearance, is selected, the system prompts the nurse with the list of appropriate responses. The nurse then enters the numbers next to the appropriate phrases.

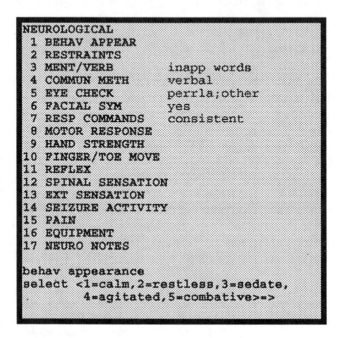

FIGURE 1. Neurological assessment primary menu.

```
HOURLY CHECKS
  1 ASSESS UNCHANGED                        PUPILS
  2 NEURO CHECKS        pupils              1 R PUPIL SIZE   pinpt
  3 CV CHECKS           pulses              2 R PUPIL REACT  slug
  4 VASCULAR ACCESS                         3 R PUPIL SHAPE  regular
  5 RESP CHECKS         C & DB              4 L PUPIL SIZE   pinpt
  6 GI CHECKS                               5 L PUPIL REACT  slug
  7 GU CHECKS                               6 L PUPIL SHAPE  regular
  8 WOUNDS & DRAINS
  9 ACTIVITY
 10 MISC
 11 REAC TO TREATMENT
 12 CODE 5
 13 HOURLY NOTES
 14 DOC NOTIFIED
```

FIGURE 2. Hourly checks menu.

4. Data Structure

The prompts and responses are defined in a data dictionary. There are a variety of data entry modes available depending on the nature of the data being collected. The types of screen presentations include direct entry, sub-windows, tables, and free text. In figure 1 behavioral appearance is an example of direct data entry. Selecting eye check and then entering "other" will bring up a window with specific pupil evaluations (see figure 2). The pain evaluations (selection 15 in figure 1) are made in tabular format to allow for the fact that the patient may experience pain in more than one location (see figure 3). Free text data entry is available in each section to allow nurses to include information that can not be captured through the menus.

The data entry structure consists of a frame of major systems or categories, each of which points to layers of coded evaluations and coded responses. The screen definitions and data definitions are located in a distinct sections of the data dictionary. The screen definitions point to the appropriate data entry selections or back to another screen definition. The data definition section of the dictionary points to the appropriate responses in the dictionary. For the example in figure 1 the dictionary would contain a neurological screen definition that pointed to 17 data definitions. The first

```
PAIN
  LOCATION  DEFINER  INTEN  TYPE   RAD-FROM  RAD-TO  RELIEVED
1 flank     right    9.5    sharp                    med
2 back      lower    2      dull
```

FIGURE 3. Pain data entry screen (sample table format).

data definition for behavioral appearance would then point to the appropriate coded data phrases in yet another section of the dictionary. This separation between the different sections of the data dictionary allows flexibility in modifying the pointers to make additions and modifications to the assessment content.

The assessment is organized in a hierarchial structure which allows the nurse to branch on details of the patient condition. For example if it was noted that a patient was experiencing a reaction to a treatment, the nurse would be prompted to answer detailed questions as to the nature of the reaction. If no reaction was noted, she would continue with the assessment. There is no limit to the level of detail (number of branches) available, although most items do not go beyond 5 levels of detail.

5. Development

The initial vocabulary set was completed in the summer of 1988. For the next year the dictionary was revised and the TMR program was modified to handle some of the special situations that arose. When the nurses began testing the electronic charting system, they found that they had excluded a large number of variables that they normally had collected. These items dealt with checks and procedures that were performed as part of their patient care, but not as part of the initial assessment. In addition, they found that the body system organization was appropriate for the initial assessment, but that for updates the data should be organized differently. Figure 3 shows the hourly checks menu that was added. This menu combines items from the individual body system menus and adds specific questions relating to updates of the original assessment. It is important to note that you could go to the neurological menu and update pupils from there, as well as from the hourly checks menu. New menus were also added to capture the procedures that were performed. These menus include items such as intubation and line placement. In addition, the nurses audited the free text notes that were being entered in order to code evaluations that were originally excluded.

The major design modification dealt with the ability to handle shift boundaries and the implementation of electronic transcription. The SICU nurses are on two 12 hour shifts per day, a 7 am shift and a 7 pm shift. At the beginning of each shift, the nurse is required to complete a full assessment of the patient, which is then annotated as the patient's condition changes throughout the shift. On admission to the unit, a nurse enters a full assessment on the patient. Each nurse on subsequent shifts was required to reenter the base assessment. The nurses requested that the system be designed to bring forward the previous nurse's assessment, excluding hourly update type information. The data was organized to distinguish data that should be transcribed from shift to shift and that which should not. Examples of data that were brought forward included the current vascular

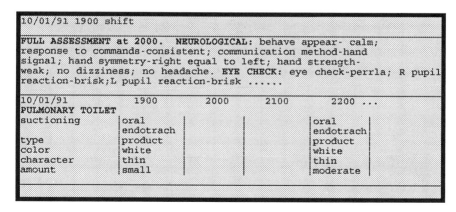

FIGURE 4. Sample nursing assessment report sections.

lines and location of wounds and drains. Examples of data that was not transcribed included therapies given and dressing changes. It takes a nurse 8 to 15 minutes to complete an initial assessment without the preload feature. With the preload feature a nurse simply updates the data from the last shift as appropriate.

6. Reports

There are two reports available to review the nursing assessment. The first is a flow sheet format. The second is a narrative report. Figure 4 shows a sample of both reports. In general a nurse reviews the flowsheet format on-line throughout the day as necessary. A chart copy is generated at the end of the shift.

7. Training and Implementation

Nurses replaced their written note with the computer generated note in the winter of 1989. This event was preceded by extensive training, a portion of which was from the TMR staff, but the majority of which was done by the nurses. The TMR staff trained the nurses on the design committee. The committee members then trained the other nurses on the unit. They developed check-off sheets to track the staff's familiarity and levels of competence with different computer functions. A TMR test system was available for the nurses to practice entering assessments and to familiarize themselves with the different functionality. The nursing staff developed various levels of users. Work schedules were created so that a highly trained user was available on all shifts [2].

The electronic assessment was initially turned on room by room so that nurses could adapt to the new system. Double documentation was not required in any phase of this implementation. Nurses could also voluntarily enter their assessment on-line. By the time the eighth room was scheduled to come on-line, the nurses had voluntarily turned on all sixteen rooms.

8. Evaluation

A study was done to compare the number of evaluations made and the time taken to complete an initial written assessment versus a computer assessment (without using the preload feature). Initial studies show that there is a slight time savings with the computerized note and there is a significant increase in the amount of data being collected in the computerized assessment. The time per evaluation was reduced once the break even point was exceeded. There were no time savings for the first 50 evaluations made. There was a substantial savings in time for the computerized assessment after the first 50 evaluations. The average computer generated assessment ranges between 180–350 evaluations depending on patient acuity [3]. In a time-study analysis reported by Bradshaw, nursing documentation on a thoracic ICU was monitored both prior and post installation of a nursing charting system. The system described by Bradshaw included clinical data and nursing plans; it did not include nursing assessments. Bradshaw was not able to report any time savings [4]. We attribute our ability to show a time savings to the fact that the assessment portion is complete and separate from the other nursing documentation tasks. Our system does not require interaction with the paper chart, whereas the nurses using the system de-

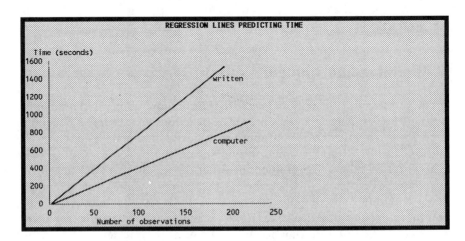

FIGURE 5. Time versus number of observations.

scribed by Bradshaw "often charted the same information both manually and at the computer" [4].

9. Uses of Coded Nursing Data

The creation of a coded standardized vocabulary allows us to manipulate and use the nursing data in a manner not possible in the paper system. Coded nursing data is now used to create a glasgow coma scale and monitor quality assurance functions. The nursing variable used to create a glasgow coma scale is used to passively calculate an apache score for the patient. In addition assessment data is used to flag quality assurance violations. Examples of these flags include reintubation within 48 hours of extubation and complications in swan-Ganz catheter insertions.

10. Conclusion

Initial surveys of nursing satisfaction show that an overwhelming number of the nurses prefer a computerized unit over a manual unit. In addition the majority of nurses are satisfied with the system. The success of the computerized assessment can be linked to the time savings associated with the preload feature and with the immediate familiarity the nurse gains with the patient's case. It can also be associated with the fact that prompted data entry is easier than pages of handwritten narratives. It is important to note that some habits can not be changed. Nurses who previously wrote very detailed narrative assessments tend to have longer more complete computerized assessments. These nurses also tend to overuse the free text capability in the system.

References

[1] Stead WW and Hammond WE. Computer-based Medical Records: The Centerpiece of TMR. *MD Computing* 1988,5:48–62.
[2] Blaufass J. Promoting the Nursing Process Through Computerization. In: *MEDINFO 1986*. Amsterdam: Elsevier, 1986:585–6.
[3] Minda S. Marshal & Computer Recorded Nursing Assessments. Masters Thesis (Duke University School of Nursing) 1990.
[4] Bradshaw KE, Sittig DF, Gardner RM, Pryor TA, and Budd M. Computer-based Data Entry for Nurses in the ICU. *MD Computing* 1989,6:274–80.
[5] Grewal R, Arcus J, Bowen JJ, Fitzpatrick K, Hammond WE, and Hickey L. Bedside Computerization of the ICU, Design issues: Benefits of Computerization versus Ease of Paper & Pen. In: *Proceedings of the Fifteenth Annual Symposium on Computer Applications in Medical Care*. New York: McGraw-Hill, 1991:793–97.

29
The Patient Problem/Nursing Diagnosis Form: A Computer-Generated Chart Document

Colleen M. Prophet

Introduction

In a era of cost constraints, patient-centered computing enhances communication of patient data among disciplines, facilitates efficiency and, most importantly, fosters quality patient care. The patient-centered care approach organizes diagnostic activities and care protocols based upon the particular patient's needs [1]. Computerized patient records which focus upon patient problems/nursing diagnoses can demonstrate linkages between patient conditions, interventions, and outcomes.

The American Nurses' Association (ANA) encourages nurses in the development of Nursing Information Systems (NISs) that support the nursing process [2,3]. Criteria for automated systems that facilitate this process include capabilities to accommodate the following nursing data elements: (1) assessment data, (2) nursing diagnoses with etiologies, (3) interventions for each problem, (4) outcomes for each problem, and (5) progress notes detailing an evaluation of the care plan and actual patient outcomes [4]. However, a review of an 18-year span of development of six NISs revealed that only one allowed charting against care plans whereas four accommodated recording vital signs [5]. This focus on task fulfillment charting gives the appearance that nurses' responsibilities suit a technical rather than professional model of nursing [6].

Furthermore, the recent effectiveness initiative of the Health Care Finance Administration (HCFA) magnifies the need for automated systems to provide data for patient outcomes research [7]. It therefore behooves system designers to create information systems that are patient-centered and, through the online documentation of clinicians, provide the data required to investigate patient care effectiveness.

Reprinted with permission from *Proceedings: Seventeenth Annual Symposium on Computer Applications in Medical Care: Patient-Centered Computing*, Miller, R.A. (Ed.). 1993. Pp. 332–336. © 1994, American Medical Informatics Association: Bethesda, MD.

The University of Iowa Hospitals and Clinics (UIHC)

The UIHC is a 891-bed tertiary-level health care facility providing services to approximately 2,500 patients each day. The most recent annual data reveal more than 465,600 ambulatory care visits and 28,400 acute inpatient admissions. Of the hospital staff complement of 7,560 members, the Department of Nursing includes 1,500 registered nurses, 55 clinical nursing specialists, 80 licensed practical nurses, and 330 nursing assistants.

At the UIHC, the INFORMM system operates on an IBM 3090-500J with 126 billion characters of online storage. A locally distributed network contains 1,100 cathode ray terminals (CRTs), 200 personal computers (PCs), and 200 terminal printers which includes IBM 3812 page printers installed on the inpatient care units to produce chart quality documents on demand. While the daily transaction volume on INFORMM exceeds 1.3 million, the average response time is less than 0.2 seconds.

Informm Nursing Information System (NIS)

Developed entirely in house at UIHC, the INFORMM NIS was implemented in 1988. The INFORMM NIS encompasses interdisciplinary communication of individualized patient care based upon current professional standards of care [8]. In the patient care planning component of the NIS, patient critical data, patient problems/nursing diagnoses, and patient care orders are entered and updated. The patient care planning data generate the patient acuity profile as a system by-product. Maintained by nursing personnel, the NIS data base contains content specific to patient populations, patient care units, and therapeutic modalities.

The INFORMM NIS is being developed and implemented in three major phases. In Phase I, Patient Case Planning was installed on 41 general inpatient care units. Currently, Phase II: Patient Care Documentation is being designed and established on the same general inpatient care units. Phase II involves revision of documentation practices as well as replacement of existing manual documentation and creation of new chart forms. Following an integrated and logical development plan, each computer-generated chart document is being designed, piloted, and implemented separately.

At this time, two computer-generated chart documents are in use: the patient problem/nursing diagnosis form and the patient discharge referral form [9]. During Phase III of the INFORMM NIS, Patient Care Planning and Documentation will be enhanced and implemented on the ambulatory care units.

Available to more than 2,350 nursing users, INFORMM NIS functions account for an average of 50,000 transactions daily. Of these transaction totals, approximately 8,000 relate to problem/nursing diagnosis functions which are accessible to nearly 1,000 registered nurses and generate 300 patient problem/nursing diagnosis chart forms daily. The patient discharge referral functions, available to 1,200 nursing users, account for approximately 3,000 transactions and 230 patient discharge referral chart forms per day.

Patient Problem/Nursing Diagnosis Functions

Reflecting UIHC Department of Nursing policy, the patient care plan must be initiated for a patient admitted for greater than 24 hours. Although policy requires that a patient be assessed by a registered nurse, it does not mandate that a patient problem/nursing diagnosis be identified. However, for each identified patient problem/nursing diagnosis, the registered nurse must audit, i.e., evaluate, the patient's progress toward outcome achievement at least every six days and at discharge.

The content data elements contained in the problem/nursing diagnosis functions are:

- problem/nursing diagnosis number (assigned chronologically at the time of computer entry);
- problem/nursing diagnosis name (label from the date base of more than 900 or entered free-text);
- defining characteristics (signs and symptoms from a table of more than 940 or entered free-text);
- etiologies/related factors (causes/contributing factors from a table of more than 910 or entered free-text);
- patient outcomes (patient behavior statements from a table of 330 or entered free-text); and
- patient care orders (assessments and interventions from a data base of more than 3,000 or entered free-text).

Patient Problem/Nursing Diagnosis Printouts

In the INFORMM NIS care planning system, two printouts contain problem/nursing diagnosis data: the care plan problem list and problem/nursing diagnosis/order sheet. The care plan problem list contains the patient's active problems/nursing diagnoses with the associated etiologies/related factors, projected patient outcomes, and several dates: date activated, audit due date, and last audit date. Additionally, the initials of the registered nurse who completed the "add" and last "audit" functions are printed.

The second printout contains similar information as well as associated defining characteristics and a compilation of associated patient care orders.

These different printouts attest to divergent patient care delivery systems. The care plan problem list and separate order sheet are useful in organizing care to reflect distinctions in the care provided by different levels and functions of nursing staff, whereas the problem/nursing diagnosis/order sheet is preferred by nursing staff who conduct problem-focused care planning and documentation.

However useful these printouts are, neither suffices as official documentation in the patient record. Therefore, the computer-generated patient problem/nursing diagnosis form was created.

Patient Problem/Nursing Diagnosis Form: Objectives

The objectives for the patient problem/nursing diagnosis chart form were:

1. to generate a patient record form to replace manual recording of all patient problem/nursing diagnosis activity from problem identification to problem resolution;
2. to facilitate manual review and retrieval of patient problem/nursing diagnosis and patient outcome data in the paper patient record;
3. to facilitate continuity of care by providing an online display of the patient problem/nursing diagnosis history to authorized members of the health care team;
4. to enhance patient outcome achievement by providing capabilities to review previous clinical notations and reactivate patient problems/nursing diagnoses; and
5. to capture patient problem/nursing diagnosis and patient outcome documentation for quality improvement, and clinical and administrative research.

Patient Problem/Nursing Diagnosis Form: Implementation

As occurred with the implementation of the patient care planning system, the patient problem/nursing diagnosis chart form was implemented on the general inpatient care units in three waves: a pilot on one unit, an expanded pilot on nine additional representative units, and finally, hospital-wide implementation. Prior to system activation on a unit, registered nurses were provided a one-hour educational session. Although "hands-on" training was not indicated since the "print" was the only new function, the registered nurses were provided a review of the enhanced problem/nursing diagnosis functions.

Patient Problem/Nursing Diagnosis Form: Chart Document

The patient problem/nursing diagnosis chart form is divided into three sections: the list, the discharge audit summary, and the history. For the current inpatient stay, the list contains all the patient problems/nursing diagnoses—first the active, then the inactive patient conditions. For each identified patient problem/nursing diagnosis, the date and name of the registered nurse who added and last audited or inactivated the patient problem/nursing diagnosis are included.

Following this list, the discharge audit summary is printed. In this section, the registered nurse documents the patient's overall health status and outcome achievement at the time of discharge. Obviously, this section does not appear on the patient record form until the registered nurse has completed the discharge audit online.

Following the list and, at discharge, the discharge summary, a complete history of each active and inactive patient problem/nursing diagnosis is printed in chronological sequence, beginning with problem number 1. The history contains the name of the patient problem/nursing diagnosis with associated etiologies/related factors and projected patient outcomes as well as the results of each update and audit. Audit data indicate whether the patient met the projected outcomes and include the registered nurse's free-text comments about the patient's status.

Patient Problem/Nursing Diagnosis Form: Evaluation of Objectives Achievement

The automated patient problem/nursing diagnosis form has achieved its stated objectives and the registered nurses report that documentation of patient problems/nursing diagnoses has improved.

Automated Patient Record Form

The automated patient problem/nursing diagnosis chart form replaces all forms of manual documentation detailing the registered nurse's assessment and evaluation of the patient's status in terms of identified clinical conditions. In the previous manual system, the majority of patient problem/nursing diagnosis documentation was entered in chronological sequence on narrative nurses' notes interspersed with other notations. In some instances, these particular notes were preceded by a heading of the germane patient problem/nursing diagnosis. Also, a separate chart form—the patient problem list—was available to provide an overview of the entire set of patient problems/nursing diagnoses.

In addition to replacing manual documentation, the computer generation of the patient record form has been accompanied by an increase in the number of patient problems/nursing diagnoses identified for each patient. In 1988, a study was conducted which compared the number of patient problems/nursing diagnoses in the manual system (one month prior to the installation of Patient Care Planning) with those identified six months post-implementation.

In the manual system, 91% (eighty two of the ninety patient records) had zero patient problems/nursing diagnoses and zero records had two patient problems/nursing diagnoses. Six months post-implementation, 88% (71 of the 81 patient records) had zero patient problems/nursing diagnoses, 9% had one, and 3% had two.

Subsequent analysis of archived data reveal that the percentage of patients with any patient problems/nursing diagnoses identified decreased from 69% in 1989 to 63% in 1990. With the automation of the record form in June 1991, the percentage rose to 82% and to 93% in 1992. From January to July 1993, the percentage increased to 94.5% with a shift in the mode of patient problems/nursing diagnoses from one to two per patient record.

Although policy still did not require it, the identification of patient problems/nursing diagnoses did increase with the implementation of Patient Care Planning. However, the achievement of greater than 90% fulfillment occurred only after the computer generation of the patient record form.

Cumulative Patient Record Form

In addition to eliminating manual documentation, the computer-generated patient problem/nursing diagnosis chart form enhances manual review and retrieval of associated clinical notations. In contrast to the manual method, one patient record form contains all data pertaining to the history of identified patient problems/nursing diagnoses and the status of patient outcome achievement. Moreover, this cumulative patient record form contains all previous data as well as the most recent updates. In this manner, the new chart form replaces the previous version thereby reducing paper bulk in the patient record.

Continuity of Care

Available to all authorized health care team members in inpatient and ambulatory care settings, the online display of the patient problem/nursing diagnosis documentation enhances the continuity of care both before and after hospital inpatient stays. Also, during an inpatient stay, the patient problem/nursing diagnosis data are transferred when the patient moves to a different unit.

In addition, the list of active patient problems/nursing diagnoses is included in the patient discharge referral form. In this way, the patient problem/nursing diagnosis information facilitates continuity of care with receiving agencies and facilities.

Patient Outcome Achievement

The patient problem/nursing diagnosis functions provide capabilities to review all previous germane clinical notations and to copy a prior note when documenting patient status. In this way, registered nurses are reminded of the patient's previous outcome status and may minimize free-text data entry by copying and updating pertinent prior comments. Moreover, any inactive patient problem/nursing diagnosis may be reactivated at any time, thereby retaining the previous problem/nursing diagnosis number and providing congruency within documentation.

Quality Improvement and Research

The capabilities to store and retrieve patient problem/nursing diagnosis data are identical to those for care planning data. Patient and nursing data are retained online for 42 days post-discharge, then transferred to an archival file. With requisite approvals, quality improvement studies and clinical and administrative research can be conducted on the active and archived data.

With the automation of the patient record form, the documentation of clinical data related to patient problems/nursing diagnoses and patient outcomes has been captured. Stored in the nursing archive, these data can be retrieved and analyzed in order to conduct outcomes effectiveness research. These analyses for patients and patient populations are greatly facilitated by the ready availability of data concerning the efficacy of nursing interventions and clinical treatments.

Summary

In addition to achieving the stated objectives, the INFORMM patient problem/nursing diagnosis online documentation and computer-generated patient record form have satisfied the criteria for a computer system design that supports the nursing process and professional nursing practice. Moreover, the patient-centered focus of documentation enhances patient care delivery as well as capturing clinical data critical to the examination and provision of quality patient care.

References

[1] Tarte, J., and Bogiages, C. (1992). Patient-centered care delivery and the role of information systems. *Computers in Healthcare. 13*(2), 44–46.

[2] American Nurses' Association. (1980). *Nursing: A social policy statement.* Kansas City, Missouri: ANA.
[3] American Nurses' Association. (1986). *Development of computerized nursing information systems in nursing.* (Resolution No. 24). Kansas City, Missouri: ANA.
[4] Zielstorff, R, McHugh, M., and Clinton, J. (1988). *Computer Design Criteria for Systems that Support the Nursing Process.* Kansas City, Missouri: ANA.
[5] Hendrickson, G., and Kovner, C. (1990). Effects of computers on nursing resource use. *Computers in Nursing.* 8(1), 16–22.
[6] Turley, J. (1992). A framework for the transition from nursing records to a nursing information system. *Nursing Outlook.* 40(4), 177–181.
[7] Roper, W., Winkenwerder, W., Hackbarth, G., and Krakauer, H. (1988). Effectiveness in health care: An initiative to evaluate and improve medical practice. *New England Journal of Medicine.* 319(18), 1197–1202.
[8] Prophet, C. (1989). Patient care planning: An interdisciplinary approach. *Proceedings of the Thirteenth Annual Symposium on Computer Applications in Medical Care (SCAMC).* 823–826. Washington: IEEE Computer Society Press.
[9] Prophet, C. (1992). Patient discharge referral: Interdisciplinary collaboration. *Proceedings of Sixteenth Annual symposium on Computer Applications in Medical Care (SCAMC).* 332–336. New York: McGraw-Hill, Inc.

30
Information Management in Ambulatory Care: The Nurse and Computerized Records

ROBIN STOUPA, JUDITH J. WARREN, JUNE E. BONK, and
JAMES R. CAMPBELL

Description

COSTAR V, originally developed at the Massachusetts General Hospital and now in the public domain, [1] has been extensively modified by users to fit specific practice needs. Our implementation in the Department of Internal Medicine at the University of Nebraska Medical Center (UNMC) has been no exception, with major changes over the last six years primarily designed to better support what we believe must be an interactive use of computerized medical information.

COSTAR was initially designed for implementation on the Digital Equipment Corporation (DEC®) family of minicomputers, but in recent years has come available through the COSTAR Users' Group (CUG) on a variety of platforms, including mainframes and microcomputers of the IBM® family. Due to new hardware options and the low cost of the software, recent surveys by CUG have demonstrated that a majority of new users are installing microcomputer systems in small and medium size offices. These trends have necessarily led to changes in the appearance and function of the system nationwide.

Computerized ambulatory medical records have been in use in our Internal Medicine Clinic, since 1983 and more extensively in the medicine specialties and remote sites since 1987. We first installed COSTAR on a DEC PDP® 11/34. Computer expansion to a Microvax® 3900 with 2.0 gigabytes of computerized patient records has been necessary as acceptance and use of the system has grown.

Successful use of COSTAR in ambulatory care at our site has led to implementation of enhanced versions of the software in Medicine Specialty, Cancer Center, and Surgery/Transplant clinics. Connections to other cam-

Reprinted with permission from *Proceedings: Fifteenth Annual Symposium on Computer Applications in Medical Care: Assessing the Value of Medical Informatics*, Clayton, P.D. (Ed.). 1991. Pp. 941–942. © 1992, American Medical Informatics Association: Bethesda, MD.

pus information systems for capture of laboratory and radiology information has dramatically increased the utility of COSTAR for clinic staff. These wide area network links are available through a hybrid network architecture across a token ring campus-wide superhighway.

Computerized patient records offer accessibility to information which is impossible with a paper record, thereby promoting efficiency and creating new possibilities for practice management. [2] Past research [4,5,6] has demonstrated that nurses spend substantial amounts of time managing and coordinating information for patient care both in clinic and via telephone. Due to their interest as high volume users of COSTAR, our nurses and technicians have been key participants in our users group, constantly offering ideas for developments and novel uses of the computer.

The bulk of recent program changes at our institution has focused upon facilitation of *interactive* ambulatory record keeping using the basic COSTAR data structure. Nursing staff input has been key to the evolution of user friendly data entry features, and improved the quality of record maintenance. Program development tools written in Medical Query Language (MQL®) have sped this process, allowing a freer interaction between health care providers and programming staff, thus allowing more rapid change.

Past demonstrations [3] have acquainted attendees with interactive exam room developments for COSTAR V. This demonstration will focus on nursing enhancements in use in our clinics which have developed a functional environment for interactive ambulatory nursing management. Clinical features to be presented will include:

1. *nursing encounter data capture*—definition of a minimal nursing ambulatory data set by clinic and patient problem. These data are recorded during the intake exam by the nurse in the exam room.
2. *rule driven nursing history and management*—medical logic modules (MLM) designed and implemented by a nursing practice committee are the basis for this forward chaining rule system which organizes nursing history taking and assures follow-up on needed nursing interventions.
3. *prescription refill functions*—includes prescription writing, documentation of patient complaints and drug allergy checking at the time of entry.
4. *nursing telephone module*—an interactive recording system for management of telephone encounters and facilitation of staff communication.
5. *nursing case management features*—nurse managed care for patients taking oral anticoagulants. Custom features support review of case data, recording of treatment decisions and disposition and communication with the patient.

The majority of these developments employ custom features of MQL, which has been critical for rapid prototyping and development of unique nursing information sets. MQL has been modified to support an interactive environment, and has given us the tools we have needed to support this evolution of nursing information management.

COSTAR and MQL are registered trademarks of Massachusetts General Hospital. PDP and VAX are registered trademarks of Digital Equipment Corporation.

References

[1] Barnett GO. Computer Stored Ambulatory Record. *Research Digest Report of the NCHSR*; US DHHS Publication HRA 76-3145, National Center for Health Services Research, 1976.
[2] Campbell JR, Givner N, Seelig C, Greer A, Patil K, Wigton R, Tape T. Computerized Medical Records and Clinic Function. M.D. Computing. 1989; 6(5):282–287.
[3] Campbell JR, Stoupa R. The patient, the provider, the processor: Information management in ambulatory care. Proceedings of the Fourteenth Annual Symposium of Computer Applications in Medical Care: 939–940, 1990.
[4] Greenlick MR, et al. Determinants of medical care utilization: The role of the telephone in medical care. Medical Care; 11(2):121–134, 1973.
[5] Robert Wood Johnson Foundation. Medical practice in the United States. Princeton, NJ: Robert Wood Johnson Foundation, 1981.
[6] Miller E, A conceptual model of the information requirements of nursing organizations. Proceedings of the Thirteenth Annual Symposium of Computer Applications in Medical Care: 784–788, 1989.

31
A Data Model for an Automated Nursing Tool to Support Integrated Rapid Care Planning in a Multiple Patient Assignment

Linda L. Lange and J.A. Rossi

1. Introduction

We will describe a long-term research program that has the following aims: to describe the process of integrated rapid care planning (IRCP), to identify information requirements of the process, to describe existing information management tools used to support IRCP, and to build and evaluate the effects of automated systems to meet those requirements. Work completed to date includes a description of staff nurses' supplemental information-seeking activities [1], identification and analysis of clinical nurses' beginning-of-shift planning processes [2], and description and analysis of one information management tool, the nurses' shift worksheet. In this paper, we will describe our analysis of shift worksheets and propose a data model to support a computerized tool for integrated rapid care planning. The objectives of the study were (1) to identify and describe the content of nurses' shift worksheets, and (2) to identify data elements and derive a data model for a computerized tool for integrated rapid care planning by nurses.

2. Background

2.1 Classification Systems for Nursing Care

In 1986, Werley [3] proposed the development of a Nursing Minimum Data Set (NMDS) that would establish agreement on the concepts used to describe nursing phenomena. This effort would require identifying uniform definitions for nursing diagnoses, nursing interventions, nursing outcomes,

Reprinted from *Nursing Informatics: An International Overview for Nursing in a Technological Era*, Grobe, S.J., Pluyter-Wenting, E.S.P. (Eds.). 1994. Pp. 710–714, with kind permission from Elsevier Science—NL, Sara Burgerhartstraat 25, 1055 KV Amsterdam, The Netherlands.

and intensity of nursing care. Not only would the NMDS assist nurses in communicating their unique practice domain, but it would facilitate the encoding and storage of large amounts of nursing data in computerized databases.

Bulechek and McCloskey [4], who direct the Classification of Nursing Interventions research team at the University of Iowa, define a nursing intervention as: "any direct care treatment that a nurse performs on behalf of a client, which includes nurse-initiated treatments, physician-initiated treatments, and performance of daily essential functions" [4, p. 290]. An inductive research method was used to identify intervention labels, group discrete nursing activities, and attach a conceptual label. Input from nurse experts was solicited to group the 134 labels into a standardized language. Identifying and classifying intervention labels is the first phase of their research; organizing labels into a conceptual framework that will lead to a taxonomy will be the second stage.

The work toward identifying standardized language for nursing is critical to subsequent development of computerized tools that support nursing practice. However, to date the various taxonomies have not been integrated in a clinically applied tool. It would seem that classification schemes and taxonomies will be useful categories within a data model, but that both higher- and lower-level categories will be needed in a system that supports the rapid care planning process. Specifically, at a higher level, the data model must reflect the subprocesses within the care planning process, and at a lower level it must include "atomic-level" terms that unambiguously reflect clinical phenomena. In the present paper, we address the higher-level data model, which, we believe, must incorporate organizational and environmental contexts that impose requirements on the implementation of interventions. Nurses practice in multidisciplinary settings and they provide nursing care within the time-capsule of a single shift. Nurses usually care for more than one patient. And finally, a significant percentage of patient care stems from interdependent and dependent nursing functions.

2.2 Traditional Nursing Care Planning

For more than 50 years, the written care plan has been promoted as the technology to support and verify traditional nursing care planning [5]. Traditional nursing care planning follows a systematic and deliberate process of collecting and analyzing data; setting priorities among nursing diagnoses, stating goals in terms of measurable patient outcomes, and selecting nursing interventions to meet the goals. Unlike the spontaneous and sometimes intuitive process of IRCP, traditional nursing care planning is a thoughtful, reflective activity that culminates in a carefully written plan of care. Written care plans are developed for individual patients, and, typically, they are limited to independent nursing functions [6].

In recent years, considerable attention and effort have been given to automating traditional nursing care planning technology. For example, a search of *Cumulative Index to Nursing and Allied Health Literature* identified 30 articles published since 1983 related to computerized nursing care plans. The July, 1992, issue of *Nursing Management* listed more than 40 vendors who market computerized nursing care planning programs. However, the positive effect of written care plans, computerized or manually developed, remains unproven [7, 8].

2.3 *Integrated Rapid Care Planning*

Integrated rapid care planning (IRCP) is the process of designing a set of nursing care activities for multiple patients to be accomplished during a single work shift or episode of care. IRCP is distinguished from traditional care planning in that it (1) is done under conditions of clinical urgency, (2) is done with the expectation of immediate action, (3) involves organizing care and setting priorities for multiple patients, and (4) requires incorporation of interdependent and dependent nursing actions. IRCP involves the processes of clinical judgment—observation, inference, and decision-making [9]—concerning a group of assigned patients. It requires skill in using information created by other providers, in being aware of actions of other providers and how those actions impact one's own plan of work. Finally, and perhaps most complex of all, it requires the ability to integrate information about multiple patients into a seamless plan that allows everything to get done on time, and without error.

Technology to support integrated rapid care planning has received minimal attention from vendors or in the literature. Hinson, Silva, and Clapp [10] described and automated system that integrated the treatment Kardex, nursing care plan, and nurse's notes into a one-page printout for each patient. Called the Patient Care Profile, the form provided a comprehensive picture of the nursing care requirements for a single patient on a single shift. Nurses could write notes directly on the form, which was filed as a permanent record in the patient's chart at the end of each shift. Updates were made during the shift by handwriting information on printed profiles and by entering the new information into the computerized profile for use during subsequent shifts. Data from Patient Care Profiles were available for use by the patient classification system and for DRG-related administrative studies. Hujcs [11] described the development of an integrated charge nurse report from data existing in a computerized hospital information system. For each ICU patient, the report lists identifying data, current IV infusions, vasopressors, arterial blood gas reports, ventilator status, Glasgow Coma Score, and level of consciousness. The aim of the report is to reduce time required by charge nurses to collect data and report on patient status at the end of each shift.

We believe that one technology Presently used to support IRCP is the nurse's shift worksheet. Despite the enduring use of shift worksheets by nurses, we could locate no reported studies of worksheet structure, content, or function. The worksheet is usually initiated during shift report and serves as the basis for planning, scheduling, and documenting patient care throughout the coming shift. Nurses use worksheets to integrate data from the Kardex, the medication schedule, medical orders and progress notes, nurses' notes, and shift report and to create a plan of care activities for all assigned patients during the shift. In effect, the personal shift worksheet is a representation of available information about patients and plans for patients care.

2.4 Conceptual Framework

Information processing theory [12] was used to develop the conceptual framework for the study. The theory suggests that problem solving occurs within an information processing system, which is composed of long-term memory (LTM), short-term memory (STM), and effectors and receptors which communicate with the environment. Problem solving is assumed to involve manipulation of task-oriented symbols within STM, in a problem space that is an internal representation of the task environment. A third type of memory, external memory (EM), may be constructed to augment the limited capacity of STM.

Human problem solving behavior is determined by the demands of the task environment and the psychology of the problem solver. Problem solving behavior is constrained by limitations on human memory structures. LTM has a large, perhaps infinite, storage capacity, but STM capacity is much smaller, varying from two to nine symbol structure, or chunks. Items in STM are available for immediate processing, but its limited capacity means that only a very few, perhaps not more than two, chunks can be retained if the processing task is interrupted. Both LTM and STM capacity and read–write times are related to meaning and similarity of chunks, and to environmental distractions.

In our research program, the process of developing integrated rapid care plans for multiple patients is the problem solving task of interest. IRCP is assumed to occur as manipulation of task-related symbols within STM and LTM. Performance of IRCP should be enhanced when LTM contains symbol structures, or knowledge, relevant to the task and performance should be limited by distractions that cause competition for space within the limited capacity of STM. The nurse's shift worksheet has an effect on IRCP performance as an EM device that is used to augment STM capacity.

2.5 Summary of Background

In summary, the written nursing care plan is the principal technology advocated to support nursing care planning. However, the written care plan provides minimal support for the process of IRCP for a multiple patient assignment. IRCP is an information process in which the nurse's shift worksheet is used as an external memory device to enhance performance. Although considerable work has been done to develop language systems for nursing interventions and other nursing processes, these systems have not yet been integrated and applied in a computerized tool that reflects the clinical reality of hospital-based nursing practice. The aim of the present study is to lay the groundwork for the development of such a tool.

3. Methods

3.1 Sample

The sample was comprised of 12 registered nurses (RNs) who had worked full-time for at least one year on one of four medical-surgical units at a teaching hospital in the western United State. The subjects averaged 35 years of age, 9 years as RNs, and 6 years on their present units. Most were baccalaureate graduates and only one also had a master's degree in nursing. The number of patients assigned to subjects ranged from 1 to 4 (mean = 2.8, SD = .72). Over all the units, the patient census on days when data were collected averaged 26.0 (SD = 6.87), the patient acuity averaged 3.4 on a 5-point scale (SD = .27), and the number of direct care staff averaged 9.0 (SD = 1.76). Even though each unit had a specialty designation (cardiovascular, orthopedic, oncology, and general surgery), all units usually had all types of medical and surgical patients in addition to patients in the specialty area. A total of 33 patients was assigned to the 12 subjects during the data collection period. Patients' length of present hospitalization ranged from an average of 4 days on the cardiovascular unit to 19 days on the oncology unit, which included a bone marrow transplant subunit.

3.2 Data Collection and Analysis

Data for the present study consisted of subjects' shift worksheets. Each subject was observed before, during, and for one hour after morning shift report to determine how an when worksheets were developed and supplemental information-seeking behaviors. A photocopy was made of each worksheet immediately after shift report and each subject was interviewed to determine what plans the subject had made for assigned patients. Detailed findings from the interviews have been reported elsewhere [2].

A worksheet data unit was defined as a word or phrase that could have meaning from a clinical perspective. Meaning was determined in part by context and by location on the worksheet. Data units were extracted from worksheets by a nursing graduate student who also worked as a clinician in the hospital where data were collected. The data were entered into a computerized database for coding and analysis. Data units were first coded according to subject, patient, and worksheet heading (if any). Next, the data were grouped into categories according to the type of elementary-level content they represented. The elementary-level categories were then aggregated into higher-level groups which were used to construct an entity-relationship data model. Two nurse researchers independently coded the elements at each data level, and achieved agreement of 95% or better at each level.

4. Results

4.1 The Content of Nurses' Personal Shift Worksheets

In all, 497 data elements were identified from the 12 worksheets (mean = 41.4, SD = 17.3). From the raw data, 26 elementary-level categories were derived. Ten elementary-level categories had nequencies of 20 or more: signs and symptoms (n = 70), medical diagnosis (n = 48), vital signs (n = 47), diet (n = 35), IVs (n = 35), medications (n = 32), medical service or physician name (n = 29), intake and output (n = 25), and laboratory tests (n = 21).

The elementary-level data had both content and time dimensions, and both dimensions yielded several higher-level categories. Higher-level content categories included contextual identifiers, observations and assessments, and future care events. Within the contextual identifier category were such elementary-level data as patient's name, age, diagnosis, room number, and allergies. Observation-and-assessment-level data included signs and symptoms, vital signs, and diagnostic test results. Planned-care-event-level data included activities such as monitoring intake and output, medications, changing dressings, oxygen therapy, specimens to be collected, and discharge planning. In the time dimension, elements were categorized as past, existing, or future conditions or events. Future care events were further categorized as not scheduled or PRN, scheduled by the nurse, or scheduled by other (eg, surgery or medications).

4.2 Data Model for Integrated Rapid Care Planning

IRCP concerns all activities the nurse expects to accomplish for multiple assigned patients within a work shift. As reported elsewhere [2], IRCP process involves three major processes: Setting the Context, Reviewing Information, and Making Plans. IRCP involves coordinating care among the assigned patients, as well as between patients and environmental constraints. By integrating findings about the process of IRCP derived from interviews of subjects with findings about the content of shift worksheets, it is possible to propose a data model for the IRCP process. Each planned care activity can be described by answering five questions: (1) What activity is planned? (2) What actions are required? (3) Who is involved in the activity? (4) When is it to be done? (5) What follow-up is needed?

For example, the planned activity might be patient teaching; the required actions would be to assess the patient's knowledge, assemble materials, and conduct the teaching; the persons involved could be the nurse, the patient, and a family member; the time when teaching is to be done would be scheduled by the nurse; and the follow-up would be to report the teaching by documenting it in the medical record and to make a new plan to evaluate the teaching at a later time. Another planned activity might be to administer a pre-operative medication; the action required would be to determine the drug to be given, the dose, and the time; the nurse and the patient would be involved; the administration time might be scheduled by the physician, or it might be "on-call;" and the follow-up would be to document the action in the medical record. Figure 1 illustrates an entity-relationship model for rapid care planning.

5. Discussion

The findings of the study present a description of an information management tool used by nurses in medical-surgical clinical settings. On the basis of personal experience and conversations with colleagues, we suspect that the shift worksheet is used by most nurses in most acute care settings, yet it has received no attention in the literature or from computer system vendors.

We suggest that the shift worksheet serves as an external memory device to augment short term memory during the rapid care planning process. It contains detailed information about activities the nurse intends to accomplish during a work shift. The content focus of the worksheet is heavily weighted toward interdependent and dependent nursing actions, perhaps because such time-linked, required activities are processed in short term memory. In contrast, independent nursing action plans are more likely to be constructed from knowledge existing in long term memory, thus no external memory device is needed to augment such planning.

We have proposed a data model that might be incorporated into a computerized shift worksheet. The model consists of patient-related entities and entities that describe the rapid care planning process. Contextual identifiers describe enduring characteristics of patients, such as age, room number, and medical diagnosis. Observation and assessments describe dynamic characteristics such as vital sign laboratory test results, and signs and symptoms. Rapid care plans are described by five entities: type of plan, required actions, persons involved in the action, schedule for the plan, and follow-up actions. The model is parsimonious and can be used in a relational database design.

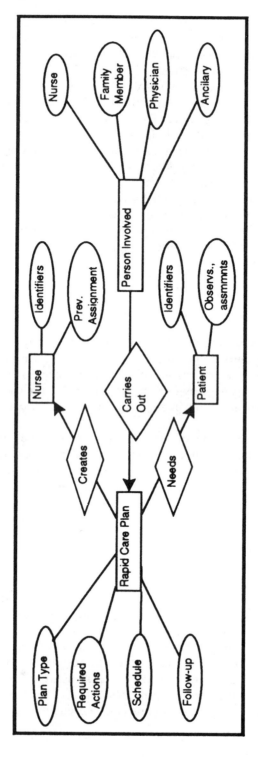

FIGURE 1. Entity-relationship model for rapid care planning.

Future studies will be designed to test the adequacy of the model as a database design to support rapid care planning in a medical-surgical clinical environment.

References

[1] Lange LL. Information Processing and Information Seeking by Nurses During Beginning-of-Shift Activities. In Frisse ME (Ed.). *Proc 16th SCAMC*, McGraw-Hill 1992; 317–321.

[2] Lange LL. Information Processing and Management by Nurses during Beginning-of-Shift Activities. *Research in Nursing and Health* 1993. (under review).

[3] Werley HH and Lang N. *Identification of the Nursing Minimum Data Set.* Springer 1986.

[4] Bulechek GM and McCloskey JC. Defining and Validating Nursing Interventions. *Nurs Clin N A* 1992, 27:289–97.

[5] Henderson V. On Nursing Care Plans and Their History. *Nurs Outlook* 1973, 21:378–379.

[6] McFarland GK and McFarlane EA. *Nursing Diagnosis & Intervention: Planning for Patient Care.* CV Mosby 1989.

[7] Holzemer WL and Henry SB. Computer-supported Versus Manually-generated Nursing Care Plans: A Comparison of Patient Problems, Nursing Interventions, and AIDS Patient Outcomes. *Comp Nurs* 1992; 10:19–24.

[8] Aidroos N. Use and Effectiveness of Psychiatric nursing care plans. *J Adv Nurs* 16:177–181.

[9] Kelly K. Clinical Inference in Nursing: I. A Nurse's Vie point. *Nurs Research* 1966; 15:23–25.

[10] Hinson I, Silva N, and Clapp P. An Automated Kardex and Care Plan. *Nurs Management* 1984; 15:11:35–43.

[11] Hujcs M. Utilizing Computer Integration to Assist Nursing. R. A. Miller (Ed.) *Proc 14th SCAMC*, IEEE Computer Society Press. 1990; 894–897.

[12] Newell A and Simon H. *Human Problem Solving.* Prentice-Hall 1972.

32
Information Seeking by Nurses During Beginning-of-Shift Activities*

Linda L. Lange

A core purpose of clinical nursing information systems (CNISs) is to assist in the management and processing of nursing data, information, and knowledge [1]. Central to achieving that purpose is the identification of information and data used by nurses not only to document nursing events, but also to give patient care. The literature suggests several approaches to identifying data and information of interest to nurses. Some writers identified data elements from computer or paper-based documentation systems used by nurses [2,3,4], while others have derived data elements by analyzing nursing textbooks and other written sources [5].

Information needs can also be identified by directly observing nursing practice in a clinical setting. In two papers, Graves and Corcoran [1,6] described the supplemental information sought by cardiovascular nurses in order to make decisions about patient care. Forty-six volunteer RN subjects from three hospitals were observed in 178 separate instances of supplemental information seeking (SIS) behavior. A questionnaire was developed to describe SIS behaviors by determining what information was sought, the purpose of the information, the source used and why, and success and difficulties encountered in obtaining the information. Data were collected on all shifts and all days of the week. Observation of each subject continued until 5 SIS instances had occurred or until 2 hours elapsed, whichever came first. Content analysis procedures were used to place the SIS behaviors into groups and categories. The 175 SIS observations were grouped into 4 categories: patient-specific information (49%), institutional policies (27%), domain knowledge (21%), and procedures (3). The authors noted the similarity of SIS instances across the three hospitals, despite differences in the information milieu of each. Also observed was the significant amount of

Reprinted with permission from *Proceedings: Sixteenth Annual Symposium on Computer Applications in Medical Care: Supporting Collaboration*, Frisse, M.E. (Ed.). 1992. Pp. 317–321. © 1993, American Medical Informatics Association: Bethesda, MD. *Supported in part by a University of Utah Research Grant.

time on all shifts spent searching for information, indicating that "a CNIS that does not provide information *to* nurses is going to be accompanied by some sort of auxiliary paper system" [1, p. 363].

The findings reported here were part of a larger study that described the cognitive processes involved in rapid intervention planning by nurses during beginning-of-shift activities. One part of that study was a follow-up of the earlier work of Graves and Corcoran [1, 6] in that it examined information seeking behavior of nurses as they began their shifts of work. In addition, the larger study extended into a new area by describing how nurses created and used worksheets to manage the information needed to give patient care. This paper reports findings based on an analysis of information-seeking behavior of nurses during beginning-of-shift activities.

Methods

Subjects

Subjects were registered nurses who had been RNs and had worked on their present nursing unit at least one year, and were considered full-time employees. Subjects were recruited from four medical-surgical units of a teaching hospital in a western state. Fifteen potential subjects were nominated by head nurses and then were contacted by the graduate research assistant to invite participants; all agreed to participate. Subjects gave written informed consent at the time of data collection. One subject was ill on the scheduled data collection day and was unable to be rescheduled during the data collection period. Two other subjects did not complete all phases of data collection, one because of pressing clinical demands and one because of problems with recording equipment, leaving a final sample of 12 subjects.

The subjects ranged in age from 24 to 57 years, and averaged 35 years of age. They had practiced nursing an average 9 years, but experience ranged from 1 to 36 years. Experience on their present unit ranged from 1 to 17 years and averaged 6 years. Eight were BSN graduates, 3 were graduates of ADN programs, and one held a diploma in nursing. None held advanced degrees or certification.

Setting

The four medical–surgical patient care units from which subjects were drawn were considerably different from one another in terms of type of patients served, usual census, patient acuity, and number of direct care staff. The smallest unit served hematology, oncology, and bone marrow transplant patients and had a usual census of 13 patients, an average acuity of 3.4 (4-point scale), and usually had 7 RNs or other direct care staff on day shift during the data collection period. The largest unit, a general medical–surgical unit, had a usual census of 31, average acuity of 3.1, and typically had 11 direct care staff on day shift. The third unit served orthopedic patients, had a typical census of 27, average acuity was 3.3, and usually had 9 direct care staff. The fourth unit served medical and surgical cardiovascular patients, including patients on telemetry, had a usual census of 25 patients, an average acuity of 3.6, and usually had 11 direct care staff. Even though each unit had a specialty designation, all units usually had all types of medical and surgical patients in addition to patients in the specialty area.

Despite these differences, the units were similar in their information management practices. Shift report on three of the units was given one-to-one: the departing nurse gave a report directly to the arriving nurse who would be caring for the patient that day. On the fourth unit, the entire oncoming staff heard a brief report on all patients, followed by one-to-one reports as described above. On all the units, each patient had a Kardex folder, a medical chart, a bedside chart, a nursing assessment and care plan folder, and a medication administration record (MAR). As in most settings, the Kardex was used as a record of current medical and nursing treatment and included information about the patient's diet, fluid restrictions, vital signs, activity, elimination, allergies, daily and special lab studies, and so on. Kardex folders were stored at the main desk of the nurses' station in a large file folder. Medical charts were the "official" patient record, where physicians wrote orders and progress notes for their patients. The bedside chart contained nurses' notes, the graphic sheet, intake and output records, and various flow sheets; it was kept in a plastic holder mounted on the wall outside the patient's room. The MAR consisted of two pages for each patient, one for PRN medications and one for regularly scheduled medications. It was used as the listing of current medication orders and as the form on which nurses charted medications that had been given. All MAR sheets were kept in a loose-leaf notebook on the medicine cart in the medicine room. Only one nurse at a time could use the MAR to retrieve or enter information. Finally, each nurse also developed a personal shift worksheet and used it throughout the shift to keep track of tasks to be done and to jot down observations and actions for later reference or permanent documentation.

Patients

A total of 34 patients was assigned to the 12 subjects during the data collection period. The number of patients assigned to subjects ranged from 2 to 4, and averaged 3 patients. The average patient length of stay on the units ranged from 4 to 19 days. Patients were rated by subjects in terms of how difficult they were to care for (1 = not difficult, 5 = very difficult), how similar they were to patients the subject usually cared for

(1 = very similar, 5 = not similar), and acuity level (1 = not acute, 4 = very acute). Overall, subjects rated patients as slightly difficult to care for (2.67), somewhat similar to previous patients (3.00), and moderately acute (3.19).

Procedures

The larger study involved collection of verbal data about intervention planning, collection of shift worksheets, and observation of information seeking behaviors after shift report. Only the latter data are reported here. Subjects were observed by the investigator for one hour following shift report to determine what information sources and documents were used to support the intervention planning process. Data collection occurred during the day shift; subjects were not observed while they were in patients' rooms. Each instance of information seeking was documented on a form similar to that used by Graves and Corcoran [1]. Information sought, source of the information, and start and stop times for each information seeking event were recorded at the moment and then validated with the subject at the end of the observation period. Content analysis procedures were used to identify categories and elements of information from the information seeking data forms. After the information seeking data were analyzed, categories and frequency distributions were compared with those identified by Corcoran-Perry and Graves [6].

Results

Information Seeking Behavior

For the 12 subjects, a total of 69 information seeking events was observed. The time required for each event ranged from 30 seconds to 25 minutes. Fifteen (22%) of the observed events involved using multiple sources to obtain the needed information. Over all the subjects the total time required for information seeking instances was 3 hours and 10 minutes, or 26% of the 12 hours of observation. In other words, each subject spent a little more than 15 minutes of the first hour after shift report looking for and retrieving information needed for patient care.

Types of Information Sought

After reviewing the types of information sought and deriving an initial coding scheme, it was determined that the data could be grouped into the categories identified by Corcoran-Perry and Graves [6]. As shown in Table 1, only two of the major categories identified earlier, PATIENT SPECIFIC INFORMATION (90% of information seeking instances) and INSTITU-TION SPECIFIC INFORMATION (10%), were identified in the present

TABLE 1. Comparison of types of information sought: Lange data vs. Corcoran–Perry & Graves data

Information Type	Lange Data	Corcoran-Perry & Graves Data
Patient specific	90%	49%
Institution specific	10%	27%
Domain Knowledge	—	21%
Procedural Information	—	3%

study. No instances of seeking DOMAIN KNOWLEDGE or PROCE-DURAL INFORMATION were observed.

Table 2 shows a comparison of distributions for subcategories of PA-TIENT SPECIFIC INFORMATION for the two studies. For the present study, data elements could be grouped into several of the subcategories identified by Corcoran–Perry and Graves: medications, physicians' orders, lab data, cardiovascular status, and diet. Compared to the earlier data, there were more instances of seeking information about medications and physicians' orders and fewer instances of seeking information about diet and cardiovascular status.

Most items in the MEDICATIONS subcategory involved seeking infor-mation about what medications were scheduled for subjects' patients dur-ing the shift. The second largest category included instances of seeking

TABLE 2. Comparison of subcategories of patient care information: Lange data vs. Corcoran–Perry & Graves data

Patient Care Information	—Lange Data— n = 62	Time (min.)	CP&G Data [6] n = 185
Medications	34.4	61	18.8
Physicians' orders	18.0	22	8.2
Lab data	9.8	11	15.3
Cardiovascular status	3.3	3	12.9
Diet	1.4	1	4.7
Interdepartmental information	13.1	12	—
Nursing information	9.8	50	28.0
New information update	6.6	19	—
Preop. preparation	4.9	3.5	—
Other	—	—	9.0

TABLE 3. Examples of information sought for most frequently used subcategories of patient specific information

Subcategory	Example
Medications	Med schedule for my patients. Pre-angiocath medication for patient—angio came early for the patient.
Physicians' orders	Pre-op and pre-cath orders for patient. New orders and orders missed on the night shift.
Lab data	Blood gas report. Whether blood is ready for my patient.
Interdept. information	When is my patient's appointment in the clinic. Will social worker talk with the patient's family about financial concerns.
Nursing information	Patient's temperature last night. Whether bowel care was done last night and what was done about patient's elevated temperature.
New information update	New Kardex information to copy onto worksheet. Patient's history and any new orders.

information about physicians' orders, many of which involved questions about medications. Table 3 gives examples of information types in the PATIENT SPECIFIC category. The present study identified several sub-categories of patient specific information that were not reported earlier. For example, 8 of the 62 instances (13%) were classified as INTERDEPART-MENTAL, seeking information about other departments' plans or activities concerning subjects' patients. Six instances (10%) involved seeking NURSING INFORMATION, such as nursing assessments or care plans recorded by nurses on earlier shifts. Four instances (7%) occurred in which subjects consulted several sources, such as the medical chart, Kardex, and MAR, in order to update their knowledge about the patient and the treatment plan. Finally, 3 instances involved seeking information about PREOP PREPARATION, including reviewing the preoperative checklist and identifying preoperative medications.

Patterns of Information Seeking Behavior

Every subject sought information about medications at least once during the one-hour observation, and 8 of the 12 subjects sought information about medical orders. When questioned about their information seeking patterns, every subject described a personal, consistent routine that was used to gather information before beginning patient care activities. Although the order of search activities varied among subjects, all subjects said they routinely obtained patients' medication schedules from the MAR, checked the medical charts for new or missed orders, reviewed and updated the Kardex, checked for lab results, and reviewed nurses' notes and assessments. Since many of these activities routinely occurred after the rush of AM care, all were not captured during the 1-hour data collection period.

Time Required for Information Seeking

Table 2 also shows the time across all subjects required for each PATIENT SPECIFIC subcategory. As could be expected, seeking medication information required the largest block of time (61 minutes overall). Surprisingly, seeking nursing information about patients required the next largest block of time (50 minutes), although there were only 6 such instances. The nursing information, such as assessments and care plans, was text-based and often located in more than one document, which may account for the longer time requirement. In contrast, the 6 instances of seeking lab results, which were usually available via computer terminal or printout, required only 10.5 minutes.

Sources of Information

Because some information seeking instances required the use of more than one source of information, a total of 83 sources was used by subjects. Sources were easily grouped into the major source categories developed by Corcoran-Perry and Graves [6], as shown in Table 4. The earlier study found that verbal and written sources were used equally by cardiovascular nurses. In contrast, the present study found much greater use of written sources (59% of instances) by the 12 subjects. Verbal sources of informa-

TABLE 4. Comparison of information sources: Lange data vs. Corcoran-Perry & Graves data

Information Source	Lange Data (%) n = 83	Corcoran-Perry & Graves Data (%) n = 175
VERBAL	*36*	*45*
Other nurses	12	25
Other personnel	24	20
WRITTEN	*59*	*45*
Patients' charts	22	25
MAR	20	—
Kardex	7	—
Bedside chart	6	—
References	1	15
Other documents	—	5
TECHNICAL	*5*	*10*
Computer output	5	8
Cardiac monitor	—	2

tion were used only 36% of the time, with other personnel accounting for twice as many sources as other nurses.

Discussion

The information seeking behaviors observed in this study are similar to those described by Corcoran-Perry and Graves [6]. Most of the information sought by subjects could be described within the PATIENT SPECIFIC information category, which is not surprising given that all observations were made during the first hour after morning shift report. During that period, subjects were gathering information necessary to begin the day's patient care activities. Every subject's morning routine included quick reviews of medical charts, Kardexes, and lab results in order to create or update the nurse's personal store of information about assigned patients. Given these commonalities, it was also found that each subject sought a unique constellation of information types, perhaps based on rapid intervention plans made during and immediately after shift report.

The most frequently used sources of information were documents, and among those, the MAR was the most common source. Non-nurse personnel were more frequently used sources of information than other nurses, perhaps because during the early part of the shift, other nurses are also busy gathering information needed for patient care.

The results of the study can make an important contribution to the design of clinical nursing information systems (CNISs). To support the information needs identified in the study, future CNISs should draw information from a variety of sources and integrate it into a real-time data and information source. Given a common database of patient information, users should have the capability of designing interfaces to fit their own unique needs. Further, patient information should be available to nurses at all times, and should be immediately accessible, wherever the nurse happens to be. In short, future CNISs should provide mobile, customizable information management tools to nurses. Future research by the investigator will test the utility of the new pen-based "notepad" computers in meeting the information management and processing needs of nurses.

References

1. Graves, J. R. & Corcoran, S. (1988). Identification of data element categories for clinical nursing information systems via information analysis of nursing practice. In R. A. Greenes, *Proceedings of the Twelfth Annual Symposium on Computer Applications in Medical Care, pp. 358–363.* Los Angeles: Computer Society Press.
2. Saba, V., O'Hare, P., Zuckerman, A., Boondas, J., Levine, E., & Oatway, D. (1991). A nursing intervention taxonomy for home health care. *Nursing & Health Care, 12,* 6, 296–299.

3. Romano, C. McCormick, K. & McNeely, L. (1982). Nursing documentation: A model for a computerized database. *Advances in Nursing Science, 4*, 2, 43–56.
4. Werley, H. & Lang, N. (1988). *Identification of the Nursing Minimum Data Set.* New York: Springer.
5. Bulechek, G. M. & McCloskey, J. C. (1990). Nursing intervention taxonomy development. In J. C. McClskey & H. K. Grace (Eds.). *Current Issues in Nursing (3rd Ed.)* (23–38). St. Louis: Mosby.
6. Corcoran-Perry, S. & Graves, J. (1990). Supplemental-information-seeking behavior of cardiovascular nurses. *Research in Nursing & Health.* 119–127.
7. Korpman, R. A. (1990). Patient care automation: The future is now. Part 2. The current paper system—Can it be made to work?. *Nursing Economic, 8*, 4, 263–267.
8. Graves, J. R. (1989). The study of nursing informatics. *Image: Journal of Nursing Scholarship, 21*, 4, 227–23.

33
The Patient-Oriented Bedside Terminal

N.K. Meehan

1. Nurse's Role in Design of a Patient-Oriented Interface

Nurses have been patients' advocates for decades. Nurses act as patients' representatives to hospital administration and ties to the health care team. Presently, nurses function as patients' communication link with the bedside terminal. Nurses also fulfill many other roles. Nurses are educators who assess patients' needs for information about their diseases and supply necessary information. Nurses also provide direct care to patients. Patients generally choose to share their fears and anxieties with nurse members of the health care team.

Basically, nurses are "information managers," managing data pertinent for patients' return to health. Nurses interact with patients in many ways and are familiar with their information needs. Therefore, nurses should be involved in the design of a patient-oriented interface.

Nurses should also encourage patients to have input into the design of a patient-oriented interface. Nurses can include patients by asking them to assist with information system committee duties. Yet patient representatives seldom have the commitment necessary to remain with the committee until completion. Therefore, nurses should be the primary patient representative when designing and selecting a patient-oriented interface for the bedside terminal.

Reprinted from *Nursing Informatics: An International Overview for Nursing in a Technological Era*, Grobe, S.J., Pluyter-Wenting, E.S.P. (Eds.). 1994. Pp. 246–249, with kind permission from Elsevier Science—NL, Sara Burgerhartstraat 25, 1055 KV Amsterdam, The Netherlands.

2. Definition of a "Patient-Oriented" Interface for the Bedside System

The question, "What defines a 'patient-oriented' interface for the bedside system?" is an interesting one. The single most important component of a patient-oriented interface is the ability of patients to interact with the computer. First, consider the information patients desire. Patients want to learn about their disease or condition and the possibility of future illness. They want to know if their test results are normal. Patients have questions concerning their level of activity or pain medication. They want to understand medical procedures and to obtain a daily schedule of meals, diagnostic tests, and treatments. The type of information frequently requested by patients falls into three categories: (1) information patients can access directly from their computer record, (2) information in patients' records that necessitates interpretation, and (3) information not available from the computer record.

2.1 Data Directly Available from Record

Patients frequently request information they could obtain directly from their medical record. Many patients want access to information in their medical record. Patients have a right to this information. Putting a medical record on a computer system should not affect that right. With a patient-oriented interface, patients can directly access parts of their medical record. However, allowing patients direct access to information from the medical record introduces new problems.

The first problem that arises is safeguarding the privacy of patients' records. Nurses have always been concerned with patient privacy. Traditional methods for insuring privacy do not work with the computerized record. Faaoso [2] states that an increase in the number of terminal locations has multiplied the possibilities for access. If patients are allowed access to their records, the sheer number of individuals having access to patient data increases the chances of a breach of privacy.

The next problem is identifying parts of the record to which patients can be allowed direct access. Certain parts of the medical record are self-explanatory. Patients could access their demographic information with the ability to mark errors for correction. Patients could access charges and give the medical facility input about these charges. Allowing patients direct access introduces the issue of accuracy. If patients are given direct access to their medical records, who should be responsible for the accuracy of the record? Should the patient, the medical facility, or the nurse assume this responsibility? These are just a few of the problems introduced when patients have direct access to their data.

2.2 Data Indirectly Available from Record

A second type of information the patient frequently requests is information that necessitates interpretation. Certain information obtained from patients' records requires interpretation by a medical professional. The legal ramifications of patients directly accessing this information without some form of interpretation are staggering. Patients want information about their medication. Listing the medication, dosage, and administration times does not provide patients enough information. Patients want to understand their test results. Lab results alone mean nothing to patients. Most lab results need some explanation of the findings. A patient might misunderstand that a negative finding on a biopsy means cancer was not found.

A patient-oriented interface for the bedside terminal could access patients' medical records and then present this data in a way to educate patients about their diseases. Patients could be given an interpretation of the data. For instance, patients could request information about blood tests for hemoglobin. A patient-oriented interface could give patients their hemoglobin results, explain the normal range for their particular gender and age, and then explain problems associated with a high or low hemoglobin. The patient-oriented interface could incorporate the results of tests with a "lay" explanation of the findings.

2.3 Data Not Available from Record

The last category of information that patients desire is data that is not available from their medical record. Patients want information about their diagnoses. They want to understand their illness and the treatment options available to them. Patients want to know about any special diet or exercise limitations. One method of providing this data is similar to that suggested by Blue Cross/Blue Shield [3]. The company developed a "Shared Decision Making" system composed of a laser disk system which gives patients information about the treatment options available to them. The system gives information about patients' illness and pros and cons available for those treatments. In this way, patients are able to make better decisions about their own care.

3. Patients' Utilization of a Patient-Oriented Interface

Another area of discussion is the utilization of a patient-oriented interface. Today almost all individuals have interacted at some time with a computer. ATMs (automated teller machines) and grocery store bar code readers are just a few examples of how computers are incorporated into our everyday life. Most people do not realize that they deal with computers daily.

These interactions seem too commonplace to be considered computer interactions.

For patients to get medical data from their bedside terminals, systems must be user-friendly. A patient-oriented interface should encourage patient interaction with the bedside terminal. If a computer interface is appealing and easy-to-use, patients are more likely to use the system to participate in their health care.

One suggested method of providing information meaningful to patients while allowing a user-friendly interface is to have a question/answer component. Richards et al. [4] developed a computer system that contained a section called "Personalized Dialogue." The dialogue section allowed patients to enter into a conversation with the computer in the same way they would talk with a nurse or doctor. However, answers would be available 24 hours a day and patients would not have to wait for physicians to make rounds before they could get answers.

Sometimes patients have questions they find too embarrassing to ask nurses or physicians. A dialogue section could enable patients to ask questions they feel uncomfortable asking a health care professional. A study by Van Cura et al. [5] found some interesting results concerning information patients consider personal. The study found that the majority of patients would rather give personal information to a computer than share it directly with nurses or physicians.

The way the system presents data to patients is a second component important in defining a patient-oriented interface. For years, health educators have been using visual images to teach patients about their illnesses. Patients learn more when they visualize an abnormality or disease. One research study by Hinohara et al. [6] used the computer's color graphic capability to educate patients about their cardiovascular risk factors. Color graphics were used to plot an individual's risk factors within a circle. The further the plotted points fell from the center of the circle, the fewer the significant risk factors.

Another major area of consideration is that some features of a patient-oriented interface might discourage patient utilization. One study by Robinson and Walters [7] looked at a computer network called Health-Net. The network was made available to graduate and undergraduate students at Stanford University.

Health-Net provided an electronic mail system, an electronic bulletin board, an information and referral listing, and a self-help/health information library. However, only students with computer experience used the system often. Other students said Health-Net was intimidating and too difficult to learn to use. They also said they did not have convenient access to a computer terminal, they did not know how to use computers, and they did not trust computers.

Computers are still too complex and frightening for average patients. And, until using bedside terminals becomes as easy as using the ATM, most patients will probably avoid using a patient-oriented interface for the bedside terminal. To encourage all patients to interact with their bedside terminals, voice recognition abilities are essential. The patient-oriented interface should provide language options and multiple data entry methods to accommodate handicaps. In this way, the patient-oriented bedside terminal could meet the needs of most patients.

4. Suggestions for Development of a Patient-Oriented Interface

In summary, suggestions for development of a patient-oriented interface for the bedside terminal must address three areas. First, the nurse must identify information important to patients. Nurses are the likely health care professionals to be involved with the design of a patient-oriented interface.

The second suggestion for development concerns operationally defining a 'patient-oriented' interface for the bedside system. This category must consider two types of data: data available from medical records and data not available from medical records. Data from patients' records are necessary to educate patients about their particular disease, medication, etc. Patients need to understand their lab results in relationship to their disease process. Patients also want other educational tools to guarantee the understanding of their illness.

The third area for development targets the use of the patient-oriented interface. This interface should be so inviting that patients would choose to utilize the system to participate in their health care. The patient-oriented interface should allow patients 24-hour access, the ability to share in decision-making, and easy-to-understand graphic capabilities.

In summary, the bedside terminal is coming. In the future, patients *will* have some interaction with bedside terminals. The type and quality of that interaction is the responsibility of nursing. Representing patients on an information system committee, nurses can provide input on the best methods to encourage patients' utilization of their bedside terminals.

References

[1] Packer CL. Point-of-Care Terminals: Interest Abounds. *Hospitals* 1987, 61: 72.
[2] Faaoso N. Automated Patient Care Systems: The Ethical Impact. *Nurs Management* 1992, 23: 46–48.
[3] Patients Hit Computer Age. *The Greenville News*. Friday, March 05, 1993.
[4] Richards B, Cadman J, Farmiloe H, Leong F and Wong K. The Value of Computer-Aided Patient Education For Nurses In General Practice. In: *Proceedings of the Fourth International Conference on Nursing Use of Computers and Information Science*. Hovenga EJS, Hannah KJ, McCormick KA and Ronald JS (eds). New York: Springer-Verlag, 1991: 545–549.

[5] Van Cura LJ, Jensen NM, Greist JH, Lewis WR and Frey SR. Venereal Disease. Interviewing and Teaching by Computer. *Am J Public Health* 1975, 65: 1159–1164.

[6] Hinohara S, Takahashi T, Uemura H, Robinson D and Stehle G. The Use of Computerized Risk Assessment for Personal Instruction in the Primary Prevention of Ischaemic Heart Disease in a Japanese Automated Multiphasic Health Testing and Services Center. *Med Inf* 1990, 15: 1–9.

[7] Robinson TN and Walters PA. Changing Community Health Behaviors with a Health Promotion Computer Network: Preliminary Findings from Stanford Health-Net. In: *SCAMC '87.* November 1987: 514–520.

34
Benefits of Bedside Terminals— Myth or Reality?

EVELYN J.S. HOVENGA

To completely realize their benefits, bedside terminals need to be part of a fully integrated hospital-wide information system. Such a system is capable of consolidating all patient data from admission to discharge and beyond. Furthermore, an integrated system requires all data to be entered only once. The use of bedside terminals alone does not determine whether benefits become a myth or reality; the effectiveness of the system plus the organizational climate within which it is used determine this. Bedside terminals provide the greatest benefits when they are used by all health care professionals delivering a patient service, to access the patient's computerized medical record and to document their observations and treatment/care provided at the point of care.

Packer (1987) reported a survey which found that two out of every three hospitals in the United States were interested in information systems that collect and retrieve data at the patient's bedside. As a result of this level of interest, more vendors are directing their research and development activities into designing or expanding their systems to meet this demand. But what are the real benefits?

Mowry and Korpman (1987) list potential benefits of automated systems as: a significant reduction in nursing time spent on clerical activities; enhancement of the quality of documentation; elimination of error prone telephone communication between departments; elimination of costly errors of duplication and omission; incorporation of both physician orders and nursing orders within the patient care schedule; the ability to trace patient outcomes to interventions; the possibility of creating improved on-line quality assurance programs using extensive, system provided audit trails; extensive clinical and management research capabilities; automatic calculation of patient acuity and suggested staffing patterns; the ability to

Reprinted with permission from *Nursing Informatics '91: Proceedings of the Post Conference on Health Care Information Technology: Implications for Change*; Marr, P.B., Axford, R.L. & Newbold, S.K. (Eds.). 1991. Pp. 99–104. Heidelberg-Berlin, Germany: Springer-Verlag.

track labor and material costs by patient and DRG; and scheduled or ad hoc management reports derived by use of a query language. Zielstorff, McHugh, and Clinton (1988) add that automated systems can be used to help structure the care planning process; to support the nurse's clinical decision-making skills; to guide future nursing decisions; to help detect or prevent certain types of nursing errors; and to increase the body of nursing knowledge. Value-added projected benefits include reductions in length of stay through improved patient scheduling throughout the hospital stay and reduced complication rates due to improved data accuracy, timeliness of test results and documentation responsible for timely and appropriate responses. These improvements in the quality of care are likely to result in improved outcomes for individual patients. In addition, it is anticipated that there will be more opportunities for health service consumers to become more informed and to assume a more active role in their care.

Bedside terminals, used in conjunction with fully integrated health care systems, (i.e., integration beyond the hospital), permit the consolidation of factual clinical and other data about the health and health care services of a nation, creating large databases. The use of these facilitates more accurate evaluation of government policies and should lead to the development of better targeted health and social policies determining government expenditure. The ultimate benefit of which should be a reduction in the nation's morbidity. Ideally this data is also used to assure equity in access to and quality of health services.

Potential benefits of fully integrated systems may be grouped into a number of categories. Some are considered cost benefits, others are perceived as service benefits. Notwithstanding, the bottom line usually is to be able to demonstrate savings to justify purchase and maintenance costs. Potential benefits are generally perceived to consist of improved productivity and an improvement in the quality of care delivered. Savings from the improvement in quality are realized by the elimination of costs resulting from complications or errors during care delivery.

Staggers (1988) organized direct benefits, as perceived by a number of authors, under the two main categories of accountability and efficiency. Each potential benefit mentioned, requires its own management strategy to ensure benefit realization. Clearly, strategies need to be employed and incorporated as part of planning and implementation processes to ensure that anticipated benefits will ensue. The extent to which benefits are realized by the provider, the industry, the patient, and the nation as a whole depends on how well automation is planned for and implemented within each organization; that is, benefits are not automatic (Barry & Gibbons, 1990).

Organizational Impact

An important impact of automated systems and the use of bedside terminals is the amount and timeliness of available information. Information is power. Thus a group previously powerless due to a lack of timely information has the potential to redefine its power base. The benefits for some may be at a cost to others within an organization.

There needs to be an understanding of what is preventing apparently logical changes to occur prior to the development of management strategies aimed at realizing anticipated benefits. There are a number of issues. Automating existing inefficient practices will not result in improved productivity. Good system design, data and data base structures, together with optimum use of technological advances, are necessary prerequisites to a potentially successful system. Successful implementation requires an understanding of the organizational climate, a good assessment of the likely impact of the system upon existing work practices, power bases and communication channels. Frequently the introduction of an efficient fully integrated system within an organization leads to major organizational changes (Warnock-Matheron & Plummer, 1988).

Not only do people have to become familiar with new technology, but their work practices and roles are redefined. Everyone has their own expectations about what the system will or will not do. In short, it can be very traumatic. However, a system may be successfully implemented in terms of its ability to automate functions and to provide timely information without realizing other anticipated benefits.

Peters (1987) predicted that a successful firm in the 1990's and beyond would have fewer layers within the organizational structure, have more autonomous units with more local authority, be oriented toward differentiation, be quality and service conscious, more responsive, faster at innovation and use highly trained, flexible people as the principal means of adding value. This is a major change for most nursing divisions and most hospitals.

Nothing is more threatening to individuals than uncertainty, coupled with role and organizational changes. In such circumstances, human behavior becomes unpredictable. Controlling the flow of information is a common strategy by individuals to maintain power. Some will go to extremes to safeguard their power bases and the status quo. Peters talks about empowering people and advocates that all information be shared, thus diluting the power bases. Fully automated integrated systems make this readily achievable.

An additional benefit is therefore a better understanding of everyone's contribution to the process of care and outcomes. It also means that the activities of some individuals will be under greater scrutiny. The nursing profession needs to be aware that the control of nursing information by nurses is crucial to the control of nursing practice. Thus the issue here is who owns what information. This needs to be clearly identified and incorporated in the system's design and maintenance.

Staggers (1988) has conducted an extensive literature review to identify the documented benefits of computer usage in nursing. This led to the question of whether perceived benefits have in fact been demonstrated by empirical studies and whether the effects of computer systems on nurses' work activities support the statements and service benefits. More studies have been conducted, but it is difficult to access the findings.

An empirical measurement study by MacArthur (1988) of the expected benefits following the implementation of the Clinicom system demonstrated that all anticipated benefits had been realized. However, these results were made available to the system vendor and hospital client only, as the study was commissioned from a private consulting organization. Such study results are usually considered confidential. Another anecdotal article regarding the benefits of bedside terminals was published by Yero (1988).

Noehr and Bernstein (1989) assert that one needs to understand the tasks, the working methods, and the organizational environment in which the systems are to be used before selecting or designing an integrated system. These authors talk about the final product as being not just another technical system but an organizational change. They identify as the most significant obstacle to realization of potential benefits "the lack of concepts for capturing the application oriented perspective, and models for capturing working routines and communication structures in a modern hospital." They argue that it is crucial to develop user knowledge about the technology to produce new conceptions. This can be achieved through user involvement in system development and implementation. Further, effective integration requires standardization. Currently we have many systems which are department, or at best, health agency specific.

Increasingly, efforts are being directed toward first interfacing and later integrating these existing systems. Data integration generally works only between application packages supplied by the same development team since it requires the use of a "common language" not to be expected when attempting to combine software from different vendors (Bakker, Kouwenberg, & Ottes, 1989).

One of the American Nurses Association's criteria for automated systems is that "the system should be designed to permit nursing data to be transported electronically to other systems" (Zielstorff et al., 1988). They consider that this would eliminate the re-keying of data and provide a much broader database than any one agency could produce. Not only does this require application standardization but also data element standardization. That is, all data elements used in databases need to have a standard meaning to permit the creation of a regional, national, or even international nursing database. These authors state that "systems that can promise transportability of data across hardware environments will, in the future, have a distinct advantage." Standard data meanings are emerging from work done in various countries aimed at establishing nursing minimum data sets. The lack of a comprehensive uniform coding format to describe clinical nursing data renders current and future technological capabilities useless (Simpson & Waite, 1989). A priority for the nursing profession is to adopt a national, and possibly an international, taxonomy describing nursing (i.e., clinical indicators, interventions and outcomes).

Are benefits of bedside terminals just myths or can they become reality? To answer this question, we also need to examine how staff time saved is actually used. Can nurses handle spending more of their time interacting directly with patients? This may require a re-orientation to nursing.

Hovenga's studies (1988, 1989, 1990a, 1990b, 1990c), conducted in eighteen hospitals between 1981 and 1989, indicate that nurses spend between 20% (nursing home type patients) and 40% (acute general medical/surgical type patients) of their time on activities which would benefit from the use of bedside terminals. These studies also showed that the introduction of additional non-nursing staff to perform non-nursing duties in ward areas did not result in a change in the amount of time nurses spent in direct patient interaction.

A common finding from five empirical studies (Staggers, 1988) addressing work activity changes and actual service benefits was that extra nursing time available after computerization was not usually spent in direct patient care as the authors had originally hypothesized, but was channelled into other areas. A later study conducted in an intensive care unit (Kalbach & Kalbach, 1988) supports these findings. Yet the potential to help nurses improve their productivity has been reported by several authors (Cook, Fleming, & Buchanan, 1981; Edmunds, 1984; McHugh 1986; & Hughes, 1988).

Conclusion

In theory, there are significant savings to be achieved. To realize these potential benefits will require new management styles, considerable effort by all concerned, and union co-operation. Saving nursing time is only one side of the equation; the other question to be answered is, what will nurses do with this extra time? Unless the time saved is equivalent to one nurse on any shift, this saving will not translate into a cost saving unless sicker patients are cared for with the same staff thus reducing the cost of treating specific patient types. Savings are greatest where the information processing needs are greatest, i.e., in acute care settings with a high patient turnover where most patients require complex care.

Another projected saving is through improved patient scheduling throughout the length of stay, improved data accuracy, timeliness of test results and documentation leading to timely and appropriate responses, resulting in a reduction in complications, reduction in average length of stay, and improved outcomes for individual patients.

More studies are required, both pre- and post-implementation of any integrated system, to conclusively determine the extent of the benefits of bedside terminals.

References

Bakker, A., Kouwenberg, J.M.L. & Ottes, F.P. (1989). HIS and PACS integration aspects. In *Proceeding of Medinfo'89*, p. 379.

Barry, C.T. & Gibbons, L.K. (1990). Information systems technology: Barriers and challenges to implementation. *Journal of Nursing Administration, 20* (2), 40–42.

Cook, M., Fleming, J.J., & Buchanan, N.S. (1981). El Camino hospital: Ten years later. *Computers in Hospitals, 2* (4), 22–25.

Edmunds, L. (1984). Computers for inpatient nursing care. *Computers in Nursing, 2*, 102–108.

Hovenga, E.J.S. (1988). Work sampling at Peter MacCallum Cancer Institute. Northcote, Australia.

Hovenga, E.J.S. (1989). Comparison of the Resident Classification Instrument (RCI) with other measures of care and resources in Victorian Nursing Homes. Department Victoria, Melbourne, Australia.

Hovenga, E.J.S. (1990a). The origins of the Patient Assessment and Information System (PAIS). Northcote, Victoria, Australia.

Hovenga, E.J.S. (1990b). PAIS for Midwifery Patients. Northcote, Victoria, Australia.

Hovenga, E.J.S. (1990c). PAIS in Extended Care. Northcote, Victoria, Australia.

Hughes, S. (1988). Bedside information system: State of the art. In M.J. Ball, K.J. Hannah, U. Gerdin Jelger & H. Peterson (Eds.), *Nursing informatics: Where caring and technology meet*. New York: Springer-Verlag.

Kalbach, P.J. & Kalbach, L.R. (1988). Effects on the distribution of nursing care time after implementation of a computerized patient monitoring system. In *Proceedings of the Third International Symposium on Nursing Use of Computers and Information Science*. Dublin, Ireland.

MacArthur (1988). Pre-Conference Workshop. In *Proceedings of the Third International Symposium on Nursing Use of Computers and Information Science*. Dublin, Ireland.

McHugh, M.L. (1986). Increasing productivity through computer communications. *Dimensions of Critical Care Nursing, 5* (5), 294–302.

Mowry, M.M. & Korpman, R.A. (1987). Evaluating automated information systems. *Nursing Economic$, 5* (1).

Noehr, C. & Bernstein, K. (1989). Can HIS be developed without organizational change? The creative potential in user participation. In *Proceedings of the Sixth Conference on Medical Informatics*, p. 335.

Packer, C.L. (1987). Point-of-care terminals: Interest abounds. *Hospitals, 61* (18), 79.

Peters, T. (1987). *Thriving on Chaos—Handbook for a Management Revolution*. New York: Alfred A. Knopf.

Simpson, R.L. & Waite, R. (1989). NCNIP's system of the future: A call for accountability, revenue control and national data sets. *Nursing Administration Quarterly, 14* (1), 72–77.

Staggers, N. (1988). Using computers in nursing: Documented benefits and needed studies. *Computers in Nursing, 6* (4), 164–170.

Warnock-Matheron, A. & Plummer, C. (1989). Introducing nursing information systems in the clinical setting. In M.J. Ball, K.J. Hannah, U. Gerdin Jelger & H. Peterson (Eds.), *Nursing Informatics: Where Caring and Technology Meet*. New York: Springer-Verlag.

Yero, M. (1988). St. Francis Hospital goes bedside and beyond. *Health Care and Costs*, January, p. 48.

Zielstorff, R.D., McHugh, M.L. & Clinton, J. (1988). *Computer design criteria for systems that support the nursing process.* Kansas City: American Nurses Association.

35
Point of Care Terminals: A Blessing or a Curse?

JUDITH SHAMIAN, BETTY HAGEN, RUTH BRENNER, and PHILIP LOHMAN

Introduction

Nursing is an information intensive profession: nurses constantly assess, plan, and evaluate patient status and care. Nurses gather and organize patient data in order to make clinical decisions and maintain detailed documentation that follows the patient throughout the hospital stay. As in other information-intensive professions, the more the nurse can close the gap between the source of the information and the place where she must store it, the more effective she is and the more efficiently she can work. Hence, the growing interest in point-of-care computer systems.

Bedside, or point-of-care, terminals are an important option to consider when attempting to create a positive working environment. In the literature, there are a number of reports on current experiences with point-of-care systems (POCS). St. Joseph Hospital in Milwaukee, is one of the hospitals that has evaluated the potential benefits of POCS. The financial pay back benefit was estimated at 28 full time equivalents (FTEs) or $1,218,000 on the low end. On the high end: $2,094,000 of saving was predicted (K. Kahl, 1990). In Salt Lake City, G. Halford, M. Burkes, and T.A. Pryor (Halford, Burkes, Pryor, 1989) compared bedside terminals with pod, or workstation terminals. A second study of bedside terminals was conducted by Peat Marwick Main and Co. of Baltimore, Maryland and reported by F. Cerne (1989). The study was conducted at Nebraska Methodist Hospital, in Omaha, Nebraska; Saint Joseph's Hospital in Atlanta, Georgia; and Frankford Hospital in Philadelphia, Pennsylvania. A review of these two studies revealed that the use of bedside terminals affected the professional nursing environment in five ways: decreased

Reprinted with permission from *Nursing Informatics '91: Pre-Conference Proceedings*; Turley, J.P. & Newbold, S.K. (Eds.). 1991. Pp. 26–30. Heidelberg-Berlin, Germany: Springer-Verlag.

workload, improved quality of care, increased positive public relations, improved communication, and increased positive perception of administration. These findings and others led to a growing interest in POCS.

Before a hospital makes a decision on the acquisition of a point-of-care system, it should consider a number of factors very carefully. In this paper we discuss seven factors that should be considered prior to commitment to point-of-care technology.

Factors to Be Considered Prior to the Acquisition of Point-of-Care Terminals

Functionality

What do you want the system to do? Does it fit the organizational goals for automation? Most of the following functions can be done by most point-of-care systems, but not all systems can perform all functions. It is important to determine which applications are necessary. Those functions to consider include: patient assessment; nursing diagnosis; care planning; order entry; medication administration record; kardex; clinical flow records; planned activity list; nursing documentation; nursing progress notes; chart management; patient education; and, for intensive care environments: instrument/monitor interface, cardiac and neuro flow sheets, and ventilator monitoring.

Location

Where do you want to put the terminal? Different systems are designed for different types of placement, and allow different degrees of flexibility. The Critikon Vitalnet, Clinicom/Cliniview and IBM 7690 (with Hill-Rom mounting) can only be located on the wall. The IBM has to be placed at or near the headboard, because it uses the Hill-Rom Datalink. Other systems allow more freedom—the MedTake system uses a small, proprietary terminal which is relatively easy to move around the room, although your options may be limited by cabling.

Check to make sure that the terminal has been approved for UL 544 for current leakage and placement at the bedside. Not all terminals have yet received this approval. Consider patient confidentiality policies when choosing the location of POCS. Patients will occasionally attempt to log on to the system, so it must be password-protected and the nurse should make sure that the patient cannot see her enter her password. Otherwise, it is not necessary to place terminals so the patient cannot see them. Research findings indicate that many patients become quite interested in the clinical system and enjoy watching the nurses use it.

Integration

To what extent will you require that your POCS be integrated with the hospital's existing or planned patient care system? Most POCS vendors comply with the HL-7 interface standard, which eases interfacing. Integration at the bedside will be *functional* integration in most cases, i.e., the nurse is able to access the order communications system without having to log off of the POCS and log onto the Patient Care Information System (PCIS).

POCSs can, of course, be installed stand-alone at first, if the hospital has, or is in the process of obtaining, a new, non-POCS-capable Hospital Management Information System and if Nursing wishes to automate the bedside early. This requires manual entry of some ADT data and tracking orders at the nursing station, as the hospital will probably be doing already. The full range of nursing functionality is available regardless of whether the POCS is integrated with the patient care information system; it is just that more data has to be handled manually until the interface is completed. When evaluating systems integration, the hospital should be certain that the vendor reference sites are on the current releases of both the PCIS and POCS involved, and that reference sites are *production* sites.

POCS Benefits

What are they and how are they achieved? Our experience suggests that clinical and financial benefits should be assessed when exploring POCS. We have also found that the highest clinical benefit of a fixed point-of-care terminal is in intensive care units, as the nurse spends many hours with a few patients, relies continuously on information and there is a large amount of information that must be managed on each patient.

An identification of expected benefits should be outlined. The following points should be considered during this identification process:

Caution should be taken about vendor claims for time saved and other quantitative benefits (such as reduced med errors). The hospital will need to talk directly to people at the reference sites, rather than asking questions through the vendor.

Caution should also be taken in managing expectations: Do not let the administration, or the board, get the idea that overtime is going to go to zero the day after the POCS is implemented; it will not. Rather, a realistic schedule (eight weeks, for example) should be worked out for overtime reduction and then care should be taken that this schedule is enforced.

Spending more time at the bedside is not always a desired benefit. Many nurses report that they feel isolated unless they can spend some time at the nursing station.

Some benefits are hard to quantify, but they are real nonetheless. These include: (1) reduced medication errors. This is a key quality-of-care indicator, (2) improved quality of documentation, with Unit Managers and Head Nurses spending much less time in Medical Records trying to decipher charts for Medical Record Technologists, (3) improved morale (which leads to easier recruitment and retention of nurses), (4) reduced risk and liability exposure, (5) easier, faster patient education (applicable only if your POCS has a patient education module), and (6) cost benefit. Many of the vendors and users claim a real time savings with POCS. The hospital should decide ahead of time what it will do with the predicted savings so it can be converted to real dollars if so desired.

When determining an analysis of benefits achieved, the hospital must distinguish between:

1. Benefits derived from bringing nursing capabilities (charting, assessment, etc.) to the *nursing station*.
2. Benefits derived from bringing these capabilities to the *bedside*.

Before reporting benefits, the hospital must also be certain they are sustainable benefits.

Implementation Staging

What is the best sequence of implementation activities for your hospital? The hospital will probably want to bring up a pilot unit initially, rather than converting the entire Medical/Surgical service at once (for example). Clearly, the choice of a pilot site should be made with training in mind: Which unit has been most receptive to new ideas and change in the past? Which is likely to be the easiest to train? The hospital may then wish to make the *next* unit be the unit which has been the *hardest* to train in the past.

If there are separate systems for POCS and PCIS, it may be necessary to train on both systems. This is confusing and could inhibit consistent adoption by staff. The hospital should work toward one operational system so one training system will prepare nurses to perform on all information systems. The system chosen should be as user-friendly as possible, with clear prompts.

Physician Acceptance

How will the physicians react to the POCS? Our experience with various hospitals in North America suggests that usually five to ten percent of doctors oppose the POCS and refuse to have anything to do with it. Another five to ten percent are highly motivated, and the remainder are moderately and benignly interested. At some hospitals, many physicians are active participants and want to see what they can do with the system.

Some factors which influence physician acceptance are how the POCS is introduced to the physicians and whether provision has been made for physician involvement in the POCS procurement. Have the benefits to them been pointed out and have their concerns been addressed?

Financial

What are the financial implications of the POCS project? This is a matter of comparing costs to benefits. To achieve a correct financial projection, it is important to conduct a joint clinical and cost analysis. With healthcare funding shrinking, there is an increasing demand for solid cost justification. It is becoming increasingly apparent that POCS benefits are there—however, in many cases, costs have been higher than estimated. While it is common to find cost overruns in adapting to new technology and costs are normally brought under control as an industry's experience with a technology matures, the hospital should be careful to examine the experience of a vendor's production sites in this regard.

Some vendors, such as IBM, have stated POCS product design requirements will save one hour per nurse per shift. If a POCS costs $5,000 per bed, the payback time will be approximately two years. But these are merely goals; it is important that the hospital validate any claims of time saved with production references—and by looking at hospitals where the product is installed, but look at those not cited as references.

As the battle over clinical quality and the cost of care intensifies, nurses can find that the POCS, if carefully selected and properly managed, gives them a powerful tool. Institutions also have the responsibilities to collaborate with industry in further developing and strengthening the POCS systems.

In summary the POCS could become a curse or a blessing. In this paper we have attempted to offer you, based on our experience, factors to consider. If these factors are considered before and during POCS implementation, you have good potential to have a POCS which is a blessing. Any form of technology adoption to a clinical site requires collaboration among numerous groups. The more you anticipate and preplan as a project team the more blessed you will be.

The seven factors we have discussed in this paper are the main issues to consider. The examination and response to these factors should take place in a collaborative fashion between all stakeholders. Some of the key stakeholders are nurses, physicians and information systems experts. Institutions should be realistic in anticipating benefits. Whether a POCS system is a curse or a blessing is strongly dependent on the upfront work and conclusions by the key stakeholders.

References

Cerne F: Study finds bedside terminals prove their worth. *Hospital* 1989: 63(3) 72.
Halford G, Burkes M, Pryor TA: Measuring the impact of bedside terminals. *Nursing Management* 1989: 20(7) 41–44.
Kahl K: Hospital budgets bedside savings down to the FTE. *National Report on Computers & Health* 1990: 11(16).

36
Information Systems in Critical Care: A Measure of Their Effectiveness

D. Kathy Milholland

1. Introduction

The PDMS Effectiveness Measure evaluates, from a clinical nursing perspective, the effectiveness of patient data management systems (PDMS) and is designed to be non-vendor-specific. This paper describes the development and testing of this measure.

PDMS are computer-based information systems which facilitate the collection, integration, retrieval, and interpretation of the tremendous quantities of multi-source, multi-variant data found in critical care units. They are intended to improve clinical data collection and to support clinical decision making by providing meaningful data organization, manipulation and display [1]. PDMS are expensive in time and capital resources to install, implement, and maintain. Thus their effectiveness for critical care nurses, the primary users of PDMS, is important in today's limited resource and cost-conscious health care environment.

2. Background

The PDMS evaluation literature is primarily anecdotal, focusing on staff and organizational responses to the computer system [2–4]. In the few formal evaluations, the focus is on the system's effect on discrete nursing tasks or patient morbidity and mortality [5–8]. The reliability and validity of the instruments and methods used in these studies are limited or not reported at all; the results, therefore, cannot be applied to other systems and environments. The reported research does not examine how PDMS affect clinical nursing practice. Nursing, when it is studied, is viewed as a collec-

Reprinted with permission from *MEDINFO '95: Proceedings of the Eighth World Congress on Medical Informatics*; Greenes, R.A., Peterson, H.E. & Protti, D.J. (Eds.). 1995. Pp. 1068–1070. Edmonton, Alberta, Canada: Canadian Organization for the Advancement of Computers in Health (COACH).

tion of sequential tasks requiring efficiency techniques and automation to ensure their completion. Nursing practice, as a cognitive discipline, is more than the execution of a sequence of tasks.

To remedy the situation, this research was directed to the development of a reliable, valid measure that would address information management from a clinical nursing practice perspective. The design of the measure was focused on assessing the effectiveness of computer information systems in assisting critical care nurses to manage information activities and processes.

The interaction between a PDMS and a critical care nurse is viewed as two open systems connected via a human-device interface with a shared, overlapping area within each systems' functions. The patient care unit environment is shared. Each system, however, operates independently of each other. Because there is a shared area, one system's functions may influence the functions of the other.

Evaluation research utilizes scientific methods in the study of how effectively knowledge has been applied. It identifies the working of a program or compares different programs [9]. Effectiveness can be the achievement of progress towards a goal rather than 100% fulfillment [10].

Critical attributes of effectiveness were identified as goals, achievement, and degree. System goals are viewed as progressing along a continuum of achievement. Degree is the extent of goal progression at a given point in time.

3. Instrument Development

A norm-reference approach was used to develop the measure [11]. PDMS design goals and system user goals were derived from an examination of the research and descriptive literature on PDMS. From this examination, 8 PDMS goals were identified: improve data management (MANAGE), improve data analysis (ANALYZE), help the staff (HELP), improve data quality (DATA QUALITY), improve access to data (ACCESS), provide savings (SAVINGS), improve the quality of patient care (CARE), and totally computerize the patient chart (COMPUTERIZE).

The theoretical definition of PDMS Effectiveness was developed: the degree to which the system has achieved these goals in terms of the experiences and perceptions of the nurses who interact with the system. A highly effective PDMS has a high degree of achievement for all goals.

PDMS Effectiveness was operationally defined through development of definitions and observable indicators for each goal, through specification of goal achievement criteria, and through establishment of the measure's objectives. Then items were written along with scoring and administration directions. Items were oriented to principles of data management in general. The goal was to use the cumulative score to determine system effectiveness, rather than asking explicitly about computer systems. A total of 79 items comprised the PDMS Effectiveness Measure.

4. Instrument Testing (Methods and Results)

Two critical care units with functioning PDMS and two medical-surgical units with no computer systems were the sites for instrument testing. The hospitals ranged from a university health center to a rural, community hospital. The sites were chosen to provide significant contrasts between units with PDMS and units without PDMS. A non-random sample of 71 nurses was obtained with an approximately equal distribution between the units. Two rounds of measure administrations were conducted with a six week interval between rounds.

There were no significant differences in demographic characteristics. There were significantly higher comfort levels with computers among the respondents from the critical care units.

The range of possible scores for the PDMS Effectiveness Measure was 79 to 395 if all items were answered. The total sample's range was 210 to 339 with a mean score of 272.24. The first critical care unit (Unit 1) had a range of 217 to 339 and a mean of 283.95. The second critical care unit (Unit 2) achieved a mean of 295.53 and a range of 264 to 329. The first medical-surgical unit (Unit 3) had a mean score of 260.35 and a range of 233 to 298. A mean score of 224.33 and a range of 210 to 260 was achieved by the second medical-surgical unit (Unit 4).

Most of Unit 1's scores and all of Unit 2's scores were in the upper half of the possible scoring range. Most of Unit 3's scores were also in the upper half of this range. Most of the scores for Unit 4 were at or below the halfway point of the possible range of scores. The systems for managing data in all of these units are at least moderately effective, and in the units with PDMS, they are very effective.

Measurement testing included assessment of: internal consistency via calculation of alpha coefficients; test-retest reliability through the Pearson Product Moment Correlation Coefficient; content validity with use of the content validity index (CVI); and construct validity through contrasted groups analysis. An *a priori* acceptance level was set at 0.62 for the internal consistency, test-retest, and content validity estimations. The analysis of contrasted groups employed an *a priori* significance level of .05.

Internal consistency reliability was estimated at .9098. Alpha coefficients for each PDMS goal sub-scale were as follows: ACCESS (.4215), CARE (.5048), DATA QUALITY (.5359), SAVINGS (.7337), ANALYZE (.6525), MANAGE (.7578), HELP (.7400), and COMPUTERIZE (.7263). Given the very acceptable alpha value for the measure as a whole, this range of coefficients for the sub-scales may indicate that they are not independent factors within the measure. That is, the individual goals cannot be measured separately, while the entire set of items do measure PDMS Effectiveness.

A Pearson's r of .8941 (p < .05) was calculated for test-retest reliability, indicating 79.9% agreement. For a new measure, this is a very good coefficient and indicates that the measure is stable over time. There were significant correlation (p < .005) for all subscales, with a range of .6087 to .8527.

Two nurses with PDMS expertise assessed content validity. They evaluated the relevancy of the measure's items to the content domain. From their responses, a CVI of 0.65 was calculated, indicating 65% agreement between the judges. While not robust, it is an acceptable value.

The differences in mean scores of the respondents from different units (contrasted groups analysis) were assessed via one-way analysis of variance (ANOVA). This analysis revealed significant differences among the units (F = 13.0760, p < .05). Tukey's HSD range test identified the two critical care units (with functioning PDMS) as the units with significantly higher PDMS Effectiveness scores.

5. Conclusions

The PDMS Effectiveness Measure is reliable and valid. It is able to discriminate differences in the effectiveness of data management systems among nursing units. The PDMS being used in the participating critical care units are nearly fully effective in reaching their design goals. The PDMS Effectiveness Measure has potential for use in studying the impact of computer-based information systems on clinical nursing practice.

References

[1] Milholland K. Patient Data Management Systems (PDMS) Computer Technology for Critical Care Nurses. *CIN* (1988) 6: 237–243.
[2] Cook M and McDowell W. Changing to An Automated Information System. *AJN* 1975, 75:46–51.
[3] Beckman E, Cammack B and Harris B. Observation on Computers in an Intensive Care Unit. *H&L* (1981) 10: 1055–1057.
[4] Diaz O and Haudenschild C. Implementation of an Integrated Critical Care Computer. In: *Computers in Critical Care and Pulmonary Medicine.* Nair, I. (ed). New York: Plenum Press (1983).
[5] Hilberman M, Kamm B, Tarter M and Osborn J. An Evaluation of Computer-based Patient Monitoring at Pacific Medical Center. *Computers and Biomedical Research* (1975) 8: 447–460.
[6] Tolbert S and Partuz A. Study Shows How Computerization Affects Nursing Activities in ICU. *Hospitals, J.A.H.A.* (1977) 51: 79–84.
[7] Miller J, Preston T, Dann P, Bailey J and Tobin G. Charting vs Computers in a Postoperative Cardiothoracic ITU. *Nursing Times* (1978) August 24: 1423–1425.

[8] Bradshaw KE, Setting DF, Gardner RM, Pryor TA and Budd M. Improving Efficiency and Quality in a Computerized ICU. In: *Proceedings of the Twelfth Annual Symposium on Computer Applications in Medical Care*. Greenes R.A. (ed). Los Angeles, CA: IEEE Computer Society (1988) 763–767.

[9] Suchman E. *Evaluative Research*. New York: Russel Sage Foundation (1967).

[10] Rutman L. *Evaluation Research Methods: A Basic Guide*. Beverly Hills: Sage Publications (1977).

[11] Waltz C, Strickland O and Lenz E. *Measurement in Nursing Research*. Philadelphia: F.A. Davis Company (1984).

37
Bedside Computerization of the ICU, Design Issues: Benefits of Computerization Versus Ease of Paper and Pen

RUBY GREWAL, JOYCE ARCUS, JOHNETTA BOWEN, KEVIN FITZPATRICK,
W.E. HAMMOND, LIZA HICKEY, and WILLIAM W. STEAD

History

In the mid 1980's the Surgical Intensive Care Unit (SICU) staff began searching for a bedside computer system. Their goal was to find a system that would create a computerized medical record, reduce the clerical burden on the staff and provide the necessary data for patient care and research in a unique and meaningful fashion. In the process, they hoped to reduce the time spent on documentation and to improve patient care. After evaluating the commercial products available on the market, the SICU staff determined that there were no "ready to go" products that would meet their needs and be able to interface with the Duke University Hospital Information System (DHIS). In the fall of 1987, the SICU staff approached the TMR staff with a proposal to develop a bedside computer system using TMR as the platform. TMR [1] is a comprehensive computer-based medical record system developed at the Duke University Medical Center (DUMC) in an evolutionary fashion over the past twenty years.

Introduction

Computerization can provide legible records, data accessibility from multiple locations, customized and sophisticated data displays, and data interpretation and decision support tools. Yet the success of a system depends on its ability to provide these benefits with minimal interaction from the users. The most difficult task in creating a computerized medical record is capturing data that cannot be obtained electronically. Human data entry is necessary to complete the on-line record, and the implications of this must

Reprinted with permission from *Proceedings: Fifteenth Annual Symposium on Computer Applications in Medical Care: Assessing the Value of Medical Informatics*, Clayton, P.D. (Ed.). 1991. Pp. 793–797. © 1992, American Medical Informatics Association: Bethesda, MD.

be understood. The computerized medical record that replaces the paper chart will be one that requires a minimal amount of data entry and provides functionality not available in the paper format. Paper and pen are both easy to use and flexible. Despite the many disadvantages of a paper record (illegible data, a single location of data, and inability to track data over time), it continues to be the preferred method of charting.

Environment Configuration

The sixteen SICU patient care rooms were redesigned to include a workstation outside of each room. The workstation was an alcove that contained a flat work area and a terminal on a raised movable arm. A window was placed so that the nurse could observe the patient from the work area. The patient rooms were wired to the microcomputer to allow for acquisition of data from bedside instrumentation. In addition, a terminal was placed in each of the two workrooms on the unit, and a line printer was placed in a central area. It is interesting to note that the line printer had a very negative effect on the user's perception of the system due to paper jams and noise. We later upgraded to two laser printers to replace the line printer. At the time, the nurses considered the upgrade to be the best thing that happened to the system, and overall appreciation of the system increased.

Passive Data Acquisition

The decision was made to begin building the computer record with data available electronically. The focus was on downloading data from DHIS and interfacing the hemodynamic monitors. Data to be acquired from DHIS included demographic data, admission/discharge/transfer (ADT) data, and laboratory results. The linkages between TMR and DHIS were developed taking advantage of the MAPS programs [2,3] developed at Duke. ADT type data is downloaded every 20 minutes, and laboratory results are downloaded every 5 minutes. The frequency of data acquisition was chosen based on the urgency of the necessity of the data and the CPU usage necessary to facilitate the download. It was felt that lab data should be transmitted as frequently as possible without affecting response time on the system. ADT data was not considered as critical and therefore was not downloaded as often. There is a single button push in the system that allows the user to initiate the ADT download between the 20 minute cycles. An issue that arose with the laboratory dealt with the staff having no means of knowing the last time data was downloaded for their patient. A message notifying the user of the last lab draw for which results had been downloaded was added. In addition, a buffer for new data was created. The user is informed when new data is available, and a display is used to show only the new data.

An interface was written to capture data from the Mennen Horizon 2000 hemodynamic monitor. Vital signs were captured at 5 minute intervals, and the data were compressed in hour intervals for charting purposes. Cardiac output and pulmonary wedge pressure values were also obtained and time was stamped when the nurse accepted the value on the Mennen monitor. The frequency of data acquisition was selected by determining the minimum frequency necessary to adequately capture trends. Recreating the alarming functionality provided by the monitors was not a goal. Evaluations were made for data capture at 1 minute intervals and at 5 minute intervals. The 1 minute intervals did not provide enough additional data to warrant the increased sampling rate [4]. Our original design generated a chart value for an hour by taking the 5 minute data for a given hour and time stamping the compressed value on the half hour. A study comparing the compressed value generated by the computer and the nurses' charted value showed that 63.2% of the diastolic pressures and 49.7% of the systolic pressures were within ± 2 mm Mg of the nurses' values. 86.8% of the diastolic pressures and 80.9% of the systolic pressures were within ± 5 mm Mg of the nurses' values. Nurses' charts on the hour and their values could be mapped more closely by changing the compression routine to take data from half hour to half hour and time stamping the values on the hour. We expect that our numbers will be better using the new compression routine.

Nursing Assessment

The nursing assessment was the first application design that required data entry. It was selected because it was the easiest block of data to remove from the paper flow sheet without disrupting the staff. The written assessment consisted of unstructured narrative evaluations of the patient's condition. The design of the nursing assessment began with formatting the assessment by defining the items that were to be assessed and the vocabulary that was to be used in this process. The development was done by a design committee made up of a group of nurses on the unit and members of the TMR and DHIS staffs. This process took countless meetings and lasted over two years. It was extremely time consuming to take an unstructured task and attempt to organize it in a logical and functional manner. The group organized charting requirements by body systems, utilizing a standard vocabulary. This information was then compiled by the TMR staff and entered in the TMR data dictionary to create the frames and subsequent sub-frames that would be accessed in the data entry mode. The data entry structure consists of a frame of major body systems or categories, each of which points to layers of coded evaluations and coded responses (fig. 1). The data is stored by shift and there is one assessment per shift. The current

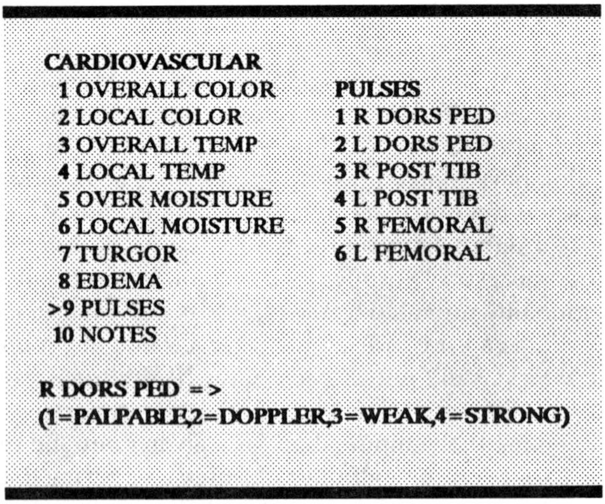

CARDIOVASCULAR
```
   1 OVERALL COLOR      PULSES
   2 LOCAL COLOR        1 R DORS PED
   3 OVERALL TEMP       2 L DORS PED
   4 LOCAL TEMP         3 R POST TIB
   5 OVER MOISTURE      4 L POST TIB
   6 LOCAL MOISTURE     5 R FEMORAL
   7 TURGOR             6 L FEMORAL
   8 EDEMA
  >9 PULSES
  10 NOTES


  R DORS PED = >
  (1=PALPABLE,2=DOPPLER,3=WEAK,4=STRONG)
```

FIGURE 1. Sample nursing Assessment data screen.

design includes the ability to preload the previous shift's assessment and check lists for common tasks; a hierarchial data structure which prompts for more specific data when appropriate, and areas for free text notes. The preload feature allows a nurse to electronically transcribe the previous nurse's assessment into the current assessment, thereby reducing a major portion of data entry. There are over 750 evaluations that can be made, and the assessment is continually growing and changing. In general, the data entry philosophy is data entry by exception.

Training and Implementation—Nursing Assessment

Nurses replaced their written notes with the computer generated notes in the winter of 1989. This event was preceded by extensive training, a portion of which was conducted by the TMR staff; the majority was done by the nurses. The TMR staff trained the nurses on the design committee. The committee members then trained the other nurses on the unit. They developed check-off sheets to track the staff's familiarity and levels of competence with different computer functions. A TMR test system was available for the nurses to practice entering assessments and to familiarize themselves with the different functionality. Having a test database gave the nurse the security that he/she was not corrupting the real database. New features under development are made available on the test system prior to being moved to production. The nursing staff has developed various levels of users. Work schedules were created so that a highly trained user is always available on each shift. An "expert" nursing staff member is also on call during the night shift, and it is an "expert" user that decides when it is necessary to call the TMR staff.

The on-line assessment was initially turned on room by room so that nurses could adapt to the new system. Double documentation was not required in any phase of this implementation. Nurses could also voluntarily enter their assessments on-line. By the time the eighth room was scheduled to come on-line, the nurses had voluntarily turned on all sixteen rooms. Currently, we are in the process of redesigning the data entry screens to place more selections on a screen at once and to reduce the number of screen changes required. The training procedure that was developed is taken advantage of whenever new functions come on-line. New nurses become familiar with the system within their first shift on the unit and nurses from other units in the hospital are often brought in on a temporary basis without any major problems.

Timing Studies—Nursing Assessment

Initial studies show that there is a slight time savings with the computerized note and that there is a significant increase in the amount of data being collected. The average assessment ranges between 180–350 evaluations depending on patient acuity [5]. An initial assessment may take a trained nurse anywhere from 10 to 15 minutes out of a 12 hour shift. Updates are made as needed. The success of the computerized assessment can be linked to the time savings associated with the preload feature and with the immediate familiarity the nurse gains with the patient's case. It can also be associated with the fact that prompted data entry is easier than pages of handwritten narratives. It is important to note that some habits can not be changed. Nurses that previously wrote very detailed narrative assessments tend to have longer, more complete computerized assessment. These nurses also tend to overuse the free text capability in the system. It is important for the nurses to have this flexibility and not feel limited by the system.

Computer Use—Lack of Expected Dependence

By early 1990, the SICU TMR record contained patient demographics, laboratory results, vital signs, a problem list, and nursing assessments. There was not a reliance on the system as a whole, although there was a dependence on the computer system for the nursing assessment functionality. The remaining data was still available on the paper flow sheet, and it was reviewed there. Reasons why the SICU staff weren't using the computer included that the data was considered to be harder to access in the computer, the displays were not fast enough, or the data was not in the format in which the staff was accustomed to viewing it. Clearly it was easier

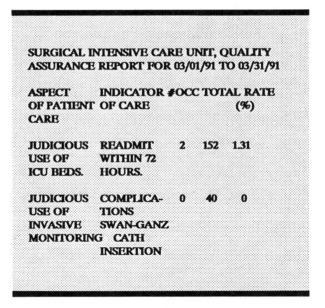

FIGURE 2. Sample segment of monthly QA report.

and faster to pick up a flow sheet, glance in the area that contained the desired data and review the data. It was evident that the system would need another level of redesign before a reliance on the system would develop.

In the spring of 1990, the redesign of the displays and access to those displays was completed. In addition, multiple new reports were added to the system. Two reports of significance were the rounding summary and the quality assurance (QA) report. Rounding summaries contain basic demographic data, a problem/procedure list, vital signs and selected lab results. These reports are printed prior to morning rounds and can now be found in the coat pocket of all physicians on the unit. Physicians will complain if the report does not print or if data is missing (suggesting that the computer chart has made a mark), but the extent to which they depend on the data is still being studied. The second report was a QA report that took advantage of data from the nursing assessments and combined it with admission and laboratory data. It is generated prior to rounds on a daily basis and monthly for administrative purposes. The QA reporting has been growing and the latest addition was problem specific concurrent QA definitions (fig. 2).

Paperless Experiment

With the new displays and reports in place, it was decided to remove laboratory data from the paper flow sheet. With the willingness of the staff, laboratory results were no longer transcribed on the flow sheet. There are an average of 90 lab results downloaded on each patient per day. The time savings in the transcription of that data should have proven to be beneficial. Instead chaos broke out, due to situations that were never anticipated. It began with the fact that DHIS could go down for long periods of time and thus render the computer record incomplete until DHIS was available again. The nurse was calling the lab and writing results on a scrap of paper (or back on the flow sheet). The location of the data was split between the computer record and the reintroduced paper record. Downtime was further complicated when the Cerner lab system was installed at Duke. With the installation of Cerner, lab orders went from DHIS to Cerner, and results went from Cerner to DHIS, and finally to TMR. Cerner and DHIS nightly downtimes were not synchronized, so the night staff on SICU was left without lab results on TMR through both the systems' downtimes. Other complications included nurses getting stat lab results over the phone, treating the patients based on those results, and then realizing that the results were not the values entered into the lab computer system and finally passed to TMR. The lab had corrected the results prior to the data entry step. The paper system allowed for this type of situation but the computer path was never aware of the existence of the incorrect result. Our experiment ended as the laboratory results went back on the flow sheet. New lab data reviews, trend analyses, and unique comparisons were done on-line. Often a nurse actually looked at the computer for new lab results and then transcribed them onto the flow sheet.

The downtime of DHIS and Cerner was synchronized and changes were made to speed up the availability of results. Our proposal to deal with the call-in values is to enter them in the nursing note along with the treatment given. Lab results will be removed when the paper flowsheet is replaced with the electronic record.

Respiratory Therapy

A data entry routine similar to the nursing assessment was developed for the respiratory therapists on the unit. The data entry routine included coded variables wherever possible, and also provided a feature to accept the previous settings in order to eliminate repetitive data entry. It was necessary to design a validation and electronic signature routine for the therapists because the therapists rotate patients and duties throughout the day, and because the therapists are not available when the chart copy of the respiratory therapy is generated. The validation and signature step required the therapist to enter his/her TMR username and password, review all the data for a given time and then accept that data. Validated data could not be modified. In the design of the electronic signature, a representative of the Risk Management department was brought in to approve of our implementation. The therapists began charting in the computer and generating a daily respiratory therapy summary. The system was successful in doubling the therapists' documentation time on the unit. They first walked into the patient room, wrote the respiratory parameters on a scrap of paper; then they walked to the terminal and entered their results, and finally they validated the current data. Having the respiratory data available on-line was an obvious benefit, but unfortunately it was not worth the effort required on the part of the therapists. It was determined that if the computer was interfaced to the ventilator, the system could chart respiratory data at regular intervals and that the therapist could then append any additional data and validate the electronically acquired results. The later scenario would both reduce the documentation burden on the therapist and make the results available as part of the computer record. The Puritan Benett 7200 ventilator was interfaced and data was collected at hourly intervals as well as on demand, thus allowing ventilator settings to be captured when a specific procedure was performed (e.g., an ABG blood sample was drawn).

Completion of the Computerized Chart

The majority of the data available in the system was acquired passively from DHIS and bedside instrumentation. Other than the nursing assessment, we had not required the staff to do much data entry. The decision was made to replace the whole flow sheet, not just sections of it. This meant that intake/output (I/O) data and medication data needed to be charted on-line, and that hemodynamic data acquired from the monitors had to be validated. Currently we are finishing this phase of the design stage of our implementation.

The design of the I&O data entry screens began with the nurses. Initial requirements included the ability to enter results for multiple hours at once, the ability to create an I/O profile from a list of over one hundred possible choices, and automatic calculations of subtotals and a running balance. As prototypes were made available, it became obvious that the ability to indicate quickly that the volume delivered was the same as the previous hour, and the interfacing to infusion control devices and electronic urimeters would be beneficial. Both devices have been interfaced, and data acquired electronically is validated by the nurse by entering a username and password, selecting the appropriate times, reviewing data for that time period, and then validating it. In order to acquire intake data correctly from the infusion devices, the nurse is required to identify the pump and the fluid running through the pump. I/O documentation on the paper flow sheet required the nurse to list all intakes and outputs once a day, to make an entry on the flow sheet when necessary, and to calculate a running balance. Data entry of I/O data requires the nurse to select the I/O data entry function, update the list of intakes and outputs when an item is added or deleted, move the cursor to correct position on the screen, and enter a value. Although data entry is slightly more cumbersome than the flow sheet method, it was determined that the calculated balances and review features would make the computer desirable.

Documenting medications on the flow sheet involved writing the name and strength of the medication at the beginning of the shift and then making the appropriate tick mark or notation when a medication was given, not given, or given at a different dosage. Because a data entry routine could not be as efficient as the flow sheet, there is very little motivation to enter medications other than to complete the computer record. One solution would be to download pharmacy data from DHIS. Unfortunately, most medications are given before the paper trail is completed and the data is available on DHIS. Another problem is that the Duke Unified Medical Language (DUML) that allows systems to identify uniquely laboratory results does not contain pharmacy information as of yet. Other more general design issues deal with the ability to step through the computerized medical record efficiently. A nurse who had entered data on a fairly specified evaluation in the nursing assessment should not have to step backward through the previous screens to exit that function and begin a new one (an hourly I/O entry, for example). With 1 or 2 keystrokes, the nurse should be able to switch functions and enter the I/O data. A new intern who walks up to a terminal that was left in a nursing function should be able, with 1 or 2 keystrokes, to get to a menu that he/she is familiar with and then get to the data of interest. A patient overview should be the default screen of the system. This provides the users a summary of the patient's conditions without any interaction whatsoever. The user should be able to access the detailed information with minimal effort. The design changes over the past three years have shown that a cumbersome or awkward flow will cause the system to fail, regardless of how rich the data in the system may be.

Conclusion

Some of the lessons we have learned up to now include the fact that an insignificant change to a developer may actually be a major improvement to the user. It is important to understand the interaction between different systems and functions, and the effects they have on each other. But most importantly, one must acquire data directly from the source whenever possible, and wherever possible, this should be done electronically. The design of a data entry routine should never require the user to make an effort without some sort of payback. The time required in data entry should be given back to the user by making some other task less time consuming. The flow of the system must be easy and consistent. Data should be available in flexible and meaningful displays. Once all the necessary data is available in the bedside system, much can be done to pay back the user for his/her efforts. Alerts, work lists and careplans, and expanded QA functions are just a few examples of the advantages of a computerized medical record.

The benefits of computerization can not be realized until there is a complete medical record available on-line—there is a dependence on that data.

Acknowledgment. This work was supported in part by the National Library of Medicine Grant G08LM04613, awarded by the National Institutes of Health, Department of Health and Human Services.

References

1. Stead, W.W., Hammond, W.E.: Computer-based Medical Records: The Centerpiece of TMR. MD Computing 5:48–62, 1988.
2. Kirby, J.D., Pickett, M.A., Boyarsky, M.W., Stead, W.W.: Distributed Processing with a Mainframe-based Hospital Information System: A Generalized Solution. Proceedings of the Eleventh Annual Symposium on Computer Applications in Medical Care (IEEE) 1987. 764–770.
3. Hammond, W.E., Grewal, R., Straube, M.J., Stead, W.W.: Networking Data Sources for Intensive Care Monitoring. Proceedings. Eighth Annual AAMSI Congress 1989. 227–281.
4. Veltman, G.: Comparison of Pulmonary Arterial Pressure Recordings. Student Project 1990.
5. Minda, S.: Manual & Computer Recorded Nursing Assessments. Masters Thesis 1990.

38
Using the Actigraph to Measure Activity-Rest in the Acute Care Setting

E.M. Wykpisz, N.S. Redeker, D.J. Mason, and B. Glica

1. Introduction

Patterns of activity-rest, are of central importance in acute care nursing. Alterations in activity-rest may be symptomatic of disease. Activity-rest patterns "can play significant roles in the prevention, cause, and alleviation of fatigue,"[1,p.192] a common symptom of illness and treatment. Improvement in activity is an important component of recovery and quality of life.[2,3] Studies have shown that an improvement in activity after surgery is related to greater perceived health status and enhancement in quality of life.[4,5] Redeker, Mason, Wykpisz, Glica, and Miner[6] found that rhythm and positive linear trend in activity predicted self-reports of dysfunction and length of stay in women who had undergone coronary artery bypass surgery. In another study[7], adherence to the critical path for activity was an important determinant of length of hospital stay in coronary bypass patients.

There has been relatively little systematic research into the outcomes of activity or its use as an intervention, and few instruments available to objectively measure activity. Researchers have relied on subjective methods, such as observation and questionnaires, or polysomnography, which is cumbersome and expensive, to measure sleep. None of these methods allows continuous measurement of the complete activity spectrum.[8,9] Recent advances in electronic technology and computers have made objective measurement of activity-rest practical in the acute care setting.

Reprinted from *Nursing Informatics: An International Overview for Nursing in a Technological Era*, Grobe, S.J., Pluyter-Wenting, E.S.P. (Eds.). 1994. Pp. 484–490, with kind permission from Elsevier Science—NL, Sara Burgerhartstraat 25, 1055 KV Amsterdam, The Netherlands.

2. Wrist Actigraph

The wrist actigraph or motionlogger[(tm)], distributed by Ambulatory Monitoring, Inc., Ardsley, New York, is an electronic accelerometer. It senses motion via a ceramic bimorph beam arranged to generate a signal or charge when subjected to the force of acceleration; it processes and quantifies the sensed motion over a pre-programmed period of time; and stores that information. It operates on a lithium battery that is easily replaced and can last from days to weeks. Two forms of the motionlogger are available: the 16K actigraph (2.5 × 3.5 × .75 inch; weight 3 ounces) and the 32K Mini-Motionlogger (about the size of a divers' watch –1.5 × 1.3 × .375 inch; weight 2 ounces). Both actigraphs produce equivalent measurements and have event markers that allow marking of the activity record to note timing of events, such as preparation for sleep, onset of specific activities, or symptoms.

The actigraph is sensitive to movement ranging from 0.05 to 0.10 g ($g = 9.81$ meters/second^2) at sea level and senses movement in three dimensions. Two units of measurement are produced: The zero crossing mode counts the number of times that the displacement of the sensor beam generates sufficient voltage to cross a pre-set zero point during a pre-programmed epoch of time. The threshold mode indicates the amount of time per epoch that activity above a certain threshold is sensed. Units of measure in the threshold mode are seconds of activity per epoch length of time, while units of measure in the zero-crossing mode are number of movements/epoch of time. Use of the threshold mode is helpful for eliminating fine movement, such as tremors, or vibrations from an automobile.[8,10] The zero crossing mode is used for general activity monitoring and is required for use with available sleep algorithms. The motionlogger contains a microcomputer that permits programming of start-stop times, data collection intervals, or epochs, and storage of data.

3. Reliability and Validity

The motionlogger is highly reliable and valid. Reliability is demonstrated by the virtually identical measurements produced by recording the repeated swings of a laboratory pendulum. Validity is determined by comparing the decay in the amplitude of the pendulum swing with the data recorded by the actigraph.[10] Validity in healthy human subjects was demonstrated in a recent series of studies.[11] In the first study, fifteen healthy, young adult males and females wore actigraphs on the non-dominant wrist while performing a set of non-sedentary and a set of sedentary activities. Differences between actigraph counts among treadmill levels and speeds and among two levels of stair stepping were statistical significant ($p < .0001$). Differences among various sedentary activities were also significant ($p < .0001$). Although overall differences between actigraph counts for the sets of sedentary and non-sedentary counts were statistically significant, the author noted that sedentary activity requiring a great deal of wrist activity (eg. playing video games) produced higher activity counts than knee bends or stair stepping. This finding highlights the importance of considering the site of attachment when planning activity studies or interpreting the results. The authors also found that average and high levels of activity computed from an activity diary were correlated with activity counts ($r = .81$ and $r = .80$, respectively, $p < .0001$). The 16K actigraph has also been reported to have higher subject acceptability than an activation-deactivation checklist.[12]

The actigraph has been shown to be a valid measure of sleep in the sleep laboratory and in health persons. Computerized programs for calculating sleep parameters from actigraphic data have been developed. Most recently, Cole, et al.[13] reported that their sleep algorithm distinguished nocturnal sleep parameters from wakefulness (as defined by polysomnography) approximately 88% of the time. Actigraphic sleep percentage and sleep latency estimates were correlated $r = .82$ and $r = .90$, respectively, with parameters obtained from polysomnograms ($p < .0001$). Several researchers have reported that actigraphy overestimated sleep time.[13,14] However, this may be due to methods of scoring of polysomnography and the presence of a sleep onset spectrum.[10]

4. Site of Attachment

Site of attachment will influence the type of data obtained.[10] The actigraph can be used on the wrist, waist, ankle, or trunk. Webster et al.[15] compared the sites of attachment of a piezo-ceramic accelerometer over 22 nights of activity recording. They found that the non-dominant wrist reflected the greatest amount of bodily activity. This site has become the standard site for distinguishing sleep/wake and activity using actigraphy.

5. Downloading of Data

Data are retrieved, and the motionlogger is programmed through an interface unit that connects to an IBM compatible personal computer. Action(tm) software is available from Ambulatory Monitoring Inc., Ardsley, N.Y. This DOS-based program is used to manipulate and partition data; calculate descriptive statistics; perform sleep analysis; and graphically display and print the data. In addition, the software is used to initialize the actigraph. A more advanced program, Action3(tm) performs full and daily cosinor analysis, autocorrelation, cross-correlation, and maximum entropy spectral analysis and multiple channels for graphically displaying and printing the data, allowing multiple parameters to be assessed simultaneously. Although marketed for use with the Actillume(tm), Action3 can be used with data obtained from motion loggers.

6. Uses of Actigraphy

Actigraphs have been used in a variety of populations, including patients with sleep disorders, children with attention deficit disorders, adult psychiatric patients, and patients involved in drug studies. Tryon[10] provides a detailed review of these studies. To our knowledge, our study of activity

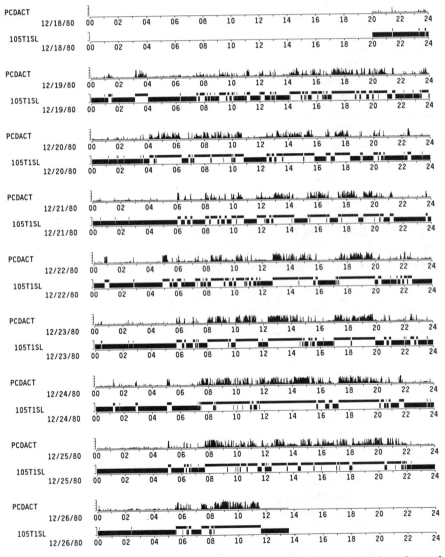

FIGURE 1. Seven day data obtained from one subject using wrist actigraphy and Action3 software.

patterns and levels in women who had undergone CABS is the first use of the actigraph in adult surgical patients. The implications of using actigraphy in critical care have been described previously.[16]

Figure 1 presents data obtained with the motion-logger actigraph and the Action3 Software program on one female CABS patient for one week from the immediate post-operative period to hospital discharge. The channel labeled "PCDACT" displays the raw activity data, measured in one minute epochs, the standard epoch length used for sleep scoring. The lower channel for each day of recording displays sleep scoring for the activity data. The scale to the left of the activity bar (Y axis) indicates activity counts. Each horizontal mark indicates 100 counts of data. The X axis, ranging from 0 to 24 indicates hours of the day. The data presented have been reduced to fit on one page. However, larger data plots are available to allow more detailed inspection of data. Evident in this display is this subjects' increase in daytime activity over the course of the week and consolidation of sleep during the night time hours as the week progresses.

7. Advantages of the Wrist Actigraph

The actigraph provides continuous, objective data on activity-rest. Measurement of the relative decrease in motion associated with sleep can be incorporated into the assessment of 24 hour rhythms and patterns as patients progress through stages of recovery and move from critical care to medical-surgical settings, and then are discharged to the home environment.

The actigraph requires minimal subject attention to data collection, an attribute of particular importance in patients who are beginning to return to normal patterns of ambulation and self-care, but may be experiencing pain, fatigue, and emotional distress. Many of the women in our study[6] preferred the 32K to the 16K motionlogger because of its smaller size and lighter weight. The unobtrusive and non-restrictive nature of the actigraph is a factor that prevents interference with post-operative activity progression such as might occur when using a larger device, direct observation, or a device involving wiring or leads (i.e., polysomnography).

The actigraph requires little manipulation by the research team, aside from initialization and downloading. The nursing staff and research team were vigilant about noting that subjects were wearing the actigraphs throughout the study period, to guard against loss. Nurses were also in-structed to avoid using the non-dominant wrist for intravenous catheter insertion. If that was impossible, actigraphs were moved further up the forearm or placed on the dominant wrist. Patients were instructed not to immerse the device in water while bathing, to guard against water damage.

8. Disadvantages of the Wrist Actigraph

The primary disadvantage of the actigraph is its cost. Currently the interface unit is listed at a cost of $4000.00. Each actigraph is $2100.00.

We experienced some data loss because of moisture accumulation inside the actigraph due to environmental humidity and perspiration. Since the completion of our study, Ambulatory Monitoring, Inc. has upgraded the device to provide a better seal against moisture. Several subjects also complained of perspiration underneath the arm band. This problem can be solved by placement of a gauze pad or terry cloth athletic wristband between the actigraph and the skin.

9. Summary

The actigraph is an effective, reliable, and valid means of measuring activity in the acute medical-surgical setting. It has the potential to greatly enhance knowledge of activity-rest patterns. The use of this new technology, along with computer hardware and the software described, will lead to the development of new knowledge that will result in more effective means of promoting recovery and quality of life in patients recovering from illness and surgery.

References

[1] Piper BF. Fatigue: Current bases for practice. In SG Funk, EM Tournquist, MT Champagne, LA Copp, & RA Wiese (Eds.). *Key Aspects of Recovery: Management of Pain, Fatigue, and Nausea* (pp. 187–198). New York: Springer, 1989.
[2] Andreoli KG. Key aspects of recovery. In SG Funk, EM Tornquist, MT Champagne, LA Copp, & R Wiese (Eds.). *Key Aspects of Recovery: Improving Nutrition, Rest and Mobility* (pp. 22–31). New York: Springer, 1990.
[3] Schron EB and Shumaker SA. The integration of health quality of life in clinical research: Experience from cardiovascular clinical trials. *Prog Cardiovasc Nurs* 1992, 7:21–28.
[4] Allen JK, Becker DM and Swank RT. Factors related to functional status after coronary artery bypass surgery. *Heart Lung* 1990, 19:49–55.
[5] Permanyer-Miralda G, Alonso J, Anto JM, Alijardo-Guimera M and Solen-Solen J. Comparison of perceived health status-conventional functional evaluation in stable patients with coronary artery disease. *Qual Life Coronary Dis* 1990, 12:779–786.
[6] Redeker N, Mason DJ, Wykpisz EM, Glica B and Miner C. Activity patterns, mood, and recovery in women after coronary artery bypass surgery: The first post-operative week. Manuscript in review.
[7] Strong A and Sneed NV. Clinical evaluation of a critical path for coronary artery bypass surgery patients. *Progr Cardiovasc Nurs* 1991, 6:29–37.
[8] Mason DJ and Redeker N. Measurement of activity. *Nurs Res* 1993, 42:87–92.

[9] Redeker NS and Mason DJ. Perspectives on Activity. Manuscript in review.
[10] Tryon WW. *Activity Measurement in Psychology and Medicine*. New York: Plenum, 1991.
[11] Patterson SM, Krantz DS, Montgomery LC, Deuster PA, Hedges SM and Nebel LE. Automated physical activity monitoring: Validation and comparison with physiological and self-report measures. *Psychophysiology* 1993, 30:296–305.
[12] Mason DJ and Tapp W. Measuring circadian rhythms: Actigraph versus activation checklist. *West J Nurs Res* 1992, 14:358–379.
[13] Cole RJ, Kripke DK, Gruen W, Mullaney DJ and Gillin JC. Automatic sleep/wake identification from Wrist Activity. *Sleep* 1992, 5:461–469.
[14] Mullaney DJ, Kripke DF and Messin S. Wrist-actigraphic estimation of sleep time. *Sleep* 1980, 3:83–92.
[15] Webster JB, Messin S, Mullaney DJ and Kripke DF. Transducer design and placement for activity recording. *Med Biol Engineering Comput* 1982, 20:741–744.
[16] Redeker NS, Mason DJ, Wykpisz EM and Glica B. Using the wrist actigraph to measure activity in critical care. Abstract presented for the National Critical Care Nursing Research Conference, May 1993.

39
Expert Systems: Automated Decision Support for Clinical Nursing Practice

ANN WARNOCK-MATHERON

Introduction

In recent years, rapid advances in data processing technology have made available new tools to assist in decision making. The more powerful of these tools rely on artificial intelligence (AI) techniques to extend and augment the problem solving capabilities of the user. The questions facing our profession are whether or not these tools are applicable to clinical nursing practice and, if so, how we should proceed in integrating them into clinical nursing practice. This paper will focus on one of these tools, expert systems, and its relation to clinical nursing practice. In particular, it addresses within this context:

The current state of expert systems and the nursing knowledge base,
The use of nursing models in expert system development,
The role of the Clinical Nurse Specialist in the development of expert systems, and
The ethical and legal considerations in the applications of expert systems.

To assess the applicability of artificial intelligence and expert systems, we must first have a clear understanding of what these tools are, the benefits that they can provide, and the limitations to their use. We must also be cognizant of any factors in our profession which may constrain our use of this technology.

Artificial Intelligence

The advent, in the mid-nineteenth century, of machines that could be preprogrammed to act independent of human intervention gave rise to the question if whether or not machines could think. In 1842, Lady Lovelace,

Reprinted with permission from *Proceedings of Nursing and Computers: the Third International Symposium on Nursing Use of Computers and Information Science*; pp. 492–505. Daly, N. & Hannah, K.J. (Eds.). 1988. St. Louis: The C.V. Mosby Company.

commenting on Charles Babbage's Analytical Engine, stated that it was incapable to thought since it had "no pretensions to originate anything. It can do whatever we know how to order it to perform." Turing (1950) suggested that rather than addressing whether machines can think, the question should be whether machines can exhibit behavior indistinguishable from that of a human. In 1956, a conference was held, at Dartmouth College, which had as its theme the simulation of human intelligence by computers. The term "artificial intelligence" originated with this conference and is used to describe "computer programs which exhibit behavior that we call 'intelligent behavior' when we observe it in human beings" (Feigenbaum & Feldman, 1963, p. 3).

A common variation of Lady Lovelace's statement is that computer generated results for a given set of input parameters are entirely predetermined by the program and that this is a limitation to the capabilities of the computer. While this is often desirable or essential, our experience has taught us that this is neither always true nor that it needs to be a limitation. The fallacy of this view is succinctly explained by Feigenbaum & Feldman (1963) who find that

> it is wrong to conclude that a computer can exhibit behavior no more intelligent than its human programmer and that this astute gentleman can accurately predict the behavior of his program. These conclusions ignore the enormous complexity of information processing possible in problem-solving and learning machines. ... And, more importantly, they presume that he can perform the same complex information processing operations equally well with the device within his skull. (p. 4)

Thus, if we are able to instruct the computer on how to solve a complex problem, it is not only feasible that it will derive the solution but that the solution will be arrived at faster and that it may be a better solution.

The unique aspect of artificial intelligence is that the programs are heuristic as opposed to deterministic or algorithmic, that is, the programs "learn" from their experience. Whereas traditional programs are algorithmic and will, given the same set of inputs, always produce the same answer, a heuristic program may produce different answers for the same inputs as its "experience" or knowledge base increases. The answers given by a program utilizing artificial intelligence are not necessarily "correct" but are the ones most optimal or acceptable given the status of the knowledge base at that time. Like a human, it can only work with what it knows. This has significant legal and ethical implications which will be discussed later.

What Are Expert Systems?

Expert systems are a branch of artificial intelligence dealing with the capture, representation, and application of human knowledge and experience with the objective of allowing the computer to make decisions based on an imitation of human reasoning. As the name implies, expert systems attempt to duplicate the role of a human expert in a particular subject area. It is this quality which distinguishes them within the broader category of decision support systems. Where decision support systems generally follow very specific rules in solving problems, expert systems attempt to incorporate the experience and rules-of-thumb employed by the human expert.

Brennan (1986) defines a decision support system as an "automated system that capitalizes on the skills of the nurse and the computer to solve problems that neither could solve alone" (p. 51). By this definition, a decision support system may be as simple as a system which allows for fast retrieval of information, a more complex modelling program which allows the user to assess the impact of certain action, or an extremely advanced system which advises the user as to what the problem is and how to rectify it. It is to this latter class that expert systems belong. "What distinguishes the expert system field is that in addition to rules, the diagnoses call for general and specific knowledge, tricks of the trade, exceptions, reasonable guesses, and reasoning from partial knowledge" (Peat, 1988, p. 81).

The main components found in most expert systems are:

1. A knowledge base consisting of
   facts
   relationships
   methodologies
   rules of thumb
   performance goals
   reasoning procedures
2. A knowledge acquisition mechanism
3. An inference engine which performs
   diagnosis
   data validation
   consistency analysis
   violation detection
   decision simulation
   pattern recognition, and
4. A user interface system (Tou, 1985).

Using the components described above, an expert system should be able to:

Solve complex problems that a human expert would be able to solve
Propose Solutions based on incomplete knowledge
Explain how the solution was derived
Elicit, structure and transfer knowledge
Integrate new knowledge into its knowledge base
Communicate with the user in a natural language manner (Walker, 1986)

Early expert systems attempted to provide a generalized system for solving many different problems. While theoretically possible, difficulties in implementation led Feigenbaum & McCorduck (1983) to propose that, in practice, separate systems be used for specific types of problems. In other words, unique expert systems should be constructed for solving problems in specific, well-defined areas of knowledge. Each area of interest has its own knowledge base and its own procedures for solving problems. Davis (1984) recommends that expert systems be used only in areas:

Which are mainly cognitive
Which are well-defined
Which have recognized experts
Which can be taught to novices
Where the performance of expert is better than that of the novice
Which have problems which experts can solve in minutes or hours
Which require no common sense or value judgments

Currently, there are numerous expert system shells commercially available. These are systems which provide the tools or mechanisms necessary to perform the four basic functions described above. It is left to the end user to define the knowledge base and the inference/recognition rules required. Thus, we have the tools but can we, or should we, utilize these tools in nursing practice? To answer this question, we must first conduct an introspective analysis of our profession.

The Nursing Knowledge Base

The prerequisites for the development of expert systems are a clearly defined knowledge base and an in-depth understanding of both the decisions required and the procedure that are used to make these decisions. Clinical knowledge has been described as "that knowledge embedded in the practice of nursing" (Benner & Wrubel, 1982, p. 11). The development of conceptual models, descriptions of what we do, is the initial step in formalizing clinical practice. However the lack of a single, unifying conceptual model for nursing practice highlights the diversity of views and practices currently found. Ozbolt (1986) describes lack of agreement regarding the domain of nursing knowledge and the nature of nursing decisions as a major obstacle to the formalization of nursing knowledge and decision-making.

It has been suggested that nursing practice, with the exception of some very restricted and narrowly defined areas, has not been (Ozbolt, 1986), or cannot be (Benner, 1982; Benner, 1983), adequately formalized to the extent required for building an expert system. Further, Benner & Tanner (1987) contend that intuition, defined as "understanding without a rationale" (p. 23), is a significant attribute of the expert nurse and that it is not possible to formalize the processes associated with intuition. In other words, they suggest that there are aspects to clinical practice which we are unable to describe in terms of formal processes and which, therefore, cannot be reduced to the set of rules, facts, and relationships utilized by expert systems.

The unmistakable conclusion that one reaches is that currently we do not have a clear, overall understanding of our profession and that our knowledge base is still developing. However, there are specific areas that are well-defined and which satisfy Davis' (1984) criteria.

The Role of the Clinical Nurse Specialist

Clearly, by definition, for an expert system to be feasible, there must exist individuals who are recognized as experts in the discipline which the expert system can emulate. Although the role of the Clinical Nurse Specialist (CNS) is still being defined, Hamric (1983) states that there is an acceptance that "the CNS is an expert clinical practitioner in a specialized area of nursing" (p. 40). Butler (1985) identifies one requirement for the development of expert systems in nursing as nurses "who are experts in their chosen specialized areas of knowledge" (p. 312). As such, the CNS is ideally suited to participate in the development of expert systems.

Ethical and Legal Considerations

The lack of fully operational expert systems related to nursing practice has minimized the need for nursing to carefully discuss and scrutinize the legal and ethical implications. However, it can be expected that these will not be all that different from those applied to medical expert systems. Adams & Gray (1987), in discussing medical expert systems, pose the following questions:

1. Who is responsible for injury caused by following the advice/directions of an expert system?
2. What theory of liability should be applied?
3. If an expert system is available, is the practioner negligent if he or she does not utilize it?

As stated earlier, expert systems do not always provide a correct answer. Unfortunately, an attitude prevalent throughout society is that if the computer produces the answer, it must be true. Where this may be valid for algorithmic systems, blindly acting upon or following the answers generated by an expert system may have detrimental or injurious results. How the legal system will respond in this situation has still to be answered. It is questionable whether current laws regarding liability are able to cover this eventuality. Under the principles of strict liability, a product must be suited for its intended purpose. However, most products do not "learn" or gain knowledge over time. At what point in time is an expert system "suited" for its intended purpose? What is the intended purpose? It is self-evident that an expert system with a minimal knowledge base is unsuited for any purpose other than developing a knowledge base. It is also self-evident that an expert system having a complete knowledge base must be suited for its purpose but that this goal is unattainable. Within these two extremes lies a gray area that the legal system has yet to explore.

In practice, the user of an expert system is caught in a double bind. What are the legal consequences where a nurse has used her own judgment instead of the advice offered by an available expert system and this course of action has resulted in injury? Particularly if the course of action recommended by the expert system proved to be the better. For the user of the system, the question becomes when is the system competent as opposed to incompetent?

The Application of Expert Systems to Clinical Practice

In most situations where expert systems are utilized, it is feasible for the user to sit down at a terminal and interact with the system. The nature of clinical nursing may make it impractical for the nurse to leave the bedside and review a problem using an expert system. This suggests that the practical applications of expert systems within clinical practice are restricted to those activities that can be conducted away from the patient. Possible applications are in the development of care plans, the providing of education, the confirmation of actions to be taken, and the recommendation of particular courses of action. In general, any situation where assistance is required either in making or in reviewing the validity of a decision may be considered. It must be stressed, however, that an expert system does not replace the decision-making responsibility of the nurse, it is only a means of obtaining another opinion.

Expert systems are particularly useful in the transfer of knowledge. Where the expert reviews and selects the solutions available almost without conscious effort, it is often difficult to explain to a novice the reasoning performed. The ability of the expert system to explain the rationale of how the solution was derived provides an invaluable tool for teaching the process followed in selecting the solution.

Conclusion

Perhaps the desire seemingly expressed by Ozbolt (1986), for an expert system which encompasses as much as possible of the nursing knowledge base, and the pessimism of Benner & Tanner (1987), that intuition prohibits us from utilizing expert systems, are the two extremes of the spectrum of possibilities open to us. The development of a single expert system which encompasses all of nursing may be an impractical task. As suggested by Feigenbaum & McCorduck (1983) and Davis (1984), it may be more practical to direct our energies to developing expert systems which deal with specific areas and practices for which we have been able to develop conceptual models.

The utilization of expert systems in clinical nursing practice opens the door to a greater understanding of our profession. However, the introduction of expert systems is not without its risks and costs. Obstacles are numerous. According to Davis (1984), the development of a "substantial expert system with real performance takes at least five man-years of effort, assuming the team already has some background in artificial-intelligence problem-solving techniques" (p. 27). The role of the Clinical Nurse Specialist, whom we see as playing a crucial part in the development of expert systems for nursing, is still being developed. We are still discussing the nature and practice of nursing. The ethical and legal implications are still to be defined. However, these obstacles are not insurmountable. The solutions to some of these problems are a natural outgrowth of the development of our profession.

The major benefits of using expert systems are obtained through the structuring and acquisition of knowledge required in clinical practice. The development of an expert system forces us to analyze and document the activities we perform and how we perform these activities. In this manner, it broadens our knowledge and understanding of our profession.

References

Adams, E. S. & Gray, M. W. (1987). Strict liability for the malfunction of a medical expert system. In W. Stead (Ed.), *The Eleventh Annual Symposium on Computers in Medical Care* (pp. 93–99). Los Angeles: IEEE Computer Society Press.

Benner, P. & Tanner, C. (1987). How expert nurses use intuition. *American Journal of Nursing, 87*(1), 23–31.

Benner, P. (1982). From novice to expert. *American Journal of Nursing, 82*(3), 402–407.

Benner, P. (1983). Uncovering the knowledge embedded in clinical practice. *Image: The Journal of Nursing Scholarship. SV*(2), 36–41.

Benner, P. & Wrubel, J. (1982). Skilled clinical knowledge: The value of perceptual awareness. *Nurse Educator, VII*(3), 11–17.

Brennan, P. (1986). DSS – A meaning behind the buzz (guest viewpoint). *Computers in Nursing, 4*(2), 51, 96.

Butler, E. A. (1985). A direction for nursing expert systems. In K. Hannah, E. Guillemin & D. Conklin (Eds.), *Nursing uses of computer and information science* (pp. 309–313). Amsterdam: Elsevier Science.

Davis, R. (1984). Amplifying expertise with expert systems. In P. H. Winston & K. A. Prendergast (Eds.), *The AI business: Commercial uses of artificial intelligence* (pp. 17–40). Massachusetts: The MIT Press.

Feigenbaum, E. A. & McCorduck, J. (1983). *The fifth generation.* Reading, MA: Addison-Wesley Publishing Co.

Feigenbaum, E. A. & Feldman, J. (1963). Artificial intelligence. In E. A. Feigenbaum & J. Feldman (Eds.), *Computers and thought* (pp. 1–8). New York: McGraw-Hill Book Company.

Hamric, A. B. (1983). Role development and function. In A. B. Hamric & J. Spross (Eds.), *The clinical nurse specialist in theory and practice* (pp. 39–56). Orlando: Grune & Stratton.

Ozbolt, J. G. (1986). Developing decision support systems for nursing: Issues of knowledge representation. In R. Salamon, B. Blum & M. Jorgensen (Eds.), *MEDINFO 86* (pp. 186–189). Amsterdam: Elsevier Science.

Peat, F. D. (1988). *Artificial intelligence: How machines think.* New York: Simon & Schuster.

Tou, J. (1985). Knowledge engineering revisited. *International Journal of Computer and Information Science, 14*(3), 123–133.

Turing, A. M. (1950). Computing machinery and intelligence. In E. A. Feigenbaum & F. Feldman (Eds.), *Computers and thought* (pp. 11–35). New York: McGraw-Hill Book Company.

Walker, A. (1986). Knowledge systems: Principles and practice. *IBM Journal of Research and Development, 30*(1), 2–13.

40
Evaluation of an Artificial-Intelligence-Based Nursing Decision Support System in a Clinical Setting

JANET E. CUDDIGAN, SUSAN LOGAN, STEVEN EVANS, and HELEN HOESING

COMMES and the Nursing Protocol Consultant

The decision support system under discussion is the COMMES system. COMMES (Creighton Online Multiple Modular Expert System) is a group of artificial-intelligence-based expert systems designed to manage the vast stores of professional knowledge necessary to make intelligent decisions about patient care. Although a number of COMMES knowledgebases and consultants have been developed, this discussion will be restricted to the Generalist Nursing Knowledgebase and the Nursing Protocol Consultant (NPC).

The Generalist Nursing Knowledgebase is a hierarchically organized, comprehensive description that defines, through a series of goals and subgoals, what a generalist nurse needs to know to provide safe, comprehensive care. This knowledgebase was originally derived from the Creighton University undergraduate BSN nursing program. Based on the recommendation of clinical users, this knowledgebase has been expanded to include some specialty content.

The NPC utilizes this knowledge base (as well as an extensive semantic network and the COMMES driver) to respond to a user's request for very specific information on patient care issues. In the clinical area, the NPC provides appropriate information to guide the nurse in the development of care plans for the patient and in the creation of standards for the institution (Evans, 1983; Ryan, 1985). Figure 1 provides an example of an NPC response to a request for information on the patient undergoing a thyroidectomy.

The NPC has undergone a USA-government-funded content validation study with favorable results (Cuddigan, Norris, Ryan, & Evans, 1987; Norris & Cuddigan, 1987). Following content validation, the COMMES

Reprinted with permission from *Proceedings of Nursing and Computers: The Third International Symposium on Nursing Use of Computers and Information Science*; pp. 629–636. Daly, N. & Hannah, K.J. (Eds.). 1988. St. Louis: The C.V. Mosby Company.

CLINICAL PRACTICE PROTOCOL:

CLINICAL PRACTICE SHOULD INCORPORATE OR INTEGRATE THE FOLLOWING:
1. NURSING MEASURES TO RECOGNIZE THE COMPLICATIONS OF SUBTOTAL
THYROIDECTOMY AND APPROPRIATE NURSING INTERVENTIONS TO CONTROL
COMPLICATIONS.

In POSTOP CARE FOR SUBTOTAL THYROIDECTOMY, consider:

assess upper airway patency		assess swallowing
check dressing	check back of neck & back for bleeding	
check dressing for tightness		
loosen tight fit & call md		daily weight
avoid over-sedation	check lung sounds	
tell pt not to hyperextend neck		assess for hypocalcemia
i&o	fluids as tolerated	food by second day
ambulate by second day	observe for dyspnea	observe for stridor
suction mouth	suction trachea	cold humidifier
cold nebulizer	suction in room	
tracheostomy setup in room		oxygen
vitals	rectal temperature every 4 hrs for 24 hours	
calcium gluconate for seizure		assess for tremor
assess hyperirrritability		
monitor for thyroid storm		
avoid cholinergic blocker		semi-fowlers position
sandbag to neck for support		
support neck on position change		cool liquids and food
pain medication	observe for hypothyroidism	
assess quality of voice		
frequent pulmonary hygiene		
teach patient to support neck		
neck exercise after suture removal		
check with md before neck exercise		chvostek's sign
trousseau's sign		

In DISCHARGE TEACHING FOR SUBTOTAL THYROIDECTOMY, consider:

teach signs of thyrotoxicosis	
teach signs of hypothyroidism	
see md at least twice yearly	
report signs of thyrotoxicosis	
report signs of hypothyroidism	rom to neck
lubricant cream to neck incision	
do not omit thyroid medication	
take as same time each day	
consult md during or before stress	
call md at first signs of infection	adequate rest
adequate food and fluid intake	avoid stress
medication teaching	

Note: Due to space limitations, information on complications, nursing diagnosis, desired outcomes and preoperative care have been deleted.

FIGURE 1. Protocol on care of the thyroidectomy patient.

nursing system was implemented in a number of sites in the United States and Canada. This paper describes the evaluation of the NPC at one of these clinical sites.

Planning and Implementation

The clinical implementation site used in this study was a 500 bed acute care facility in an American midwestern urban area. Prior to considering house-wide implementation, the system was pilot-tested with two adjacent nursing units sharing one terminal. The nursing units were chosen as the units most representative of the average hospital clientele.

Change theory was utilized in guiding the implementation of the COMMES system on these two nursing units (Bennis, 1969). The hospital's Vice President for Nursing designated an experienced staff development nurse as the "change agent" responsible for coordinating implementation and evaluation of the system.

A task force was formed representing staff nurses from all shifts on the two pilot units, as well as representing from management. After an orientation to the COMMES system, members of the task force delineated facilitating and inhibiting factors involved in implementing the COMMES system. Implementing plans were then developed which maximized facilitating factors and minimized inhibiting factors. A train-the-trainer approach was used with the change agent and task force members serving as trainers and resource personnel for the staff nurses on the pilot units.

Evaluation

Evaluation Methods

The COMMES system's impact on the two pilot units was evaluated on a quarterly basis. Evaluation focused on the following areas: (1) impact on the quality of care, (2) adequacy of the COMMES knowledge base in addressing the patient care problems encountered on these units, and (3) the level of user satisfaction.

Quality of Patient Care

The system's impact on the quality of care was measured using standard quality assurance auditing techniques. Prior to system implementation, four commonly encountered patient care issues were selected for monitoring on each of the pilot units. Unit A selected postoperative teaching for cholecystectomy patients, postoperative assessment of thyroidectomy patients, pain management in bowel obstruction patients, and postoperative assessment of diabetic patients. Unit B selected assessment of depression in cancer patients, assessment of pneumonia patients prior to discharge, and the monitoring of steroid therapy and enteral feedings. The hospital quality assurance team established monitoring criteria (Patient Outcome Indicators) for each of these patient conditions and conducted chart audits prior to system implementation and on a quarterly basis thereafter. Hospital personnel collected, organized, and calculated all data independent of any COMMES personnel. See Figure 2 for an example of monitoring criteria for the postoperative thyroidectomy patient.

Indicator	Sampling	Criteria
Postoperative Thyroidectomy Assessment	Charting through 2nd postoperative day for 10 consecutive patients having thyroidectomy	100% of patients will have documented assessment of – respiratory quality – voice quality – swallowing quality at least 2 times daily

FIGURE 2. Example of patient outcome indicators.

Knowledge Adequacy

The adequacy of the knowledge base was evaluated by monitoring the number of user requests which could be met by the COMMES system. Information was requested on all primary diagnoses for all patients admitted to the two pilot units over a one week period of time.

User Satisfaction

User satisfaction was evaluated using an investigator-designed Lickert scale evaluation tool. The tool was administered at quarterly intervals.

Evaluation Results

Quality of Patient Care

Patient record audits indicated progressive and significant improvements in the quality of care as measured by predetermined Patient Outcome Indicators (PIO's). Chi-square analysis was used to compare pre-COMMES PIO measurements with each set of quarterly post-COMMES PIO measurements. See Table 1 for a summary of these results.

When comparing pre-COMMES POI measurements (first quarter) to measurements taken three months after implementation (second quarter), no significant improvement in the quality of care was noted. At this stage of the implementation process, nurses were still gaining proficiency in the use of the system and protocols were not obtained on all patients.

Significant improvements in the quality of care were demonstrated by the third quarter. By this time, users had gained greater proficiency in using the system and the level of usage had increased. However the use of the system was not required and variability existed in the use of COMMES to support careplanning. Despite these factors, significant improvements were noted in postoperative thyroidectomy assessments and the assessment of patients with pneumonia. Two indicators showed nonsignificant improve-

TABLE 1. Comparison of patient outcome indicators before and at quarterly intervals after COMMES implementation

Indicator	Unit	Pre-COMMES vs 2nd Quarter Chisq/p	Pre-COMMES vs 3rd Quarter Chisq/p	Pre-COMMES vs 4th Quarter Chisq/p
Cholecystectomy teaching	A	.05/NS	1.26/NS	**5.01/.02**
Thyroidectomy assessment	A	.56/NS	**9.34/.001**	**17.69/<.001**
Pain management	A	.10/NS	1.43/NS	2.67/NS
Diabetic assessment	A	NA	NA	NA
Unit A analysis	A	1.33/NS	**14.19/<.001**	**29.71/<.001**
Depression assessment	B	NA	NA	NA
Pneumonia assessment	B	.23/NS	**6.15/.01**	**14.46/<.001**
Steroid therapy	B	NA	NA	NA
Enteral feeding	B	NA	NA	NA
Unit B analysis	B	.08/NS	**4.47/0.02**	**9.70/.001**
Overall	A&B	1.45/NS	19.08/<.001	40.68/<.001

$\alpha = .05$.
NS = Not Significant.
NA = Not analyzed due to insufficient sample size. All of these indicators showed a stable or positive trend over the four quarters.

ment. Chi-square analysis could not be performed on four indicators due to insufficient sample size.

Further improvements in the quality of care were noted at the fourth quarterly POI measurement interval. Significant differences were noted over pre-COMMES measurements for postoperative cholecystectomy teaching, postoperative thyroidectomy assessment, and the assessment of pneumonia patients. One indicator showed nonsignificant improvement. The positive trend in the remaining three indicators could not be analyzed due to an insufficient sample size. Prior to this measurement, significantly higher levels of system utilization increased the probability that COMMES would influence careplanning and the quality of care delivery.

For the third and fourth quarter, significant differences were noted over first quarter baseline measurements for each nursing unit and for the overall total. Patient Outcome Indicators which failed to show significant changes tended to be indicators which reflected relatively good quality in the pre-COMMES measurements. In effect, there was little room for improvement.

Knowledge Adequacy

In determining if the COMMES system could provide information on the patient problems most frequently encountered on these two nursing units, COMMES protocols were requested on all primary diagnoses for all patients during a one week period of time. The COMMES system provided information in response to 71% of the requests. The COMMES Development Team later added information on the patient care issues which were not addressed by the system during this trial week.

User Satisfaction

User satisfaction surveys yielded generally positive results. Seventy-three percent of the staff surveyed found the system very valuable or valuable. Seventy-nine percent found it very easy or easy to use. Respondents provided valuable constructive commentary and cited time limitations and limited COMMES terminal availability as obstacles to the system's use. The discharge teaching component of the system was frequently identified as a major strength.

Study Limitations

Inherent in this methodology are two unavoidable limitations which should be acknowledged. The first limitation occurs in any study measuring the effects of a computer system on patient outcomes. Because the computer system interfaces with the nurse rather than directly with the patient, the nurse's use or nonuse of the system's recommendations serves as an uncontrolled variable.

The pretest-posttest design used to measure the quality of care increases the likelihood of intervening variables. The quality of care may have generally improved on these units during the evaluative period for reasons other than the introduction of the COMMES system. To control for this limitation, several Patient Outcome Indicators (POIs) which could not be influenced by the COMMES system were monitored during the evaluative period. Although sample sizes were too small to submit to Chi-square analysis, these POIs showed very little variability during the evaluative period. The lack of variability of control POIs tends to reduce the likelihood that results were due to intervening variables and strengthens the conclusion that the improvements in quality are attributable to the COMMES system's influence.

Conclusions

The COMMES artificial-intelligence-based computer system was designed to quickly provide the professional knowledge necessary to support clinical decisions and improve the quality of patient care. A clinical evaluation of this system demonstrated a high level of user satisfaction and significant improvements in the quality of patient care as measured by critical Patient Outcome Indicators.

Acknowledgments. The development of the COMMES system was supported in part by a grant from the W.K. Kellogg Foundation of Battle Creek, Michigan.

The authors wish to acknowledge, in supporting the development and implementation of this system.

References

Bennis, W. G. (1969). *The Planning of Change.* New York: Holt, Rinehart and Winston.

Cuddigan, J. E., Norris, J., Ryan, S. A., & Evans, S. (1987). Validating the knowledge in a computer-based consultant for nursing care. In W. W. Stead (Ed.), *Proceedings of the Eleventh Symposium on Computer Applications in Medical Care* (pp. 74–78). Washington, DC: Computer Society Press.

Evans, S. (1983). Nursing applications of an expert system. In J. H. van Bemmel (Ed.), *Proceedings of the Fourth World Congress of Medical Informatics* (pp. 182–185). New Holland: Amsterdam.

Hannah, K. J. (1987). Understanding the concept of computer based decision support systems for nursing practice. In K. J. Hannah, M. Reimer, W. C. Mills & S. Letourneau (Eds.), *Clinical Judgement and Decision Making: The Future with Nursing Diagnosis* (pp. 513–518). New York: John Wiley & Sons.

Naisbitt, J. (1884). *Megatrends.* New York: Warner Books Inc.

Norris, J. & Cuddigan, J. (1987). Validating the output of computerized decision support consultant in nursing. In K. J. Hannah, M. Reimer, W. C. Mills & S. Letourneau (Eds.), *Clinical Judgement and Decision Making: The Future with Nursing Diagnosis* (pp. 562–564). New York: John Wiley & Sons.

Ryan, S. A. (1985). An expert system for nursing practice: clinical decision support. *Computers in Nursing, 3*(2), 77–84.

41
Process Control: Clinical Path Analysis

Rosa Portus

As part of an integrated patient data system, clinical path analysis becomes a unifying theme for the identification of service delivery, quality outcomes, and continuous assessment. The path analysis provides clinical data for evaluation of the appropriateness and effectiveness of nursing interventions. As clinicians, this gives us a unique new opportunity to understand and formalize processes of patient care.

Clinical pathways, a multidisciplinary problem solving system and case management tool, is appropriately designed to ensure continuity of services with predictive outcomes through a current and formalized understanding of the clinical processes. Understanding clinical processes and outcomes establishes clinical and financial outcomes within a prescribed time.

The implementation of clinical paths focuses on the development and organization of key interventions through a process of sequencing and customizing those events in a plan of care for each type of patient (casetypes) that is to be managed by this approach; the casetype may be described by the DRG label (e.g. Traumatic Stupor, Coma) or could be a subset of a DRG (e.g. Traumatic Subdural Hemorrhage patients are in the Major Diagnostic Category (MDC) of Diseases and Disorders of the Nervous System).

The clinical path is developed collaboratively by all disciplines involved in managing a particular type of patient during the episode of stay. It documents the usual length of stay (LOS) for that casetype and the major intermediate outcomes to be achieved for the final outcome (discharge from hospital) to occur on time. Intermediate outcomes could be, for ex-

Reprinted with permission from *Informatics: The Infrastructure for Quality Assessment and Improvement in Nursing: Proceedings of the Fifth International Nursing Informatics Symposium Post Conference*, Henry, S.B., Holzemer, W.L., Tallberg, M. & Grobe, S.J. (Eds.). 1995. Pp. 69–76. San Francisco, CA: UC Nursing Press.

ample, mobilization achieved on day 2, or patient demonstrates an understanding of discharge medications on day 5.

The activities of the nursing, medical, and allied health staff which are directed at getting the patient to each of the outcomes are detailed in the clinical pathway plan. Therefore, the plan is used to guide care and track and monitor patient progress on a shift-by-shift basis.

The goal of the plan is to formally document the care to be delivered by multidisciplinary groups, hospital wide, and to promote collaborative practice with appropriate utilization of resources. The clinical pathway plan enables the team to evaluate the individual patient against the proven capability of achievable expectations and standardized outcomes for a particular casetype or DRG. Individual expectations and clinical outcomes are based on the treating physician's requirements. The clinical path plan is the tool that provides for the overall, continuous, and well-coordinated delivery of care.

Clinical Pathway Model

A clinical pathway model has four major components. These are:

- Clinical paths
- Variance (variation) analysis
- Case consultation
- Shift report

Clinical Paths

The content of clinical paths consists of clinical activity to be achieved by staff providing the care. The clinical paths are the clinical management tool that organizes, times, and sequences the delivery of patient care by the multidisciplinary team providing the care. All major interventions by the team are formally documented, linking the direct caregivers across the hospital during the patient's episode of care. Major interventions or themes of care can be classified into factors, for example:

- assessment/monitoring
- consults
- procedures/tests
- medications
- fluid management
- patient/family teaching
- psychosocial needs
- discharge planning

Using the known average length of stay (LOS) for each casetype or DRG, a concise chart can be made with each day of stay listed across the page and the desired standard of practice for each factor listed down the page, as shown in the example for a Coronary Artery Bypass graft (Figure 1). This type of management tool anticipates and describes in advance the care required by a specific casetype. The progress of the patient is then compared to the expected or anticipated outcome for that hour/day. The anticipated care requirements and outcomes of specific patient populations are used as a guide or plan to the actual care being delivered. From this point, variation (variance) from the standard of practice can be observed and evaluated (Figure 2).

Variance Analysis

Variance analysis is one of the major components of the clinical pathway system. Variances from the norm may occur, with some patients being different in many complex ways. Some patients will respond to interventions in unpredictable ways and beyond any overall control. Clinicians track and monitor their own outcomes of care. If variation analysis exists, the multidisciplinary team has the opportunity to analyze the variation, use their expertise to problem solve, and either better understand the variation or determine another approach to get the patient back on track. Evaluation factors such as measurement of expected outcomes, readmission rates, mortality rates, LOS, and cost per episode of care may be analyzed through patterns of variance. Clinicians tracking and monitoring their own outcomes of care establish collaborative goals that may then be measured against the norm. This offers opportunities to understand what really works in clinical practice.

Components of variance analysis are:

- special or common cause variation
- action on clinical/hospital variation
- variation in coding charts

These components may then be broken into four groups as follows:

1. Patient/family
   - condition
   - decision
   - availability
   - other
2. Hospital
   - bed/appointment time available
   - availability of information data
   - supplies/equipment availability
   - department overbooked/closed
   - hospital/other

<table>
<tr><td colspan="2">CORONARY ARTERY
BYPASS GRAFT
DRG 225 / MDC 5</td><td colspan="4">Episode No.   Medical record No.

Surname   Specialist

Given Names

Ward   Age   Sex   D.O.B</td></tr>
</table>

CORONARY ARTERY
BYPASS GRAFT
DRG 225 / MDC 5

DAY 1
(PRE-OP DAY)

Episode No.   Medical record No.
Surname   Specialist
Given Names
Ward   Age   Sex   D.O.B

DATE:

CLINICAL PATHWAY	YES	VAR	OUTCOMES	YES	VAR
MEDICAL CONSULT / DOCUMENTATION / DISCHARGE PLANNING / FAMILY SUPPORT					
* Surgeon / Registrar consult			* Patient understands purpose, process & risks of the surgery		
* RMO check / complete: - full admission - informed consent - Group & Hold, Cross Match - pre-operative test results - pre-operative medication orders			* Pre-operative medical documentation complete		
* Whereabouts / contact No: for significant others sought			* Accessible documentation is evident for significant other contact		
* Significant others advised of level 6 facilities for day of surgery			* Significant others aware of facilities		
ANAESTHETIC & GIT PREPARATION					
* - premedication order - sedation - drugs to continue through nil by mouth period are specified			* Sedation administered as ordered		
* Weight, height, allergies & known adverse drug reactions established			* Baseline data available to assist drug & fluid administration in O.T & ITU		
* Full (low fat) diet until NBM period			* Patient adheres to diet regime		
* Bowel assessment					
* NBM 6-8 hrs pre-operative - Advise Dietetics			* Onset of fasting period noted on U4B		
CIRCULATION & RESPIRATORY SUPPORT / INFECTION CONTROL					

* Physiotherapy consultation
- assessment of pre-op condition
  # chest status
  # mobility
- db&c, Triflow use
- discussion of post-op activities
			* Patient demonstrates effective:
			- deep breathing exercises
			- cough
			
			- Triflow use
			- shoulder & ankle exercises		

* Measure for anti-thrombotic stockings			* Anti-thrombotic stockings available		
* Baseline HR, BP, RR, Temp & U/A			* Baseline observations NAD		
* Stubble shave as per protocol			* No evidence of infection		
* Patient showers with antibacterial soap			* Skin preparation completed		
MEDICATIONS					
* Pharmacist consultation - obtain history - supply medications			* Medication history documented * Allergy check attended * Essential medications continued * Appropriate medications supplied		
REFERRALS					
* Referral needs - Social Worker eg. support/counselling - Dietitian eg. obesity, diabetes - Other			* Referral (s) made - Front sheet request completed - Variance record identifies need - Required consultant contacted		

FIGURE 1. Clinical pathway example for CABG preoperative day 1. Reprinted with permission.

VARIANCE RECORD

Variance code

Patient / Family
A1. Condition
A2. Decision
A3. Availability
A4. Other

Care Provider
B5. Physician Order
B6. Decision
B7. Response Time
B8. Other

System
C9. Bed / Appt Time
C10. Information Delay
C11. Supplies / Equipment
C12. Other

Community
D13. Placement / Home Care
D14. Transportation Delay
D15. Other

Episode No.   Medical record No.
Surname   Specialist
Given Names
Ward   Age   Sex   D.O.B

DATE	DESCRIBE VARIANCE	DESIGNATION	CODE	WAS OUTCOME AFFECTED ?	DESCRIBE CORRECTIVE ACTION / RESOLUTION	INITIALS

FIGURE 2. Variance record for clinical pathways. Reprinted with permission.

3. Caregiver/clinician
    - physician order
    - caregiver's decision
    - caregiver's response
    - caregiver—other factors
4. Community
    - placement/home care
    - availability
    - ambulance delay
    - community—other

The concept of variance and the technique of variance analysis is a dynamic component of the system. Its greatest potential is in alerting the caregiver to the need for action with the aim of continuous quality improvement. It individualizes the care through the analysis and evaluation of variation. Variances are real and they reflect the way the staff respond to individual patient needs. The optimal result of clinical paths is that unnecessary variance is reduced to a minimum, whereby the control and predictability of the process can be managed.

In addition to analyzing and acting upon variation from the path at an individual level, it is possible to monitor aggregate variance across casetypes and identify systematic problems that are diminishing quality of care and efficiency. For example, review of the variance of individual patients from the Coronary Artery Bypass Graft clinical path over three months may show that the Holter monitor was not applied on Day 4 in 30% of patients because there were not enough monitors available. The manager analyzing aggregate variance in this way has a powerful tool for improving the quality and efficiency of the care delivery system.

Case Consultation

As part of the clinical pathway system, case consultation is review and evaluation of patient care undertaken due to a significant variance between the planned and actual delivery of care. For example, if a patient is on a daily clinical path and variance continues for anything longer than 24 hours, then multidisciplinary consultations should take place. This approach is the basis of a collaborative contribution towards quality. Patient and family are included in the consultation with the patient and family taking part in their own goal setting, either on an hourly, daily, weekly, or monthly basis. Patient and family responses to clinical interventions may be categorized by problem statements which transform into expectations, intermediate goals, and final clinical outcomes.

Stetler and Dezell[1] claim that four generic categories should be considered when evaluating patient and family responses to clinical interventions. These are:

- Potential for complications in self-care, i.e., patient's ability to manage.
- Potential for injury unrelated to treatment, i.e., risk factors unrelated to environmental and patient's general state of health.
- Potential for complications related to treatment, i.e. risk factors inherent in the in-hospital treatment, health safety, preventive measures, and ongoing clinical monitoring.
- Potential for extension of the disease process, i.e., risk factors endangering the patient with a potential to increase if presence of specific or pathological processes go undetected.

Shift Report

The report section of managed care provides oncoming staff with a tool that gives cues to the delivery of care required for the next shift. The purpose of the report is that nursing practice and expected quality outcomes are monitored on a shift-by-shift basis in the context of the patient's length of stay. The report section should include:

- patient's addressograph label.
- diagnosis.
- anticipated length of stay.
- DRG number.
- brief medical history.
- patient day number, e.g., day 6 of 10 day stay.
- patient's present condition.
- critical activities identified on the clinical path expected for that day.
- evaluation of clinical path compliance.
- case consultation request if variance unclear.

Benefits of a Clinical Pathway Model

Benefits of a Clinical Pathway model include:

- Focuses on the patient/family.
- Prescribes, manages, and evaluates quality.
- Provides a comprehensive protocol for an entire episode of care.
- Increases knowledge and understanding of clinical and financial outcome management.
- Offers a problem solving tool for clinician's use.
- Tracks, describes, and monitors variations in an episode of care.
- Provides quality data for the integration of health plans, and facilitates an integrated patient data information system.
- Provides expertise in transforming a set of problems into meaningful outcomes.

Organizational solutions such as bottom line management and redesigning of clinical processes by the use of case management tools such as clinical pathways should provide a clear understanding of the clinical processes of care. Information compiled from actual clinical based practice then becomes the key to optimal cost and quality outcomes. Outcome based strategies can then be developed based on the actual clinical practice.

Effects of a clinical pathway model reported by the Center for Case Management[2] include:

- Increases levels of patient satisfaction as evidenced by their comments.
- Increases likelihood that patients will receive the care desired, no matter where they are in the institution. Keeps all other care providers "in synch" with the physician's plan of care.
- Keeps control over patients care with the physician. Those activities that currently require a physician's order continue to do so. Physicians are actively involved in the development of clinical pathways, which reflect the care they have determined is needed by their patients.
- Provides nurses and other members of the health care team who are interested in and committed to the physician's practice types with insight into another's role.
- Facilitates the resolution of system issues that are often annoying and/or frustrating to clinical personnel.
- Makes communication between physician and other clinical members consistent.
- Strengthens collegiality.
- Allows research findings to be readily incorporated into practice.

Adopting case management and a clinical pathway model in Australia as a tool for clinicians to gather clinical data is providing vital information on cost and quality issues at the bedside.

Development of a Clinical Pathway

The clinical pathway is predictive, outcome based plan for patient care. It is not expected that every patient and every caregiver will follow the plan precisely, but the clinical pathway affords a cue to help ensure that all services are provided to patients in a timely manner.

Assessment

Selection of casetype:

- high volume
- high cost
- high risk

Additional considerations:

- interest of caregivers
- high variability in practice
- identified co-ordination of care issues
- predictability

Selection of the Multidisciplinary Team

One of the greatest strengths of clinical paths is the multidisciplinary collaboration that is initiated during the process. Collaboration can improve patient care through the elimination of fragmentation and/or duplication of services. Consider the role of each of the following in caring for the patient with a clinical pathway:

- Physician/Surgeon/Geriatrician/Rehabilitation
- Occupational Therapist
- Physiotherapist
- Social Worker
- Nurse Manager/Registered Nurses
- Discharge consultants
- Chaplains
- Clerical staff
- Clinical Psychologist
- Educational consultants (diabetic/renal/stomal)
- Nutritionist
- Pharmacy
- Bed allocations personnel

It is necessary to determine who should be involved and when, confirming input with the head of each discipline or department involved. Identifying a physician who may be interested in working with the team may motivate a physician to not only help, but to become a "champion" of the collaborative effort to improve patient care.

Strategies for Writing a Clinical Pathway

The clinical pathway should be developed through a combination of chart review of actual practice and interdisciplinary group discussion to review actual and preferred practice patterns.

In determining which charts to review, it is important to choose charts of patients whose length of stay (LOS) appears to be within the average range for that casetype. The Medical Records Department can help determine which patients were hospitalized with a specific episode of care in the acute care setting and this will establish the average LOS.

The team should plan to review at least 8–10 charts, which may need to be requested four days or so prior to reviewing them. Small groups of charts are usually taken from Medical Records to a central location for the group to review. Either the Project Leader of Clinical Pathways or the Clinical Leader needs to be responsible to Medical Records for charts to be returned within the approved time frame. In reviewing charts, team members look for key interventions and their timing. A clinical pathway trial may be required if clinicians are not clear on the process.

Clinical pathways are started from the compiled data collected from the chart review. Interventions occurring in 80% of the casetype population are included on the clinical pathway for that casetype. Other interventions which may have significance need to be discussed as problems or issues when the multidisciplinary group meets.

When the first draft is typed, it must be remembered that it is only a draft and may be changed during and after the pilot phase. All clinical pathways need to be continually evaluated and modified as required.

The patient's potential and actual problems related to the condition should be formalized when the clinical pathway is being developed. Discharge outcomes should be linked to the patient's condition and expected progress. Intermediate or process outcomes are related to key interventions described on the map as standards set by the clinicians. All outcomes must be measurable; therefore, the wording for outcomes and their management is vital for continuous improvement. There may not always be daily process outcomes for each discipline involved, but this will depend on the casetype being described.

Implementation

All steps in the process should be a group decision, including how to finalize the clinical pathway. Physicians who care for the casetype should be involved at all stages of implementation.

Educational needs for all multidisciplinary staff need to be identified. An educational task force needs to develop a plan of ongoing education for all staff, including new staff being oriented to the hospital setting.

Other resources and implementation issues will need to be identified and addressed by working parties that need only to meet for as long as the issues are resolved. Examples of working parties:

- Documentation team
- Operational team
- Education team

All of theses teams must have multidisciplinary input including Medical Records, Finance, and Information Systems Departments.

The plan of implementation needs to consider issues such as:

- Which units are suitable for clinical paths?
- When is an appropriate time to begin?
- Who will be the key person in the unit to act as a resource person for that unit?
- Who will be the key person to monitor the progress of clinical pathways in the area?
- Will there be rostering (staffing) issues?
- Will there be a need to evaluate the type of nursing model practiced in the unit/hospital? How may this affect the implementation of clinical paths?

Strategy for Clinical Path Design Team

The function of the design team is to write a clinical path for the specific casetype selected. Multidisciplinary members on the team are those clinicians who contribute specifically to the episode of care being developed.

Four sessions are required in development of a clinical path and its outcomes:

Session 1.   Multidisciplinary education. It may be necessary to repeat this session to cover all clinicians involved. The aim of this session is to give a sound overview of case management and its components. (Most of the clinicians' learning comes from actual experience using the clinical path).

Session 2.   Development of the clinical path. The project leader guides the process as the multidisciplinary team designs the steps in the process of an episode of care. The clinicians also define their boundaries, highlighting issues and potential problems. Process outcomes are then linked to key interventions described.

Session 3.   Review and discussion of the clinical path. The project leader meets with the multidisciplinary team to check the clinical path and the content. Modifications are done as required. Preparations are then made with the clinicians to implement trial of path. No fewer than 10–15 samples should be collected for the pilot period.

Session 4.   Review and discussion of the pilot study. When the sample size is completed, the multidisciplinary team meets to discuss the content, variance, problems, and or issues that may have been highlighted in the pilot study. Modifications are made as required, and formal implementation of the pathway is planned. The path will continue to evolve for up to 6–12 months, depending on the complexity of the casetype. All paths should be evaluated and modified every six months.

Ongoing support is required for the maintenance and stabilization of the system. Therefore, it is worthwhile to develop a resource person for each specialty or cluster area.

Variance (Variation) Analysis

Ongoing education is required for the analysis of variation. Clinicians need to be guided through the process of how they can use the data collected, thereby using the system to its great potential. Experience is proving that this is where the major infrastructure changes are taking place, for example, in theater (operating room) utilization, admission protocols, and excessive delays in the more isolated units and departments. The principles of Total Quality Management may be used successfully for these key issues.

Predictors of Nursing Outcomes

Key nursing interventions are developed and described to use as predictors for nursing outcomes. Plans are now underway on a national basis to develop tools that will help us as a profession to understand and evaluate the causal relationship between intervention and outcome. It seems the best we can do is to say that an intervention has an association with a variance and/or outcome.

Interventions such as wound care, hemodynamic monitoring, or neurological observations are providing nurses with a strong professional identity as part of their database of clinical activity. Further research needs to be done to establish that specific nursing interventions are strong predictors for nursing outcomes management. Cognitive aspects and concepts such as the art of nursing or "that caring and intuitive knowing" incorporated in an abstract way in the concept of patient focus, must also be remembered during objective evaluation linking intervention to outcome. The opportunity to evaluate and improve our service delivery and quality of care is demanding that clinicians plan, think, and manage differently.

Predictors of nursing outcomes for a casetype need to be continually monitored and evaluated, using questions such as the following:

- Are the current interventions the best predictors of nursing outcomes?
- Are the predictors providing the expected outcomes set as a standard?
- Are the predictors making a difference to the quality of care and its outcomes?
- What else could we be doing as a profession?

The formalization of roles and responsibilities established in the clinical pathway system is providing nursing with an opportunity to create a strong professional identity, equality, independence, and, in turn, a synergy with other professionals never before experienced. The clinical pathway system is requiring us to come to terms with the direct relationship between the service we provide and the effect it has on quality outcomes.

References

[1] Stetler C. Case Management Plans: Designs for Transformation. Boston: New England Medical Center Hospitals, 1987.
[2] The Center for Case Management. Definitions. Boston: The Center for Case Management, Inc., 1990.

Part III
Nursing Administration

This section focuses on the administrative tasks necessary to implement computerization within a clinical environment. The first two articles focus on minimum data sets. Sermeus and Delesie report on Belgium's six-year experience with collecting, collating, and analyzing nursing data. Werley and Leske then report on the collection and standardization of data across populations and settings. Finally, Seipp and O'Donnell provide a framework for the collection of functional information as a prelude for determining the suitability of off-the-shelf packages for patient classification.

The second dyad of articles focuses on data management processes and application. Hannah describes the various aspects of data management and how each component contributes to the business of health care. Newbold, on the other hand, explores the processes of using automation for Nursing QA activities.

The final group of articles on explore the cost of automation, both from an initial investment perspective and the advantages of automation on productivity. Bakker, van Gennip, and Roelofs explore the benefits of computerized technology at the bedside. This article reviews the costs associated with the implementation of such a system. Sermeus discusses the relationship between Diagnostic Related Groups (DRGs) and the Minimized Nursing Data Set (MNDS). Lubno attempts to cast out nursing care and remove it from the traditional "room charge" category. Finally, Weaver and Fredericksen look at automation not as a panacea for increased productivity, but as an instrument, which combined with other systems, could enhance productivity.

In summary, these articles on nursing administration explore the necessity for developing objective criteria for evaluating nursing's contributions to improving patient outcomes. Additionally, it offers some elements to be considered when analyzing cost factors associated with automation.

42
The Registration of a Nursing Minimum Data Set in Belgium: Six Years of Experience

WALTER SERMEUS and L. DELESIE

1. Introduction

On April 18, 1986, Belgium got its new hospital law which gave the legal basis for the registration of patient data in the broadest sense. Since then, some royal decrees have been implemented the law. A Royal Decree of August 14, 1987 started to monitor as of January 1, 1988 a minimum number of variables, called the Nursing Minimum Data Set (NMDS).

The construction and implementation of such a Nursing Minimum Data Set nation-wide goes slowly. In this process, each step is a challenge. The first step is the translation of nursing practice to nursing data. The second step is the translation of these nursing data into information. The third step is the use of this information for communication and decision making. The last step is the transformation of nursing practice based on decision making. The process will be illustrated by the use of the Nursing Minimum Data Set in Belgium which is collected in all general Belgian hospitals since 1988.

2. From Nursing Practice to Nursing Data

To transform nursing practice in nursing data, a "uniform nursing language" is necessary. In a lot of countries, nurse researchers are developing nursing languages to describe patient problems from a nursing perspective. Examples are the Nursing Diagnosis list from the NANDA[1], the development of a nursing taxonomy in the Netherlands, in Scotland, in Denmark and in the UK. Similar research work is done in the field of nursing interventions. Examples are the research work of Bulechek & Mc Closkey[2],

Reprinted from *Nursing Informatics: An International Overview for Nursing in a Technological Era*, Grobe, S.J., Pluyter-Wenting, E.S.P. (Eds.). 1994. Pp. 325–333, with kind permission from Elsevier Science—NL, Sara Burgerhartstraat 25, 1055 KV Amsterdam, The Netherlands.

Grobe[3], Saba[4] in the USA, Ehnfors[5] in Sweden. The International Council of Nurses (ICN) is developing a overall framework for a international Classification of Nursing Practice. These languages are necessary to communicate among nurses all over the world.

Most countries put a lot of scientific effort in this first step. In Belgium this step was handled in a very pragmatic way. In 1985, the Belgian Nurses Association[6] developed a list of 111 nursing interventions. This list has been used as the nursing language to describe nursing practice in Belgium.

3. From Nursing Data to Information

While most countries concentrate on the first step, in Belgium most effort has been put in this second step. Eight conditions have to be fulfilled to transform data into information.

The first condition is the use of samples instead of populations. The idea of sampling is integrated in the concept "Minimum" data set. Minimum means that not all aspects of nursing care have to be described but that a selection of the most relevant aspects has to be made. This has been done by the reduction of the whole list of 111 nursing interventions to a selected list of 23. These 23 nursing interventions are selected on statistical and professional grounds and contains 80% of the statistical information of the whole list of 111.

Secondly, samples have been introduced in delineating the registration frequency. The nursing minimum data set does not have to be collected each day but only 4 times a year during a 15 days sampling period. Out of this series of 15 days, 5 random days are selected and are sent to the Ministry of Public Health.

A second condition is the multivariate approach. All attempts so simplify the complex process of patient care into an overall measure have failed. The length of stay, the medical diagnosis, the medical activities, the severity, the nursing interventions, the total cost of care, the intensity of the care, the drug consumption, the nursing workload, etc. all tell something about the patient and the care he receives. No one variable though is capable to give a full answer. How tempting this search for the holy grail may be to some, it is of no avail.

Some of these measures deal with the patient himself—his demand for care—some measures deal with the care that the patient receives—the care provided: hence, the diversity of the patient population on the one hand and the variability in the practice patterns on the other hand. In Belgium, data about the diversity of the patient population (medical diagnosis, age, degree of dependency on daily activities) and the variability of the practice variations (23 nursing interventions, length of stay, number of nursing staff, level of qualification of the nursing staff) are registered.

A third condition is the systematic approach of the data collection. All the data are collected on a similar way in all Belgian general hospitals. Each year about 1.2 million data records are collected by the Ministry of Public Health.

The interrater-reliability of the Nursing Minimum Data Set was controlled in 70 Belgian Hospitals for 4000 records[7]. The global reliability of the data collection is 79%. The basic care and technical interventions are very reliably collected (more than 80%). Interventions such as emotional support, patient teaching are only weakly reliable. Their impact on the global reliability figure is however limited.

A fourth condition is the way these samples are taken: cross-sectional or longitudinal. Belgium has chosen a cross-sectional approach. The argument is that nursing is not characterized by an individual interaction between an individual patient and an individual nurse but consists in many-to-many interactions[8]. The time that nurse X spend on patient Y, depends on the demands of the other patients assigned to nurse X and the presence and competence of the other nurses on a nursing unit. The care for an individual patient can only be discussed if you know something about the nursing care on all other patients.

A fifth condition is a micro/macro- design. It means that the data set must hold the necessary detail to describe a nursing speciality (oncology, intensive care, geriatric care) but is not too specific so that it also can be discussed on a more general level. A micro/macro design enforces both local and global comparison and at the same time, avoids the disruption of context switching[9].

This micro/macro design is built in the Belgian NMDS on a twofold way. Firstly, the number of combinations based on this 23 nursing interventions far exceeds 1.7 million of possible combinations. It means that 23 nursing interventions are enough sensitive to describe very specific care combinations. Secondly, in the presentation of the information, two presentation techniques have been used: the fingerprint and the national map. The fingerprint gives all detailed information within a general frame of reference and is meant for the inside world of the nursing unit. The national map presents a summary of this information for all nursing units and is meant for the outside world.

The fingerprint consists technically in horizontal bar charts for each of the 23 nursing interventions. The fingerprint of the nursing unit's practice compares the interventions of every nursing unit with the same interventions of some reference nursing unit: the sum-nursing unit in Belgium in 1988 or the theoretical nursing unit which we obtain by lumping together all data for all nursing units in Belgium. Figure 1 gives a example of such a fingerprint. A deflection to the left means that the intervention grades lower in the nursing unit than in the sum-nursing unit. A deflection to the right means that this interventions grades higher than in the sum-nursing unit. Moreover, these deflections are standardised for the whole country. Utmost

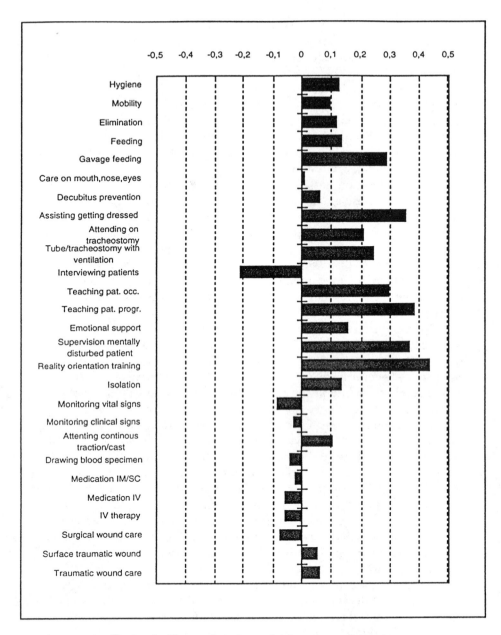

FIGURE 1. Fingerprint of a geriatric care nursing unit.

to the left and to the right, we find the most extreme deflections which are observed in Belgium in 1988. If a particular nursing unit would not differentiate itself whatsoever from the sum-nursing unit, no deflections would be visible. The fingerprint puts equal emphasis on nursing interventions that

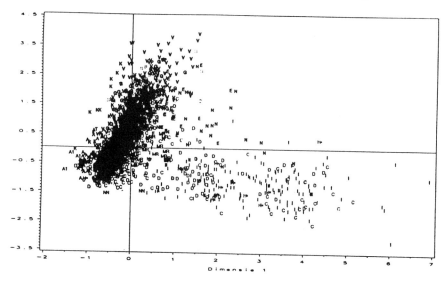

FIGURE 2. National statistics—national map: localization of all Belgian nursing units 1988.

are present as on nursing interventions that are absent in each nursing unit. Although most people accentuate the positive, often one learns as much from the things one does observe as from the things that do not occur.

The national map (Figure 2) uses a specific graphic projection technique to show the position of all 2757 nursing units in Belgium with respect to all other nursing units on the basis of their fingerprint of nursing practice. Each nursing unit has its location on the map. Symbol I (right down) stands for intensive care nursing units. Symbols V and G (at the top) stand for geriatric care nursing units). Symbols C and D (in the middle) stand for surgical nursing units and internal medicine nursing units respectively.

The national map also indicates to what extent the NMDS allow to group nursing units with a similar nursing practice. Figure 2 shows that intensive care nursing units are not very homogeneous.

Defining the 2 dimensions, helps in understanding the national map (figure 3). The first dimension (from the east to the west) is related to the conceptual framework of Orem[10]. A deflection to the east means that nursing interventions are characterised by "doing for." A deflection to the west means that nursing interventions are characterised by "doing with or self-care." The second dimension (south to the north) indicates a balance between care and cure activities. More to the north means that the nursing care profile is dominated by care activities. More to the south, means that the nursing care profile is dominated by the cure activities supporting medical diagnosis and treatment. A strong relationship (68%) has been

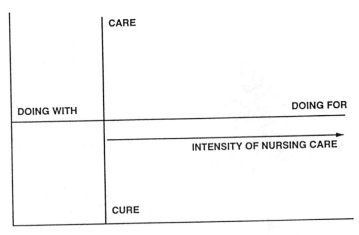

FIGURE 3. Frame of reference national statistics.

found between the first dimension and nursing intensity, based on the traditional patient classification systems such as the San Joaquin system. Moving in an eastern direction is associated with an increasing intensity of the nursing care.

A sixth condition is the feedback. People can only be motivated to collect data if they have timely results. This feedback is realised on different ways. First of all, a booklet "National Statistics"[11] is published by the Ministry of Public Health, which gives the general framework of nursing practice in Belgium. Secondly a computer diskette is developed which makes it possible for each hospital and nursing unit in Belgium to produce its own fingerprints right after the data collection in comparison with the stable reference point of 1988. Thirdly, education programs have been developed in co-operation with the 7 Belgian universities to teach nursing directors, head nurses to work with the program and to learn to read the fingerprints and national map.

A seventh condition is the degree of aggregation. In the "National Statistics" nursing data are aggregated at the level of the nursing unit. By lumping together all the units, we do obtain the location of hospital. Figure 2 points out that this "point of gravity" is just theoretical. A hospital is not very homogeneous concerning nursing care. It is however a fallacy to believe that a nursing unit is more homogeneous with respect to nursing care. The nursing care also varies from patient to patient and even from day to day. That is why ways have been sought to zoom in the world of the nursing unit and to describe individual patients and patient days within the general framework set-up on the level of nursing units[12]. Again on all different levels of aggregation, fingerprints and national maps can be

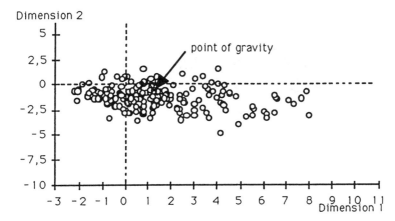

FIGURE 4. Projection of the nursing profile on the national map of 207 inpatient days from a coronary care nursing unit.

derived. Figure 4 shows the location of 207 inpatient days for a coronary care nursing unit. The black cross indicates the "point of gravity" which corresponds with one of the symbols in the "National Statistics." The figure makes clear that the variability of care in this nursing unit is very high. Some patient are intensive care patients, while other patients are self-care patients.

A eighth condition is the common denominator used to present the information. In the national statistics, the common denominator is the nursing unit. All patients hospitalized on the same nursing unit are taken together. But patients have other characteristics in common: their medical diagnosis, age, day of admission. Again it is possible to change the perspective to choose another common denominator e.g. medical diagnosis. Even more interesting are Diagnosis Related Groups (DRGs). Since 1982 a lot of research has been done all over the world to show the homo(hetero)geneity of DRGs in relation to nursing care. Several research studies reveal that DRGs explain only about 20–30% of the variation in nursing intensity[13][14][15]. Based on the NMDS the homogeneity of DRGs in relation to nursing care can be shown. Figure 5 shows the location of 182 inpatient days for the DRG014 "specific cerebrovascular disorders except TIA." The figure makes clear in a spot that this DRG is not homogeneous in relation to nursing care. Some patients are intensive care patients, some patients have high emphasis on basic care, some patients are self-care patients. For a selection of DRGs in one Belgian hospital, the variability in nursing care has been calculated. DRGs explained about 25% of the variability in the intensity of nursing care (first dimension NMDS-framework).

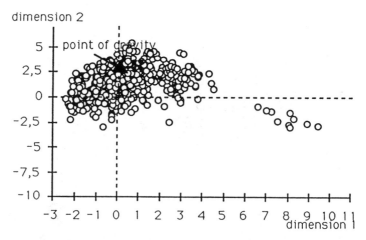

FIGURE 5. Projection of the nursing profile on the national map of 182 inpatient days for patients in DRG014: Specific disorders except TIA.

4. From Information to Decision Making

Despite the fact that the introduction of the NMDS was situated in a new hospital financing scheme in Belgium, the process goes very slowly. Data have to be collected. Then policy makers have to "trust" these data. Confidence is more than just reliability. In the national statistics of 1989 and 1990, the national map of Belgium has hardly changed for 0.2%. It means that the frame of reference is stable. It means that in 2 years time Belgium has not become sicker. At the micro level, at the level of hospitals and nursing units, changes are more noticeable. A study investigating the dynamics over the period 1988–1991 has started. The stable frame of reference has strengthened the confidence in the information. At this moment a governmental work group is preparing a proposal to use the NMDS-information to determine the hospital's budget.

Besides this use by the government, these data are used within the hospital for management purposes. A first purpose is budgeting. Once the hospital's budget is determined, the budget has to be divided to departments, nursing units and finally to how many nurses you need to care for how many patients. This process is mainly a process of communication. The nursing director uses by preference a top-down approach to calculate fair budgets for each nursing unit. The head nurses use predominantly some bottom-up approaches in showing how many patients they are admitting, how long they stay, with what problems they are dealing, what they are doing with these patients, what they want to do next year, their workload etc. All these expectations mostly far exceed the budget which means that priorities have to be made. NMDS-information can be very helpful to support this communication process. Information is also needed to monitor the budget the top management and the head nurses have agreed upon. We call them dashboard instruments, because you need them while driving your nursing unit in the good direction. Several dashboard instruments have been developed based upon this NMDS: controlling nurses' workload by comparing this NMDS with patient classification systems[16]; controlling material consumption[17].

The development of Minimum Data Sets has just begun. More and more, other processes are monitored such as social processes, drug administration etc. All these process data finally will lead to patient outcomes and quality of life indicators. Finally that is what it is all about: Delivering good patient care to a reasonable cost.

Reference

[1] NANDA, *Taxonomy I—revised 1990—with official nursing diagnoses*, NANDA, St. Louis, 1990.

[2] McCloskey JC & Bulechek GM (Eds). *Nursing Intervention Classification*, St. Louis, Mosby, 1992.

[3] Grobe SJ. Nursing intervention lexicon and taxonomy study: language and classification methods, *ANS Adv Nurs Sci*, 13(2), 1990, pp. 22–34.

[4] Saba V. et al, A nursing intervention taxonomy for home health care, *Nurs Health Care*, 12(6), 1991, pp. 296–299.

[5] Ehnfors M. et al, Towards basic nursing information in patient records, *Var i norden*, 21(11), 1991, pp. 12–31.

[6] AUVB-UGIB, *Profiel van de verpleegkundige zorgverlening en de minimale verpleegkundige gegevens, cahiers 1 en 2*, AUVB-UGIB, 1985.

[7] Sermeus W, Delesie L. Betrouwbaarheid van de registratie van minimale verpleegkundige gegevens, *Acta Hospitalia*, 32(2), 1992, pp. 39–54.

[8] Halloran EJ, Conceptual considerations, decision criteria, and guidelines for the nursing minimum data set from a administrative perspective in Werley HH & Lang NM (Eds), Identification of the nursing minimum data set, Springer Publ. Co, New York, 1988, pp. 48–66.

[9] Tufte ER. *The visual display of quantitative information*, Graphic Press, Cheshire, 1983.

[10] Orem DE. *Nursing: concepts of practice 3th ed.*, Mc Graw Hill, New York, 1985.

[11] Ministerie van Volksgezondheid en Leefmilieu & Centrum voor Ziekenhuiswetenschap. *Medische Activiteiten in algemene ziekenhuizen: Nationale Statistieken 1988*, Brussel-Leuven, 1991.

[12] Sermeus W. *Variabiliteit van verpleegkundige verzorging*, Ph.D. thesis, Leuven, 1992.

[13] Atwood JR et al, Relationships among nursing care requirements, nursing resources and charges, in Shaffer FA (ed.), Patients & purse strings: patient classification and cost management, NLN, New York, 1986, pp. 99–120.

[14] Green J et al. Severity of illness and nursing intensity: going beyond DRGs, in Scherubel JC & Shaffer FA (eds). Patients & purse strings II, NLN, 1988, pp. 207–230.

[15] Halloran EJ. Nursing workload, medical diagnosis related groups and nursing diagnoses, *Res Nurs Health*, 8(4), 1985, pp. 421–433.

344 W. Sermeus and L. Delesie

[16] Vanden Boer G & Sermeus W. Linkage of NMDS and patient classification systems, Nursing Informatics San Antonio, USA, 1994 (submitted).
[17] Vandewal D & Vanden Boer G., Using NMDS-information for the allocation of budgets to nursing units, Nursing Informatics San Antonio, USA, 1994 (submitted).

43
Standardized, Comparable, Essential Data Available Through the Nursing Minimum Data Set

HARRIET H. WERLEY and JANE S. LESKE

Introduction

It is a pleasure to be participating in this preconference workshop on Standards and Minimum Data Sets, for it is important that nurses move forward in their work on developing nursing information systems (NISs) and computerization of data in such a way that their systems will provide access to comparable data across clinical populations and settings—locally, regionally, nationally, and internationally. It also is a pleasure to be participating in this program with colleague speakers, who represent a vendor, an information network of a United States consortium of university hospitals, the Project Director for the Australian Community Nursing Minimum Data Set, and others working on data sets in health care. Discussion among the workshop leaders and attendees should provide a rich learning experience.

Comments on standardization, comparable data, and essential core data will pertain, in the main, to the U.S. Nursing Minimum Data Set (NMDS). In this way, there will be some tangible content to refer to for discussion. To make certain that workshop participants are thinking about the same content and context, and their pertinence to the workshop topic under discussion, some background on the concept of uniform minimum health data sets (UMHDSs) and the development of the NMDS will be presented. However, because much of the work on the NMDS has been published previously (Devine & Werley, 1988; Werley, 1987; Werley, Devine, & Zorn, 1988; Werley, Devine, & Zorn, 1989; Werley & Lang, 1988a; Werley, Lang, & Westlake, 1986a, 1986b; Werley & Zorn, 1989), background presented initially will be limited but can be expanded as indicated by questions and discussion.

Reprinted with permission from *Nursing Informatics '91: Pre-Conference Proceedings*; Turley, J.P. & Newbold, S.K. (Eds.). 1991. Pp. 95–106. Heidelberg-Berlin, Germany: Springer-Verlag.

Standardization of Data

In the U.S., the need for quantitative information to support health policy formulation, program planning, management, and evaluation in health at all levels of the health care system is widely recognized. But through the years it also has become apparent that health data are diminished because of lack of comparability of definitions, codes, classifications, and terminology used. Therefore, within the Department of Health and Human Services (DHHS) a program of standards and guidelines was established in 1979. This program provides for the consideration of UMHDSs. For purposes of the standards program, a UMHDS is defined as "a minimum set of items of information with uniform definitions and categories, concerning a specific aspect or dimension of the health care system, which meets the essential needs of multiple data users" (Health Information Policy Council, 1983, p.3). Thus nursing and nurses profit by this emphasis on standardized data that will enhance the comparability and uniformity of health information and statistics. Minimum health data sets play a large role in the program of Health Data Standards and Guidelines. This was kept in mind as the developmental work on the NMDS was done.

The Health Information Policy Council (HIPC) is the principal internal advisory body to the DHHS Secretary on health data policy matters, and the National Committee on Vital and Health Statistics is a public body that advises the secretary on all statistical matters, including minimum data sets. The NMDS has been presented to both of these groups; and the research potential of the NMDS was recognized readily, with the suggestion that funds be sought for further development and research. For some of this, nurse researchers should be encouraged to conduct research using the NMDS in their clinical interest areas.

The NMDS Definition Based on the UMDHS Concept and Definition

Built upon the concept and definition of the UMHDSs, the NMDS is defined as a minimum data set of items of INFORMATION WITH uniform definitions and categories concerning the specific dimension of nursing, which needs the information needs of multiple data users in the health care system. It includes those specific items of information that are used on a regular basis by the majority of nurses in any care delivery setting. It is an abstraction system, or tool, designed for the collection of uniform, standard, comparable, minimum nursing data for use across various types of settings and clinical populations. These data also are useful to other health professionals and researchers, if the total health care picture is to be represented in clinical and health policy decision making.

Underpinnings of the NMDS: The Nursing Process and the UMDDS

First, the nursing process is a systematic problem-solving methodology that nurses use to deliver patient care. Bulechek and McCloskey (1985), in their book on *Nursing Diagnosis and Interventions*, did an excellent job of tracing the early work on the nursing process; this work was initiated in 1967 at the Catholic University of America in Washington, DC, where four phases of the Nursing Process were identified; these were assessment, planning, implementation, and evaluation (Yura & Walsh, 1978, 1982, 1983). Through the years, the four-step model became a five-step model by adding nursing diagnosis and changing implementation to intervention. Thus in the present model the steps are assessment, diagnosis, planning, intervention, and evaluation. The nursing process constitutes professional nursing practice, that is, the diagnosis and treatment of health problems for which nurses are responsible (Bulechek & McCloskey, 1985).

The NMDS includes 16 elements that have been divided into three categories: Nursing Care, Patient or Client Demographics, and Service Elements. Three of the five-step nursing process phases are included in the NMDS, these are: Nursing Diagnosis, Nursing Intervention, and Nursing Outcome (sometimes referred to as nursing-sensitive patient outcome). Included also under the Nursing Care Elements is the Intensity of Nursing Care. This element should not be confused with "patient acuity," for Intensity of Nursing Care pertains to the allocation of nurse resources to provide care.

Nursing Diagnosis

Through the nursing process, care is standardized while individual service is provided. Part of the standardization comes from the classification of nursing diagnoses in accordance with the work that has been ongoing since 1973 (Gebbie & Lavin, 1975), when the National Conference Group for Classification of Nursing Diagnoses was formed. The Group met biennially since then, with nine conferences conducted to date. The purpose of these conferences has been the development of a diagnostic taxonomy for nurses, that is, "the definition of a standard nomenclature for describing health problems amenable to treatment by nurses" (Kim & Moritz, 1982, p. xvii). There are currently 100 nursing diagnoses that have been approved by the North American Nursing Diagnosis Association (NANDA) for clinical testing; these are listed in NANDA's (1990) Taxonomy I Revised. Efforts have been made to have the categorized nursing diagnoses included in the tenth revision of the International Classification of Diseases (ICD 10). Work done to translate nursing diagnosis into the ICD code is available in the literature (Fitzpatrick et al., 1989). This movement will require the support of nurses internationally, and it would be a great step forward for nursing as it moves toward standardization of its nursing care language.

Nursing Intervention

After having made the nursing diagnosis comes the decision about what to do with or for clients, that is, what nursing intervention or nursing action is the appropriate treatment for the nursing problem or diagnosis. Bulechek and McCloskey (1985) defined the term: "A nursing intervention is an autonomous action based on scientific rationale that is executed to benefit the client in a predicted way related to the nursing diagnoses and stated goals" (p. 8). Interventions are what nurses do with and for clients to solve a patient problem, or prevent a possible problem. Their definition has been broadened somewhat more recently, during their work on developing a classification system for nursing interventions.

Unlike what happened with nursing diagnosis, there is no organization to work on a classification of nursing interventions. The most unique and the best work being done in this area, to date, is that of McCloskey and Bulechek at the University of Iowa College of Nursing, where they have a large team of people developing a classification of nursing interventions. Their team consists of nurse faculty, hospital personnel, and two statisticians who are valued for their contributions and want to be part of the team. The team has done extensive work on this project for several years without external funding. Fortunately, they were funded in June 1990 by a federal grant; therefore they will be able to work more productively. The funding will facilitate completion of their work on the classification system in a shorter period of time, so the coded interventions can be shared with the profession and used, as for example, in the NMDS. McCloskey and Bulechek brought in their project Advisory Committee in November 1990 to review their work on the classification system to date, react to it, and to offer advice or suggestions as indicated. The Advisory Committee was most impressed with their work and urged them to carry on.

Nursing Outcome

Another aspect of the NMDS that requires further work is that of nursing-sensitive outcomes. Marek (1989) conducted a pilot project to identify outcome indicators found in the nursing literature that were used or proposed for use in measuring the effectiveness of nursing. She then classified these indicators into 15 categories, but they were not mutually exclusive nor exhaustive. Later, in two articles on patient outcomes Lang and Marek (1990, 1991), from the University of Wisconsin-Milwaukee, focused on the end results of nursing and health care, pointing up the absence of nursing data in various data bases. In essence, these are review articles covering the historical and contemporary influences on the work of outcomes, the American Nurses' Association role, and the establishment of the new, federal Agency for Health Care Policy and Research that focuses on effectiveness initiatives. There also is a Nursing Services Administration Research Team—a faculty group at the University of Iowa, led by Marion Johnson—whose members are exploring work being done on patient outcomes, in order to identify the nursing-sensitive outcomes. Their effort may eventually lead to the development of a classification system for nursing outcomes. This developmental work will be watched very carefully by all who are interested in the nursing process, which is the mode of professional nursing practice.

Until such time as a nursing-sensitive outcome classification is further developed, the proponents of the NMDS have coded the outcomes for nursing diagnoses as "resolved," "not resolved," or "not recorded" (Werley, Devine, & Zorn, 1988, 1990). And, the coding for nurse documentation of the NMDS element labeled "Disposition of Patient or Client" might reflect "Discharged to home with referral to organized community nursing service" (Werley & Lang, 1988b, chap. 31, p. 410). This could be discharge to a home health care agency or to a nursing home for short- or long-term care.

Intensity of Nursing Care

This element is to reflect the nurse resources required to provide patient or client care, as measured by the two sub-elements: Hours of Care and Staff Mix. To some extent, this element makes available costing of nursing care provided.

Second, as to the influence of the Uniform Hospital Discharge Data Set (UHDDS), ten of the NMDS elements in the demographic and service categories have been drawn from the UHDDS, which already is being collected for all hospitalized patients receiving Medicare benefits. In addition, the UHDDS serves as a linkage to other data sets within a facility. Thus, access is provided to additional client data that may serve as correlate or predictor variables when studying nursing practice or conducting research. This system linkage with the UHDDS "is valuable not only because of the information it contains but more importantly as the key to enter other data sets. Thus, through the UHDDS one can obtain an almost complete picture of the total period of hospitalization for a variety of uses" (Thompson, 1988, p. 284). Use of the NMDS can enhance the management of health care data, not only within hospitals, but also across settings in various long-term care, public health, and geographical locations, because of the inclusion of specific nursing care data.

Early Beginnings to Develop a Basic Nursing Data Set

The NMDS effort is a follow-through on earlier work that was done at the University of Illinois. In a Nursing Information Systems Conference held in 1977 at the University of Illinois College of Nursing in Chicago (Werley & Grier, 1981), an effort was made to stimulate nurses to move toward computerization of nursing services data and toward submission of proposals for research and development of NISs. In addition, one of the small work groups was given the challenge of identifying a basic nursing data set. Their effort was reported by Newcomb (1981) in the Werley and Grier (1981) *Nursing Information Systems* book. However, the timing for movement in this direction apparently was not right for nursing at that time, and nurses did not move forward in this area. This was so despite the fact that in the 1970s federal funding was available for research and development of information systems, and physicians and hospital administrators developed medical and hospital information systems that today are well known throughout the country. Most of those investigators received several rounds of funding. Unfortunately, however, most of their information systems were and are silent on nursing documentation whereby nursing practice and outcomes can be assessed in nursing's terminology. Nurses, too, should have been developing their NISs to complement and supplement the other data sets.

The NMDS Conference: Its Characteristics and Participants

Later, the subject of NISs was opened again, and in May 1985, a national, invitational NMDS Conference was held at the University of Wisconsin-Milwaukee School of Nursing to identify the NMDS. A national group of 64 experts participated in a three-day conference. Approximately 30 papers were commissioned to identify and discuss the issues involved in developing the NMDS, from the various authors' perspectives. These papers were assembled and distributed three months before the conference, to be studied prior to the conference so the participants would be ready to participate actively, in six task forces, to identify the elements for the NMDS.

The numerous conference participants included nurse experts in a variety of areas; health policy spokespersons; information systems, health data, and health records specialists; governmental and proprietary agency personnel; and persons knowledgeable about the development of the previous minimum health data sets (HIPC, 1983).

The first day of the conference, seven discussants, in turn, presented a brief synthesis of the issues identified in their block of assigned papers; then the discussant led a discussion of these issues among the total conference group. That evening, the charge was given for the next two workshop days, when the six task forces would be deliberating and identifying the NMDS elements. There was discussion of the task force plan, with the conferees having an opportunity to suggest changes. Consensus was reached to have everyone assigned to task forces in accordance with aspects of the nursing process, that is, nursing assessment, diagnosis, intervention, outcome, intensity of nursing care, and one on demographics. The resulting work then was reviewed by a Post-Conference Task Force several months later for agreement, modification, filling in nursing content, and approval for further work. Hence, the NMDS was consensually derived by this group of 64 experts at a national, invitational NMDS conference involving task force work (6 task forces) and consensus building—both within their separate task forces and across all task forces, or, the total group, followed with additional work by the Post-Conference Task Force. Thus, there was an element of validity.

Comparable Data

You will recall from the U.S. DHHS Program of Health Data Standards and Guidelines, discussed earlier, that in order to have comparable data collected, there must be decisions on what essential data are to be collected for what purpose. Special attention must be focused on definitions, codes, classifications, and terminology used, if comparability of data is to be enhanced.

Agreement on Data Elements Required

To have comparable data means that there is agreement on what data nurses will want to collect to portray their practice, and on standardization of language as they identify and define the elements to be collected for specific purposes. McCormick (1988) has written on the subject of the need for a unified nursing language system, indicating that the profession could or should define this language, that the language system should be seen as a part of health care language system developments generally, and that there should be clarity about frameworks and criteria for selecting content in a unified nursing language system. She also commented on advantages of a unified nursing language system, as well as on considerations essential to integrating clinical, scientific, and management data in meaningful ways. This latter point ties in somewhat with a statement made at the 1982 Cleveland conference on NISs regarding clinical and administrative data (Study Group on Nursing Information Systems, 1983). This Study Group stated that "management and practice data are interrelated or complementary and should be so perceived; ultimately, both kinds of information could be obtained from the same data" (p. 104).

To be assured of having comparable data, nurses also must learn to trust good work that has been done previously by others, without having each person start all over. There should be testing of this earlier work in a variety of settings in order to build on the work, changing things only as warranted by research and new developments. New knowledge is built in this way, that is, previous work is tested, research is conducted, and the results are shared as small accretions of new knowledge that add to the body of nursing and health care knowledge. It should be recognized that documentation of nursing diagnoses and interventions are the major building blocks of new nursing knowledge.

Adherence to the Definitions of the NMDS Elements

The NMDS elements were defined as can be found in the Werley and Lang (1988a) book and the Werley, Devine, and Zorn (1988, 1990) data collection manual. But, in order to advance the work on the NMDS, there must be testing, implementing, retesting, modifying, and developing further the data set. And then, research must be conducted to test further the true potential of the data set, in terms of both the projected benefits, the purposes of the NMDS, as well as the effectiveness of nursing care and patient outcomes.

Nurses should realize that information systems are improved with implementation and use; so they should move along with the research and development work, as well as testing and implementation. They could well take a lesson from the statement made in 1972 by the editors of the final report of the Uniform Hospital Discharge Data Demonstration. Hodgson and Kucken (1972) stated, "Hospital discharge data will be more valuable to users when they learn to manipulate the data to its fullest potential and to determine their own precise data requirements. . . . A uniform hospital discharge abstract data system will increase in value when data sets are developed and linked together for nursing homes, home health agencies, physician's offices, and other delivery sectors. The uniformity of data is also likely to enhance the worth of the hospital discharge information. The benefits to a medical community in adopting a basic data set increase proportionally to the number of hospitals in the area that collect uniform data" (p. 205). The essence of the above statement also will be true for nursing, once nurses implement and use the NMDS and then conduct comparative research across both units within facilities and across types of settings. Nurses, then, could make their own statement as it applies to the use and benefits of the NMDS implementation.

In addition, it must be recognized that, fortunately, more nurses prepared in informatics are beginning to contribute to nursing's growth in developing information systems and data bases. In recent years, since Judith Graves' completion of a two year post-doc in health informatics, Graves and Corcoran (1988a, 1988b, 1989) have been enriching the literature with articles on: designing NISs, identification of data element categories for clinical NISs, and the study of nursing informatics. These are excellent references that will help to advance the work on information management and computerization in the field of nursing; the first two articles mentioned are research-based. No doubt, these authors would welcome being called upon for consultation and assistance in promoting the forward movement of nursing's information systems.

Essential Core NMDS Elements per the Nursing Process and the UHDDS

Within the broader concept and definition of UMHDSs, HIPC saw minimum data sets as groupings of data items with standard definitions pertaining to a specific aspect of the health care system. These data sets have the potential to be powerful tools in meeting the purposes of the specific data set and of supporting a program to enhance comparability of data. And, this is as the proponents of the NMDS saw it when the data set was developed.

NMDS Elements

The NMDS includes 16 items, or elements, that have been categorized in three general groups: nursing care, patient or client demographics, and service elements, as shown below:

Nursing Care Elements
1. Nursing Diagnosis
2. Nursing Intervention
3. Nursing Outcome
4. Intensity of Nursing Care

Patient or Client Demographic Elements
*5. Personal Identification
*6. Date of Birth
*7. Sex
*8. Race and Ethnicity
*9. Residence

Service Elements
*10. Unique Facility or Service Agency Number
11. Unique Health Record Number of Patient or Client
12. Unique Number of Principal Registered Nurse Provider
*13. Episode Admission or Encounter Date
*14. Discharge or Termination Date
*15. Disposition of Patient or Client
*16. Expected Payer for Most of This Bill (Anticipated Financial Guarantor for Services)

*Elements marked with an asterisk are included in the UHDDS.

Ten elements of the NMDS are components of the UHDDS already being collected for all hospitalized patients receiving Medicare benefits; six items are new to the set. When health information systems are computerized and linked across different types of settings, only the new items would need to be recollected for hospitalized Medicare recipients.

Through this powerful, small data set (the NMDS), nurses can describe patient problems across types of settings, clinical populations, geographic areas, and time; identify the nursing diagnosis made; learn what nursing interventions or nursing actions were taken; observe nurse sensitive patient outcomes; and assess what nurse resources were used to provide nursing care. If the data from this set were part of ongoing nurse documentation, and computerized in such a way that the data could be retrieved readily, nursing would for the first time be in an excellent position to compare and contrast nursing practice locally, regionally, nationally, and internationally; offer pertinent, data based testimony on critical nursing and health care issues; develop data bases needed to conduct research on many aspects of clinical care; assess the cost effectiveness of nursing interventions for the respective nursing diagnoses; assess the cost of nurse resources used to provide care; and provide data to influence health policy making. Further, through the linkages between nursing's and other professional's data bases, nursing could share data with various health providers and researchers and at the same time have access to their data. This should be a challenge and opportunity toward which all nurses will wish to direct their efforts. Examples of what some nurses in the U.S. are doing about moving forward with the NMDS, are listed in the Werley and Leske (1991) paper to be presented during the main conference here at the Fourth International Conference on Nursing Use of Computers and Information Science.

References

Bulechek GM, McCloskey JC: Nursing diagnosis and intervention. In Bulechek GM, McCloskey JC (Eds.): *Nursing interventions: Treatments for nursing diagnoses* (pp. 1–18). Philadelphia: W. B. Saunders: 1985.

Devine EC, Werley HH: Test of the nursing minimum data set: availability of data and reliability. *Research in Nursing and Health* 1988:11, 97–104.

Fitzpatrick JJ, Kerr ME, Saba VK, Hoskins LM, Hurley ME, Mills WC, Rottkamp BB, Warren JJ, Carpenito LJ: Translating nursing diagnosis into ICD code. *American Journal of Nursing* 1989:89, 493–495.

Gebbie KM, Lavin MA (Eds.): *Proceedings of the First National Conference: Classification of Nursing Diagnoses.* St. Louis: Mosby 1975.

Graves JR, Corcoran S: Design of nursing information systems: Conceptual and practice elements. *Journal of Professional Nursing* 1988a:(4) 168–177.

Graves JR, Corcoran S: Identification of data element categories for clinical nursing information systems via information analysis of nursing practice. In Greenes RA (Ed.): *Proceedings of the Twelfth Annual Symposium on Computer Applications in Medical Care.* New York: Institute of Electrical and Electronics Engineers Computer Society Press, 1988b 358–363.

Graves JR, Corcoran S: (1989). The study of nursing informatics. *Image: Journal of Nursing Scholarship* 1989:(21) 227–231.

Health Information Policy Council: *Background Paper: Uniform Minimum Health Data Sets* (Unpublished). Washington, DC: U. S. Dept. of Health and Social Services, 1983.

Hodgson DA, Kucken LE (Eds.): *Uniform Hospital Discharge Data Demonstration: Final Report-Vol 1. Technical Report.* Chicago, IL: Health Services Foundation, 1972.

Kim MJ, Moritz DA (Eds.): *Classification of Nursing Diagnoses: Proceedings of Third and Fourth National Conferences.* New York: McGraw-Hill, 1982.

Lang NM, Marek KD: The Classification of patient outcomes. *Journal of Professional Nursing* 1990:6(3), 158–163.

Lang NM, Marek KD: The Policy and politics of patient outcomes. *Journal of Nursing Quality Assurance* 1991:5(2), 7–12.

Marek KD: Outcome measurement in nursing. *Journal of Nursing Quality Assurance* 1989:4(1), 1–9.

McCormick KA: (1988). A unified nursing language system. In Ball MJ, Hannah KJ, Jelger UG, Peterson H (Eds.): *Nursing informatics: Where caring and technology meet.* New York: Springer-Verlag, 1988.

Newcomb BJ: Issues related to identifying and systematizing data—Group discussions. In Werley HH, Grier MR (Eds.): *Nursing information systems.* New York: Springer Publishing, 1981.

North American Nursing Diagnosis Association: *Taxonomy I Revised 1990: With official diagnostic categories.* St. Louis, MO, 1990.

Werley HH: The nursing minimum data set: status and implications. In Hannah KJ, Reimer MR (Eds.): *Clinical judgment and decision making: The future with nursing diagnosis.* New York: Wiley, 1987 540–555.

Werley HH, Devine EC, Zorn CR: Nursing needs its own minimum data set. *American Journal of Nursing* 1988:(88) 1651–1653.

Werley HH, Devine EC, Zorn CR: Nursing Minimum Data Set: An abstraction tool for computerized nursing services data. In Saba VK, Rieder KA, Pocklington DB (Eds.): *Nursing and computers: An anthology.* New York: Springer-Verlag, 1989 187–195.

Werley HH, Devine EC, Zorn CR: *The Nursing Minimum Data Set Data Collection Manual* (reprinted). Milwaukee, WI: University of Wisconsin-Milwaukee, School of Nursing, 1990. (Original work published 1988)

Werley HH, Grier MR (Eds): *Nursing information systems.* New York: Springer Publishing, 1981.

Werley HH, Lang NM (Eds): *Identification of the Nursing Minimum Data Set.* New York: Springer Publishing, 1988a.

Werley HH, Lang NM: The consensually derived nursing minimum data set: elements and definitions. In Werley HH, Lang NM (Eds): *Identification of the Nursing Minimum Data Set.* New York: Springer Publishing, 1988b, pp 402–411.

Werley HH, Lang NM, Westlake SK: (1986a). Brief summary of the nursing minimum data set conference. *Nursing Management* 1986a:17(7), 42–45.

Werley HH, Lang NM, Westlake SK: (1986b). The nursing minimum data set conference: executive summary. *Journal of Professional Nursing* 1986b:2, 217–224.

Werley HH, Leske JS: *Use and implementation of the Nursing Minimum Data Set.* Paper presented at the Fourth International Conference on Nursing Use of Computers and Information Science, Melbourne, Australia, April 1991.

Werley HH, Zorn CR: The nursing minimum data set and its relationship to classifications for nursing practice. In *Classification systems for describing nursing practice.* Kansas City, MO: American Nurses' Association, 1989, 50–54.

Yura H, Walsh MB: *Human needs and the nursing process.* New York: Appleton-Century-Crofts, 1978.

Yura H, Walsh MB: *Human needs 2 and the nursing process.* New York: Appleton-Century-Crofts, 1982.

Yura H, Walsh MB: *Human needs 3 and the nursing process.* New York: Appleton-Lange, 1983.

The Blanke Foundation is acknowledged gratefully for continued partial support of ongoing work on the Nursing Minimum Data Set.

44
An Evaluation Study of Off-the-Shelf Patient Classification Systems

K.A. Seipp and J.P. O'Donnell

1. Introduction

Although an evaluation of commercial systems can examine many characteristics, functionality is usually given the highest priority. Functionality encompasses not only the range of functions performed, but the specific way the system accomplishes those functions (Pivnicny & Carmody, 1989). Before committing to expensive, time-consuming testing, it is essential to identify the systems that will produce the desired outcomes in a satisfactory manner. The evaluation model used in this study provided a framework for the collection of functional information to identify suitable systems for further consideration.

A 3-phase plan was developed to expedite identification of suitable systems using readily available information. Respectively, the objectives were to: (a) identify and collect information on commercially available, off-the-shelf PCSs, (b) organize pertinent information using an adapted evaluation model, and (c) identify the PCS's meeting predetermined selection criteria.

2. Methodology

Eighty-nine potential PCS sources were identified from lists in nursing administration and hospital automation references (*Software Guide*, 1991; Rowland & Rowland, 1989; *Directory of Consultants*, 1990). A data collection form guided the telephone interviews. Written materials on PCS methodology were also requested. Information was sorted using an adapted model which organized data according to system content, input, process and product. Preestablished selection criteria identified suitable systems.

Reprinted from *Nursing Informatics: An International Overview for Nursing in a Technological Era*, Grobe, S.J., Pluyter-Wenting, E.S.P. (Eds.). 1994. Pp. 82–86, with kind permission from Elsevier Science—NL, Sara Burgerhartstraat 25, 1055 KV Amsterdam, The Netherlands.

The views expressed in this article are those of the authors and do not reflect the official policy or position of the Department of the Army, Department of Defense, or the U.S. Government.

2.1 Phase I

The majority of the PCS sources were consultant or information systems companies. Most firms referred the inquiries to registered nurses on their staff who functioned as members of the design, research, and/or implementation teams. Occasionally, questions were answered by marketing personnel. Although the information received from marketing personnel may not be totally accurate or complete, it was not unreasonable to expect them to provide accurate product information to potential clients. This was considered an acceptable limitation, as the purpose of the study was to identify functionally suitable systems for further review, not to make a final selection. Fourteen sources were eliminated due to lack of response from the companies.

Fifty-seven sources were eliminated for various reasons. Some rejected sources did not have a PCS methodology. These included nursing information systems without PCS modules, software programs that automate a hospital's existing PCS, management applications of acuity data, and firms that only provided consultative services. Eight of the eliminated sources had PCSs used in only one specialty area. Other sources eliminated from further evaluation had PCSs that were one module of an extensive automated system and could not function as a stand-alone system.

Product information was provided by fifty-nine of the sources. To reduce selection bias in the event several suitable systems were identified, code numbers were assigned to the information for the remainder of the study.

2.2 Phase II

The context-input-process-product (CIPP) model is an evaluation tool proposed by Stufflebeam (1987) for use with educational programs. Context, input, process and product are the four parameters evaluated in the model (Stufflebeam et al, 1971). Information about objectives, needs, and expectations is obtained through context evaluation. Input evaluation yields information regarding procedural designs as well as strengths and limitations. Process evaluation provides information regarding implementation and monitoring. Product evaluation allows decision makers to assess information about results, reactions, and deficiencies.

After synthesizing information from the literature regarding patient classification systems, the researchers constructed a framework comprised

TABLE 1. Adaptation of the CIPP evaluation tool

I.	PCS tool code number

II. Operating context
   a. Purpose
   b. Setting—Size and type of hospitals/clinical units
   c. Historical information—Year developed, length of time in use
   d. Intended and realized information needs generated—Acuity, scheduling, productivity monitoring, audit procedure

III. Input or system capabilities
   a. Design
   b. Research
   c. Procedures for use
   d. Resource requirements for implementation

IV. Process or implementation design
   a. Monitoring system—Audit procedures
   b. Program/System redesign—Customizing, maintenance
   c. Defects
   d. Cost

V. Evaluation or outcomes
   a. Customer satisfaction
   b. Changes in patient assignment, staffing, productivity, etc
   c. Problems
   d. Benefits
   e. Additional studies on tool

of four parameters: operating context, system capabilities, implementation design, and outcomes. See Table 1 for an outline of the adaptation.

A CIPP evaluation matrix was completed from the information from each source. PCS sources were eliminated from the study as soon as they were identified as meeting one of the rejection criteria. This occurred at various stages of the study. Some sources remained in the study through phase III, while others were eliminated after the first telephone call.

2.3 Phase III

Selection criteria for a major system requires clarity about the strategic goals of the organization as well as the needs of customers at all levels. Therefore, selection criteria were developed before data collection to identify systems meeting functional requirements. The predetermineded selection criteria required: (a) reliable & valid tool(s) for seven clinical areas, (b) tool(s) requiring minimal or no adaptation, (c) standardized categories used across clinical specialties, (d) information for rating patients accessible in hospital records, (e) in use in multiple sizes and types of hospitals, (f) an audit, or interrater reliability system, and (g) a predictive daily staffing system.

3. Findings

Eighteen sources were identified as having commercially available PCSs and were evaluated using the CIPP matrix. Four sources were subsequently deleted when they were found to provide duplicate tools. Two of the 14 systems met all selection criteria described earlier. Both are reported by their companies as well-researched, valid and reliable PCS tools reflecting current nursing practice. Developed in the 1970's, both tools are used nationwide in many teaching and nonteaching acute care facilities of various sizes. Factor evaluative, or checklist-type tools, they use standard categories across all units. The acuity values are weights, not time. Interrater reliability is determined from information in the medical record.

The number of patients per acuity category is reported and therefore available for development of acuity-based staffing standards. Translating acuity weights to full-time equivalents by the staffing systems requires some customizing by the companies to identify the needs and philosophy of the facility or multi-hospital system. The staffing systems project staffing requirements as numbers of each skill mix per shift.

Additionally, both companies have other management applications that use the acuity and staffing data. The cost of the two systems is flexible and dependent on the amount and type of support requested from

TABLE 2. Differences between PCS A and PCS B

Criteria	PCS A	PCS B
Basis of acuity	Amount & complexity of care	Risk, complexity, skill level, & time
Number of indicators	36	70
Time/frequency of acuity rating	Daily	Every shift
Tool modification	None required	Minimal
Face validity for nursing staff	Total nursing domain not shown	Total nursing domain is shown
Number of categories	6	7
Staffing system	Projects staffing 3 shifts based on planned care	Projects staffing 1 to 3 shifts based on actual care
Input used to determine staffing	Direct and indirect time, operating constraints	Direct and indirect time, short length of stay patients, outpatients, operating constraints
Number of hospitals using the tool	300	70
Automation	Multiple options available	Currently manual
Access to civilian data base	Yes, annual reports	No
Maintenance of system	Comprehensive support & maintenance	Annual updates

the companies. Implementation time appears about the same for both systems.

Despite the similarities between the two systems and the fact that they both meet the selection criteria, there are significant differences. These differences between the two PCSs provide a mechanism for selecting a system to replace the current system, if an off-the-shelf option is deemed acceptable. The differences are detailed in Table 2.

4. Discussion

The sense of urgency felt by users and top management to replace an obsolete system is understandable. "If problems with an existing system are serious enough to justify spending tens of thousands of dollars to find a new system . . . how can a hospital spend years waiting for a new system to be in place?" (Doyle, 1990). The process of identifying a system that meets organizational needs is necessarily time consuming.

However, there are strategies for meeting the goals of the search for a system and reducing time delays. First, senior management must define its expectations. The requirements of the system should be derived from the organization's strategic plans (Doyle, 1990). Selection criteria can then be developed that identify the purpose of the system and set priorities on customers' needs in accomplishing that purpose. The next major step is to identify systems for thorough review and pilot testing. Missteps can result in expensive delays by implementing and testing systems that do not meet functional requirements.

Adapting the Stufflebeam CIPP model resulted in identification of relevant data in a systematic manner, facilitating the judgement process. Clearly identifying systems that meet functionality requirements from readily available information reduced both the time and cost of the selection process. Examining system functionality does not eliminate the need for further evaluation. Other aspects of purchasing a system must be explored to insure valid performance in any practice setting. The differences between systems provide a mechanism for final selection.

References

[1] Pivnicny VC and Carmody JG. Criteria Help Hospitals Evaluate Vendor Proposals. *Healthc Financ Manage* 1989, 43:38–47.
[2] Software Guide. *Nurs Manage* 1991, 22:65–92.
[3] Rowland H and Rowland B. *Hospital Software Sourcebook*. Rockville, MD: Aspen Publishing, 1989.
[4] Directory of Consultants to Nursing Administration. *J Nurs Adm* 20:43–81.
[5] Stufflebeam DL. Planning Evaluation Studies. In: *Handbook in Research and Evaluation*. Isaac S, Michael W (eds). San Diego, CA: Edits Publisher, 1987.

[6] Stufflebeam DL, Foley WJ, Gephart WJ, Guba EG, Hammond RL, Merriman HO, and Provus MM. *Educational Evaluation and Decision Making*. Itasca, IL: Peacock, 1971.
[7] Doyle O. Making the Most of Information System Consultants. *Healthc Financ Manage* 1990, 44:34–44.

45
The Role and Scope of Data Management in a Changing Health Services Delivery Environment

K. Hannah and J. Curry

1. Definition of Data Management

Data Management is the analysis and definition of data which is to be captured to produce the required information, and the identification of the processes needed to capture data most effectively. Data Management must be done in a coordinated way, led by data and information management specialists, in order to maximize the value of the data and minimize the cost of data capture for the entire health services delivery system. Data Management includes identifying standard data definitions and the corresponding data capture processes as well as facilitating the more complex information and data management responsibilities. Integrated information systems require new management processes to ensure that data is of sufficient quality, is adequately secure, is used for the purposes agreed to, and is disposed of appropriately when no longer required. The more data is used for productive purposes, the more its value increases and the unit cost of capture decreases. Data standards ensure comparability across many diverse sources and enhance administrative processes, accountability measures, service provider information exchange, and security provisions. A minimum set of standard data also ensures that information providers are not burdened by redundant data requests.

2. Relationship Between Data Management and Business, Application, Technology, and Methodology

What is the relationship among the domains and what is the Data Management relationship with the domains? Data Management is literally within the intersection of all the intersections. It is the last piece of the puzzle.

Reprinted with permission from *MEDINFO '95: Proceedings of the Eighth World Congress on Medical Informatics*; Greenes, R.A., Peterson, H.E. & Protti, D.J. (Eds.). 1995. Pp. 475–477. Edmonton, Alberta, Canada: Canadian Organization for the Advancement of Computers in Health (COACH).

The history of Data Management mirrors the evolution of how information systems are used by Business and by the increase in understanding how information systems support the Business. At first, these domains were considered to be separate and independent. Gradually, the awareness dawned that these domains were not independent at all but rather were highly interdependent.

Historically, data belonged to an application; they had no independent existence. An application was the means by which data were created, updated, and used; these were the traditional roots of Data Management. Thus the modern day Application domain is linked to Data Management in terms of data capture and data use. This link reflects the move to separate the original, tightly coupled bond between Data and Application.

Similarly, Applications were dependent on the technology that ran them. Those two domains have been traditionally coupled. Hardware is useless without an Application to go on it; one is useless without the other. Therefore, the Hardware domain is strongly bound to the Application software domain. But Data Management also has its own technology implications, i.e., the need to track where data exist in a dispersed technical environment. Therefore, the Hardware domain is also bound to the Data Management domain. However, the links between Data Management and Hardware are not as great as those between Data Management and Application. This illustrates the evolution of the focus known as data administration.

Methodology became a factor in the process because the building of Applications evolved. Methodology overlaps with both Applications and Technology because the building of Applications is dependent on the Technology, as the capability of the Technology constrains how an application can be implemented. The advent of software development and data structure—from batches flat files to on-line direct access files to relational databases to object orientated uses of data—has as much Technology implication as Application implication. Consequently, Methodology has a strong overlap with Data Management because Data Management requirements change as the Methodology changes.

The most important domain is the Business. The Business dictates the Data requirements. Data Management serves the Business. Data Management does NOT exist to serve the Application or Technology developers. The role of Data Management is to serve the Business; consequently there is a strong bond between these two domains. In addition, the relationship between Data Management and Business also has a strong link with Methodology. This link is a consequence of the Business Methodology. There is a close relationship between the Business Methodology (such as TQM or Business Process Re-Engineering) and Application Development Methodology; this is in addition to the link between Business and Application because the Business is implemented through its Applications.

Business also has a strong relationship with Technology because of the networks which have been developed. Today, the system is the network and the network is the system. Networks are enablers which allow businesses to have a virtual organization. Until recently, the various communication barriers imposed by distance and time made concrete physical organizations essential and dictated that management structures be partitioned to allow each individual geographical location to be managed independently. Today, management of virtual organizations is possible because the technology ties the various components together with communication networks. Distance, time, and location all become almost irrelevant. However, Data Management must consider all of the domains. To focus on one domain to the exclusion of the others, or to exclude any domain rapidly, creates an imbalance and exposes the Business to unnecessary risk. Data Management is by definition within the intersection of all the intersections. The evolution of Data Management is the evolution of the intersections— the recognition of the impact of the intersections and that the various domains are interdependent.

3. History of Data Management

The original stand-alone systems characterized by the intrinsic bond between application and data were followed by the interfacing era. During this era, Data management was considered to be data administration and originated because of the need to monitor the data exchange within and between applications in the interfacing mode (taking the output of data from one application as input to another). Gradually, the concept of integration evolved. Integrated systems have different views of the same data. Integration requires much more careful attention to methodology and data design. Therefore, the need for Data Management became apparent. The need for Data management became even more pronounced when Methodology (both Business and Application) was impacted by Technology. For example, the Technology evolution from the main frame box to client server networks required an entire new Application Development Methodology paradigm. This Technology shift also impacted what Business could do in terms of sharing information and transferring information; this contributed to the dissolution of the barriers of time and space and the feasibility of the "virtual" organization, e.g., the hospital without walls and a seamless healthcare delivery system.

The result is technology dependent information and an associated expansion of what constitutes data. In the beginning, data appeared as an administration record form with little fields and little records. Now, everything is data. Wave forms, images, videos, digitized landsat maps, virtual human bodies. Anything that can be reduced to an electronic form and translated back to some human perceivable form is data. Applications that actually capture and manage the data in their various forms are essential, but what is being captured is data. The role of Data Management is to manage data as a resource in ALL its various forms so as to avoid escalating the cost of data capture and the use of such data beyond affordability.

Data are not information unless presented in context. Data are a collection of facts captured within a specific context, e.g., the policy framework and healthcare situation at the time. For example, in isolation a wave form means nothing. In order to make some sort of clinical judgment one needs to know: a wave form of what, for whom, who ordered it, why was it ordered, what else was going on? Information can be defined as relevant knowledge for a specific purpose. Data can be transformed into information by selecting, collating, aggregating, and presenting pertinent data. However, when data are taken out of context, often *misinformation* rather than *useful information* is created. Improvements in the quality of data are required in order to give decision makers access to more appropriate information. This is why data must be managed, and data must be managed in context. Data Management can be considered the management of the connections between data and the context in which they are captured (the Business, Application, and Technology domains) in order to transform data into appropriate information in a different context.

4. Conclusion

Data Management is complex because the world that data represent is complex. Let us add dynamic change over time to that little picture. The definition of what is data has been expanding. The way in which applications are built, and the capabilities of those applications, is changing; the technology that enables those applications are changing and the business that takes advantage of those new capabilities are not only changing, but also rapidly dissolving the barriers of space and time. The only constant is change. Methodology manages business change and methodology is impacted by and impacts the technology and the business changes. We are just beginning to learn how to harness the power of Technology and Methodology to manage the complexity of the dynamic environment surrounding Data Management. As the delivery of health services (i.e., the "business") changes, and as the technology enabling characteristics change, the importance of Data Management grows. The responsiveness of the health services delivery system (i.e., the capacity, capability and flexibility) to change provides a competitive advantage either to an organization within the health services delivery system or to a country which can then devote fewer scarce national resources to achieving the health benefits for its citizens. The often repeated statement that information technology is an enabling factor really means that the capability of transferring and sharing information is a competitive advantage. The technology enables the organization to overcome the barriers of distance and time. Data Management is the means of coordinating data to ensure that the data provide useful information for the purpose of supporting the delivery of health services.

46
Nursing QA—Standard-Setting Forces and Automation

SUSAN K. NEWBOLD

One of the prime aspects of Nursing responsibility is the assurance of quality patient care. The objective of this paper is to highlight the standard-setting forces that influence Nursing quality assurance (QA) and discuss how automation can be used for Nursing QA activities.

Nursing QA—Standard Setting Forces

There are a number of entities which influence quality assurance standards in healthcare. Many of the standards are suggestions and guidelines but others are rules and regulation to which Nurses have no choice but to adhere.

In the United States (U.S.), the Joint Commission on Accreditation of Healthcare Organizations (JCAHO) introduced QA standards in 1979 and suggested that audit is one approach to evaluating quality assurance. Currently three Nursing Service standards focus on standards of patient care. New standards expected to be published in 1991 will promote the use of computers in handing patient care data (Patterson, 1990). JCAHO is revising the method in which it conducts surveys of healthcare organizations in a major research and development project "The Agenda for Change." The goal is to change from a "meets standards" situation to a method that will allow the organization to judge the effectiveness of its care. There are three major aspects to the Agenda for Change. Clinical indicators are developed to determine the quality of care in hospitals; a national database will collect data and offer feedback on performance compared to other facilities; and organizations will use this information to introduce quality improvements. The Australian healthcare arena, particularly the Austra-

Reprinted with permission from; *Nursing Informatics '91: Proceedings of the Fourth International Conference on Nursing Use of Computers and Information Science*; Hovenga, E.J.S., Hannah, K.J., McCormick, K.A. & Ronald, J.S. (Eds.). 1991, pp. 378–381. Heidelberg-Berlin, Germany: Springer-Verlag.

lian Council on Healthcare Standards is also working to introduce a care evaluation program.

Specialty Nursing organizations such as the Oncology Nurses Society, Post Anesthesia Nurses Association, Rehabilitation Nurses Association, and the American Academy of Ambulatory Nursing Administration are examples of organizations that have written standards of practice to guide the Nurse in providing care. A specialty multi-disciplinary organization, the National Association of Quality Assurance Professionals, also focuses on suggesting standards as well as holding annual meetings and publishing the *Journal of Quality Assurance*.

Expert Nurses developing the Nursing Minimum Data Set (Werley, 1988) seek to standardize essential nursing data that can be used by Nurses across the U.S. in all care delivery settings. Research on the data will assist in studying the outcomes and quality of Nursing care as well as the cost for providing that quality.

The American Nurse's Association (ANA) publishes many varieties of Standards of Nursing Practice (1978). Among these are standards for Medical/Surgical Nurses, Home Health Nursing Practice, Gerontology, Maternal-Child, Nurse Practitioners, and Psychiatric-Mental Health Nurses. The ANA has produced several QA publications, although they date in the mid 1970's. A more recent document provides peer review guidelines and several items on credentialing of Nurses which can be viewed as QA material.

The National League for Nursing supports a program known as CHAP (Community Health Accreditation Program). This accrediting body is dedicated solely to quality in the home care industry.

Individual hospitals and other healthcare facilities set standards which may include Nursing policies and procedures, position descriptions, and organization-wide policies.

Expert witness testimony is another force that sets standards for Nursing practice. Nursing experts are called upon in legal cases where the Nurse must testify as to what a reasonable and prudent Nurse would do in a similar circumstance.

Common law guides the way decisions are made regarding QA. Nurses are being held legally accountable for their actions and past legal judgments guide Nurses in their practice.

State and Federal requirements drive Nursing practice in determining QA guidelines. Examples include licensure standards, changes in Health Care Financing Administration requirements, Professional Standards Review Organizations for Medicare and Medicaid, maternal and child health programs, and Peer Review Organizations. Third Party Payors provide reimbursement for Nurse Practitioners and therefore their guidelines determine the quality of care patients should receive. The Omnibus Budget Reconciliation Act of 1987 includes a host of regulatory requirements to enforce minimum quality standards in the Federal Government. In the United States, the National Practitioner Data Bank will record every

Doctor and Nurse who pays a patient for a malpractice claim, is disciplined by a state Medical or Nursing licensing board or whose clinical privileges are revoked by a hospital. Hospitals are required to check to see whether a Physician or Nurse's name is listed.

Formerly QA focused on operational performance and now the focus is moving toward consumer response to performance or consumer opinion (Beyer, 1988). Strasen (1988) agrees that "patient satisfaction indicators are emerging as a dominant and critical outcome measure for quality of care."

Nursing QA and Automation

A related discussion analyses how automation can be used to assist Nursing QA. Not all QA activities need to be automated, but a review of how quality assurance can be assisted by automation follows:

Data Collection, Tracking, and Transmission

Assembly of data in either a stand-alone or integrated information system can improve the quality of data. Reminders and edits can be built into the computer software which check the quality of the data as they are being entered. Hospitals will look to its software vendors to provide a means of capturing and submitting data electronically to comply with the JCAHO Agenda for Change program. Automation can assist in quality assurance related to personnel. Items that can be tracked include degree programs, post-graduate training, continuing education, professional licensure certification, professional appointments, presentations, publications, honors, malpractice payments, disciplinary action, and community activities.

Identification of Potential Problems

Risks can be identified and managed before they become problems. An example of how computer technology has been used to identify potential problems is the U.S. Department of Defence (DoD) Composite Health Care System and occurrence screening. A Medical Treatment Facility defines clinical practice criteria (occurrences) and events such as patient falls and medication errors requiring further investigation are identified, tracked and documented (U.S. DOD, 1985).

Statistics

Arithmetic calculations, frequencies, percentages, means, medians, and standard deviations are frequently used statistics used in QA studies. Data manipulation is made significantly easier by use of a computer. Statistics can be trended over time to reflect if a specific criteria is improving or declining.

Presentation Mechanisms and Reports

Statistical results that are graphically displayed enable the reviewer to readily visualize improvements or departures from quality care. Various charts such as pie, bar, and graph can be easily drawn and updated with the use of automation. Reporting such as cardiac arrest critiques, operating room and emergency room audits, nosocomial disease reports, incident summary reports, and professional licensure reports can be readily compiled, maintained, and trended with the aid of automation.

Case Identification

Automation can be used for fast and accurate case identification and retrieval. Criteria can be input and the computer is instructed to retrieve all cases matching that criteria. Case identification can readily extract specific data—physical parameter readings, Nursing diagnosis, treatment, room number, specific care provider, etc. for analysis purposes. Data for quality assurance studies may be easily extracted from a variety of sources provided they are on-line. These sources could be infection control and incident reports, medication error reports, patient care plans, patient classification data, Nurse staffing and scheduling systems, patient satisfaction surveys, diagnosis related groups, census, and other patient records.

Random Selection of Criteria For Evaluation

Some quality assurance studies require only a subset of the potential number of cases. Automation can select random cases in which to conduct studies without bias.

There are numerous influences upon quality assurance in healthcare that were highlighted in this paper. Also discussed is how the use of automation can assist with quality assurance activities.

References

American Nurse's Association 1978. Standards of Nursing Practice.
Beyer, Marjorie. Quality: the banner of the 1980s. *Nursing Clinics of North America* 1988;3:617–623.
Joint Commission on Accreditation of Healthcare Organizations. Accreditation Manual for Hospital 1978 and 1990 editions.
Omnibus Reconciliation Act of 1987.
Patterson, Carole H. Quality assurance, control, and monitoring. *Computers in Nursing* 1990;3:105–110.
Public Law 99–660 Title IV, Health Care Quality Improvement Act of 1986.
Standards of Nursing Practice. American Nurse's Association, 1978.
Strasen, Leann. Incorporating patient satisfaction standards into quality of care measures. *Journal of Nursing Administration* 1988;11:5–6.

U.S. Department of Defense, Functional Descriptions for the Composite Health Care System and Nursing, 1985.

Werley, Harriet H., Lang, Norma M. *Identification of the Nursing Minimum Data Set.* New York: Springer Publishing Company, 1988.

47
Bedside Nursing Information Systems; Quantities and Costs

A.R. Bakker, E.M.S.J. van Gennip, and W. Roelofs

Introduction

The attractiveness of support of the nursing profession by means of bedside terminals has widely been described and has raised a lot of interest in this way of applying information technology in the heart of the hospital. Both the quality, the effectiveness and the efficiency can be expected to benefit. The expcted effects are listed here briefly:

- up-to-date information on history, present state and goals will become available immediately at the bedside, in a presentation geared towards the specific tasks to be performed;
- communication between the members of the team is supported (also across shifts);
- planned activities both for the patient and the nurse will be recorded in a coherent way and can be coordinated; quality of care can be monitored directly
- the system will take into account consequences of planned activities;
- communication with supporting departments will be improved and accelerated.

When the bedside terminals are incorporated in an integrated Hospital Information System (HIS) the functions of the HIS will add to the benefits listed above, leading to support of mangement, research and education. On the other hand the HIS will gain in value through the process information supplied by the NIS. In view of the benefits to be expected it is not surprising that several projects were started to realize bedside nursing information

Reprinted with permission from; *Nursing Informatics '91: Proceedings of the Fourth International Conference on Nursing Use of Computers and Information Science*; Hovenga, E.J.S., Hannah, K.J., McCormick, K.A. & Ronald, J.S. (Eds.). 1991, pp. 398–407. Heidelberg-Berlin, Germany: Springer-Verlag.

systems, primarily in the USA, but also in Europe. Although the realization and implementation is not proceeding as rapidly as initially expected the first prototypes and early products are available and operational in several hospitals. Now that the concept has demonstrated to be feasible, the following two questions have to be answered:

1. do these bedside nursing information systems fulfil the expectations; what are the benefits really achieved (both in qualitative and in quantitative sense)?
2. what are the costs to be expected for the hospital when introducing these systems?

Well documented answers to both questions are required to convince hospital management that the introduction of bedside nursing information systems is worthwhile. The studies should be set up in a way that they will be of help for institutions in making a sound decision. Since the circumstances will vary between institutions, already within countries but even more between countries, special attention should be given to the presentation of the results in a form that allows for projection on the own situation. Just presenting overall data on costs/savings and benefits will be of little help, the components and the reasoning behind the figures are essential.

In this paper the question about the costs will be dealt with. The paper does not pretend to give final answers to this most important question, it hopefully can contribute to a well-structured discussion in this field that is confronted at present with a confusion of tongues. First the various cost categories will be identified. Next a global quantification will be given of the volumes of transactions and data to be expected in a bedside NIS. In the next section the cost categories will be confronted with the results found and the presently available technology. To make the considerations more concrete as a case the costs to be expected for the bedside NIS of the BAZIS foundation in the Netherlands [Bakker 90] are considered for a hypothetical 1000 bed teaching hospital. Finally some concluding remarks are presented.

Cost Categories

Introduction to Costs of NIS

Costs for a bedside NIS are caused by the utilisation of resources of different type. In the next paragraphs the various resources needed to realise a NIS are considered. To be able to compare costs we need a common yardstick, so all costs will be expressed as annual costs. Investments in equipment and software will be depreciated, loss of interest is taken into consideration.

Costs of Equipment

The equipment needed can be subdivided into:

1. bedside equipment and other terminals or workstations on the nursing ward,
2. shared equipment; in general an HIS computer and possibly a departmental computer,
3. network facilities.

As bedside equipment we find a wide range of "solutions" comprising portable terminals, normal terminals, terminals with special facilities (e.g. for user identification) and special PC-based workstations. The categories a and b can be depreciated in 5 years, leading to annual costs equal to 25% of the investment if the interest rate is taken as 10%. For category c in general a period of 10 or 15 years is used leading to annual costs of 15 or 12%. The annual equipment costs can be expressed in the following formula: $\$ = A * (1/N + I/200)$, with A the invested amount, depreciation in N years with interest percentage I, $ the annual cost. Sometimes a nonlinear depreciation is applied since computer equipment is losing its value quickly because alternatives with better price/performance are introduced. A scheme for 5 years depreciation with 30% in the first year and 25%, 20%, 15% and 10% respectively in the following years seems more appropriate.

Apart from the capital costs we also have to consider costs of maintenance. For central computer equipment there is in general a maintenance contract. The annual costs range from 6 to 12% of the investment, depending on the type of maintenance. For 24 hours coverage one should calculate with at least 10%. For duplicated systems a one shift maintenance contract seems justified (costs 6–8%).

Since in a bedside NIS many terminals will be in use, it is often cheaper not to choose a full maintenance contract but to buy some spare items that can replace defective equipment. The defective items are collected and offered for repair with a low priority (and at low cost). The annual costs for maintenance of terminals in that situation will not exceed 4%. For the network the maintenance costs are relatively low, 1–3% is a reasonable range.

When computer equipment is shared with other applications as will in general be the case when the NIS is integrated with the HIS, a part of the cost of shared equipment should be counted. Often an accounting system will be in place for the computer facility. The outcome of such an accounting system should be handled carefully, the costs of operating the system should be dealt with separately.

Costs of Software

As far as costs for software are concerned, there are basically two different situations: it comes from a vendor or it is a homebrew. The vendor mostly charges an annual license for the use of the software. Often maintenance is included, in some situations maintenance is charged separately. In this "ideal" situation we directly know the annual costs. When there is an initial charge to be paid to the vendor this can be depreciated as for hardware; a depreciation period of 5 years seems reasonable. For homebrew software one should calculate the number of hours spent, multiply it with a realistic integral rate and depreciate this amount (again over 5 years). Maintenance should not be forgotten since per year this may easily amount to 10–20% of the initial development costs. It should be born in mind that software licences may well depend on the intensity of use foreseen, e.g. estimated from the size of the hospital, the number of nurses using the system or the number of terminals.

Costs of Support

One of the requirements of an NIS is user friendliness, nevertheless the system and its users will need support from time to time. Typical activities are:

- answering questions of users who are confronted with unusual situations;
- file maintenance (e.g. extension when the number of standard careplans increases)
- loading new versions of the software;

Support should be expressed in the number of manhours needed. When the support is supplied by a vendor the costs can directly be determined by multiplication of this number with the manhour rate. When the support is supplied by own staff a realistic manhour rate has first to be determined.

Costs of Training

Training costs contain both costs of the users of the system and of the teachers. When the system is first introduced all personnel have to be trained. But also when the system is in operational use, training will be needed not only for new personnel, but also for experienced users. Training will be needed to make them aware of new functions that can be expected to become available (further evolution of NIS).

The number of manhours for training should be estimated and multiplied by the average hourly rate. Initial training costs might be depreciated e.g. over 5 years. The amount of training needed depends heavily on the user friendliness of the system (e.g. help texts) and on the level of familiarity with computer applications that can be expected from the nurses.

Costs to Let the System Operate

Although computer applications are often indicated by the word "automated" one should realize that information systems in general do not run by themselves; they need care. Typical activities needed are:

- making safe-copies of the databank to allow for recovery in case of corruption or loss
- distributing of centrally printed output
- replacing defective terminals
- scheduling preventive maintenance
- signalling technical problems and calling for maintenance
- mounting magnetic tapes

The costs are primarily related to manhours spent. When the central equipment is installed in the computer center of the hospital, that organization will take care of all these activities. In case the NIS is based on a departmental computer, these activities have to be done as well and will need extra manpower that should be taken into account (estimated number of manhours * rate). A complication is that problems do occur at unexpected moments, someone should be available (at least on-call) to handle these.

Apart from manhours we need energy, floor space and supplies to let the computer system run. The costs involved should not be forgotten. They are often contained in the charges of the computer center. For a departmental system they should be counted separately.

Costs of Using the System by Nurses

Using the system to enter and retrieve data will take nursing time. Of course these actions form part of their daily work and are expected to pay-off either by replacing manual information handling or by contributing to the quality of care (efficiency and effectiveness). One should realize that the percentage of time to be spent using the system will not be negligible. If it is counted explicitly it should be balanced with the number of hours that will be saved.

Apart from the time spent on using the system for daily routine we should bear in mind that some files will need nursing attention, e.g. standard careplans and nursing instructions. Moreover the access rights of each nurse should be identified and monitored, the nursing management will have to spend some time on this.

Global Quantification of the Volume of Transactions and Data

A bedside NIS by nature requires interactive equipment at the bedside. One may choose a terminal/workstation at each bed, but one might also choose one terminal in each room. Portable terminals are another option. Apart from equipment in the patient rooms, additional terminals will be needed at the nursing desk (with printing capabilities) and in some other places (e.g. in the corridors, outside the patient room). If one chooses to have a terminal at each bed the total number of terminals can be estimated at 1.3 * #beds. When a terminal per room is judged to be sufficient this figure may go down to .7 * #beds. When portable terminals are applied the number of these devices will at least be equal to the number of nurses in the prime shift, in addition to that "normal" terminals will be needed.

Apart from the terminals, communication facilities will be needed to connect them to the databank where the data are stored. Computer capacity will be required for the storage of the data and the processing of the required transactions. To be able to make an estimate of the capacity needed we need to estimate the number of transactions to be performed and the amount of data to be collected. A study at Leiden University Hospital [Heemskerk '88] yielded an estimated 80 transactions per patient per day of which 65% in the day shift. The number of nursing data items to be recorded per patient per day was estimated between 140 and 270 (av 200). The total volume of data to be stored might be estimated as follows:

- store the data during the stay of the patient plus one week
- assume as an average 10 bytes per item
- assume overhead in databank of 100%
- realize that the average history of a hospitalized patient is larger than half the average length of stay since "patients with a longer stay stay longer." Taking the full average length of stay seems a reasonable estimate. If we consider a 1000 bed acute hospital with an average length of stay of 10 days and 90% bed occupancy, we arrive at a total volume of data to be stored of $1000 * .9 * 10 * 200 * 17 * 2 = 600 M$ bytes

Confrontation of Cost Categories with Quantities in NIS

Introduction

In this section the various cost categories are considered again with the quantities in mind as indicated in the previous section and with a look at current technology. The actual situation as to the realization of HIS can be taken as a reference, giving confidence that bedside NISses are feasible, although the number of terminals may be twice as high as in a current HIS.

Equipment

The number of terminals/workstations needed depends on the solution chosen, this number may easily vary by a factor 2. Later in this paper it will be found that the terminal costs are a significant percentage of the total cost. The cost contribution can directly be determined when the type of terminal/ workstation is chosen. In estimating the costs, one should realize that the printing terminals that will be needed at the nursing desk will have an increasing effect on the average cost per terminal. For each (nonportable) terminal, a network connection will be needed. The cost of cabling will depend heavily on the architecture and facilities (ducts?) of the building. The network solution chosen may also influence the costs.

The volume of data as estimated is substantially lower than in current HIS implementations and will yield no problem at all. Even when the storage facilities are fully duplicated the storage costs will be small when compared to terminal costs.

To process the transactions a powerful computer system should be available. This might be realized by embedding the NIS in the HIS or by linking one or more dedicated NIS computers to the HIS. For an integrated HIS the total number of transactions is several times higher than predicted in the previous section, so no serious technical limitations have to be expected. Estimating the costs for computer capacity will not be easy when equipment is to be shared. It will be necessary to specify the various cost components of the central computer system and try to determine the NIS share for each component.

A Hypothetical Case

To make these considerations more concrete a hypothetical case will be considered. The present bedside NIS as being developed by the BAZIS foundation in the Netherlands [Nieman89] will be projected on a 1000 bed teaching hospital. Data are derived partly from the prototype implementation of this system at Leiden University Hospital, partly they are derived from cost analysis studies for the BAZIS HIS [Bakker90].

Costs are estimated per bed and the total is expressed as equivalents of the average annual cost of one nurse, this to make them more or less independent of local currency. This effect will be achieved only partly since the ratio between manhour cost and equipment cost shows a significant variation between countries. In the USA this ratio is lower than in Western Europe (a factor between 1.5 and 2), the difference with Eastern Europe is even larger.

It is assumed that there will be a "normal' terminal (keyboard/screen) for each bed; printing terminals and terminals for general use amount to 30% of the number of beds. The price of such a simple terminal is at present about Dfl 1000, however a factor 1.3 is taken into account for printer facilities. In this way we arrive at an annual cost per bed of about Dfl 500 (1000 ∗ 1.3 ∗ 1.3 ∗ .29).

The costs for cabling can be estimated at Dfl 1000 per connection, in addition to that data communication equipment is needed, another amount of about Dfl 1000. This leads to annual costs of about Dfl 300 per terminal for DC and network. For the application software we can estimate for a full NIS an annual software license of Dfl 150,000, so per bed per year Dfl 150. In addition to that there will be a charge for system software (OS, DBMS) of about Dfl 100 per bed per year.

It is estimated that support and training together will require 3 fte, leading to annual costs per bed of Dfl 250. The time nurses need to be trained is not considered here. It is assumed that the NIS will be embedded in the HIS and will use the hospital HIS computer centre, based on presently available computer configurations the central equipment costs would be about Dfl 300,000, so per bed per year about Dfl 100. Although it is expected that the computer centre staff will need extension with 1 fte, however the cost of operations are calculated in an integral way leading to an amount of 250,000 per year, so Dfl 250 per bed.

The various cost components are summmarized in the table below, that indicates that the cost per bed will be equal to between 2 and 3% of a nurse fte

hardware:	terminal equipment	500
	dc and network	300
	central equipment	100
software;	application	150
software;	system	100
support and training		250
operational		250
total annual costs per terminal		1650

It can be observed that the major part is formed by costs for equipment, 55% of the total. Costs for software are about 15% and almost equal to those of training/support and operations.

Concluding Remarks

Although costs of a bedside NIS will depend heavily on the technical solution (hardware and software), on the local situation and on the moment of introduction, a common approach to cost calculations will be helpful to pave the way for such systems. This paper may be a stimulus for IMIA working group 8 to try to develop a uniform cost model.

Contrary to what is often assumed hardware costs at this moment will form the largest cost component even when a simple terminal per bed is used. When sophisticated workstations are to be used these costs may easily double. Because of developments in technology, hardware costs can be expected to decrease. Over the past 20 years we have seen an improvement in price/performance of 20–30% per year. The hardware costs for a state of the art NIS will not decrease at that pace since the technological progress will lead to demands for more functionality. Nevertheless the share of hardware in total NIS costs can be expected to decrease gradually and slowly. Network and DC show hardly a tendency to decrease and may become the largest single cost component in a bedside NIS.

One might think that the wide-spread use of bedside NIS-ses will lead to a reduction of software costs. This will most probably not be the case. This wide-spread use will lead to a high demand for extended functionality and user friendliness. At best we can hope that the software costs will be stable.

Since equipment costs are the largest cost component it can be expected that the cost/savings balance will yield different results for different countries. Costs are only one aspect of a bedside NIS, the benefits to be obtained are the primary motivation to implement an NIS. Systematic assessment of the effect of NIS implementation is needed to justify the investments and efforts needed to realise a successful NIS implementation.

References

Bakker AR: An Integrated Hospital Information System in The Netherlands: Clinical Computing Vol 7, No 2, 1990, pp 91–97.

Bakker AR, Willemsen W: HIS cost modelling; a suggestion for uniformity; Procs Medical Informatics Europe '90; R. O'Moore et al, Eds; Springer Verlag, 1990, pp 143–148.

Heemskerk- van Holtz PRB: Data Handling in a Nursing Unit. Proc 3rd Int. Symp. on Nursing Use of Computers and Information Sciences, Dublin, june 1988; Daly N, Hannah KJ, Eds; The C.V. Mosby Company, St. Louis ISBN 0-8016-3235-8; pp 796–802.

Nieman HBJ, Bakker AR, Heemskerk- v Holz PRB, Roelofs W: Bedside Nursing Information Systems: Vision and Experiences: Procs MEDINFO 89 Singapore. Barber B et al Eds: North Holland, 1989, pp 654–657.

48
Savings and Other Benefits Experienced from Use of a Computerized Bedside Documentation System

Lois Nauert

Economic constraints and the nursing shortage are forcing nursing services to re-evaluate many current practices. One such practice, documentation of nursing care, requires a substantial amount of nursing time each day and is not the favorite task of nurses. This paper describes the savings and other benefits achieved by the Division of Nursing Services at University Hospital and Clinics (UHC) after installation and implementation of a computerized bedside documentation system, on all general care departments.

Charting Overtime

This is a benefit that we have not been able to quantify because of the difficulty that exists in separating charting overtime from all other types of overtime. We know that charting overtime no longer exists on the departments with computerized bedside documentation because the nurses are all gone by shift end.

Nurse Satisfaction

A survey of staff using the computerized bedside documentation system was conducted in January of 1990. The "Bedside Computer Survey" questionnaire was distributed to 306 RNs and LPNs on eight nursing departments using the system. One hundred seventy-two (172) surveys (58.5%) were returned.

Reprinted with permission from; *Nursing Informatics '91: Proceedings of the Fourth International Conference on Nursing Use of Computers and Information Science*; Hovenga, E.J.S., Hannah, K.J., McCormick, K.A. & Ronald, J.S. (Eds.). 1991, pp. 408–411. Heidelberg-Berlin, Germany: Springer-Verlag.

Simple descriptive statistics were used to analyze the responses. Overall, 129 (78.1%) "Like" or "Strongly Like" the bedside computer, while 15 (9.1%) "Dislike" or "Strongly Dislike" the bedside computers. Sixty-seven and one-half percent (67.5%) of the staff perceive that it takes less time to document patient care tasks using the bedside computer compared to 19.1% perceiving it takes more time to chart, while 13.4% perceives it takes the same amount of time to chart. More than 75% of the staff perceived it took less time to document both vital signs and intake and output measurements, while more than 70% of the staff perceived it took less time or the same amount of time to document nursing assessment and treatment.

The last question on the survey was, "Please take this opportunity to share any thoughts you have on using the bedside computers." The most frequent themes were: (1) difficult to get on terminal; need to enter comments at the bedside, (2) screens need more features; screens need to be unit specific, (3) saves time; makes me keep charting current; efficient, (4) documentation more accurate, clearer. In general, the comments related to how the system can be improved.

Time Savings

A research study to evaluate the time spent charting on one unit, pre- and post-implementation of the computerized bedside documentation system was completed in 1989. The actual time spent in nursing functions, including nine charting functions, was measured by a trained nurse observer using the tool "Monitoring Nursing Functions Observation Records" previously developed and used at UHC. One hundred eighty four (184) two or three hour observations were completed pre-implementation and 191 observations were completed post-implementation.

The study showed that nurses spent an average of one and one-half minutes more per hour on the nine charting functions post-implementation. Although this slight difference was not statistically significant, more time spent charting was not an expected result.

As a result of the unexpected outcome, a decision was made to analyze other variables, such as census, workload, and nursing hours, that could effect charting time on this nursing department.

That analysis showed census had increased 23%; workload, as measured by the Medicus Type 5 Patient Classification System, increased by 27%; and actual hours per workload index had decreased 8% during the time of the post-implementation study. After all changes were evaluated, a decrease of 18.12 staff hours was achieved each day. Annualized, this represents a savings of 6,613.8 hours. Using an average salary figure of $15.40 per hour an annual savings of $101,852 would be realized.

Improved Quality of Documentation

A study to evaluate the quality of nursing documentation was completed in 1990. "Quality charting" for the study was defined as documentation according to institutional policy. Fifty charts were randomly selected both pre- and post-implementation of the bedside computer system. Charts from the pre-implementation phase were selected from the two month period prior to having the bedside computers on the nursing units. The post implementation phase was not started until four months after the computers had come on-line in order to ensure staff competency with the system. Charts were again selected from a two month period. Each chart review was done by a Registered Nurse and consisted of three separate reviews: 1) the day of admission, 2) the day of discharge, and 3) a random day. Fifty items were evaluated for each of the three reviews. Charting responses were reported as: present, absent or not applicable for each of the 50 items.

Results of the study showed seven (7) items, with statistical significance, were better pre-implementation and twenty-three (23) items, with statistical significance, were better post-implementation.

The study also identified areas in which nursing documentation was deficient both pre- and post-implementation and provided some direction for correcting those deficiencies.

Increased Reimbursement Fees

The nurse who reviews charts in patient accounts has told managers within the Division of Nursing Services that fewer charges are being questioned by third party payers. Nurses are charting the use of chargeable equipment (i.e., special beds, IV pump cassettes, etc.) because it is simple to do on the computerized documentation system.

Improved Legibility

Since all charting is printed, it is more legible. People doing chart reviews (utilization reviewers, staff doing QA, lawyers, etc.) have stated it is easier to read charts and to find particular items because it is printed in an established order.

Accessibility of Patient Information

Anyone who needs information included in nursing documentation can access the information immediately on-line. There is no need to find the nurse or wait until a chart is returned to the nursing unit if it was sent with the patient to some other hospital department.

In summary, the benefits achieved include: (1) elimination of charting overtime, (2) improved nurse satisfaction, (3) reduction in the time required to document care, (4) improvement in the quality of documentation, (5) increased reimbursement fees from third party payers, (6) improved legibility of documentation, and (7) constant accessibility to patient information.

Based on the above benefits, UHC plans to continue development of the computerized bedside documentation systems and extend bedside computers into the intensive care departments.

49
Comparing Information on Medical Condition and Nursing Care for the Management of Health Care

WALTER SERMEUS

Introduction

In order to manage health care, appropriate information systems have to be developed. The extension of insurance coverage to the majority of the population, the rapid growth in the number of physicians and hospital facilities, important progress in medical technologies and health care sciences have led to high and still rising costs. They reach 5 to 9% of the GDP in most European countries (OECD, 1990)

All governments are concerned. They are amending cost-containment programs and introducing new financing methods. The best known system is the Prospective Payment System (PPS) and Diagnosis Related Groups (DRGs) developed and introduced in the USA. Belgium has also introduced a new hospital financing system, that is less cost and more budget oriented.

Essentially, hospital care operating costs are subdivided in 2 parts: part one, all logistic costs including administration; part two, non-physician care costs, called costs of departments, primarily nursing costs. For part one and two, a national prospective hospital budget is provided yearly and is subdivided amongst all hospitals.

Therefore an allocation procedure is required. Several allocation models have been suggested until now. A constant feature in all these models, is that budgets must be allocated on the basis of activity indicators rather than costs.

For the clinical departments, it was proposed to define this activity "on the basis of the patient's medical diagnosis, age of the patient, special medical procedures and the workload of the nursing staff generated by the degree of dependency of the patients (Dehaene, 1985)."

Reprinted with permission from; *Nursing Informatics '91: Proceedings of the Fourth International Conference on Nursing Use of Computers and Information Science*; Hovenga, E.J.S., Hannah, K.J., McCormick, K.A. & Ronald, J.S. (Eds.). 1991, pp. 144–149. Heidelberg-Berlin, Germany: Springer-Verlag.

In September 1985, a research project was commenced at the Catholic University of Leuven to develop one national nursing care registration instrument. For two months, data were collected in 13 Flemish hospitals, 92 nursing units and about 12000 patients (Delesie a.o., 1989). At the same time, a similar research project was conducted in the French speaking part of Belgium by a research team of the Faculté Notre Dame de Paix, Namur (Meunier a.o., 1986). Both studies converged in one national nursing care registration instrument consisting of a list of 23 minimal nursing activities which were approved by the General Association of Belgian Nurses (table 1).

The study resulted in a Royal Decree of 14 August 1987 "determining the rules on how hospitals have to collect and communicate statistical data to the Minister of Public Health." These statistical data include patient data (age, sex, length of stay), medical diagnosis and the 23 nursing minimal nursing data.

This "Nursing Minimal Dataset" (NMDS) has to be collected in every Belgian hospital 4 times a year during a 15-day sampling period pointed out by the Minister of Public Health. These Nursing Minimal Data (NMDS)

TABLE 1. List of 23 minimal nursing activities

1.	Hygiene care	no help, assistance, partial help, complete help
2.	Mobility care	no help, assistance, partial help, complete help
3.	Elimination care	no help, assistance, partial help, complete help
4.	Feeding care	no help, assistance, partial help, complete help
5.	Gavage feeding	Yes/no
6.	Complete care on mouth, nose, eyes	times/day: 0–99
7.	Decubitus preventive care	times/day: 0–99
8.	Assisting in getting dressed	Yes/no
9.	Attending on tracheostomy or ventilation	2 categories
10.	Interviewing patient or relatives	Yes/no
11.	Teaching indiv. patients or relatives	2 categories
12.	Supporting patient/highly emotionally disturbed	Yes/no
13.	Supervision to mentally disturbed patient	2 categories
14.	Isolation	Yes/no
15.	Monitoring of vital signs	times/day most frequent parameter: 0–99
16.	Monitoring of clinical signs	times/day most frequent parameter: 0–99
17.	Attending on continous traction or cast	Yes/no
18.	Drawing of blood specimen	number/day: 0–99
19.	Medication I.M., S.C.	number/day: 0–99
20.	Medication I.V.	number/day: 0–99
21.	I.V. therapy	number of lines: 0–99
22.	Surgical wound care	number of wound care/day: 0–99
23a.	Surface of the traumatic wound	4 classes 0–20%, 21–45%, 46–70, 71–100%
23b.	Traumatic wound care	number of wound care/day: 0–99

have to be collected daily for every patient hospitalized during this 15-day period.

Recently, in the Royal Decree of 21 June 1990, the minister of Public Health has ordered the hospitals start collecting complementary to this MNDS also "Minimal Medical Data" including medical diagnosis, medical therapy (surgery, different procedures), patient characteristics and characteristics about hospital stay.

These 2 regulations provide Belgium with an unique experience regarding the availability of health care information. Nationwide information is available on medical as well as on nursing activities in hospitals. E.g. for 1988 national statistics on nursing activity (based on this NMDS), patient characteristics, medical diagnosis are currently available on a random sample of patient days covering 15% of all inpatients. For 1988, data of about 1.3 million patient days are available.

Aim of the Study

The aim of our research is to investigate the complex relationship between medical condition (as measured by DRGs) and nursing care (as measured by the Minimal Nursing Data set). The DRG system in the U.S.A. does not specifically address nursing care requirements. Length of stay was selected as the proxy for resource use (cost) because it was the only readily available and consistent measure that could be derived for a large sample size (Mowry, 1985). The DRG-model uses patient days to apportion nursing costs and to calculate the budget for nursing care. This does not allow for variation in intensity of nursing resource use by patient nor by patient day. Medical diagnoses may be valid indicators of the medical interventions that are needed, but they do not necessarily relate to requirements for nursing care. It is obvious that two patients with the same DRG, could have substantially different nursing care requirements, depending on many factors that are not accounted for in DRGs, e.g. need for emotional support.

Since 1982, much research has been done to investigate the association between DRG's and nursing care (Grimaldi & Micheletti, 1982; McKibbin a.o., 1985; Mowry & Korpman, 1985; Fosbinder, 1986; Sovie a.o., 1984; Lagona & Stritzel, 1984; Halloran, 1985; Thompson & Diers, 1988). Different measures have been reported such as the coefficient of determination (Halloran, 1985), the percentage of the cost of nursing care in total cost of the hospital (McKibbin a.o., 1985; Fosbinder, 1986; Sovie a.o., 1985), average hours of nursing care per patient day by DRG (Lagona & Stritzel, 1984), variations in NCH per patient day during the hospital stay (Lagona & Stritzel, 1984; Grimaldi & Micheletti 1982; Caterinicchio, 1984).

In this study, the coefficient of determination (R^2) is used to describe the relationship between DRGs and the amount of nursing care. Two more questions are addressed in this study; the first question deals with the problem whether nursing care is related to the patient or rather to the nurse or the characteristics of the nursing unit. Wennberg (1982) reported large "cultural" differences in medical practice among small areas. Many authors stated that DRGs are not at all homogeneous in resource consumption. Different reasons have been suggested. Fetter (1986) stated that heterogenity is a feature of an instable process. Non-homogeneous DRG-groups should be studied and organized so that it can be lead to a stable process. Other explanations are variations in severity of illness (Horn, 1985) or variation in physician practice (McMahon & Newbold, 1986). The object in this study is to investigate the variation in nursing practice. The second question surpasses previous research which is oriented in studying the total amount of nursing care. The amount of nursing care is important for such issues as staffing and financing but what about the content of nursing care? Maybe even while there is little difference in the total amount of nursing care between 2 DRG-categories, the content of the care can be totally different.

Design of the Study

The data collection took place from September 1988 until December 1988 in the University Hospitals of Leuven. It is a multi-center complex of 4 hospitals with a total capacity of 2055 acute hospital beds, 85 nursing units and about 2500 nurses.

The Minimal Nursing data file and Minimal Medical Data file were merged. Data of 7515 patients on 52578 patient days were collected. Data on medical diagnosis, medical therapy and several patient characteristics were converted to U.S.A.–DRG's using the GROUPER algorithm. 416 DRG groups (out of 477) were observed in the University Hospitals of Leuven. For the study, we selected 5 groups which were clinically relevant and for which there were more than 50 patients and 500 patient day observed.

DRG125   Circulary Disorders exc. AMI with card. cath.
DRG373   Vaginal Delivery w/o complications
DRG209   Major joint & limb attachment procedures
DRG082   Respiratory Neoplasm
DRG107   Coronary bypass w/o cardiac Cath
DRG014   Specific cerebrovascular disorders exc. TIA

The Nursing Minimal Dataset was treated in 2 ways. First patients were classified in 4 categories according to their amount of care by selecting from the NMDS the 5 criteria also used in the SAN JOAQUIN patient classification system (Murphy a.o., 1978). Theoretically, a ratio of about 1:2:3 of nursing care time per 24 hour period between category 1, cat 2 versus 1, category 3 versus 1 can be hypothesized. These ratios were found in the U.S. study (Murphy a.o., 1978) and also in a Belgian study in the University Hospitals of Leuven (Desmit, 1986). For this study, we dropped some of the assumptions usually made and we treat the data strictly ordinal. The second approach is the multidimensional scaling approach (Wish & Carroll, 1982) in which the total set of 23 nursing minimal data are treated in globo. The interrater reliability of the NMDS was tested in 8 of the 85 nursing units for 965 registrations. A reliability score of 91.9% was obtained.

Results of the Study

An analysis of variance (ANOVA) shows that DRGs (all groups) explains about 45% of total variance in lengh-of-stay (LOS). In the analysis the logarithm of LOS was used because of normality conditions.

Applying an analysis of variance on the average amount of nursing care per patient day, as measured by the SAN JOAQUIN classification, DRGs explain only 22% in total variation. It means that DRGs are hardly homogenous according to the amount of nursing care. Our analysis confirms the research results already attained by Halloran (1985).

A second conclusion is that large differences have been seen between nursing units in length of stay and the amount of nursing care within various DRGs (factor 3:1). E.g. Unit A has an average LOS of 8.95 days for patients of DRG125 (circulatory disorders exc. AMI with card. cath.). Unit B has an average LOS of 3.18 days for patients from the same DRG-group. The difference in LOS rates can be explained by the fact the Unit B closes during the week-end. Before the week-end the most severe patients are transferred to Unit A or to other units.

Similar differences (factor 3:1) were seen for the amount of nursing care. These differences were mostly related to organizational aspects such as the use of intensive care units, site. E.g. the average amount of nursing care is significantly higher in the main location of the University hospital than at the nursing units at off-site locations for DRG-125 (circulatory disorders exc. AMI with card. cath.).

Analysing the first 5 subsequent days of hospitalization separately, we see some differences in the amount of nursing care per patient day for DRG-125 (circulatory disorders exc. AMI with card. cath.) and DRG-373 (vaginal delivery). For subsequent days, the amount of nursing care does not differ for DRG082 (major joint procedures) and DRG-107 (coronary bypass surgery). For DRG-125 (circulatory disorders exc. AMI with card. cath.) the first 5 subsequent day pattern also differs from one nursing unit to another.

We do not know if this is determined by the natural process of healing, patient characteristics or some nursing practice variation. Further research in comparing different health care settings will give some answer to this difficult but interesting question.

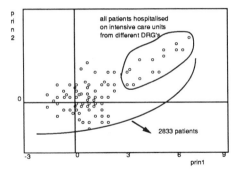

FIGURE 1. Plot of all 2833 patients.

The global nursing care profile is analyzed by using a multidimensional scaling technique to display the underlying structure of the data matrix. This technique resulted in 2 pictures: A graphical projection which shows the position of all the 23 activities from the NMDS (see fig. 1) and a projection which shows in the same plot the position of every patient (see fig. 2). It becomes clear that the nursing care profile for various DRG-groups is not quite homogenous (see fig. 3) with one exception for DRG-373 or vaginal delivery w/o complications. It means that only these patients, follow a highly predictable and clearly understood critical path of nursing care. For all other DRG-categories of interest is it not so obvious. Quite some research has to be done in analysing these nursing care profiles.

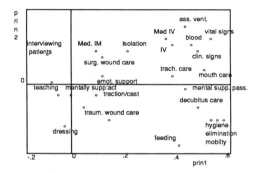

FIGURE 2. Plot of the nursing minimal dataset.

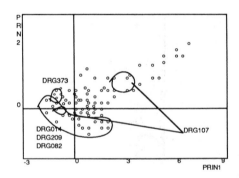

FIGURE 3. Plot of the patients indicating various DRG-groups.

Conclusions

For this research project, we have concentrated on the relationship between the medical condition (as measured by Diagnosis Related Groups) and nursing activities (as measured by the Minimal Nursing Dataset).

The study was conducted at the University Hospitals of Leuven. In 1988, September, 1–15 and December, 1–15, data of about 7515 patients were collected on 41775 registration days. Six DRG groups of interest were selected for further analysis. Our limited research, in just one hospital and just for a selected group of patients of interest, reveals however a very rich world where procedures and structures serve the organization of healthcare, in which patients have some needs, nurses and physicians make decisions, set priorities. In this world, DRGs are an oversimplification. Bearing in mind the words of Einstein: "make things as simple as possible, but not simpler."

References

Caterinicchio (P.): A debate: RIM's & the cost of nursing care, *Nursing Management*, 1983; vol. 14, 36–39.

Delesie (L.), P. Debecker & W. Sermeus: Hospital care financing, *Hospital Management International '89*, International Hospital Federation, 1989; 219–226.

Desmit (P.): *Patintenclassificatie, een instrument voor personeelstoewijzing: beschrijving van de eerste analytische resultaten in het Academisch ziekenhuis te Leuven*, Niet-gepubliceerde eindverhandeling K.U. Leuven, 1985; 126 pp.

Fetter (R.) & J. Freeman: Diagnosis Related Groups: Product Line Management within hospitals, *Academy of Management Review*, 1986; 41–54.

Fosbinder (D.): Nursing costs/DRG: A patient classification system and comparative study, *Journal of Nursing Administration*, 1986; vol. 16, 11, 18–23.

Grimaldi (P.) & J. Micheletti: RIM's and the cost of nursing care, *Nursing Management*, December 1982; 12–22.

Halloran (E.): Nursing workload, medical diagnosis related groups, and nursing diagnoses, *Research in Nursing and Health*, 1985; 421–433.

Horn (S.): Measuring severity: how sick is sick? How well is well? *Health Care Financing Management*, 1986; 21–32.

Hornbrook (M.): Review Article. Hospital case mix: its definition, management and use: part 1: Conceptual framework, *Medical Care Review*, Spring 1982; vol 39, 1–43.

Lagona (T.) & M. Stritzel: Nursing care requirements as measured by DRG, *Journal of Nursing Administration*, 1984; vol. 14, 15–18.

Levine (E.) & F. Abdellah: DRGs: A recent refinement to an old method, Inquiry 21, 1984; 105–112.

MC Kibbin (R.) a.o.: Nursing costs & DRG payment, *American Journal of Nursing*, 1985; 1353–1356.

MC Mahon (L.) & R. Newbold: Variations in resource use within diagnosis-related groups, the effect of severity of illness and physician practice, *Medical Care*, 1986; vol. 24, 388–397.

Meurisse (A.) a.o.: *Case-mix for prospective hospital financing in Belgium: data collection and basic descriptive data*, Paper presented at Medical Informatics Europe, Glasgow, August, 1990; 19–23, 8 pp.

Mowry (M.) & R. Korpman: Do DRG reimbursement rates reflect nursing costs?, *Journal of Nursing Administration*, 1985; vol. 15, 8, 29–35.

Murphy (L.): *Methods for studying nurse staffing in a patient Unit*, DHEW, USA, 1978; 226 pp. OECD, *Health Care Systems in Transition, The search for efficiency, OECD Social policy studies*, Paris, 1990; 204 pp.

Sermeus (W.): Hospital care financing and nursing in Belgium, in Roger-France a.o. (Eds), *Diagnosis Related Groups in Europe*, Goff, Ghent, 1989; 224–228.

Sovie (M.) a.o.: Amalgam of nursing acuity, DRGs and costs, *Nursing Management*, vol. 16, 22–42.

Thompson (J.) & D. Diers: Management of nursing intensity, *Nursing Clinics of North America*, September, 1988; vol. 23, 473–492.

Wennberg (J.) & A. Gittelsohn: Variations in Medical Care, *Scientific American*, 1982; 246, 100–112

Wish (M.) & J. Carroll: Multidimensional scaling and its applications, in Krishnaiah (P.) & L. Kanal (Eds.), *Handbook of Statistics*, Vol. 2, North-Holland Publishing Co, 1982; 317–345.

50
Nursing Care Cost and Resource Consumption Management

Mary Ann Lubno

Introduction

Diagnosis Related Groups (DRGs), Prospective Payment Systems (PPS), and reimbursement for nursing services continue to be issues that affect nursing practice. DRGs were first developed as a research tool for utilization review at Yale University in the late 60's and early 70's. They were intended to classify hospital admissions for statistical purposes and planning. The groups were designed according to the pattern of care received, length of stay, and overall use of services. DRGs are assigned on the Uniform Hospital Discharge Data Set which includes diagnoses (from the International Classification of Diseases-9th revision-Clinical Modification [ICD-9-CM]), surgical procedures, patient age, and length of stay. DRGs are intended to be exhaustive and mutually exclusive.

In April 1983, PL 98-21, a social security amendment was passed that mandated DRGs be used in a Prospective Payment System (PPS) for Medicare patients. PPS reimburses hospitals a standard amount of money based on the DRG assigned to the patient. The reimbursement may be more or less than the actual hospital charges billed to the patient. If the hospital can deliver care for less then the PPS reimbursement, then the hospital is able to keep the profit. However, if the hospital charges exceed the PPS reimbursement, the hospital either has to obtain the money from the patient directly or absorb the loss. PPS was implemented October 1, 1983.

The hospital component of the standard reimbursement is derived from the hospital's operating costs per case as evidenced in the patient's hospital bill. Operating costs, for the purpose of prospective pricing, includes all costs except depreciation, interest, capitalized lease costs, return on equity

Reprinted with permission from *Proceedings of Nursing and Computers: The Third International Symposium on Nursing Use of Computers and Information Science*; pp. 651–656. Daly, N. & Hannah, K.J. (Eds.). 1988. St. Louis: The C.V. Mosby Company.

for investor owned hospitals, and the direct costs of medical, nursing, and allied health professions education programs operated by the hospital.

DRGs are not treatment protocols nor a categorization of patients depending on a stage of illness. Rather, DRGs are a measure of resources consumed. DRGs are based on some of the operating costs per case and these operating costs reflect some of the resources consumed. The resources consumed are reflected in a patient's bill and the cost report for that particular hospital. In the PPS, length of stay (LOS) was used as a proxy for resource use (cost) because it was the only readily available and consistent measure that could be derived for a large sample size (Mowry and Korpman, 1986). Variation in LOS also had been linked previously to variance in cost in hospital settings (HHS, 1982). Since under retrospective reimbursement mechanisms hospitals were not required to keep accurate cost data, LOS was virtually the only cost related element of information available. Specific and detailed cost accounting was not done for each DRG. It is the purpose of this DRG resource comsumption model to determine a more accurate estimate of resources consumed and to compare the total cost of the resources consumed for a particular DRG to the actual reimbursement allowance for that DRG. Inherent within this purpose is to more accurately determine the costs of nursing services per DRG.

Cost Accounting and the Resource Consumption Model

Texas Tech University Health Sciences Center, through a three year, 1.5 million dollar W.K. Kellogg Foundation Grant, is using computer technology to demonstrate that information linkages between an academic health sciences center and community health care delivery sites will positively impact patient care. This demonstration project is also supported by hardware donations from AT & T.

One primary means of accomplishing the information linkages is through the development of an interdisciplinary automated health care record. Inherent within the automated record is the capability to program a model to determine cost effectiveness, resource utilization, and consumption management that will identify the various costs, including nursing service costs, contributing to specified DRGs.

Cost accounting is a system of identifying all labor, supply, equipment, and overhead costs of a product or service. In this case, the DRG is the product. A hospital's costs are assumed to be a function of two elements: (1) the cost of its individual resources, and (2) the complexity of the cases that the hospital treats. The complexity of a hospital could be measured by a case mix index, which is the sum of the weighting factors assigned to the DRGs treated at that particular hospital (Morgan and Kappel, 1985). Lubbock Genera Hospital (LGH) is a 297 bed acute care (tertiary care) county owned hospital. It is the primary teaching hospital for a health sciences center that offers medical, nursing, and allied health education programs. LGH is classified as a Level 1 trauma center. The case mix index for LGH is Medicare—1.2956 and Medicaid—1.0209.

The model for DRG resource consumption consists of nursing care costs (NCC), room charge (RC), ancillary services charges (ASC), supply/equipment charges (SEC), and indirect costs (IC). In determining costs, both product costs and period costs are considered. Product costs usually include direct labor, direct supplies/materials, and overhead (indirect and variable). Overhead (indirect and variable) includes costs for heating and lighting, repairs and maintenance on equipment, and all other costs associated with producing the product.

Period costs (allocated, fixed overhead) include the cost of non-revenue producing departments such as marketing and administration. These costs are not directly associated with producing the product. Period costs are generally allocated to revenue producing cost centers either directly or by the step down method. The actual costs of non-revenue producing departments are found in the same way as revenue producing departments. Direct labor, direct materials, and overhead are computed and then allocated to other departments. Once all service/product units are identified and product and period (allocated) cost elements are determined, the costs of all service units comprising a product are accumulated to determine the product cost.

A cost accounting system attempts to compare actual cost to standard cost. There are four techniques to develop standard costs: microcosting; input/output costing; patient acuity costing; and cost-to-charge ratio. Microcosting is accomplished through management engineering studies. Input/output costing relies on an average over many hospital's per service unit costs. Patient acuity costing is a subset of input/output costing. This technique applies standard nursing costs based on patient acuity. Cost-to-charge ratio is a standard cost determination technique used in Medicare cost reporting.

LGH generally uses a cost-to-charge ratio in determining costs. The standard ratio used by Medicare is 60:100 where for every $0.60 in cost, $1.00 is charged. The $0.40 accounts for the period costs which are allocated from non-revenue producing cost centers and is included in the IC in the model. However, the hospital has done some initial cost accounting studies and has determined specific cost-to-charge ratios for the ancillary services. These ratios can be found in the hospital's financial statement.

Traditionally, the room charge has lumped together nursing, dietary, housekeeping, laundry, and overhead costs. Nursing, in this arrangement is viewed as an expense item rather than as an income item. By partitioning out nursing costs from the room charge, the contribution nursing makes to the recovery of the patient can be better represented.

LGH is currently using a patient classification system (PCS). Reliability and validity data are being collected on the PCS. The PCS categorizes patient needs associated with the following elements of care:

feeding
bathing
elimination
respiration
mobility
comfort
teaching/counseling/planning
wound care
medications and I.V. fluids
monitoring/observation
discharge/transfer
activities for other departments
procedures
whole patient

Points are assigned to each element of care that reflect the extent of nursing time needed to perform the care. This PCS groups patients into five categories of acuity which reflect different nursing time requirements for the elements of care. For example:

14 points = Class I
15–28 points = Class II
29–42 points = Class III
43–56 points = Class IV
57–70 points = Class V

The time requirements reflect both direct nursing time and indirect nursing time. Direct time is that time that is spent one-to-one with the patient to provide care. Indirect time is that time when the nurse is doing something related to patient care but not one-to-one such as documentation, consultation with the lab, consultation with the physician, etc. Additionally, the direct and indirect time is calculated for each shift. Calculating nursing time for each shift reflects more accurately the dynamic nature of a patient's illness and leads to a more refined estimate of nursing care requirements.

The PCS reflects only the nursing time associated with those nurses who give direct care. It does not account for other personnel who may also staff the unit who do not regularly provide direct care such as the charge nurse, patient care coordinator, clinical manager, or ward clerk. The cost for these personnel are included in indirect costs.

The formula for calculating nursing care cost (NCC) is as follows:

1. Determine the patient classification
2. Determine the shift associated with the classification
3. Determine the direct and indirect time for the classification according to the shift from Table 1.
4. Identify the primary R.N. caring for the patient on each shift. (Only R.N.s are used in this model as this unit uses the Primary Care Model for nursing care delivery.
5. Multiply the identified R.N.'s salary plus fringe benefits plus shift differential (for 3-11 and 11-7 shifts) by the hours of care provided for the patient according to the classification and shift.
6. Add each shift total to arrive at the cost for providing nursing care to the patient for the 24 hour period.
7. Subtract the NCC from the room charge. On this particular nursing unit, the room charge is $162.00. The resulting cost (indicated by RC in the model) is assumed to cover the dietary, housekeeping and overhead costs of the room. These two elements (NCC and RC) are then summed for the patient's LOS.

As previously stated, the hospital has done some initial cost accounting studies and has determined specific cost-to-charge ratios for the ancillary services. Therefore, the cost for ancillary services is calculated by multiplying the charge to the patient for the ancillary service (from the patient's bill) by the specific cost-to-charge ratio. The product costs for ancillary services is represented by ASC in the model. Ancillary services include the laboratory, pharmacy, radiology, etc. The difference between the charge to the patient and the cost for ancillary services is considered period costs and is included in IC in the model.

Supplies and equipment are items directly charged in the patient's bill. Again, it is assumed that the charge for each item is based on the product and period costs associated with the particular department that furnishes and/or maintains the supplies/equipment. In the case of supplies and equipment, the standard cost-to-charge ratio (60:100) is used. Therefore, the

TABLE 1. Time determination per shift per classification

Classification	7-3 (D+I)	3-11 (D+I)	11-7 (D+I)
I	1.77	1.13	.83
II	1.73	1.25	1.25
III	3.31	2.50	2.63
IV	7.04	5.13	4.75
V	8.05	5.88	5.40

Thus, a patient classified as Class II on every shift would require 4.23 hours of nursing care during the 24 hour period (1.73 [7-3], 1 1.25 [3-11] 1 1.25 [11-7]).

charge to the patient (from the patient's bill) is multiplied by .60 and then added into the model. The product cost (charge X .60) is then substracted from the charge and the resulting number is considered the period cost for supplies and equipment. The period cost is added into the IC in the model. Items from central sterile, central supply, and I.V. fluids are considered part of the supply/equipment charge. Supply/equipment charge is represented by SEC in the model.

The indirect costs (IC) include overhead (indirect/variable—yearly salary plus fringes for the clinical manager, patient care coordinators, head nurses, clinical nurse specialists, ward clerks, administrative costs, and other costs associated with running the unit); period costs (allocated/fixed costs); and direct and indirect medical education costs. The IC is calculated by summing all components previously identified, dividing by the number of patient days for the year, and multiplying by the LOS of the specified patient.

Therefore, the resource consumption model reflects the following equation: (NCC $\times$ LOS) + (RC $\times$ LOS) + ASC + SEC + IC = calculated DRGRC (DRG resource consumption). The calculated DRGRC is then compared to the actual DRG reimbursement.

Several analyses and interpretations can be made with the data collected in the model that will assist Nursing Service Administrators or Hospital Administrators in developing and monitoring the budget. For example, total cost of resources consumed compared to reimbursement patterns, cost of nursing resources within DRGs, patterns of nursing resource use by acuity within and across DRGs, cost of ancillary services within DRGs, patterns of use of ancillary services within and across DRGs, patterns of supply and equipment usage within and across DRGs, and the effects of indirect costs on total DRG resource consumption. With this information, administrators will be better able to manage the consumption of the limited resources needed to deliver patient care.

Currently, data is being entered as the patient is discharged and a bill is available. However, as the automated health care record is fully developed, the information necessary for the model will come directly from the record. For example, the acuity data is not currently automated. However, several nursing documentation screens have been developed and are operational (activity, medications, I.V. fluid administration, vital signs, daily care, intake and output, teaching screens, etc.). Acuity data relative to the PCS in relation to these nursing functions can be made a part of the screens so that the data is automatically downloaded to the resource consumption model. Additionally, there is currently a table to identify all personnel authorized to enter the system and to enter data on the screens. Therefore, when a nurse enters data on one of the nursing documentation screens, that nurses's salary can be automatically entered into the resource consumption model in relation to the identified acuity data.

This resource consumption model hold promise for identifying specific costs per DRG and for costing out nursing services consumed in the delivery of care. Data are being collected on the patients that are participants on the Kellogg automated health care record. Analysis and interpretation of these data can be obtained from the author.

References

Department of Health and Human Services. (1982). *Report to Congress: Hospital payment for medicare.* Washington, D.C.: U.S. Government Printing Office.
Mowry, M. & Korpman, R. (1986). *Managing health care costs, quality, and technology.* Rockville, MD: Aspen Publishers, Inc.

51
The Relationship of Automation to Expectations for Increased Productivity: Doing More with Less

Charlotte A. Weaver and Lynnette Fredericksen

Full automation of the health care industry is an inevitable outcome of the socioeconomic conditions impacting health care internationally. However, despite a few notable exceptions, heavy investments in information technology by hospitals over the past 20 years have yielded disappointing productivity results. Largely, this was due to hospitals using HIS systems to automate old ways of doing business and leaving existing processes intact (Gardner 1990a). The industry tended to view automation's value as improving information processing control, but not as a means to decrease operational costs (Childs 1986). The consequence to Nursing is a poor track record for achieving staff reductions or cost savings with full hospital automation (Staggers 1988).

The methodology for achieving benefits realization with an HIS implementation was originally developed, tested and demonstrated by El Camino Hospital, Mountain View, California in 1974 (Fleming et al. 1975). El Camino lowered their operating costs 40 percent below all comparable hospitals in their community. These savings have been maintained through the 1980's (Buchanan and Norris 1985). El Camino Hospital's experience clearly shows that automation alone is not enough to achieve savings. El Camino discovered that it had to eliminate layers of management and push decision making down to those responsible for collecting, managing, and responding to information. El Camino also found that in automating manual procedures, major changes had to be made. How work was done and who performed the tasks had to be redefined to avoid redundancy and waste. Almost twenty years later, this same approach characterizes the successful benefits realization efforts of St. Joseph's Hospital, Milwaukee, Wisconsin in their implementation of a bedside terminal Nursing information system (Kahl 1990; NRCH 1990).

Reprinted with permission from; *Nursing Informatics '91: Proceedings of the Fourth International Conference on Nursing Use of Computers and Information Science*; Hovenga, E.J.S., Hannah, K.J., McCormick, K.A. & Ronald, J.S. (Eds.). 1991, pp. 250–254. Heidelberg-Berlin, Germany: Springer-Verlag.

Why so few success stories in twenty years? The reason is largely because restructuring of management organization, practices, and work procedures are painful and difficult to achieve. We have found that even when top management are in agreement for the need to change and on the changes to be made, implementing the changes is often undermined by the powerful need to maintain the status quo. In our experience and that of others, the inability of a hospital Nursing organization to change is due to its Nursing leadership and conditions internal to Nursing, more than external influences (Barry and Gibbon 1990).

Increasingly, vendors are selling and hospitals are buying information systems based on the expectation that the system "will pay for itself" (Gardner 1990b). The potential savings are based on three major categories: labor cost avoidance; labor reductions; and, materials and equipment savings. For example, major labor savings for Nursing can be gained in converting from a manual to an automated system for the preparation of a new chart and processing of a new medical order. Manually the task usually requires 13–15 steps to complete. These steps include chart assembly, addressographing forms, transcribing forms, transcribing orders, requisition/order forms, kardex, telephoning ancillary departments, and verifying orders. In a manual system, new chart preparation and medical order processing is heavily burdened with paper and repetitive, redundant communication of the same data items.

Figure 1 shows the same work flow in an automated system. Fifteen steps have been reduced to five. Importantly, data is entered at its point of capture and the system generates the patient chart. Telephone communication is replaced by system generated new medical orders notices to ancillary departments. In this functionally rich HIS environment, the system is capable of generating a complete electronic medical record and supporting physician order entry. Labor reduction and cost avoidance projections are calculated based on this streamlining of work principal.

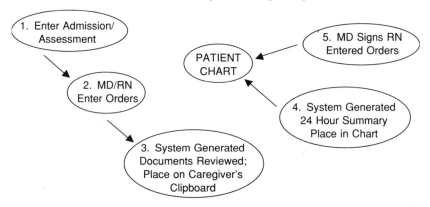

FIGURE 1. New chart preparation and processing of new medical order in an automated system.

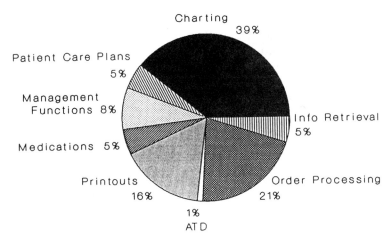

FIGURE 2. Benefit identification: nursing service potential.

The literature and our experience show that over 50 percent of benefit savings with automation come from reductions in manual tasks performed by Nursing (Figure 2) (Fleming 1975; Blask et al. 1984). Within these functions, major savings stem from elimination of manual forms, patient data logs, recopying of data, and manual transfer of data. Work streamlining impacts all the key Nursing information processing tasks: charting, patient care planning, physician orders, monitoring test status and results, and interdepartmental communications. Work avoidance results from reduction in telephone communications, hunting for charts, and capability to chart at point of action.

Table 1 lists the Nursing savings realized by example Hospitals that have implemented functionally rich HIS systems and/or undertaken benefits re-

TABLE 1. Examples of nursing labor or cost avoidance savings with HIS automation

Hospital	Country	Beds	Nursing Savings/Yr
St. John's Regional	New Brunswick, Canada	730	$750,000
Foothills	Alberta, Canada	1149	$1 mil*
El Camino	California, USA	377	$2+ mil
Kenosha Memorial	Wisconsin, USA	250	10–15%+ Productivity
Sacred Heart	Wisconsin, USA	321	$500,000
St. Joseph's	Wisconsin, USA	293	$1.2–2 mil*
			$91k Pilot Unit
St. Mary's	Illinois, USA	400	$750k*
			$43k Pilot Unit
Waukesha Memorial	Wisconsin, USA	304	$635,076 (23 FTE's)
Arrow Park	Merseyside, England	900	$150,960* (107 FTE's)
St. Mary's	London, England	650	$148,850* (70 FTE's)

*Projected Savings

alization programs. Table 1 also includes the projected savings for other example hospitals that are currently in the process of implementing functionally rich systems and/or beginning benefit realization programs. The savings range from $1.5 thousand (USD) to $2 million. The magnitude of savings realized reflects the extent to which Nursing organizations are able to streamline work and their management structure.

Nursing will carry increasing responsibility for achieving benefits with HIS automation because the potential for Nursing labor savings are so great. To achieve benefit savings, Nursing leadership will be expected to effect a radically changed Nursing Division with simplified management structures and work procedures. Nursing, like all other industries, needs to look to automation as a needed friend. Socioeconomic pressures will not allow Nursing to continue maintaining the status quo. Nursing needs to move to the forefront and proactively embrace the work and cost reduction concepts. Nursing can do more with less by streamlining work and using information technology to its fullest.

References

Barry CT, Gibbons LK: DHHS nursing roundtable: redesigning patient care delivery. *Nursing Management* 1990;21(9):64–66.

Blask D, Cleary J, Dux L: A computerized medical information system sustaining benefits previously achieved. *Healthcare and Computers* 1985;(Dec):60–64.

Buchanan NS, Norris J: A businesslike hospital gets business's attention. *Health Cost Management* 1985;2(3):1–10. Vol. 2, No. 3.

Childs BW: The myth called H.I.S. cost benefits realization. *Health Care and Computers* 1986;4(11):32–34.

Fleming JJ, Gall JE, Jr., Norwood DD, Cook M, Rydell R, Watson R: Demonstration and Evaluation of a Total Hospital Information System. Final Project Report (Contract number HSM 110-71-128), National Center for Health Services Research, Department of Health, Education, and Welfare, Rockville, MD, 1975.

Gardner E: Computer's full capabilities often go untapped. *Modern Healthcare* 1990a;(May 28):38–40.

Gardner E: Quantifying system benefits an elusive task. *Modern Healthcare* 1990b;(Feb 26):26–27.

Kahl K: Identifying the savings potential from use of bedside terminals. Paper presented at the Wisconsin Computer Applications in Nursing (WI-CAN) Conference, May 1, 1990, Milwaukee, Wisconsin.

NRCH: Management engineering study cost-justifies bedside terminals. *National Report on Computers & Health* 1990;11(6), 1, 6–8.

Parker R: Realizing benefits: the role of management and the computer. *Computers and Healthcare* 1988;(March):36–37.

Staggers N: Using Computers in Nursing: Documented benefits and needed studies. *Computers in Nursing* 1988;6(4):164–170.

Zander K: Nursing case management: strategic management of cost and quality outcomes. *JONA* 1988;18(5):23–30.

Part IV
Nursing Research

The use of computers in clinical nursing research will expand exponentially by the beginning of the twenty-first century. This section on nursing research builds a strong case for this union of technology and nursing practice. This section is divided into six groups, each delineating another element in this process.

The section begins with a theoretical and philosophical approach. Abraham and Fitzpatrick delve into the issue of nursing knowledge and how to emulate that knowledge with systems technology. Turley offers a slightly different perspective by looking at the effects of differing professional cultures and types of sciences on clinical decision making. Gassert then offers a model for defining the elements necessary for creating this expert system. Completing this triad of articles is a study by Graves and Corcoran that identifies the additional data/knowledge nurses need to make clinical decisions.

The second group of articles focuses on the importance of minimum data sets to nursing research. Foster and Conrick present an historical perspective on the development of Nursing Minimum Data Sets (NMDS). Delaney, Mehmert, Prophet, and Crossley delve into the research value of NMDS.

The third group of articles explains the use of computer-generated decision in the clinical arena. Henry's article evaluates the relationship between computer simulation and other evaluative methods, specifically cognitive examination and self-assessment. Thompson, Ryan, and Baggs explore the use of the Creighton Online Multiple Modular Expert Systems (COMMES) as a mechanism for maximizing nursing efficiency. Woolery, VanDyne, Grzymala-Busse, and Tsatsoulis develop an expert system prototype to assess preterm delivery in pregnant women.

Evaluative research comprises the fourth group of articles. Spranzo presents an adaptation of Schwirian's Nursing Informatics model as a tool for the evaluation of activities and responses surrounding computerized generation of nursing care planning. Holzemer, Henry, and Klemm compare computerized plans with hand-generated nursing care plans. And finally,

Holzemer, Reilly, Henry, and Portillo offer a perspective on inclusion of patients perceptions in the Computer Based Patient Record, as an essential part of the evaluative process.

The fifth set of articles explores the use of data management in nursing research. Hudgings describes efforts to establish a repository for nursing information needs on a worldwide level. Steve Paul provides an overview of both data management systems and techniques. Reilly, Holzemer, and Henry describe the use of a relational database program for arranging and analyzing technical data. Finally, Chang and Gilbert report on a portable system for collection of patient interview and exam data.

The final group of articles describes the use of computers for data analysis. Meintz describes the use of supercomputers for analysis of mega and tera data sets. Paul, on the other hand, explores computer use for determining power analyzes.

In summary, the articles in this section cover a broad spectrum of information from theoretical and philosophical perspectives to specific techniques of data manipulation. The scope of the information is so broad that there is a little "something for everyone."

52
Knowing for Nursing Practice: Patterns of Knowledge and Their Emulation in Expert Systems

Ivo L. Abraham and Joyce J. Fitzpatrick

The relationship between knowledge and expert systems, and the related issue of how to emulate the former in the latter, is perhaps the most central issue in artificial intelligence research efforts in many fields, including nursing. Most often the issue is phrased as one of *how* to emulate knowledge, which is a question pertaining to the technical feasibility of knowledge representation. Thus, there is debate about the relative merits of different modes of knowledge representation in artificial intelligence (e.g., production rules, frames, semantic networks, etc.), and, relatedly, about different methods of knowledge acquisition (e.g., conventional knowledge engineering, induction from example, etc.). It speaks to the progress being made in the field of artificial intelligence that problems surrounding knowledge acquisition and knowledge representation are so well described and documented in the literature, attesting to the detail with which these problems are being addressed (Buchanan, 1982; Buchanan & Shortliffe, 1984; Hayes-Roth, Waterman, & Lenat, 1983a; Kulikowski, 1980). With the emergence of artificial intelligence in nursing, a similar focus on issues related to knowledge acquisition and representation can be observed (Abraham, 1986; Abraham & Krowchuk, in press; Abraham & Schultz, 1986; Abraham, Schultz, Ozbolt, & Swain, 1984a, 1984b; Grosso & Abraham, 1987; Laborde, 1984; Ozbolt, 1986; Ozbolt, Schultz, Swain, & Abraham, 1985; Ryan, 1983).

While important progress continues to be made in the areas of acquisition and representation of knowledge, it is remarkable that an even more fundamental issue has remained largely untouched in the work of AI researchers (including our own!): the issue of knowledge itself. Knowledge acquisition and representation presume that there is something to be acquired and to be represented. Little attention has been paid to how we

Reprinted with permission from *Proceedings: Eleventh Annual Symposium on Computer Applications in Medical Care*, Stead, W.W. (Ed.). 1987. Pp. 88–92. © 1987, American Medical Informatics Association (formerly SCAMC): Bethesda, MD.

know for what we do, and it can be argued that the validity of expert systems depends on the extent to which the knowledge emulated in them is defined and elucidated. This is of particular importance to expert system development for nursing practice, because of the complexity of nursing practice and the different kinds and sources of expertise needed for providing expert clinical care. The purpose of this paper, then, is to address the issue of knowing for nursing practice, and, relatedly, the feasibility of emulating this knowing into knowledge systems technology. Thus, while the *technical* question of "how-to-emulate" (see above) remains as important as ever to the *effort* of expert system development, we argue here that the *conceptual* question of "what-to-emulate" is pivotal to the *validity* of any development effort.

This paper is structured as follows. In a first part, we present a conceptual discussion of patterns of knowing for nursing practice based on the work by Carper (1978). This is followed by a review of the characteristics and capabilities of expert systems. In a final part, we link the patterns of knowing for nursing practice with these characteristics and capabilities. This is done in the form of identifying the boundaries of expert system technology for nursing, and the extent to which they can emulate the different patterns of knowing. As such, this paper is concerned with both the features and limitations of expert system technology for nursing practice. It is intended to contribute to the clearer delineation of the contributions that artificial intelligence can make to nursing practice; and to serve as a caution against the naive perspective of blindly and uninformedly adopting artificial intelligence-based technology in nursing.

Knowing for Nursing Practice

Carper (1978) reviewed the literature in nursing and delineated four fundamental patterns of knowing in nursing: empirics, esthetics, ethics, and personal knowledge. *Empirics*, also labeled as the science of nursing, consists of the general laws and theories about the empirical world, formulated as abstractions of universals. Thus, this pattern of knowing embraces knowledge that is verifiable, and that can be described and delineated.

Esthetic knowledge in nursing, also termed the art of nursing, comprises those subjective expressions of imagined possibilities or realities that resist translation into the discursive form of language. Carper (1978) emphasizes that the individual perception of the nurse is highly important in esthetics, and that this perception is focused on the abstraction of particulars (as opposed to the abstraction of universals in the empiric pattern of knowing). While empirics is a predominantly, if not solely, cognitive mode of knowing, which moreover can be explicated in generalizable formulations, esthetic knowing blends cognition with affect. Knowing esthetically is a cognitive experience within a context of appreciation.

Ethical knowledge has its base in normative judgments, both particular and regular, and is focused on the determination of what is good, what is just, and what is right. This pattern of knowing is based on the moral judgments and the value judgments of the discipline. One should recognize that in Carper's (1978) work the notion of normativity refers to the moral sphere, and provides structure for decisions about what is good, just, and right. It should be distinguished from the notion of normativity embedded in logic (as well as the mathematical and physical sciences) where it denotes accuracy and correctness of inference. This latter notion of normativity belongs to the empiric pattern of knowing. Ethics, as defined by Carper (1978), is an aggregate of cognition and affect.

Personal knowledge is knowledge about the self as it is applied to the practice of nursing. This knowledge is in first instance about the self, yet should be seen as a state of being that is known in relation to other human beings. Personal knowledge is self-actualization in the Maslovian (1956) sense, and also involves what Polyani (1964) refers to as a risk of commitment through passionate participation in the act of knowing. Personal knowledge goes beyond cognition, and includes many instances of self- and other-appreciation.

Chinn (1987) has further developed the conceptualizations of these four patterns of knowing. She introduced product and process dimensions that are particularly useful to our discussion on the emulation of modes of knowing in nursing as they refer to tasks associated with each pattern. Thus, empirics is characterized by describing, explaining, and predicting. Esthetics implies representing, interpreting, and envisioning. Ethics includes clarifying, valuing, and advocating. Finally, personal knowledge is characterized by experiencing, centering, and realizing. Empirics finds its expression in the scientific method, esthetics in art, ethics in codes of conduct, and personal knowledge in the authentic self.

Knowledge in Expert System Technology

In their authoritative text on expert system development, Hayes-Roth et al. (1983b) offer a definition of knowledge in a given domain derived from Barnett and Bernstein (1977): "Speaking abstractly, knowledge consists of descriptions, relationships, and procedures in some domain of interest" (Hayes-Roth et al., 1983b, p. 12). We cite this definition here on purpose, for it poignantly illustrates how a focus on the "hows" of knowledge acquisition and representation colors how people will define the "what" of it.

This definition of knowledge is mostly one in function of the technology, and less for the sake of definition itself. From it can be derived the boundaries of what knowledge can be emulated in technology, and inferences can be made quite readily about the emulation of nursing knowledge. The definition implies that knowledge can be delineated as a knowledge base composed of objects and classes of objects, both of which can be explicated if not operationalized accurately and unambiguously. Thus, the knowledge base identifies and differentiates objects and their classes "in some language whose elementary components consist of primitive features or concepts" (Hayes-Roth et al., 1983b, p. 12). The knowledge base also contains a particular category of descriptions known as relationships, which "express dependencies and associations between items in the knowledge base" (Hayes-Roth et al., 1983b, p. 12). The associations described by relationships can be taxonomic, definitional, or empirical. Finally, a knowledge base contains procedures for drawing inferences or for initiating actions.

The Hayes-Roth et al. (1983b) perspective on knowledge is widely held among AI researchers. The implication is clear, namely that in artificial intelligence research (including nursing) one can only work with knowledge that is so-to-speak "known operationally": knowledge that can be broken down into items, classes of items, relationships among items and among classes, and procedures for inference or action. The knowledge of expert systems is bounded by the extend to which their knowledge referent is of an operational nature. From an artificial intelligence point of view, "knowledge consists of (1) the symbolic descriptions that characterize the definitional and empirical relationships in a domain and (2) the procedures for manipulating these descriptions" (Hayes-Roth et al., 1983b, p. 13).

Artificial intelligence researchers recognize that the operational perspective on knowledge restricts what expert systems can do. Hart (1980) points out that these systems can only do what they are taught to do, and that they cannot tackle problems outside of the scope of their knowledge. With the current predominant technology, focused on serial processing, extrapolation to analog problem situations is indeed largely impossible (although neural-network computer technology might bring about some change in this regard in the future). Further, they are unable to monitor the accuracy of their knowledge, and are largely unable to check whether their conclusions are reasonable. Similarly, while expert systems may be construed such that they are able to explain why they arrived at a certain conclusion (i.e., a so-called "explanation facility" through reproduction of the embedded reasoning process), these explanations are only as deep and fundamental as the knowledge base is designed to be. Buchanan (1982) added that the domain of expertise of expert systems is narrow, and that these systems are so highly stylized that natural reasoning behaviors and processes are seldom emulated in their human form. Expert systems, in the words of prominent expert system researchers, might be "more akin to *idiots savants* than to real human experts" (Brachman, Amarel, Engelman, Engelmore, Feigenbaum, & Wilkins, 1983, p. 55).

Emulation of Patterns of Knowing Through Expert System Technology

While one might conclude that by virtue of being perhaps nothing more than *idiots savants*, expert systems are of minimal applicability to nursing practice, such a global and undifferentiated view is unwarranted from the perspectives of both artificial intelligence and nursing. There is nursing knowledge that can be validly emulated in expert systems. However, their are distinct boundaries to them, and it is our intent to elucidate these here.

Given the restrictions in what expert systems can emulate, as described above, how can these systems be applied to nursing practice? This is a question as to the relative congruence of, on the one hand, knowing for nursing practice; and, on the other hand, the knowledge that feasibly can be embedded in expert systems. For purposes of this discussion, this question can be phrased as follows: what patterns of knowing in nursing (Carper, 1978; Chinn, 1987) are similar to the operational mode of knowing that characterizes expert system technology? In other words, what knowledge can be explicated clearly and unambiguously as objects, classes, relationships, and procedures?

The first requisite for such explication is that the knowledge can be broken down into discrete units that minimally overlap with other units. Thus, object A should be clearly distinguishable from object B. Similarly, class X should feature objects that are different from those categorized under class Y. The relationship among objects C and D should describe only their mutual association, and not that of objects E and F (unless of course it holds that C = E and D = F). The procedures embedded in the system should be object and class specific as well. While, admittedly, absolute discreteness may prove impossible, there should be enough clarity nonetheless so as to permit accuracy. Or, in technical terms, the overlap between units should be manageable within the models of fuzzy set theory (Zadeh, 1965, 1979).

The second requisite follows from the first, and that is that quantification can be achieved to some degree. It is important that values can be ascribed to objects, and that the association between objects can be described in gradation. This quantification may range from nominal (e.g., presence/absence) over ordinal (low to high rank) to interval/ratio (distribution of values with constant increments/decrements).

A final requisite pertains to generalization. Since expert systems are intended to serve many users, the knowledge should be sufficiently general so as to apply to many. Thus, idiosyncrasy cannot be emulated; nor would its emulation be acceptable for it presumes, perhaps paradoxically, the generalizability of idiosyncrasy.

It could be concluded that the knowledge reproducible through artificially intelligent technology must be primarily cognitive. Cognitive processes can be studied and analyzed much more easily than affective processes, including in the clinical domain (Abraham, 1986). It is generally accepted that current expert system technology is unable to represent affective processes.

Given these constraints, which patterns of knowing (Carper, 1978; Chinn, 1987) are amenable to emulation in expert system technology? Personal knowledge, with its emphasis on affect-oriented experience and self-realization, may prove most difficult to break down into relatively discrete units. The highly individualized nature of this pattern of knowing cannot be generalized across nurses. Its blending of cognitive and affective processes places this pattern beyond the constraint of cognition imposed by expert system technology. Consequently, personal knowledge will prove most difficult to emulate.

Ethics is knowledge incorporating judgments and values, many of which are grounded in structured beliefs about what is good, just, and right; but many of which are also grounded in intuition and emotion. Thus, ethical knowledge is in part amenable to emulation in expert technology, namely to the extent that it can be translated into rules of conduct. This implies that the premises and antecedents governing these rules can be defined.

Esthetic knowledge, with its emphasis on the individualized abstraction of particulars, reliance on personal perception, and premise of appreciation, is a pattern of knowing that, when asked, nurses may have difficulty in detailing and describing. While perhaps the art of nursing can be enriched by the acquisition of skill, these skills do not make the art of nursing. Thus, the emulation of esthetics may be limited to the incorporation of skill. We question whether including the level of skill truly represents the concept of art, given that skill has been defined as possessing the right knowledge and applying it effectively (Lenat, Hayes-Roth, & Klahr, 1979).

It is with the empirical pattern of knowing that expert systems may prove most helpful. Empirics is characterized by describing, explaining, and predicting (Chinn, 1987), and in doing so seeks to derive generalizations from particulars. Empirics emphasizes analysis of phenomena into constituant elements, with quantification of the latter. It has a goal of (relative) clarity and (relative) lack of ambiguity. Empirics is a function of logical understanding as the basis for action. Thus, empirics as a pattern of knowing is most amenable to emulation in artificially intelligent decision-support.

Conclusion

There is a naive assumption about artificial intelligence that states that technology based on AI is capable of most aspects of human reasoning and problem-solving. Similarly, in nursing it is not uncommon to hear the "uncontestable virtues" of artificial intelligence applications for nursing proclaimed at conferences and workshops, as well as through other forums for dissemination. In our respective capacities as artificial intelligence researcher (Abraham) and nurse-theorist (Fitzpatrick), we believe that most of this (over) enthusiasm is unjustified and will prove to be to the detriment of both nursing and artificial intelligence (not to speak of the funding for artificial intelligence research in nursing!). While we strongly advocate the integration of artificially intelligent technology into nursing practice, with equal if not more vigor do we wish to emphasize the need for careful assessment of options and capabilities.

It should indeed be stressed that the integration of technology into nursing is not a matter of blind adoption, but one of careful consideration of how the technology will further nursing. As our own work in the development of expert system technology has taught us, artificial intelligence in nursing is in first instance an issue of nursing science, and only in second instance an issue of artificial intelligence (Abraham, 1987a). Instead of manipulating nursing so as to fit artificial intelligence, one should manipulate artificial intelligence to serve the needs of nursing within a context predicated by nursing (Abraham, 1987b).

In sum, it was our purpose here to clarify how nurses know what they know and how they apply this knowing to what they do; and to examine, given the state-of-the-art in artificial intelligence, what of this knowing can be emulated. A global overenthusiasm is certainly not in order, yet a due enthusiasm about how expert system technology may facilitate certain aspects of knowing in nursing is more than justified.

Acknowledgments. Preparation of this manuscript was supported by the Artificial Intelligence in Nursing Project, a joint venture of Case Western Reserve University and University Hospitals of Cleveland (I. Abraham, Principal Investigator); and by a grant from the Cleveland Foundation (D. Neuhauser, Principal Investigator). Address correspondence to the first author, Case Western Reserve University, Frances Payne Bolton School of Nursing, 2121 Abington, Cleveland, Ohio 44106, USA.

References

Abraham, I. L. (1986). Diagnostic discrepancy and clinical inference: A social-cognitive analysis. *Genetic, Social, & General Psychology Monographs, 112,* 41–102.

Abraham, I. L. (1987a). Linking health care and information technology: The future of computer applications in nursing. In J. Roode (Ed.), *Changing patterns in nursing education.* New York: National League for Nursing.

Abraham, I. L. (1987b). (Nursing and informatics in the United States.) (In Dutch). In H. Dierickx, G. Evers, F. Hein, H. Nieman, & W. Sermeus (Eds.), *Verpleegkundige informatica: Van idee naar werkelijkheid.* Leuven, Belgium: Acco.

Abraham, I. L., & Krowchuk, H. V. (in press). Heuristic aspects of clinical inference in nursing. In K. Smyth & D. Neuhauser (Eds.), *Advances in clinical decision analysis.* New York: Elsevier-North Holland.

Abraham, I. L., & Schultz, S. (1986). Knowledge representation in clinical inference in nursing: Structures and their application to expert systems. In R. Salamon, B. Blum, & M. Jorgenson (Eds.), *Medinfo 86,* Volume I. Amsterdam: North-Holland.

Abraham, I. L., Schultz, S., Ozbolt, J. G., & Swain, M. A. P. (1984a). A multivariate mathematical algorithm for diagnostic information systems: I. Data acquisition and storage procedures. In F. H. Roger, J. L. Willems, R. O'Moore, & B. Barber (Eds.), *Medical Informatics Europe 84 (Lecture Notes in Medical Informatics, Volume 24).* Berlin: Springer Verlag.

Abraham, I. L., Schultz, S., Ozbolt, J. G., & Swain, M. A. P. (1984b). A multivariate mathematical algorithm for diagnostic information systems: II. Procedures for clinical inference. *Proceedings of the Eighth Symposium on Computer Applications in Medical Care.* (Silver Springs, MD: IEEE Computer Society).

Barnett, J. A., & Bernstein, M. I. (1977). *Knowledge-based systems: A tutorial.* Report TM-(L)-5903/000/00 (NTIS: AD/A-044 833). Santa Monica, CA: System Development Corp.

Brachman, R. J., Amarel, S., Engelman, C., Engelmore, R. S., Feigenbaum, E. A., & Wilkins, D. E. (1983). What are expert systems? In F. Hayes-Roth, D. A. Waterman, & D. B. Lenat (Eds.), *Building expert systems.* Reading, MA: Addison-Wesley.

Buchanan, B. G. (1982). New research on expert systems. In J. E. Hayes, D. Michie, & Y. H. Pao (Eds.), *Machine intelligence,* Volume 10. Edinburgh: Edinburgh University Press.

Buchanan, B. G., & Shortliffe, E. H. (1984). *Rule-based expert systems.* Reading, MA: Addison-Wesley.

Carper, B. A. (1978). Fundamental patterns of knowing in nursing. *Advances in Nursing Science, 1,* 13–23.

Chinn, P., Jacobs, M., & Huether, S. (Eds.) (1987). *Theory and nursing: A systematic approach (2nd ed.).* St. Louis: Mosby.

Grosso, C., & Abraham, I. L. (1987). On knowledge-based systems for the domains of nursing. In A. H. Levy & B. T. Williams (Eds.), *Proceedings of the AAMSI Congress 87.* Washington, DC: American Association for Medical Systems and Informatics.

Hart, P. E. (1980). *What's preventing the widespread use of expert systems?* Paper presented at the Workshop on Expert Systems, San Diego, CA.

Hayes-Roth, F., Waterman, D. A., & Lenat, D. B. (1983a). *Building expert systems.* Reading, MA: Addison-Wesley.

Hayes-Roth, F., Waterman, D. A., & Lenat, D. B. (1983b). An overview of expert systems. In F. Hayes-Roth, D. A. Waterman, & D. B. Lenat (Eds.), *Building expert systems.* Reading, MA: Addison-Wesley.

Kulikowski, C. A. (1980). Artificial intelligence methods and systems for medical consultation. *IEEE Transactions on Pattern Analysis and Machine Intelligence,* 464–476.

Laborde, J. (1984). Expert systems for nursing. *Computers in Nursing, 2,* 130–135.

Lenat, D. B., Hayes-Roth, F., & Klahr, P. (1979). *Cognitive economy.* Report HPP-79-15, Heuristic Programming Project, Computer Science Department. Palo Alto, CA: Stanford University.

Maslow, A. H. (1956). Self-actualizing people: A study of psychological health. In C. Moustakas (Ed.), *The self.* New York: Harper & Row.

Ozbolt, J. G. (1986). Developing decision support systems for nursing: Issues of knowledge representation. In R. Salamon, B. Blum, & M. Jorgenson (Eds.), *Medinfo 86*, Volume I. Amsterdam: North-Holland.

Ozbolt, J. G., Schultz, S., Swain, M. A. P., & Abraham, I. L. (1985). A proposed expert system for nursing practice. *Journal of Medical Systems, 9*, 57–68.

Polyani, M. (1964). *Personal knowledge.* New York: Harper & Row.

Ryan, S. (1983). Applications of a nursing knowledge-based system for nursing practice: Inservice, continuing education, and standards of care. *Proceedings of the Seventh Symposium on Computer Applications in Medical Care.* Silver Springs, MD: IEEE Computer Society.

Zadeh, L. A. (1965). Fuzzy sets. *Information and Control, 8*, 338–353.

Zadeh, L. A. (1979). A theory of approximate reasoning. In J. E. Hayes, D. Michie, & L. I. Mikulich (Eds.), *Machine intelligence*, Volume 9. New York: Wiley.

53
Professional Culture Models of Science and Data Types for Computerized Health Records

JOHN P. TURLEY

1. Introduction

This paper will discuss aspects of professional culture known to address clinical decision making [1] and aspects of science that impact on the practice of professionals [2] in order to examine how these elements can be combined and addressed in the Computerized Health Record (CHR). The overall goal of this process is to better understand how professional decisions utilize data. This will allow the designers of the CHR to optimize the displaying, indexing, and storage of data to enhance the decision making of the various professionals who will utilize the CHR.

Much of the work related to the development of the CHR has focused either on the conceptual design of the CHR itself or on the functional aspects of the data recording and display that must be part of the development of the CHR. Connelly et al. [3] and Tang et al. [4] have discussed the need to focus on the development of the Clinicians Workstation (CWS). The CWS had demanded that the focus of the CHR shift from being simply a documentation repository to a position where clinical decision support is an integral part of the CHR. With a more active CHR, there must be an understanding of elements that are not considered in evaluating the paper record.

As a concept model of the Computer Based Patient Record has evolved, the model separated the data stored in the record and the applications that utilized that data. Under the proposed concept model, the applications range from very passive (storing and displaying data) to very active. Active applications may compare patient specific data with rules and care maps developed by entities external to the care delivery organization. For example, profession-specific standards of care could be used to suggest

Reprinted with permission from *MEDINFO '95: Proceedings of the Eighth World Congress on Medical Informatics*; Greenes, R.A., Peterson, H.E. & Protti, D.J. (Eds.). 1995. Pp. 1584–1587. Edmonton, Alberta, Canada: Canadian Organization for the Advancement of Computers in Health (COACH).

protocols and interventions. Final decision making authority would rest with the care providers, but decision suggestions could arise from the automated record itself.

The notion of decision making in health care is a complex one. Elstein [5] in medicine and Corcoran-Perry and Narayan [6] in nursing have focused on the complexities involved in the clinical decision making process. They both recognize that the traditional distinctions of novice and expert do not adequately describe the range of situations necessary to describe the clinical decision making of clinicians in a variety of health disciplines. Corcoran-Perry and Narayan [6] have discovered an interesting phenomenon related to nurses' views of their decision making. They asked nurses to describe a number of the recent decisions that they have made. Many of the nurses remarked that they had not made any decisions. Upon reflection, they were able to elucidate a number of rather complex decisions that they had addressed during the shift prior to the interview. Nurses were not able to identify that decisions and decision making were an essential part of their practice.

Preliminary investigations have shown that health processionals' decision making is more complex than is apparent. Johnson [7], in examining knowledge acquisition for expert systems, found that professional experts were among the least able to articulate their decision making. Johnson found that the data and information used by professionals is so "chunked" that the professionals were not able to decompose the knowledge, let alone discuss how decision making used the knowledge.

Before discussing how the elements of this discussion will have an impact on the data types of the CHR, it is necessary to summarize the discussions related to professional culture and the discussions related to the types of science. Following the discussion will be a model proposing data types that must be included in the CHR in order to meet the elements of professional culture and types of science.

2. Professional Culture

Professions have developed distinctively different cultures. These cultures reflect the operational workings that the profession is attempting to achieve. The development of the culture has occurred over a substantial period of time. Yet, we are involved in an era of rapid change and rapid shift of duties, goals, and expected outcomes. This change is occurring within the society as a whole. The impact of this change in the culture has had complex implications for the practice of health care, as well as for the individual professions within the health care arena. Turley & Connelly [1] have summarized some of the cultural differences between Medicine and Nursing. The development of a Clinicians Workstation (CWS) necessitated examination of different professional cultures.

In examining the cultural differences between Medicine and Nursing, it is clear that the goals, focus of practice, and values are different. The following table will summarize the key points.

Both professions are joined in the overall goal of helping the patient attain improved health. The information that each profession uses and the way that the profession structures that data will have an impact on the design of the CWS.

This table compares just two professional disciplines. Similar analyses must eventually be done for other professions working in health care. For the purposes of this paper, examples will be drawn from medicine and nursing. This is not to minimize the importance to other disciplines; it is a matter of convenience.

3. Science

Turley, Corcoran-Perry, & Narayan [2] discussed the impact on the different models of science, and how that impacts role integration and decision making within Nursing. This work derives from the insights of Levi-Strauss [8]. In the *Savage Mind*, Levi-Strauss was trying to reconcile the insights of Western science with the underlying assumption that science progresses in a linear and additive progression. In examining the history of science and technology, Levi-Strauss found that there were large gaps in the linear progression of science and technology in the West. It appeared that there was a linear progression of science followed by gaps. These gaps were then again followed by a period of linear progression in science and technology. Levi-Strauss then examined what was occurring during these gaps. He found, during this time, that there was a period of continued evolution, but not in the formal abstract sciences; rather it was the evolving of what he referred to as *concrete science*.

Abstract science has become synonymous with what we refer to as western science. Abstract science derives from formalizations or laws, postulated relationships among laws, and relationships among the elements that comprise the law. These elements are abstractions from the world of daily events. The relationships are postulated with a mathematical certainty (mathematics being one of the abstract sciences par excellence). This set of formalisms and the exploiting of their relationships allowed for generalizability. Lessons learned in one part of science could be imputed into another domain. The true knowledge in abstract science is separate from the situation in which it occurs.

By contrast, concrete science is imbedded in the context where the knowledge is an integral part of being able to do or to perform. This sense of praxis completely separates concrete science from abstract science. The stone mason works using a knowledge of how stones feel, knowing where to crack or break it, and the limitations of the usefulness of a single piece of stone. This is embodied knowledge that has been developed in the actual performance of actions. Levi-Strauss found that it was necessary for concrete science to evolve and form a basis before abstract could generalize from the embodied experiences and generate a new layer of abstract science.

In summary, the evolution of the total aspects of science formulates a complex interaction between the evolution of concrete and abstract sciences. Medicine is currently in a pattern of rapid growth of its abstract science. Nursing, by contrast, has functioned on the strength of its concrete science and is only beginning to evolve its abstract science.

4. CHR and Record Types

The evolution of the CHR will bring together multiple professions in ways that were not possible using the traditional paper record system. The CHR will allow professions to communicate with each other using their native language. That language can be translated, for discussions across professional lines. Inter-professional communications can be enhanced by presenting views of the data and information that more clearly reflect the professional culture of the person accessing the information. The electronic format of the CHR is inherently more versatile and flexible than the paper record of old. The paper record had a number of inherent limitations. The paper record allowed for restricted forms of data input, the most common being hand written text. Some low-level charting and graphing could be accomplished by using pre-formatted graphs. Free hand drawings could be added to the text, with the quality of the drawings relying heavily on the drawing capabilities of the person entering the data. Photographs, EKG tracings, and other external data forms could be added to the record. However, the additions of these data forms are restricted to being "paper clipped" to the record. The permanence and consistency of these additional data types remain suspect.

With the advent of multimedia computing, the ability to add multiple electronic data types to the records needs to be explored. Most concept models of the EMR or CPR have embraced the notion of multimedia data storage. Currently, work is underway examining aspects of size limitation, compression, loss, integration, and other aspects that must be researched before there is broad inclusion of other data types. In most cases, this research has been undertaken in order to store health related data in its native format. EKG wave tracings, radiographs, heart sounds, etc. could be then stored in their native capture format to be preserved with the patient record; the interpretation applied to these elements by professional interpreters can also be stored. In the paper record, it is usually only the interpretation that becomes a permanent part of the paper record, the original being kept in radiology or in the record keeping system of the interpreter.

Insights gained from research into different data types should allow the CHR even greater flexibility. Abstract science data types are the most easily stored because they are abstract and their key knowledge content is independent of the patient specific situation; they represent a more compact data than does concrete science data. It is possible using multi-media for more complex data types to capture health related information that is not currently part of the health record. McGuiness [9] is exploring the usefulness of capturing wound photographs in addition to narrative information about the wound. Preliminary analysis seems to indicate that nurses use and understand more complex data from the photographs than what they abstract to be written in the text based record. Other work by Turley has also documented that nurses do not record much of the information that they consider to be critical about the patient and/or patient situation, because of the difficulty in representing the knowledge in a textual narrative format.

Some elements are critical to nursing. In the paper record, some of these concepts have not been allowed to function in ways which would help the clinical decision making of nurses. For example, much of the data is entered in terms of event episodes. Time and date recording is necessary for legal concerns (what occurred and when did it occur), but this may not may not be the best representation of "Patient Centered" data. The use of an electronic storage format will allow for modeling of different data displays for different purposes. While the legal record may still wish to retrieve the time and data approach to information, the patient centered approach may need to look at representation of information across time and/or across professions.

Nursing's focus on "Illness" as opposed to "Disease" may require a more contextual view of information. Patient responses, in terms of ADLs and IADLs, can be displayed in combination with the physical parameter changes which are the results of or indications of a disease process. This approach to displaying information will assist nurses in the process of their decision making, in ways that time and date ordered displays could not address.

The ability to display "hands on" information or "praxis" may require elements of Virtual Reality displays. In this arena, there will be exploration of new more complex data types. These data types may require more complex display formats than is currently available with the present state of electronic records. The CHR can allow for the embodiment of these data types in a way not possible with other record systems.

Recognition of the contextual nature of nursing data may require that audio, video, and photography be necessary to capture complex relations among data elements. In the realm of concrete science, data points out of context have relatively little meaning in contrast to meaningful data which is independent in abstract science.

The nature of "human response patterns" may require video and/or time lapse photography in order to record changes in the patient. The change occurs continuously and so subtly that traditional recordings may not capture the meaning of the data.

Nursing, like surgery and other performance disciplines, needs to explore new data types that can capture the phenomena of concern to that discipline. Nursing shares much of the abstract data used in medicine for the diagnosis and treatment of disease. However, nursing also has a greater element of concrete science as part of its discipline. The evolution of the CHR will allow for the capture, storage, and display of data types; this would not have been possible using existing record systems. If those developing current EMRs and CPRs do not explore the wider range of issues related to profession specific knowledge and culture, the CHR will neither be able to become an active participant in the professions' decision making nor create a scenario for improved patient centered care.

References

[1] Turley J. & Connelly D. "The relationship between nursing and medical culture: implications for the design and implementation of a clinician's workstation." *Proceedings of the 17th Annual Symposium on Computer Applications in Medical Care.* New York: McGraw-Hill (1973) 233.

[2] Turley J., Narayan S., & Corcoran-Perry S. "Practice disciplines, cognitive science and the other sciences the role of decision making." *Proceedings of QUARDET '93.* Barcelona (1993).

[3] Connelly D., Werth G., Dean D., Hultman D., & Thompson T. "Physician use of an NICU laboratory reporting system." *Proceedings of the 16th Annual Symposium on Computer Applications in Medical Care.* New York: McGraw-Hill (1992) 8.

[4] Tang P., Annevelink J., Fafchamps D., Strong P., Suermondt H., Young C., Ratib O., Heimendinger L., Schirato P., Ligier Y., & Perrier R. "Development of an integrated physician's workstation." In Lun K., Degoulet P., Piemme T., & Rienhoff O. (eds). *Medinfo '92.* Amsterdam: North Holland (1992) 1596.

[5] Elstein A., Shulman L. & Sprafka S. *Medical Problem Solving.* Cambridge, MA: Harvard University Press (1978).

[6] Corcoran-Perry S. & Narayan S. Lines of reasoning used by triage nurses in cases of varying complexity: a pilot study. *Perspectives on Judgment and Decision Making.* Locke W. (ed). Metuchen, NJ: Scarecrow Press (1993).

[7] Johnson P. "What kind of expert should a system be?" *The Journal of Medicine and Philosophy* (1983) 8: 77–97.

[8] Levi-Strauss C. *The Savage Mind.* Chicago: University of Chicago Press (1962).

[9] McGuiness W. *Master's Thesis* (in process). LaTrobe University, Bundora, VIC, Australia (1994).

54
Validating a Model for Defining Nursing Information System Requirements

Carole A. Gassert

Information systems are being installed to expedite the management of information in health care and nurses are being placed on information system committees to evaluate and select these systems. Nurses may have limited experience with information technology (Hoffman, 1985; Powell, 1982; Weaver & Johnson, 1984) and have difficulty identifying nursing requirements for systems. To assist with the process a graphic Model for Defining Nursing Information System Requirements (MDNISR) was developed (Gassert, 1989).

The MDNISR was developed using structured analysis techniques (Gassert, 1990) and validation techniques that will be described in this paper. The MDNISR has five elements: nurse users, information processing, nursing information systems, nursing information, and nursing system goals. Each model element has inputs, processes, constraints and outputs. The output from one element serves as an input for the next element, suggesting a sequencing of model elements. Collectively, the model element outputs of nursing information functions, nursing information processing requirements, nursing system outputs, nursing data requirements, and nursing system goals form a document for stating what an information system must include.

Content Validity of Model

Validation for the MDNISR included establishment of content validity and testing of the model's completeness, usefulness, and clarity. To establish content validity a matrix was used to compare inputs/outputs for the

Reprinted with permission from; *Nursing Informatics '91: Proceedings of the Fourth International Conference on Nursing Use of Computers and Information Science*; Hovenga, E.J.S., Hannah, K.J., McCormick, K.A. & Ronald, J.S. (Eds.). 1991, pp. 215–219. Heidelberg-Berlin, Germany: Springer-Verlag.

five model elements with existing literature guidelines for deciding about nursing information systems (NISs) (Ball & Hannah, 1984; Berg, 1983; Cook, 1982; Drazen 1983; Hoffman, 1985; McAlindon, Danz & Theodoroff, 1987; McCarthy, 1985; Powell, 1982; Reider & Norton, 1984; Romano & McNeely, 1985; Romano, McCormick & McNeely, 1982; Weaver & Johnson, 1984; Zielstorff, 1975). All but one of the 13 sets of guidelines include inputs/outputs from each of the five elements. The remaining guidelines include inputs/outputs from four of the five model elements (McCarthy, 1985). Thus the matrix established content validity for the MDNISR.

To establish further content validity the MDNISR was submitted to a panel of six experts in nursing informatics in the United States. Each expert had experience selecting, evaluating, enhancing, developing, or implementing NISs, had at least a masters degree, had spent an average of 7.2 years in their current position, and had published in nursing informatics. Five experts were responsible for information technology and one expert was a professor.

The panel judged the model's content validity by completing a questionnaire about the model. On a visual analog scale (VAS) of 0 to 10 experts indicated the extent to which each of five model outputs was essential to consider when deciding about NISs. Mean scores for each model element output (MEO) exceeded the minimal score of 7.5. On a second VAS the experts indicated the extent to which they had used each MEO in deciding about NISs. Again, mean scores for each MEO exceeded the minimal score of 7.5. When asked what additional data needed to be added to the model, no new model elements were suggested. The panel review supported content validity of the MDNISR.

User Validation of Model

The MDNISR was tested for completeness, usefulness, and clarity with 75 registered nurses who have made decisions about NISs. Nurses completed a self-administered questionnaire about the model and provided information about their informatics experiences and information systems in their agencies.

The questionnaire was developed using an item form/item frame technique to obtain the same information about each MEO. Two separate VASS were used for testing model completeness and usefulness. On the first scale participants indicated how essential they felt each MEO was to consider when deciding about NISs. Completeness was also tested by having subjects indicate additional data they considered when deciding about NISs and whether anything was missing from the model. On a second scale subjects were asked to what extent they used each MEO in deciding about NISs. To validate clarity of the model, subjects listed three examples for each MEO. In addition subjects judged the clarity of two sample sets of requirements developed using MEO definitions. Finally, clarity of the model diagram itself was judged.

The questionnaire was judged to have both content and face validity by the panel. A pilot test established instrument reliability. Three decision makers completed a second questionnaire two weeks after the first was returned to the investigator. The mean percent of agreement for the demographic portion of the questionnaire was 94%. A Spearman who calculated on the second portion of the questionnaire was .89. Thus test–retest reliability of the questionnaire was established.

A purposive sample of registered nurses who had made decisions about NISs was used to validate the MDNISR. Names of 148 potential subjects were obtained from query letters sent to directors of nursing departments, nursing colleagues, and software vendors located throughout the United States. A total of 75 subjects (50.6%) returned questionnaires in two months. All subjects had planned for, selected, implemented, evaluated, enhanced or developed NISs.

Subjects had a mean age of 40.4 years, almost all were female, and three-quarters held a baccalaureate or higher degree. Positions held by subjects were grouped as follows: information technology nurses (39%); middle managers (32%); top managers (24%); and staff nurses (5%). Information technology nurses included information nurse specialists, nurse educators for computer systems, and managers of information technology systems or projects. The five most frequently performed job responsibilities of 53% of subjects included nursing information system activities, e.g., writing RFPs, implementing systems, educating nurses to use systems, testing software and serving as a liaison to problem solve for systems. The majority had held their current positions for one to five years and were employed by nursing.

NIS experiences were examined. A majority used NISs to enter or retrieve data at least weekly. More than 70% served on NIS planning committees or were enhancing an NIS. A majority were involved in educating other nurses to use a system. In addition, more than half were currently evaluating, designing or implementing systems. Only 32% of subjects had had previous involvement with NISs. Most first learned about NISs on their jobs. When rating their level of expertise in comparison to other agency nurses, 40% felt they were well above average and 39% felt they were above average.

Subjects were employed by 44 hospitals in 20 different states within six geographical regions of the United States. Hospitals ranged from 200 to 1250 beds with the majority between 251 and 500 beds. Subjects reported that 88% of agencies had systems up and running and 12% were currently planning for, developing, or installing NISs. The most commonly used NISs included patient acuity (59%) and staffing and scheduling systems (52%).

Results

Clarity of the MDNISR was validated by asking subjects to list examples of MEOs. Examples were compared with lists of items previously compiled from the nursing informatics literature, the panel of experts, and the pilot study. Two graders independently scored examples on 10% of randomly selected questionnaires with 98% agreement. The mean percent correct for examples listed for each MEO was 78.7 or higher. This exceeded the minimally acceptable score of 66% correct. More than 60% of subjects listed all examples correctly for the five MEOs. In addition most subjects felt examples developed according to the definitions were clear and helped to understand the model. Almost three-quarters of subjects indicated the model diagram was understandable. These findings supported model clarity.

Model completeness was also supported. No new model elements could be inferred from additional data that subjects considered in deciding about NISs. Most subjects either stated that nothing was missing from the model or did not respond to the question. In addition mean scores for all five MEO on the VAS were 8.6 or greater, well above the minimal score of 7.5.

Finally, the MDNISR's usefulness was supported. Mean scores for all five MEOs on the VAS for extent used were 8.1 or higher indicating that participants indicated used each of the MEOs in deciding about NISs. Again these scores were well above the minimal score of 7.5.

Study findings have initially validated the MDNISR. Content validity has been established and subjects supported the model's completeness, usefulness and clarity. Additional work is needed to determine if the MDNISR can be applied in various settings.

References

Ball M, Hannah K: *Using Computers in Nursing*. Reston, VA: Reston Publishers, 1984.

Berg C: The importance of nurses' input for the selection of computerized systems. In: Scholes M, Bryant Y, Barber B eds. *The Impact of Computers on Nursing*, Amsterdam: Elsevier Science Publishers B. V., 1983; 42–58.

Cook M: Selecting the right computer system. *Nursing Management* 1982; 13: 2628.

Drazen E: Planning for purchase and implementation of an automated hospital information system: A nursing perspective. *Journal of Nursing Administration* 1983; 13: 9–12.

Gassert C: Defining nursing information system requirements: A linked model. In: Kingsland L, ed. *Proceedings of the Thirteenth Annual Symposium of Computer Applications in Medical Care*. Los Angeles: Computer Society Press, 1989; 779–783.

Gassert C: Structured analysis: Methodology for developing a model for defining nursing information system requirements. *Advances in Nursing Science* 1990; 13: 53–62.

Hoffman F: Evaluating and selecting a computer software package. *Journal of Nursing Administration* 1985; 15: 33–35.

McAlindon M, Danz S, Theodoroff R: Choosing the hospital information system: A nursing perspective. *Journal of Nursing Administration* 1987; 17: 11–15.

McCarthy L: Taking charge of computerization. *Nursing Management* 1985; 16: 3540.

Powell N: Designing and developing a computerized hospital information system. *Nursing Management* 1982; 13: 40–45.

Rieder K, Norton D: An integrated nursing information system—a planning model. *Computers in Nursing.* 1984; 2: 73–79.

Romano C, McNeely L: Nursing applications of a computerized information system: Development, implementation, utilization. In: Hannah K, Guillemin E, Conklin E. eds. *Nursing Uses of Computers and Information Science.* Amsterdam: Elsevier Science Publishers B. V., 1985: 43–49.

Romano C, McCormick K, McNeely L: Nursing documentation: A model for a computerized data base. *Advances in Nursing Science* 1982; 4: 43–56.

Weaver C, Johnson J: Nursing participation in computer vendor selection. *Computers in Nursing* 1984; 2: 31–34.

Zielstorff R: The planning and evaluation of automated systems: A nurses' point of view. *Journal of Nursing Administration* 1975; 5: 22–25.

55
Identification of Data Element Categories for Clinical Nursing Information Systems via Information Analysis of Nursing Practice

JUDITH R. GRAVES and SHEILA CORCORAN[†]

The Problem

It is a given that a clinical nursing information system (CNIS) assists in the *management of nursing data, information, and knowledge.* While there are other factors that must be taken into account in the design of an information system, the element most intimately dependent upon the domain served is the design of the data base, specifically, the identification of the data elements themselves and how the data in the system interact. Further, design of the CNIS must not only take into account data needed to document practice and record nursing diagnoses, interventions, and outcomes, the design must include information required by the nurses in order to give care.

The identification of the data elements for the nursing data base can be approached from several perspectives [1–7]. A large proportion of elements for the data set can be derived directly from the consideration of the conceptual or diagnostic system upon which nursing practice is based.

Other data needed to reflect the realities of practice, setting, and clients in a CNIS comes from three major sources: (a) analysis of the clinical decisions made in practice, (b) analysis of the decision task, and (c) identification of the supplemental information nurses seek in the course of practice in order to give care. Analysis of the clinical decisions made in practice in a domain enables one to specify exactly the data elements required to make each decision. Formal task analysis methods help to elaborate the nature of the decision in addition to identifying the knowledge component

Reprinted with permission from *Proceedings: Twelfth Annual Symposium on Computer Applications in Medical Care*, Greenes, R.A. (Ed.). 1988. Pp. 358–363. © 1987, American Medical Informatics Association (formerly SCAMC): Bethesda, MD.

of the decision task [8,9]. Still other data elements stemming from the nature of the practice and the setting itself and should, therefore, be identified for inclusion in the content of the nursing information system. These elements are best identified from an examination of practice.

Identification of data elements directly from observation of nursing practice in the clinical practice setting has received limited attention in the NIS design literature for any domain of nursing. An extensive study of 15 hospitals across the country was done by Lockheed Information Systems Division [10] to examine information handling requirements of typical hospital nursing stations. The goal was to develop a general information processing model for a total hospital information processing system. Two categories of observation were made of the nursing stations: (a) observation to determine the type and extent of information being processed and by whom and (b) collection of forms used and flow-charting of the activity involved in processing the forms. The study was done before nursing practice began to be organized around identifiable nursing diagnosis or classification systems, however, and the definition nursing has changed considerably in the 20 years since that report. Further, the emphasis on information processing to serve the professional (vs. the functional) nursing component played a minor role in the NTIS report. Its use as a model to predict data element categories for nursing information system content (vs. hospital information system content) today is therefore limited.

One way to tap the source of data elements for nursing practice is to do an information analysis of supplemental information sought by nurses in clinical practice. This can be accomplished by asking the question, "What supplemental information (or data, or knowledge) do nurses seek in order to make decisions about patient care?" To verify the clinical nature of the responses and to identify additional implications of this question for information system design, other questions can be asked to identify why the information is needed, what sources are used to obtain the needed information, and what problems are encountered in obtaining the information.

Two major purposes are served by an analysis of supplemental information seeking in practice. One is to identify specific data elements that should be included in the CNIS, including those which reflect the interdisciplinary and collaborative data that may not be derived easily from other forms of content design. A second purpose is identify information that nurses need to obtain *from the CNIS* in the course of their practice. Despite a comprehensive database of nursing data, information, and knowledge, the system will be of limited use unless nurses can obtain from the system that information they need in making clinical practice decisions.

Empiric identification of every unique data element needed in nursing practice, would, of course, be an exercise in futility. The universe of individual elements for even a single domain of nursing is large, making this approach to identify all needed data elements untenable. Also, most of the data elements can be derived logically from the diagnostic or classification system chosen for nursing practice and the domain-specific clinical decisions made. Identification of the *categories* of data elements, however, is both possible and desirable.

In order to identify nursing information that should be provided to the nurse by a CNIS, this study asked the question, "What categories of data elements are revealed in supplemental information-seeking by nurses caring for patients with coronary problems?

Definitions

Used generically in this article, *information* is considered to be an aggregate of statements, facts, and/or figures which are conceptually interrelated. When used specifically, information may categorized and referred to as data, information, or knowledge. In this case, *data* refer to discrete entities which are described objectively and without interpretation; *information* refers to data that are interpreted and organized; and *knowledge* refers to information which has been synthesized so that interrelationships are identified and formalized [11].

For this study, *data elements* are limited to items of supplemental information that nurses seek out in in the course of their practice to make patient care decisions. *Categories of data elements* are the conceptual groupings of data elements identified by qualitative content analysis. *Supplemental information* is defined as data, information, or knowledge not held in memory but required in order to give care or make a decision about care. Information obtained directly from patients or their families is excluded. What is of importance in this study is information that a CNIS can best provide, *not* information that could best be obtained through direct observation or examination of patients.

Methods

Study Design

An exploratory, descriptive design was used. The study was delimited to a single domain of clinical nursing practice in a restricted setting, i.e. hospital-based nursing care of patients with coronary problems. Beyond this delimitation, investigators designed the study to tap all the variance possible in order to identify the fullest range of supplemental information data elements. Because of the desire to identify the range of data elements, no attempt was made to sample in such a way that differences in groups would be meaningful.

Expected variability due to setting and time characteristics was tapped by collecting data across CCU, coronary step-down, and coronary rehabilitation units and across shifts and days. Three different agencies were selected to assure that the study would capture the range of information-seeking behaviors of nurses in varied coronary care environments. Expected variability due to practitioner differences was tapped by investigating educational preparation, years of experience in nursing, years of experience in the domain, and years of experience in the unit where the data was collected.

Settings and Subjects

The study was delimited to data elements revealed in supplemental information-seeking in a single domain of clinical nursing practice, cardiovascular nursing care settings. It was also limited to three different agencies in one metropolitan area. One agency was a community hospital (Hospital A), one a large private teaching hospital (Hospital B), and the third a large public teaching hospital (Hospital C). None of the agencies had a computerized nursing or patient-care or nursing information system at the time the study was conducted. Two hospitals had laboratory results available via computer terminal. The particular hospital units involved included coronary care units (CCU), coronary step-down units, and rehabilitation units or programs.

Nurses were selected from a list of interested volunteers to ensure representation or registered nurses on all shifts on each unit at each agency. Only nurses giving direct patient care were used as subjects to avoid inclusion of supplemental information relevant to administrative decisions of nurse managers. At least two nurses from each shift on each unit were recruited. No attempts were made to replace the few nurses who could not participate due to change in shift, illness, etc., as long as that type of unit and shift was represented by a nurse in at least one of the agencies.

There were 46 registered nurse subjects, 14 from Hospital A, 21 from Hospital B, and 11 from Hospital C. All but two of them were female. They ranged in age from 23 to 57 years, the average age being 33. All but one were classified as staff nurses. All were assigned to patient care for the time during which the data was collected. The general distribution of experience in nursing, experience in cardiovascular nursing and unit experience was about the same in all agencies.

Instrument

To elicit data elements related to supplemental information, a questionnaire composed of open ended questions was developed to help investigators identify and describe instances of nurses seeking supplemental information. The questionnaire was designed to be completed either by subjects or by the investigators using a combined observation-interview process. To describe each instance of supplemental information-seeking, the primary question was, "What information was sought?" Also, the purpose for seeking the information was asked. In addition, the questionnaire contained other questions to elicit related data potentially important in decisions about information system design (i.e. the source used, why the source was used, success and difficulties in obtaining the information).

Data obtained when using the questionnaire had content validity in as much as both subjects and observers agreed on overt instances of information-seeking behavior and on the information being sought as supplemental information. Reliability of the questionnaire when used alone by the subject was considered acceptable. The physical presence of the investigators at the time of data collection probably encouraged the identification of information-seeking events at the time rather than from memory. Investigators randomly checked observations against data reported by subjects. When used by an observer, the questionnaire must be combined with a follow-up interview in order to elicit reliable data. Otherwise, covert instances of information seeking will be missed. When the questionnaire is combined with follow-up interviews, unobserved searches for supplemental information could be reported by subjects. Thus, the observation-interview combination provides acceptable reliability as judged by consensual validation of information by the observer and the participant.

Procedure

Human subjects approvals were obtained from the University of Minnesota and the selected agencies. A list of registered nurse volunteers was obtained following a presentation of the proposed research program at each agency on each selected unit. Nurses representing all units and all shifts including week-day and weekend shifts were recruited by phone into the study from the volunteer list.

Data Collection

Arrangements were made by phone to meet subjects just before or as they began their shift of work. After signing the informed consent, the participant was given the demographic data form to complete. Subjects were then randomly assigned to one of two data collection groups. In one group the subjects were observed in their clinical practice for five instances in which they were seen to seek supplemental information. The observation results were shared with each observed subject in a follow-up interview to validate the interpretations of the observer. In the second group, the subjects recorded answers to questions about five different instances of seeking supplemental information during a two hour data collection period. The information requested about the supplemental information seeking was identical in each method. In addition, the investigators recorded the general atmosphere of the unit during the time of the data collection.

Procedure for Analysis

Qualitative Content Analysis was used to group similar data elements into categories that describe all item in the group. Content analysis methods have been developed in the fields of psychology and sociology and involve the use of standardized procedures to make inferences about meaning from textual data about the sender of the message, the message itself, or the audience [12].

In this study, one investigator grouped like items together and then labeled the group. Similar groups were then collected into still larger groups or categories. After agreeing on the subgroups and categories, the investigators recoded each data element together before entering the category codes into the database.

Results

Verbatim responses to questions about each instance of supplemental information seeking were entered into the relational database management system (DBMS), Knowledgeman II™. Biographical and agency data were coded, then entered into the DBMS. Using qualitative content analysis methods, the data were grouped and content analyzed to identify categories of data elements. The category into which each observation fell was then entered into the DBMS for each supplemental information-seeking instance. Descriptive analysis of the subject population was done. Following data analysis, the investigators returned to each agency to share findings with subjects to obtain consensual validation of the findings and interpretations.

Responses to the question, "What information was sought?" elicited 178 instances of supplemental information seeking. Although a set of 5 different instances of supplemental information seeking was requested from each of the 46 subjects, some did not seek information this frequently within the designated data collection time period. Therefore, only 178 instances were obtained. All 178 instances of information seeking were unique: i.e. no two instances reflected exactly the information-seeking for the same reason from the same source.

Content analysis revealed that the 178 instances fell into four categories of data elements (a) patient specific information (N = 88, 50%), (b) institutional policies (N = 39, 21.9%) (c) domain knowledge (N = 37, 20.78%), and (d) procedures (N = 14, 7.86%). See Figure 1.

The category, Patient-specific Information, was used to categorize all instances in which subjects sought supplemental information about a specific patient, Subcategories of Patient-Specific Information were: General (N = 18), Meds (N = 16), Lab (N = 13), Cardiovascular status (N = 11), MD orders (N = 7), Education (N = 7), Exercise (N = 5), Diet (N = 4),

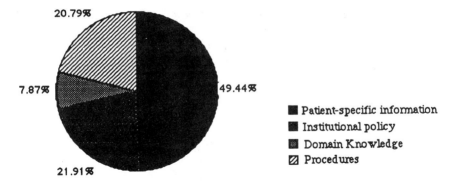

FIGURE 1. Categories of information.

Clinic (N = 2), and Other (N = 5). Examples of patient information grouped into categories are given: (GENERAL) "How a patient who underwent cardiac catheterization was doing," "The medical course since admission for a patient with a complicated MI," "(Needed) a general picture of the patient"; (MEDS) "Needed to work out IV problem (drip rate) on newly ordered IV," "Instructions on administering new medicine"; (LAB) "The time the APTT was to be drawn," "Compare previous test results with today's"; (CARDIOVASCULAR STATUS) "Patient's rhythm since admission to unit," "Family called asking for rhythm report. The patients had told them her heart was racing. There was nothing reported by monitor tech or nurse;" (MD ORDERS) "Clarification of a medication order," "Recheck dietary order"; (EDUCATION) "Dietary information about cholesterol for teaching patient," "Instruction handout about a drug and a diagnostic test"; (EXERCISE) "Patients performance record for the day (in rehab)," "Opinion of colleague as to safety and appropriateness of home exercise prescription"; (DIET) "Food likes and dislikes of patient," "Diet"; (CLINIC) "Why patient has not attended clinic lately." "Patient's previous heart rate and blood pressure during specific activities of rehabilitation"; (OTHER) "Patient's weight," "IV rate for lipids."

The Institutional Policy category was used to group *all* instances in which subjects sought supplemental information about institutional policies. Examples of this type of information sought include: "Check policy on nurse performing carotid massage," "Find out if patient can take walker home from hospital," "Policy to sue automatic compression sleeves."

The domain knowledge category was used to categorize all instances in which the nurse sought supplemental information to build their personal knowledge base. In this category, 16 instances involved learning about a prescribed medication (pharmacology knowledge), 10 involved learning more about cardiovascular physiology etc., 4 involved learning more about other diseases or pathologies (in addition to cardiovascular problems) their patients had, 3 involved learning more about clinical laboratory norms or interpretations, 3 involved learning how to use the computer, and 1 was general. Examples of patient information grouped into categories are given: (PHARMACOLOGY) "Whether or not to give isosorbide to a patient with a BP of 100/70;" "Had a question about sequence for giving (multiple) antibiotics;" (CARDIOVASCULAR PHYSIOLOGY) "What is pre-syncopy?" "What causes amyloidosis-restricted cardiomyopathy;" (NON CV DISEASE/PATHOLOGY) "Learn about effects of NA bicarb in the body," "Care plans for ETOH withdrawal;" (CLINICAL NORMS) "Normal magnesium level," "Trying to understand a decrease in Na;" (COMPUTER) "Would cardiac output info be stored in computer without recorder on?" "Function of computerized monitor system;" (GENERAL) "What is acrophagia?"

The Procedures category was used to categorize all instances in which subjects sought supplemental information about procedures for performing clinical skills. Examples include: "How to work a circle bed, Procedure for removing sutures."

There was little difference in categories of information sought by nurses in three different agencies (Figure 2), although the three agencies were substantively different and although the information milieu was notably different in each. In fact, it was notable that categories of information sought in the different agencies *were* so similar despite the differences in the three agencies. The most notable difference is that, in Hospital A, there were no instances of information seeking for enhancing one's own knowledge.

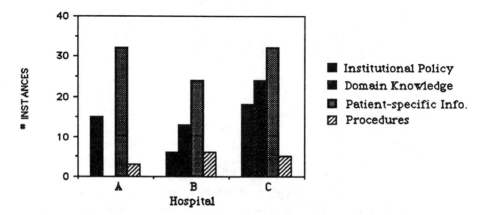

FIGURE 2. Categories of information sought in each agency.

Discussion and Future Research

The analysis of supplemental information sought for making clinical decisions was done to identify the *universe* of categories of information sought in making clinical decisions. Four main categories of data elements were identified; Patient-specific, Institutional Policies, Domain Knowledge, and Procedures. All instances obtained were unique at the data element level.

Although the sampling methods of this study do not allow for comparisons of findings between agencies, the findings are consistent with the NTIS [10] report. That report noted that, although the relative weight and discrete content of each category of information processing activity varied between nursing stations, eight major functions (of information processing) were identified that described this activity at all nursing stations in all the hospitals in the study. In addition, although not intended as a test of the framework presented in another paper by the authors, there is general agreement between the categories of data elements identified in this study and the general categories identified in the model for design of the CNIS [13]. The biggest discrepancy between categories enumerated in the CNIS design model and the categories identified in this paper has to do with the difference in data elements needed to supply domain learning needs of nurses. In the CNIS design model, the influence of conceptual structure on selection of data elements was restricted to the domain of Nursing whereas most of the instances of seeking information in order to increase one's own professional knowledge in this study involved seeking supplemental information about facts from reference disciplines. It should be noted that none of the agencies participating in this study were using any formalized system of classification of nursing problems at the time of the study. At the agency where the NANDA nursing diagnosis system was to be put into effect, there were training sessions being held and reference materials. It would be logical to expect that many nurses would be using reference materials on NANDA and nursing diagnosis generally where such a system was being introduced and used as the conceptual framework for CNIS content.

Individualized and systematic study using deliberative sampling of information-seeking behavior would be needed for any one agency to determine priorities for content of a specific CNIS. This would need to be based on the nature of the information sought and the frequency and relative cost of such searches. The methods used in the study would be valuable for this type of agency-specific data collection. All that would need to be changed would be different sampling techniques.

Further studies are needed to determine not only what information is needed most by nurses in various domains of practice within an agency but also the differences in information needed by experts, novices, and nurses practice outside of their usual domain or unit. Because the nurses in this study spent significant amounts of time on all shifts searching for information they did not keep in memory, there is little doubt that a CNIS that does not provide information *to* nurses is going be accompanied by some sort of auxiliary paper system.

References

[1] M. Gammel and P. Kretzmar, "NISS: Prelude to computerized systems." *Dimensions*, p. 18, Aug, 1984.

[2] S. Corcoran and J. Graves, "Supplemental information-seeking behavior of nurses in cardiovascular care." (in preparation).

[3] M. Kiley, E. Halloran, J.L. Weston, J. Ozbolt, H. Werley, M.J. Gordon et al., "Computerized Nursing Information Systems (NIS)." *Nursing Management*, p. 26, July, 1983.

[4] C. Romano, "Documentation of nursing practice using a computerized medical information system." In: H. Hefferman (ed), Proceedings of the Fifth Annual Symposium on Computer Applications in Medical Care. *IEEE Computer Society*, p. 749, 1981.

[5] C. Romano, K. McCormick, L. McNeely, "Nursing documentation: A model for a computerized data base." *Advances in Nursing Science*, vol. 4, no. 2, p. 43, 1982.

[6] C. Romano, L. Ryan, J. Haris, P. Boykin, and M. Power, "A Decade of Decisions: Four Perspectives of Computerization in Nursing Practice." *Computers in Nursing*, vol. 3, p. 64, 1985.

[7] E. Swenson-Feldman and P. Brugge-Wiger, "Promotion of interdisciplinary practice through an automated information system." *Advances in Nursing Science*, vol. 7, p. 39, 1985.

[8] R. Gagne, "Task Analysis: Its relation to content analysis." *Educational Psychologist*, vol. 11, p. 111, 1975.

[9] L. Resnick, "Task analysis in instructional design: Some case from mathematics." In: D. Klar (Ed.). *Cognition and Instruction*, Hillsdale, N.J.: Erlbaum Pub., 1976.

[10] Lockheed Missiles and Space Company, "Analysis of Information Needs of Nursing Stations." NTIS Technical Report # LMSC-682684, PB 186 246.

[11] B. Blum, "Medical informatics—Phase II." AAMSI CONGRESS 85 Proc Congress on Medical Informatics 3164–48, 1985 25.

[12] R. Weber, *Basic Content Analysis*. Beverly Hills, CA: Sage Publications, 1985.

[13] J. Graves and S.Corcoran, "Design of nursing information systems: Conceptual and practice elements." *Journal of Professional Nursing*, vol. 4 p. 168, 1988.

56
Nursing Minimum Data Sets: Historical Perspective and Australian Development

J. FOSTER and M. CONRICK

1. Introduction

Patient level data for medical care has been available through the International Classification of Diseases for many years. The International Council of Nurses and other groups worldwide are attempting to develop internationally agreed nursing classification systems and nursing minimum data sets which are critical to support the processes of nursing practice and to advance nursing knowledge necessary for quality cost effective and equitable health care [1] & [2]. There are a number of countries currently undertaking developments in the area of Nursing Minimum Data Sets. These developments are all at differing stages and take differing stances, with only one country, Belgium, having a Nursing Minimum Data Set accepted and information collected by the Government.

The majority of Australian Hospital Information Systems are using ICD9-CM and perhaps ICD10, DRG's and Casemix as the standard for understanding and controlling the production process of health care delivery. These standards will probably be used for future funding and resource allocation but nursing data are not adequately represented in any of these systems and cannot receive appropriate funding or resource allocation because standardised nursing data has never been collected.

2. International History of Minimum Data Sets

The pioneering development of the Data Set for nursing was undertaken by Professor Harriet Werley in the USA in the mid seventies. Professor Werley defines a Nursing Minimum Data Set (NMDS) as "a minimum set

Reprinted from *Nursing Informatics: An International Overview for Nursing in a Technological Era*, Grobe, S.J., Pluyter-Wenting, E.S.P. (Eds.). 1994. Pp. 150–154, with kind permission from Elsevier Science—NL, Sara Burgerhartstraat 25, 1055 KV Amsterdam, The Netherlands.

of items of information with uniform definitions and categories concerning the specific dimension of professional nursing, which meets the information needs of multiple users in the health care system" [3]. This is also the definition applied to the uniform minimum health data sets written by United States Health Information Policy Council. Werley & Zorn [4] emphasise strongly the need for multiple data users across all nursing practice settings to be considered in the definition of data elements. Also, central to the development of a NMDS is the development of standard uniform definitions and terminology for the data elements included [5].

The minimum data set concept was formulated in 1969 at a working conference in the USA. The aim was to collect the records of patients discharged from all hospitals and to develop a minimum set of core elements. The organizers of this conference recognized a need to order information, to contain rising health care costs, equitable distribution of services, and accountable resource use. These needs and the rapid developments in computer technology made it possible to design programs to manage large amounts of data [6].

The embryonic stage of the US Minimum Data Set was the Uniform Hospital Discharge Data Set (UHDDS) which originated from a conference attended by key health care providers and health data users. Unfortunately, a precedent was set, the UHDDS contained no nursing data. Around the same time in England, the budget shortfall for health was escalating and the National Health Service was under intense pressure, forcing Government intervention. The resultant investigation revealed problems in areas of data collection, processing, timeliness, accuracy and comparability. For this investigation the Steering Group on Health Services Information was born. This steering group identified, defined and tested those data elements to be included in a National Health Services Data Set and developed strategies for the collection of this data and this led to the "Korner Report." This report outlined the collection of data and use of information about hospital clinical activity, ambulance services, manpower, activity in hospitals and the community, services for and in the community and finance [7]. Once again no nursing data was collected. However, Wheeler [8] indicated that the "Korner Data Set" has evolved to include nursing elements, reflecting the changing role of nurses in the United Kingdom. But, once again these nursing data elements focus only on facilities and not on nursing activities. In Canada in 1990 a National Task Force on Health Information (NTFHI) was begun to develop a plan for a National System for Health Information, NTFHI, 1990. The elements were defined but again there is no clinical nursing data.

In response to the inequity in nursing data collection, the nurses in the USA have developed a NMDS, which is currently undergoing testing and evaluation. It has received a positive review by the Health Information Policy Council of the US and the National Committee on Vital and Health

Statistics. In Canada the information revolution has prompted initiatives to develop automated information systems focused on utilization of data for the purpose of resource allocation, and to facilitate the evolution of a national system for health information built on essential and comparable data [9]. According to Hannah [10], the significance of the development of the NMDS is best understood through an examination of the context within which it was developed.

In the United Kingdom the National Health Service Centre for Coding and Classification (NHS CCC) was established in 1990 and it forms part of the Information Management Group (IMG) of the NHS Management Executive (NHS ME), but has a Supervisory Board drawn from the professions. Its main functions are to maintain and develop further the Read Codes, to collaborate with the professions in the development of specialty data sets to satisfy the detailed requirements of the professions, by expanding the Read Codes (which have been the recommended standard in UK General Practice since 1990) to from a comprehensive Clinical Thesaurus by 1994. Nursing in the UK has recently completed a Scoping Project to explore nursing terminology and assess the Read Codes for their appropriateness to the nursing profession, and to liaise with the various nursing professional bodies, groups and members to establish current known work and experience in this field. The task of identifying and coding all terms required is being assessed to determine the resources needed to develop the nursing terminology in the Read Codes to be suitable across all services and sectors of the NHS [11].

Belgium has had a National Minimum Data Set of Nursing Interventions since 1987, under Royal Decree, and this allows national availability of all health information on medical and nursing activities in hospitals. The Nursing Minimum Data Set consists of a selected list of twenty three (23) nursing activities. These activities monitor basic care activities, technical activities and some very typical activities and are collected four times per year [12].

Australia has National Minimum data Set for Community Nursing (Australian—Community Nursing Minimum Data Set, CNMDSA) and this is currently in the pilot stage and results are being formulated. As there are only three NMDS available a comparison of these displays the similarities and differences in identified data elements. The USA have sixteen elements covering three main areas which are nursing care elements, patient or client demographic elements and service elements. In contrast the Belgium NMDS has twenty seven elements based on the Activities of Daily Living and the Australian CNMDS has eighteen elements. The differences between these data sets are exemplified in Table 1.

2.1 Comparison of Nursing Minimum Data Sets

Clark & Lang [14], state there is an urgent need for an international classification for nursing practice that will provide nursing with a nomenclature,

TABLE 1. Comparison of three nursing minimum data sets

Australia CNMDSA	United States of America	Belgium
1. Admission date	**Nursing care elements:**	1. Hygiene
2. Agency identifier	1. Nursing diagnosis	2. Mobility
3. Carer availability	2. Nursing intervention	3. Elimination
4. Client dependency	3. Nursing outcome	4. Feeding
5. Date of birth	4. Intensity of nursing care	5. Gavage feeding
6. Discharge date	**Patient or client demographic**	6. Care of mouth, nose, eyes
7. Discharge destination	**elements:**	7. Decubitus prevention
8. Ethnicity	5. Personal identification	8. Assisting in getting dressed
9. Sex of client	6. Date of birth	9. Attending to tracheostomy
10. Location of client	7. Sex	10. Tracheostomy with ventilation
11. Medical diagnosis	8. Race and ethnicity	11. Interviewing patients
12. Nursing intervention	9. Residence	12. Teaching patient occasionally
13. Nursing diagnosis	**Service elements:**	13. Teaching patient fixed program
14. Nursing goal	10. Unique facility or service Agency number	14. Emotional support
15. Resource utilization	11. Unique health record number of patient or client	15. Supervision to mentally disturbed patient
16. Source of referral	12. Unique number of principal registered nurse provider	16. Reality orientation training
17. Unique client identifier	13. Episode admission or encounter date	17. Isolation
18. Other support services	14. Discharge or termination	18. Monitoring of vital signs
	15. Disposition of patient or client	19. Monitoring of clinical signs
	16. Expected payer for most of this bill (Anticipated financial guarantor for services).	20. Attending on continuous traction or cast
		21. Drawing of blood specimen
		22. Medication IM/SC
		23. Medication IV
		24. IV Therapy
		25. Surgical wound care
		26. Surface traumatic wound
		27. Traumatic wound care

Adapted from Werley H et al, 1991 and National Statistics, Belgium, 1988, and The Community Nursing Minimum Data Set Australia Project, Gliddon T and Weaver C, 1993 [13].

language and classification system that can be used to describe and organize nursing data. A model which clarifies the process of this development has been identified and is encompassed on a continuum with nursing practice. This is exemplified below in Figure 1.

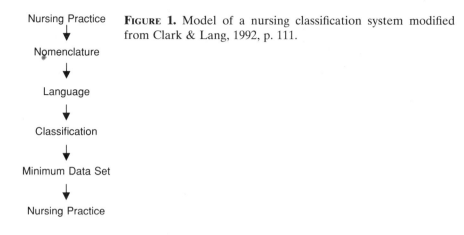

FIGURE 1. Model of a nursing classification system modified from Clark & Lang, 1992, p. 111.

3. Australian Data Set Development

Ensuring quality cost effective, equitable health care in Australia is a national priority and an appropriate information base is required for monitoring and evaluation. The development of the National Health Minimum Data Set for Institutional Care and the Australian Health Care Data Dictionary under the auspices of the Australian Health Ministers Advisory Council (AHMAC), are crucial moves in the information systems area. Nursing, a vital component of health care, is responding, by developing a National Nursing Minimum Data Set (NNMDS) for incorporation into these data sets.

The NNMDS not only offers nursing the opportunity to order its data but has profound implications for all areas of nursing. With the advent of data collection for Casemix and DRGs means that large quantities of nursing data are being collected and standards formulated by individual institutions. This will be an important complementary activity with the initial steps or the NNMDS—the development of a National Nursing Thesaurus which will collect and standardize these data.

An NMDS must standardize data both nationally and internationally and the fragmentation of data collection must be contained, but in reality we cannot set nursing apart and regard it as a separate entity from health care. It is ludicrous to suggest that we can, given that nurses are the biggest group of care givers within the Health Care System.

On several occasions we have corresponded and discussed our national and international notion and thoughts on future directions with Professor Werley. Since beginning this project some two (2) years ago, we have had many letters and corresponded with nursing groups and other interested people worldwide. The message is loud and clear—there must be integration of all health data and there must be standardized data for all health care. Not nursing in isolation—not medicine in isolation—not administration in isolation, as we are all health care givers. But, the development of the Australian Health Minimum Data Set, true to early development in other countries contains no nursing data. The revision of this project began in 1991–1992 and once more the omission was repeated! The Government has now made a priority on the development of the National Health Care Data dictionary as it became aware that standard definitions are necessary before one can develop a minimum data set [15].

At this stage we have support from many sectors of health care for this development as it is seen to be critical for health care information systems and are awaiting funding to commence development of the NNMDS. Because of the enormity of the task we have broken the project into attainable segments:

1) development of an Australian Thesaurus,
2) development of an Australian Taxonomy
3) definition of data definitions and classification,
4) data base format development
5) assembly of the NNMDS [16].

The authors see data being collected by nursing, medicine and the paramedical areas and being integrated into a National Health Minimum Data Set (NHMDS). The collection of nursing data is too important to be kept institution specific and isolated from the nursing community. We need to work together in this important area to accomplish the most efficient usage of scarce resources.

4. Conclusion

This project has the potential to be valuable in many areas yet being separate in identity and scope from all. The identification of an Australian Taxonomy and the National Minimum Data Set would be invaluable to the automation of Nursing Information and Management Systems while the Classification of nursing data would be invaluable to the Casemix project. The introduction of a NNMDS and standardised nursing data would break down one of the greatest barriers presently hindering nursing research on a national and international basis and it would support the process of nursing practice and advance the knowledge necessary for the cost-effective delivery of quality nursing care.

References

[1] Clark J and Lang N. Nursing's next advance: An international classification for nursing practice. *Int Nurs Rev* 1992, 39 (4): 109–112, 128.
[2] Wheeler M. What do we have in common. *Infor Technol Nurs* 1991, 4 (3): 12–15.

[3] Werley H, Devine E, Zorn C, Ryan P and Westra B. The Nursing Minimum Data Set: Abstraction tool for standardised, comparable, essential data. *Am J Public Health* 1991, 18 (4): 421–426.

[4] Werley H and Zorn C. The Nursing Minimum Data Set and its relationship to classifications for describing nursing practice. *Classification Systems for Describing Nursing Practice*. Kansas City: American Nurses Association, 1989: 50–54.

[5] Werley H, Devine E, Zorn C, Ryan P and Westra B. The Nursing Minimum Data Set: Abstraction tool for standardised, comparable, essential data. *Am J Public Health* 1991, 18(4): 421–426.

[6] Murnaghan J and White K. Hospital Discharge Data: Report of the Conference on Hospital Discharge Abstracts systems. *Medical Care* 1970, 8: 1–215.

[7] Hanna K and Anderson J. Background Paper: Nursing Minimum Data Set. *Unpublished paper* 1992.

[8] Wheeler M. Nurses do count. *Nursing Times* 1991, 87 (16): 64–65.

[9] Hanna K and Anderson J. Background Paper: Nursing Minimum Data Set. *Unpublished paper* 1992.

[10] Hanna K and Anderson J. Background Paper: Nursing Minimum Data Set. *Unpublished paper* 1992.

[11] NHS Management Executive. Nursing terms (scoping) project workshops. *NHS Centre for Coding and Classification—General Information* 1993.

[12] Sermeus W. Hospital care financing and drg's: How Belgium takes nursing care into account. *Inforum* 1991, 12: 31–37.

[13] Werley H, Devine E, Zorn C, Ryan P and Westra B. The Nursing Minimum Data Set: Abstraction tool for standardised, comparable, essential data. *Am J Public Health* 1991, 18(4): 421–426.
Belgium Government. *National Statistics*. Leuven: Belgium, 1988
Gliddon T and Weaver C. The community Nursing Minimum Data Set Australia: Project: Real life issues of operationalising a common data set in diverse community nursing environments. In: *HIC'93*. Hovenga E, Whymark G (eds). Melbourne: Australia, 1993: 81–90.

[14] Clark J and Lang N. Nursing's next advance: An international classification for nursing practice. *Int Nurs Rev* 1992, 39 (4): 109–112, 128.

[15] Foster J and Conrick M. A national nursing minimum data set: Challenge to alter inequity. *Health Informatics: Now and tomorrow*. Nursing Informatics Australia (Inc) (eds). Melbourne: Australia. 1992.

[16] Conrick M and Foster J. Submission to the Health Minister: National Nursing Minimum Data Set. *Unpublished submission*. 1992.

57
Establishment of the Research Value of Nursing Minimum Data Sets

Connie Delaney, M. Mehmert, Colleen M. Prophet, and J. Crossley

1. Background and Significance

Ready access to and use of nursing data are critical to implementing wise stewardship of health care resources. The US health care system faces increased costs, increased numbers of uninsured, cost-shifting, and lack of accountability for cost and outcomes. Standardized data sets provide an essential means of communication among the multiple units of this complex system. They allow comparisons across systems, sites, and settings, helping to identify areas of over utilization and underuse of resources, as well as services that are cost effective.

The development and implementation of standardized, uniform data sets in health care have been prolific. In the USA multiple federal medical and health services standardized data bases exist, including administrative, clinical, disease registries, and death registries. Other data bases have been developed.[1] Additionally, over 30 of the states in the US maintain hospital discharge data systems or collect financial data. These data systems rely at least in part on the collection of minimum data sets, including: Uniform Hospital Discharge Data Set (UHDDS), the Long-Term Health Care (LTC) Client Uniform Data Set (UDS), and the Uniform Ambulatory Medical Care Data Set (UACDS).[2,3,4] Because nursing data is absence from these data sets, critical data related to nursing's decision making and interventions are not available to monitor quality, reimbursement, and outcomes.

The development of the Nursing Minimum Data Set (NMDS) was initiated in the 1970's by Harriet Werley.[5] The NMDS, by definition, includes the essential nursing data used on a regular basis by the majority of nurses across all settings in the delivery of care. Sixteen NMDS elements are organized within three categories of patient demographics, service, and nursing care. Patient demographic elements include personal identification, date of birth, sex, race and ethnicity, and residence. The service category includes the unique facility number, unique health record number, unique number of principal registered nurse provider, episode admission and discharge dates, disposition of patient, and expected payor of the bill. Four data elements comprise the nursing care category: nursing diagnosis, nursing intervention, nursing outcome, and nursing intensity. All elements of the patient demographic and service categories of the NMDS, with the exception of the "unique number of registered nurse provider" are contained in the UHDDS and have been collected since 1975 on all Medicare patients.

Although the four nursing care elements present validity, reliability, utility, and standardization problems, the International Council for Nurses Board did approve a year of planning for the International Classification of Nursing Practice (ICN-ICNP) which includes three of the four nursing care elements of the NMDS, nursing diagnosis, intervention, and outcome. This paper addresses nursing's efforts to test the NMDS.

2. Methods

A non-experimental ex-post facto design was used to begin to investigate the research value of the computerized NMDS. Research value was defined as utility, the condition of providing usefulness within the context of a specific investigation and to the discipline of nursing.[6] Utility of the NMDS was operationally defined as the ability to (a) be a cost effective data abstraction tool for nursing, (b) produce patient profiles for each nursing diagnosis group, (c) establish retrospective validation of the defining characteristics for nursing diagnoses, (d) determine costs of direct nursing care, and (e) forecast/trend nursing diagnoses.

Two clinical sites were used for the work reported here. Site A is a 265-bed, private, midwestern, secondary acute health care center. Site B is a 1000-bed, public, midwestern, tertiary health care center. Sites A and B are nationally recognized sites which use computerized nursing care planning systems based on the NANDA approved nursing diagnosis taxonomy. Both sites have extensive ongoing educational programs and quality monitoring activities to maintain data quality.

Seven data sets containing the elements of the NMDS with the addition of defining characteristics and etiologies for each nursing diagnosis were collected from the computerized information systems of each facility. Two of the data sets (one from each site) were manually retrieved (N = 200, N = 26 respectively); five data sets were electronically retrieved (4 from Site A and 1 from Site B). The number of patient records in each electronically retrieved data set was: #1 = 704; #2 =4,248; and #3 = 1,066. The fourth electronically retrieved data set was comprised of 69,427 nursing diagnoses documented from 1987–1990 in Site A. The fifth electronically retrieved data set consisted of a stratified random sample of all patients with Diagnostic Related Group #209 (N = 211).

3. Results

Analysis of five data sets was completed to establish the availability of each NMDS element and related cost of using the NMDS as a data abstraction tool. The availability of the NMDS elements, with the exception of unique registered nurse provider number which is not available in the US, ranged from 95.5–100%. Cost analysis was completed. Cost for manual retrieval of one data set from each site ranged from $20.20–82.50 per patient record. Cost analysis related to three electronically retrieved data sets, two from Site A and one from Site B, ranged from $0.05–$.50 per patient record. Three electronically retrieved data sets have realized a cost savings of approximately $187,000.

Demographic profiles were established for all nursing diagnostic categories in all data sets. The patient demographic profile consisted of sex, age, race and ethnicity, disposition, and length of stay (determined from date of admission and discharge elements). Table 1 illustrates the patient profiles for three nursing diagnoses based on data from one data set extracted from Site A. This showed that diagnostic groups were not significantly different in sex, race, or discharge disposition. However, significant differences (p < .05) in age and length of stay were noted among the three diagnostic categories. Patients who exhibited fluid volume excess were significantly older and had significantly longer lengths of stay than patient in other categories. Patients 0–14 years old had more fluid volume deficit related to active loss compared to other fluid volume diagnoses. For patients 15–65

TABLE 1. Patient demographic profile by NDX (percent mean)

		Fluid volume deficit-regulatory mechanism	Fluid volume deficit-active loss	Fluid volume excess
Number		28	78	28
Sex	Male	44%	52%	37%
	Female	56%	48%	63%
Age		54.7	40.7	68.3
Race	White	89%	97%	100%
	Non-white	11%	3%	0%
Discharge	Home	89%	94%	82%
	Other	11%	6%	18%
LOS		6.2	6.5	16.3

TABLE 2. Sensitivity of defining characteristics of fluid volume deficit related to regulatory mechanism across datasets within site

Defining characteristics	Sensitivity	
	Dataset 1	Dataset 2
Dry skin, mucous membrane	57.0	58.3
Weakness	57.0	33.3
Increased skin turgor	39.0	33.3
Increased body temperature	32.0	16.7
Thirst	21.0	8.3

years old, fluid volume deficit related to active loss was significantly more prevalent, whereas fluid volume excess was significantly less prevalent than other diagnosis.

Retrospective validation of defining characteristics for nursing diagnoses was completed within and across datasets from within and between sites. Sensitivity was used to determine validation; levels were evaluated consistent with the North American Nursing Diagnosis Association Guidelines for major (present in 80–100% of the population) and minor (present in 50–79% of the population) characteristics. Table 2 illustrates the sensitivity measures for the defining characteristics of fluid volume deficit related to regulatory mechanism for patients selected from two different datasets extracted from Site A. Two characteristics qualified as minor in the first dataset, one of the two again qualified as minor in a second dataset from the same site. Likewise, a comparison of sensitivities for fluid volume deficit related to active loss from two datasets within the same site demonstrated that five of the six characteristics exhibited similar sensitivities. Table 3 illustrates sensitivity of one defining characteristic, dependent edema, for the nursing diagnosis fluid volume excess across two data sets from Site A and one dataset from Site B.

The utility of the NMDS for determining direct nursing care costs within a specific Diagnostic Related Group (DRG) was determined by obtaining a stratified random sample of all patients in the DRG category #209: major joint and limb reattachment procedures within a four year period (N = 211). Length of stay, average and total acuities, and frequency of

TABLE 3. Validation of defining characteristic dependent edema for fluid volume excess across sites

Defining characteristic	Sensitivity	
	Site A	Site B
Dependent edema	68.0 66.7	57.2

nursing diagnoses were quantified. The average length of stay (8.57 days) was significantly (p < .05) shorter for 1990 compared to 1988 (11.2) and 1989 (11.02). The average acuity for 1990 was significantly higher (73.24 pints) compared to 1987 (62.37) and 1988 (65.24). This sample represented a total of 826 nursing diagnoses. Two diagnoses occurred in greater than 50% of the patients in this DRG category: pain (91.9%) and impaired mobility (82%). Other diagnoses represented were self care deficit, bathing and hygiene (38.4%), knowledge deficit regarding orthopedic status (36.5%), impaired shin integrity (23.7%), and potential for infection (10%). Nursing interventions documented in the NMDS represented actual care delivered. Hours of direct nursing care per patient were consequently determined. The mean total nursing time per patient hospital stay was 68.38 hours. Using the staff mix component of the intensity element of the NMDS the mean costs for direct nursing care were calculated to be $1641.20 based on an average $24/hour pay rate. Given a Medicare DRG charge of $12,765 and a reimbursement of $8,944 per patient, 21.3% of the reimbursement was consumed for direct nursing care.[7]

The research utility of the NMDS for forecasting frequency and trends in nursing diagnoses was analyzed. The frequency of occurrence of each nursing diagnosis was compiled from 1987–1990 in Site A. Profiles of the frequency of each diagnosis for each year were established. Data analysis using multiple linear regression techniques yielded R^2 values ranging from 0.920–0.929. It appeared that it is possible to predict the frequency of occurrence of nursing diagnoses. If coupled with the cost analysis data related to direct nursing care, this approach may provide a quantifiable method for more precisely predicting consumption of nursing resources.

4. Summary

Seven studies have begun to establish the usefulness of the NMDS. The NMDS elements were available in two acute care sites. A cost efficient method for electronic data retrieval has been established. The NMDS has been used to develop patient demographic profiles within nursing diagnostic categories. Retrospective nurse validation of nursing diagnoses has occurred within and between sites. One method for demonstrating the forecasting capability of the NMDS has been demonstrated. Moreover, a method for using the *intensity* element of the NMDS to determine costs of direct nursing care has been developed.

Although the NMDS has the potential to provide the data necessary to measure patient outcomes, increased standardization of the nursing taxonomies for nursing diagnoses, interventions, and outcomes must occur. Lastly, studies to determine costs of nursing care and consumption of resources rely on the availability of the *intensity of nursing care* element as well as the other nursing care elements of the NMDS.

References

[1] Agency for Health Care Policy and Research. *Report to Congress: The feasibility of linking research-related data bases to federal and non-federal medical administrative data bases.* (AHCPR Pub. No. 91-0003), 1991. Washington, DC: U.S. Government Printing Office.

[2] National Committee on Vital and Health Statistics. *Long-term health care: Minimum data set* (DHHS Pub. No., PHS 80-1158). Hyattsvine, MD: National Center for Health Statistics, 1980.

[3] National Committee on Vital and Health Statistics. *Uniform hospital discharge data: Minimum data set* (DHHS Pub. No., PHS 80-1157). Hyattsville, MD: National Center for Health Statistics. 1980.

[4] National Committee on Vital and Health Statistics. *Uniform ambulatory medical care: Minimum data set* (DHHS Pub. No., PHS 81-1161). Hyattsville, MD: National Center for Health Statistics, 1981.

[5] Werley H, Lang N and Westlake S. (1986). Brief summary of the nursing minimum data set. *Nursing Management*, 17(7), 42–45.

[6] Waltz C, Strickland C, and Lenz E. *Measurement in research*. Philadelphia: F.A. Davis Company, 1984.

[7] *Hospital Technology Scanner*. November, 1992.

58
Clinical Decision Making in Critical Care: The Relationship among Computer Simulation Performance, Cognitive Examination, and Self-Assessment of Expertise

Suzanne B. Henry

Introduction

Although little evidence exists that supports the relationship between clinical simulation performance and performance in practice, computerized clinical simulations are currently being used to evaluate the clinical decision making skills of nursing students and may be included as part of the US National Council Licensing Examination (NCLEX) as early as the 1990's (Bolwell, 1989). The purpose of this investigation was to explore the relationship between computerized clinical simulation performance and two commonly used methods of evaluation: cognitive examination and self-assessment of expertise. The results reported here are part of a larger study which examined the relationship between patient acuity and the clinical decision making of critical care nurses with varying levels of knowledge and experience (Henry, in press).

Clinical expertise or clinical decision making in practice can be conceptualized as the construct that clinical simulation performance attempts to measure and as the criterion against which clinical simulation performance is measured. Dincher and Stidger (1972) studied the relationship between performance on a patient management problem (PMP) and evaluation of clinical decision making by clinical instructor in their investigation of eleven nursing students. Rank order correlation between the PMP and clinical evaluation was significant for simulation efficiency score, but not proficiency score. Holzemer et al. (Holzemer, Schleutermann, Farrand, & Miller, 1981) used a multitrait–multimethod approach to the exploration

Reprinted with permission from; *Nursing Informatics '91: Proceedings of the Fourth International Conference on Nursing Use of Computers and Information Science*; Hovenga, E.J.S., Hannah, K.J., McCormick, K.A. & Ronald, J.S. (Eds.). 1991, pp. 226–230. Heidelberg-Berlin, Germany: Springer-Verlag.

of the construct validity of one PMP. Proficiency score was significantly correlated with self-evaluation of clinical practice. In a related study, nurse practitioners' performance on one PMP was compared with chart audit and observation of clinical performance to explore the criterion-related validity of one PMP (Holzemer, Resnik, & Slichter, 1986). Padrick's (1990) investigation of hospice nurses revealed that there were differences between decision making in practice and on three written simulations.

Methods

Sample

The convenience sample of 68 registered nurses in this descriptive, correlational study was recruited from the critical care division of a tertiary care medical center (Table 1). The majority of the sample was female and educated at the baccalaureate level.

TABLE 1. Demographic characteristics of the study sample ($N = 68$)

Variable	Frequency	%
Sex		
Female	53	78
Male	15	22
Unit		
Surgical intensive care unit	13	19
Medical intensive care unit	12	18
Coronary care unit	10	15
Burn unit	9	13
Neurosurgical intensive care	8	12
Special care unit	8	12
Emergency room	5	7
Life flight	3	4
Nursing Education		
RN by challenge examination	1	2
Diploma	6	9
Associate degree	26	38
BSN	34	50
MS	1	2

	Mean
Age	34
Nursing experience	9
Critical care experience	6

TABLE 2. Summary statistics on BKAT, CST, and simulation proficiency scores

	Mean	SD
BKAT score	84	7
CST score	97	19
AF proficiency score	52	23
VT proficiency score	39	25

Instruments

Each subject completed three different types of instruments: a knowledge test, a self-evaluation of expertise, and two clinical simulations. The Basic Knowledge Assessment Tool for Critical Care (Ritchie, 1984). The Cardiovascular Self-Evaluation Tool is a 38 item ordinal scale consisting of task statements related to the knowledge and skills required to care for a cardiovascular patient. The ratings for each item (0–3) are summed for a total score ranging from 0–114. Tach-Man (Barrett & Power, 1985) is a computer program which generates a series of clinical simulations related to the management of tachydysrhythmias. Atrial flutter and ventricular tachycardia were the clinical simulations for this investigation. Criterion scoring was based on the Advanced Cardiac Life Support (ACLS) standards (American Heart Association, 1986) for the treatment of the dysrhythmias and was validated by a panel of clinical experts ($n = 11$). The scoring system and its validation is discussed in detail elsewhere (Henry, in press) Proficiency scores were calculated by comparing actual performance with criterion performance (Henry, LeBreck, & Holzemer, 1989). Patient outcome was a dichotomous variable determined by whether the dysrhythmia was cured or the patient died as a result of treatment.

TABLE 3. Intercorrelations among BKAT score, CST score, simulation proficiency scores, and patient outcomes

	BKAT score	CST score
AF proficiency score	47	32
	.000	.008
VT proficiency score	21	24
	.080	.049
AF patient outcome	28	22
	.006	.036
VT patient outcome	05	08
	.700	.558

Decimal points omitted on the correlation coefficients.

Results

The mean score for each instrument is shown in Table 2. Table 3 presents the correlations between the simulation scores and the other two instruments. Atrial proficiency was significantly correlated with knowledge as measured by the BKAT and with self-assessment of clinical expertise. Atrial patient outcome was also significantly correlated with both BKAT and CST score. However, in the ventricular simulation only proficiency score and self-assessment of expertise were significantly correlated.

Conclusion

The modest relationships found in this study may indicate that while clinical simulation performance is related to knowledge and self-assessment of expertise, the constructs being measured are not synonymous. This evidence provides support for the use of clinical simulations as an adjunct to other methods of evaluation.

References

American Heart Association (1986). Instructor's manual for advanced cardiac life support.

Bolwell, C. (1989). NCLEX with interactive videodisc simulations. *Nurse Educator's Microworld*, *3*, 15.

Dincher, JR & Stidger, SL (1976). Evaluation of a written simulation format for clinical nursing judgment: A pilot study. *Nursing Research*, *25*, 250–285.

Henry, SB (in press a). The effect of level of patient acuity on the clinical decision making of critical care nurses with varying levels of knowledge and experience. *Heart & Lung*.

Henry, SB (in press b). Recognition and management of computer simulated tachydysrhythmias by critical care nurses. *Heart & Lung*.

Henry, SB, LeBreck, DB, & Holzemer, WL. (1989). The effect of verbalization of cognitive processes on clinical decision making. *Research in Nursing & Health*, *12*, 187–193.

Holzemer, WL, Resnik, B, & Slichter, M. Criterion-related validity of a clinical simulation. *Journal of Nursing Education*, *25*, 286–290.

Holzemer, WL, Schleutermann, J, Farrand, L. & Miller, A. A validation study: Simulations as a measure of nurse practitioners' problem-solving skills. *Nursing Research*, *30*, 139–144.

Padrick, KP. Clinical decision making in nursing: A comparison between simulations and practice. Unpublished abstract.

Toth, JC (1984). Evaluating the use of the Basic Knowledge Assessment Tool (BKAT) in critical care nursing with baccalaureate nursing students. *Image*, *16*, 76–71.

Toth, JC & Ritchie, KA (1984). New from nursing research: The Basic Knowledge Assessment Tool for critical care nursing. *Heart & Lung*, *13*, 272–279.

59
Testing of a Computer-Based Decisions Support System in an Acute Care Hospital

CHERYL THOMPSON, SHEILA A. RYAN, and JUDITH G. BAGGS

Introduction

The increasing need for professional nursing care has emphasized the necessity of efficient use of current nursing resources. Speeding the care planning process and minimizing work load are two possible methods for improving nursing efficiency, thereby decreasing occupational stress and promoting quality of patient care. The purpose of this study was to assess the impact of a computer-based decision-support system on nursing climate and patient outcome in acute care hospital units. It was projected that a decision-support system would benefit the nursing climate by providing information needed by nurses to complete accurate and appropriate care plans for hospitalized patients. It was expected that nurse role satisfaction would increase due to decreased work load and increased confidence in quality of care. It was projected that patients would also perceive this increase in quality of nursing care.

The decision-support system selected for this study was the Creighton Online Multiple Modular Expert System (COMMES). COMMES was developed to assist with and support nursing clinical decision making about individual patient conditions, nursing care planning, discharge planning, and patient education in order to impact positively on patient outcomes (Ryan, 1985). As an expert system it is capable of processing information from a large knowledge base which supports the thinking processes of the professional nurse.

COMMES is comprised of three consultant modes. One details interventions appropriate for specific patient problems and provides information for developing quality care plans. The second allows the user to request

Reprinted with permission from; *Nursing Informatics '91: Proceedings of the Fourth International Conference on Nursing Use of Computers and Information Science*; Hovenga, E.J.S., Hannah, K.J., McCormick, K.A. & Ronald, J.S. (Eds.). 1991, pp. 769–776. Heidelberg-Berlin, Germany: Springer-Verlag.

instructional information for an identified patient situation and provides an itemized list of learning objectives. The third creates a tool for the assessment of a nurses individual learning needs.

Previous research has demonstrated the validity of output from the system. Care plans developed by COMMES have been shown to compare favorably with those developed by clinical nursing specialists and nursing educators (Cuddigan, Norris, Ryan, and Evans, 1987). Improvement in patient outcomes within six months after implementation of the system on nursing units has also been demonstrated (Cuddigan, Logan, Evans, and Hoesing, 1988).

Method: Sample, Setting

The site of the research was a 822 bed teaching hospital in the northeastern United States. One general medical and one general surgical unit were assigned as the experimental units. Two comparable units, one general medical and one cardiovascular surgical, were selected to serve as controls. A pretest/post-test control group design was utilized (Campbell and Stanley, 1963).

All full and part time registered nurses (RNs) and licensed practical nurses (LPNs) assigned to the selected units were asked to participate. Only data from RNs were analyzed and reported. Nurses joining the staff after initial data collection were asked to participate in follow-up data collection.

Patient subjects were drawn from all patients discharged to the selected units. Criteria for eligibility included being an inpatient on one of the chosen units for at least 24 hours, being capable of reading and speaking English, being at least 18 years of age, being alert and oriented to person and place, not being already included in the data set, and being scheduled for discharge within the next 48 hours.

A one month data collection period was selected after a power analysis had been completed. A sample size of 58 subjects for both the control and experimental groups is sufficient to find an effect size of 0.5, with power of 0.85 with a one tailed alpha of 0.05 (Cohen, 1988). Based upon past discharge statistics, it was projected that the required number of subjects could be recruited within a month period.

Instruments

Unit, nurse, and patient variables were measured. Unit variables included vacancy and turnover rates for staff nurse positions, stability of unit staff, and absenteeism. Nurse variables included openness to technology, organizational climate, professional confidence, and demographics. Patient variables included patient satisfaction with nursing care and demographics.

Vacancy rates for staff nurse positions were calculated as the number of budgeted, unfilled positions divided by the total budgeted positions (Prescott, 1986). Turnover rates for staff nurse positions were calculated as the number of nurses leaving during the 30 day data collection period, divided by the total full time equivalents employed at the beginning of data collection plus the number of new hires during the 30 day data collection period (Prescott, 1986). Stability was the average length of time currently employed nurses had worked on the unit (Prescott, 1986). Absenteeism was the average number of sick days per unit per staff member during the 30 day data collection period.

Openness to technology, an individual's attitude toward the use of computers, was measured to determine if a pre-existing bias towards or against computer technology might exist, on any of the units. If such a bias did exist, the ease of implementation of the system might be affected. Openness to technology was measured using Ball, Snelbecker, and Schechter's (1985) questionnaire for assessment of nurses' perceptions concerning computer use. The questionnaire consists of 24 items scored on a five point Likert Scale. The Cronbach's Alpha for this study for the complete scale was 0.85.

The term organizational climate refers to characteristics that influence the behavior and activities of members within a particular organization (Duxbury, Henly, and Armstrong, 1982). The research team postulated that access to a computerized decision- support system would impact positively on the nursing units quality of care, thereby improving the organization climate and nursing satisfaction.

One of the measures of organizational climate chosen was Form B of the Nursing Organizational Climate Description Questionnaire (NOCDQ-B) (Duxbury et. al., 1982). The NOCDQ-B is a 26 item questionnaire designed to measure six dimensions of organizational climate. The six dimensions are Aloofness, (the extent to which the leadership is characterized by formality and impersonality), Humanistic Thrust (extent to which the leader motivates subordinates by personal example), Disengagement (extent to which the staff is "not with it" in accomplishing the tasks at hand), Intimacy (extent to which the staff enjoy friendly relations with each other), Esprit (morale, the extent to which social needs are satisfied in concert with accomplishing the job), and Hindrance (extent to which routine functions and committee demands interfere with work). Each of the items is measured using a five point Likert scale. Analysis of the individual subscales by the scale's developers demonstrated internal consistency in two samples (Duxbury et al.). Cronbach's alpha for the total scale for this sample was 0.48 at baseline and 0.46 at six months.

A second measure of organizational climate is nursing job satisfaction. According to Stamps and Piedmonte (1986), this is a measure of the degree to which nurses are content with their current work. If access to a computerized source of nursing information eases the workload of staff nurses and improves the quality of their patient care, this should be reflected in their satisfaction with the work environment. Nurses' work satisfaction was measured using Part B of the Index of Work Satisfaction (IWS), which is a 44 item seven point Likert Scale with seven dimensions. The dimensions are Professional Status, Nursing Interaction, Task Requirements, Organizational Policies, Autonomy, Pay, and Physician Nurse Interaction (Stamps and Piedmonte). Analysis of the individual subscales by the scale's developers demonstrated internal consistency (Stamps and Piedmonte). Cronbach's alpha for this sample was 0.90 at baseline and 0.80 at six months.

Professional confidence is the degree to which an individual staff nurse feels capable of fulfilling her job description. Rapid access to a comprehensive, up to date knowledge base should increase the nurse's confidence in her performance. Professional confidence was measured by the Professional Confidence Scale. This five point Likert scale questionnaire measuring the individual nurse's confidence in performing seven activities specific to professional nursing practice was developed by the authors. Cronbach's alpha for this sample was 0.77 at baseline and 0.90 at six months.

Demographic data collected for nurses included gender, age, race, highest nursing degree, total number of years worked as a nurse, number of years as a nurse at current facility, and previous computer experience. Unit level data was collected on nursing vacancy, turnover, stability, and absenteeism. This information was collected from nursing administration records.

Patient data was collected from the medical record by the investigators and from computer printouts supplied by Hospital Information Systems. Data collected included gender, age, race, discharge diagnosis, data of admission, data of discharge, and destination at discharge.

Patient satisfaction is a measure of the degree to which patients perceive the adequacy of their nursing care. It was hypothesized that increased nursing role satisfaction and a decreased work load might be reflected in the quality of patient care. This improved quality of care might then be noted by patients and reflected in their satisfaction with nursing care. Patient satisfaction was measured using the Patient Satisfaction Instrument (PSI). The PSI is a 25 item, five point Likert Scale. It contains three dimensions of patient satisfaction: Technical–Professional Care, Trust, and Patent Education (Hindshaw and Atwood, 1982). Analysis of scale by the developers demonstrated internal consistency and construct, convergent, and discriminant validity (Hindshaw and Atwood). The Cronbach's alpha for this sample was 0.52 at baseline and 0.65 at six months.

Procedures

Baseline data were collected before implementation of the decision-support system to assess initial unit, nurse, and patient characteristics; for units—vacancy, turnover, stability, and absenteeism; for nurses—

organizational climate, perception of computer use, professional confidence, demographic descriptors; for patients—mortality, length of stay, satisfaction with care. Approximately six months later follow-up measurements were gathered to assess for changes. At six months the COMMES log documented that on average one person per week was using the system. The decision was made not to gather additional data.

Approval for the project was obtained from the hospital Research Subjects Review Board. All nurse subjects signed written informed consent forms.

Staff members from all four patient units were oriented to the research project during unit staff meetings approximately one month prior to the installation of COMMES. Staff members were given an envelope containing copies of all questionnaires and were asked to complete the questionnaires and return them to a designated box on the unit.

Patient entry into the study began one month prior to installation of COMMES and continued for 30 days. Unit staff informed the researchers of all patients scheduled for discharge within 48 hours. The researcher then determined if the subject met eligibility requirements. If the patient met eligibility criteria he/she was approached and the study explained. The patient was given the PSI and asked to complete it. Those subjects requiring assistance were read the questions, and the answers were recorded by the researcher. Subjects returned the questionnaire to the researcher, or if they completed it at a later time, left it in a sealed envelope with a staff member to place in a box on the unit. Patients who were unexpectedly discharged were mailed a letter explaining the study, a copy of the PSI, and a stamped, addressed envelope for return of the questionnaire.

After initial data collection, a computer terminal and printer dedicated to COMMES were installed on each of the experimental units in a location chosen by each unit's Nurse Manager. All staff members were oriented to the system via group sessions or one-on-one instruction. In addition, several key staff members were identified as unit instructors. Staff member or staff member education was encouraged. Utilization of the system was, however, voluntary and at the discretion of the nurse.

Results

Unit Statistics: Vacancy rates, turnover rates, staff stability, and absenteeism demonstrated no differences among units. This lack of difference should however be interpreted cautiously. The number of units for both control and experiment was only two, the staff for all four units was relatively small, and the data collection period of one month was too short to extrapolate long range trends.

Nurse Statistics: Fifty-five staff RNs were eligible for participation at baseline; sixty-nine were eligible at six months. Thirty-five RNs responded to at least one questionnaire at both baseline and six months.

A total of 63 nurses completed the demographic form. Three of the nurse subjects were male (4.8%) and the remainder were female (95.2%). The sample ranged in age from 21 to 54 years with a mean of 29.7 years (SD = 8.3). Fifty-nine (96.7%) of the nurses were white and two (3.3%) reported their race as "other." Twelve of the nurses reported as their highest degree in nursing a diploma (19.0%), 17 an associate's degree (27.0%), 33 a baccalaureate degree (52.4%), and 1 a master's degree (1.6%). Years experience in nursing ranged from 0.5 to 35 years with a mean of 5.9 years (SD = 7.5). Years experience at the hospital ranged from 0 to 30 years, with a mean of 3.6 years (SD = 5.8). Sixty-six percent of the sample had no previous experience with personal computers. Seventy-eight percent of the sample had not used computers previously in a clinical facility.

No significant differences in openness toward technology were found between the experimental and control units (F = 0.00, P > 0.05). Consequently, this variable was not considered during further analyses.

On the NOCDQ-B, mean total score for the control group at baseline was 64.8 (SD = 5.7); for the experimental group it was 67.2 (SD = 4.4). Mean total score for the control group at six months was 67.6 (SD = 5.8); for the experimental group it was 66.1 (SD = 5.7). There was no significant difference between the two groups at baseline (F = 1.45, P > 0.05) or at six months (F = 0.45, P > 0.05).

On the IWS, mean total score for the control group at baseline was 187.7 (SD = 17.6), for the experimental group it was 201.2 (SD = 29.6). Mean total score for the control group at six months was 200.9 (SD = 18.3); for the experimental group it was 192.9 (SD = 22.6). There was no significant difference between the two groups at baseline (F = 2.01, P > 0.05) or at six months (F = 1.31, P > 0.05).

A total score was calculated for the Professional Confidence Index by totaling the seven items. Mean total score for the control group at baseline was 29.6 (SD = 3.2); for the experimental group it was 28.3 (SD = 3.0). Mean total score for the control group at six months was 27.9 (SD = 5.5); for the experimental group it was 29.2 (SD = 3.7). There was no significant difference between the two groups at baseline (F = 1.53, P > 0.05) or at six months (F = 0.63, P > 0.05).

Patient Statistics

There were 261 patients discharged from the study units at baseline and 283 discharged at six months. Patients not asked to participate in the study included those that did not meet eligibility criteria, those that expired prior to discharge, and those who where transferred to another unit and did not return prior to completion of data collection. Of the 203 patients asked to participate at baseline, 3 (1.5%) refused outright, 29 (14.3%) did not return questionnaires, and 171 (84.2%) returned the questionnaires. Of the patients returning questionnaires, 78 (45.6%) were male and 93 (54.4%) were female. The race for 141 (82.5%) of these patients was while, for 17 (9.9%) it was black, for 1 (0.6%) it was other, and for 12 (7.0%) it was unknown. Mean age for the patients returning questionnaires was 57.7 years (SD = 16.8).

Of the 199 patients asked to participate at six months, 5 (3%) refused outright, 44 (22.1%) did not return questionnaires, and 150 (75.4%) returned the questionnaires. Of the patients returning questionnaires, 83 (55.3%) were male and 67 (44.7%) were female. The race for 108 (72.0%) of these patients was white, for 19 (12.7%) it was black, and for 23 (15.3%) it was unknown. Mean age for the patients returning questionnaires was 61.4 (SD = 17.5).

Mean total score on the Patient Satisfaction Index at baseline for the control group was 71.0 (SD = 4.2); for the experimental group it was 69.4 (SD = 4.9). This was a statistically significant difference (F = 4.85, P < 0.05). Mean total score at six months for the control group was 69.5 (SD = 6.1); for the experimental group it was 69.4 (SD = 6.6). This was not a statistically significant difference (F = 0.02, P > 0.05).

These results indicate that a 1.6 point difference existed between the patients on the experimental and the control units at baseline in satisfaction with nursing care. This was a statistically significant difference, with patients on the control units scoring higher than patients on the experimental units. This difference was no longer present at six months.

The statistically significant difference in the PSI at baseline is clinically insignificant. Total score on the Patient Satisfaction Index ranges from 5 to 125 pints. A 1.6 point difference is approximately a one percent difference and of little practical consequence. This result was statistically significant because of the large sample size and the small standard deviations (< 4.9) for the mean scores. Patients demonstrated little variance in their response to the questions.

Discussion

There were no significant findings of increased work satisfaction, improved organizational climate, increased professional confidence, or improved patient satisfaction with care after the implementation of the COMMES system. This lack of difference between control and experimental groups is contrary to the results demonstrated by Cuddigan et al. (1988). The explanations for this difference are unit, staff, and system related.

One reason for these differences is the nature of the setting for the Cuddigan et al. (1988) study. This study was conducted in a facility with a ten year history of a computerized nursing charting system, as compared to the current study where 78% of the sample had not used computers previously in a clinical setting. Acceptance of computerization might be predicated on previous exposure to similar technology.

The nurses in the study by Cuddigan et al. (1988) were required to use COMMES, i.e. printouts were provided to the staff at the beginning of each shift. Nurses were expected to incorporate the provided information into their plan of care. In contrast, the nurses in this study did not regularly consult the system. The increased patient acuity and decreased staffing levels allowed little time for the nurses to learn and assimilate a new tool into their practice.

In addition, the involved units receive a somewhat limited patient population, creating a degree of specialization within the nursing staff. The nurses considered themselves to have mastered the care required by this subset of patients. When the nurses needed more information, they were seeking a higher level of knowledge than COMMES was designed to provide. Whereas COMMES was designed to be consistent with beginning practitioner performance, the staff of these units was seeking information more compatible with advanced practice performance.

Support of the Nurse Managers was identified as essential for staff usage of the system. The managers from the experimental units were oriented to the system prior to its implementation and were initially enthusiastic. They, however, lost their enthusiasm for COMMES after implementation. They agreed with the staff, who felt that it was difficult to obtain the specific information they desired. For example, for a diabetic patient with congestive heart failure (CHF) they could obtain basic information on diabetes or CHF, but nothing about the combined problem. Printouts contained excessive, repetitive information and the output generally lacked sophistication.

Another problem with use of the system was the location of the computer terminals. The best location would have been in the nursing stations. However, the units were not designed to allow room for any terminal other than the Hospital Information System terminal. Consequently, the terminals were located at a distance from the main nurses' station. Security requirements necessitated the placement of a lock on the door of one of the rooms containing a terminal. Due to bed closings related to low level of staff on this same unit, the room for the terminal was located down an empty hall.

Down time of the computer also impacted staff usage. Hardware and then software problems made the system unavailable much of the first two months of the study. Initially, when enthusiasm for the system was at its highest, staff would go to use the system, but find that the software or printer or both were not operational. This created much frustration among the staff and decreased their desire to learn or use the system.

The research team made several attempts to increase usage of the system. All staff members were reoriented to the system once the operational problems were resolved. The research team also tried a period of generating printouts for the staff members. The goal for this intervention was to increase the staffs' perception of the usefulness of the information obtained. This strategy was most helpful when information was requested for patients whose diagnoses were atypical for that patient unit.

A final reason for a lack of demonstrable findings was the insensitivity of the instruments used. Responses to the Patient Satisfaction Index, in particular, lacked variance. Patients generally reported satisfaction with the nursing care that they received, or were hesitant to reveal their dissatisfaction on this questionnaire. Patient satisfaction also might have been too indirect a measure of changes in organizational climate and workload.

Implications

One needs to be cautious in interpreting the findings from this study. The results indicate that appropriate implementation of knowledge based systems is essential for maximizing usage and optimizing derived benefits. What these requirements are, though, is as yet unknown.

The practice of nursing is extremely complex; the sources of information for the nurse are numerous. Much remains to be discovered about how nurses coordinate information from the many available sources. Even more information is necessary about the methods used to meet knowledge needs when traditional sources of information are inadequate.

The nurses in this setting did not find a decision-support system helpful. This is not, however, a negative finding. The knowledge of why it did not work will strengthen the next inquiry. This information can be used in directing further research at answering the many questions about nursing's information requirements.

References

Ball MJ, Snelbecker GE, Schechter SL: Nurses' perceptions concerning computer uses before and after a computer literacy lecture. *Computers in Nursing*, 1985; 3: 23–31. Campbell DT, Stanley JC: Experimental and quasi-experimental designs for research. Boston, MA: Houghton Mifflin Company, 1964.

Cohen J: *Statistical Power Analysis for the Behavioral Sciences* (2nd Edition). Hillsdale, News Jersey: Lawrence Erlbaum Associates, 1988.

Cuddigan J, Logan S, Evans S, Hoesing H: Evaluation of an artificial-intelligence-based nursing decision support system in a clinical setting. In: Daly N, Hannah K, eds. *Proceedings of the Third International Symposium on Nursing Use of Computers and Information Science*. St Louis, MO: C.V. Mosby Company, 1988; 74–78.

Cuddigan JE, Norris J, Ryan SA, Evans S: Validating the knowledge in a computer-based consultant for nursing care. In: Stead WW, ed. *Proceedings of the Eleventh*

Symposium on Computer Applications in Medical Care. Washington, D.C.: Computer Society Press, 1987; 74–79.

Duxbury ML, Henly GA, Armstrong GD: Measurement of the nurse organization climate of neonatal intensive care units. *Nursing Research* 1983; 31: 83–88.

Hindshaw AS, Atwood JR: A patient satisfaction instrument: Precision by replication. *Nursing Research* 1982; 31: 170–175, 191.

Prescott PA: Vacancy, stability, and turnover of registered nurses in hospitals. *Research in Nursing and Health* 1986; 9: 51–60.

Ryan SA: An expert system for nursing practice. *Computers in Nursing* 1985; 3: 77–84.

Stamps PL, Piedmonte EB: *Nurses and Work Satisfaction: An Index for Measurement. Ann* Arbor, MI: Health Administration Press Perspectives, 1986.

60
Machine Learning for Development of an Expert System to Support Nurses' Assessment of Preterm Birth Risk

Linda K. Woolery, M. VanDyne, J. Grzymala-Busse, and C. Tsatsoulis

1. The Problem

Early and accurate detection and treatment of preterm labor can prolong gestation with improved outcomes for both the infant and family. Review of the literature provided both theoretical and empirical support for research and development of an expert system to provide decision support for nurses' assessment of preterm labor risk. Determining preterm labor risk in pregnant women and making decisions about interventions remain problematic in the clinical setting [1]. The problems related to preterm labor risk assessment include a poorly defined and complex knowledge base. The plethora of information about preterm labor risks remains disorganized and of little guidance to patients and providers of prenatal care. Review of the literature found no conceptual or theoretical models of preterm labor risk, which may account for poor reliability and validity of existing manual screening techniques [2]. Existing preterm labor risk screening instruments include factors that are not valid predictors of preterm labor and delivery risk, and fail to include factors reported in the literature that may be valid predictors of preterm labor [3,4,5]. Although existing instruments are only about 44% accurate, and are not adequately predictive of preterm delivery, current preterm labor prevention programs use these invalid, unreliable tools to intervene with pregnant women on a daily basis. This phenomenon has resulted in a trend that increasingly treats pregnant women as if they are "high risk" for preterm labor. Alternative solutions to the problem may be achieved using machine learning and expert system technology to support nurses' assessments in this complex domain.

Reprinted from *Nursing Informatics: An International Overview for Nursing in a Technological Era*, Grobe, S.J., Pluyter-Wenting, E.S.P. (Eds.). 1994, pp. 357–361, with kind permission from Elsevier Science—NL, Sara Burgerhartstraat 25, 1055 KV Amsterdam, The Netherlands.

2. Machine Learning

Machine learning is an emerging specialty in the field of artificial intelligence that developed during the 1980's [6]. Machine learning involves computer science techniques where mathematical algorithms are used to analyze patterns, frequencies, and sets within data. Using various algorithms and a variety of theoretical and mathematical approaches, machine learning offers powerful new tools for knowledge acquisition directly from nursing, and other, data.

3. Methodology

The methodology used in this study was refined from earlier knowledge base development methodology work [2,7] by using multiple large datasets (n =18,890 subjects from three databases), multiple machine learning programs (ID3, LERS, CONCLUS, and a Bayesian classification program), and simplified classification schemes for machine learning analysis. The decision analyzed by machine learning programs was preterm or full term delivery, rather than weeks of gestation at delivery. The procedure included the following steps:

1.   Acquire and load data into appropriate computers and formats. It is important to note that the data was split in half at this step. Half of the data was used for statistical and machine learning analysis. This is data that was used to generate the production rules for the prototype expert system. The other half of the data was used to test the prototype expert system with real patient cases.
2.   Conduct exploratory factor analysis for data reduction purposes.
3.   Conduct multivariate regression analyses to determine predictors of preterm labor risk.
4.   Conduct machine learning knowledge acquisition to generate production rules directly from the data.
5.   Verify production rules using content validity techniques and nurse experts.
6.   Build and test the prototype expert system.

4. Statistical Analysis Results (Methodology Steps 2 and 3)

All statistical analyses were conducted with datasets that were used for production rule generation. Descriptive statistics, exploratory factor analyses, and multiple regression analyses were conducted for 9445 subjects and

214 variables. Descriptive statistics found the average age of women in all three databases was in their late twenties. Numbers of adolescent subjects were relatively small, so this data may not reflect risk factors of adolescent pregnancy. Only three of the subjects analyzed had received no prenatal care, thus this study was unable to address preterm labor risk in women who do not seek prenatal care. Dichotomous coding and small numbers of subjects with positive responses on numerous variables produced statistical results that contradict findings in the literature. Between 10.8% and 14.2% of the subjects were smokers, but smoking was recorded "yes" or "no," and multiple regression analyses did not detect a relationship between smoking and preterm delivery. This same phenomenon was true for substance abuse and a variety of medical diagnoses that complicate preganancy. In general, conclusions drawn from descriptive data analysis were that the data was voluminous, sometimes erroneous, poorly organized, inconsistently recorded, frequently dichotomous, and data items needed were often not collected. Continued statistical analyses were conducted with caution to better understand the problems and to determine data needs for future studies.

Exploratory factor analyses that yielded the best results produced a four factor solution that accounted for 25.6% of the variance. There were no double loadings in the four factor solution, and factors were named with relative ease. Factor 1 was named "Biophysical Markers" and included data items for blood pressure, pulse, weight, and mean arterial pressures. Factor 2 was named "Age and Abortion History" and included data items for maternal age, number of pregnancies, first trimester bleeding, and several abortion variables. Factor 3 was named "Reasons and Interventions" and included information about the average number of contractions, reasons given for patient contact, and patient interventions prescribed by the nurse. Although some of the interventions required physician collaboration and orders, they were initiated by the nurse. Factor 4 was named "Preterm Labor Risk Factors" and included data items for previous preterm labor and delivery, cervical history, and pregnancy within one year of a previous pregnancy. In addition, Factor 4 included data items for years of maternal education and numbers of living children. Exploratory factor analyses partially confirmed construct validity of the data. Exploratory factor analyses was also conducted for purposes of data reduction to guide multiple regression analyses. Various factor solutions were used as models for multiple regression analyses.

Multiple regression analysis used weeks of gestation at delivery as the dependent variable and tested numerous regression models with varying configurations of the remaining 213 variables as predictors. Results found very low correlations between the dependent variable and most of the predictors tested. The inability to predict preterm delivery from the data was somewhat surprising, at first, but this finding can be clarified through several explanations. It is important to remember that the exact cause of labor, whether full term or preterm, remains unknown. The data in the perinatal database reflected risk factors [8] that are consistent with most preterm labor risk screening instruments currently in use. However, review of the literature found that preterm labor risk scoring indices have not been developed with attention to psychometric standards, and remain invalid and unreliable although they are used daily as a standard of practice in providing prenatal care [9]. The low correlations between predictor variables and the criterion variable are explained, in part, to a large volume of dichotomous data. The low correlations between predictor variables and the criterion variable may also be due, in part, to the possibility that healthcare providers continue to collect a great deal of data that has little to do with preterm labor risk. The multiple regression findings in this study may lend additional support to an earlier study [10] that found no statistically significant results for race, age, marital status, parity, or socioeconomic status and a study [11] that found no statistically significant differences in age, gravidity, parity or race. It is possible that current clinical practice operates with assumptions about risk factors for preterm labor that are invalid. Continued questions exist as to the relationship between demographic data and preterm labor risk. More work is needed to replicate and analyze preterm labor risk factors in relationship to age, race, and other items believed to predict or be strongly associated with preterm labor risk.

5. Machine Learning and Expert Verification Results (Methodology Steps 4 and 5)

Multiple approaches to machine learning were conducted using software programs named ID3, LERS, CONCLUS, and a Bayesian classification program. Examples with missing values and obvious errors, such as maternal 10 pound or 700 pound weights, systolic pressures of 14,000, and pulses of less than 40, were excluded from machine learning analysis. The details of this work are reported elsewhere [12]. LERS produced the only usable output, generating about 1600 production rules directly from the data. Expert verification of the rules was difficult due to the large volume and "unfriendliness" of the rule output. Automated features built into LERS assisted with the rule verification process and programs were written to make the rule output easier for the experts to analyze. In general, the experts indicated that individual rules did not provide enough information and that important data were missing. Considering the prototype expert system results, described in the next section, limitations of expert verification in complex and disorganized domains need further study.

6. Prototype Expert System Results (Methodology Step 6)

The prototype expert system used 520 rules in an object oriented expert system shell named "Kappa" that runs on a DOS platform in a Windows environment. Forward chaining techniques and priority encoding of the rules were used to develop the prototype. It is important to remember that none of the data used for testing was used in building the prototype. A computer program was written to "feed" each of the 9445 test subjects through the prototype expert system to analyze the system's ability to accurately predict preterm delivery. Accuracy was tested by having the expert system analyze each test case's data and predict either preterm or full term delivery. The computer program then retrieved the actual preterm or full term outcome from the database, and the expert system predication was compared with the actual patient outcome. Where the predicted outcome and the actual outcome matched, there was 100% accuracy. Accuracy rates are reported in Table 1.

While the ultimate goal of expert system development is to predict preterm *labor* risk, the definition of preterm labor and data needed to analyze preterm labor risk is less amenable to study at present. There were numerous confounding variables in the data that made prediction of preterm labor impossible. It was determined that accuracy of predicting preterm delivery was more viable, and that the purpose of this study was to determine the feasibility of using an expert system for prediction of preterm delivery. Future studies are planned to study the feasibility of using the expert system to predict preterm labor risk. Even so, the reader is reminded that existing manual systems are approximately 44% accurate in predicting preterm delivery. Each of the databases tested surpassed the manual accuracy rates. And the lower accuracy for Database 3 is still very encouraging because there were no rules used from this database. The 53.4% accuracy for Database 3 reflects data tested against rules from the other two databases.

Considering the limitations with databases used, "noisy" data, and difficulties encountered with expert verification, the accuracy rates reflected in Table 1 were both surprising and exciting. Future studies using prospective, carefully planned, and quality-controlled data collection methods should

TABLE 1. Expert system prototype accuracy rates

	Database 1	Database 2	Database 3
Number of test cases	1593	1218	6608
Total correctly classified	1415 (88.8%)	722 (59.2%)	3533 (53.4%)
Total misclassified	171 (10.7%)	456 (37.4%)	2796 (42.3%)
Total unclassified	7 (.4%)	40 (3.2%)	279 (4.2%)

improve rule generation and accuracy predictions to very high levels in a fully implemented expert system that will provide valid and reliable decision support for nursing assessment of preterm labor risk. The statistical, machine learning, and prototype expert system findings from this study validated that preterm delivery risk assessment is a complex and disorganized knowledge domain. But even with this complexity, the research methodology and machine learning techniques used in this study were able to extract rules directly from data, and use these rules in a prototype expert system that was more accurate in predicting preterm delivery than existing manual systems. The knowledge base development methodology used in this study offers a mechanism to further develop linkages between technology, nursing science, and clinical nursing practice in a variety of settings.

Acknowledgments. Special thanks for data provided by St. Luke's Regional Perinatal Center (Kansas City, MO), Healthdyne Perinatal Services (Marietta, GA), and Tokos Corporation (Santa Ana, CA).

References

[1] Rosen M, Merkatz I, and Hill J. Caring for our future: a report of the expert panel on the content of prenatal care. *Ob Gyn*, 77 (5), 782–787, 1991.
[2] Woolery L. *Knowledge Acquisition for Assessment of Preterm Labor Risk.* Unpublished doctoral dissertation. University of Kansas, 1992.
[3] Keirse M. An evaluation of formal risk scoring for preterm birth. *Am J Perinat*, 6 (2), 226–233, 1989.
[4] Alexander G, Weiss J, Hulsey T, and Papiernik E. Preterm birth prevention: an evaluation of programs in the United States. *Birth*, 18 (3), 160–169, 1991.
[5] VanDyne M and Woolery L. *An Expert System for Nurses' Preterm Labor Risk Assessment.* SBIR Phase I Summary Report, 1993.
[6] Forsyth R. *Machine Learning: Principles and Techniques.* New York: Chapman & Hall Publishers, 1989.
[7] Woolery L, Grzymala-Busse J, Summers S, and Budihardjo A. On the use of LERS-LB knowledge acquisition for expert system development in nursing. *Comput Nurs*, 9 (6), 227–234, 1991.
[8] Holbrook R, Laros R, and Creasy R. Evaluation of a risk-scoring system for prediction of preterm labor. *Am J Perinat*, 6 (1), 62–68, 1989.
[9] Keirse M. An evaluation of formal risk scoring for preterm birth. *Am J Perinat*, 6 (2), 226–233, 1989.
[10] Lockwood C, Senyei A, Dische M, Casal D, Shah K, Thung S, Jones L, Deligdisch L, and Garite, T. Fetal fibronectin in cervical and vaginal secretions as a predictor of preterm delivery. *New Engl J Med*, 315 (10). 669–674, 1991.
[11] McGregor J, French J, Richter R, Franco-Buff A, Johnson A, Hillier S, Judson F, and Todd, J. Antenatal microbiologic and maternal risk factors associated with prematurity. *Am J Ob Gyn*, 163 (5), 1465–1473, 1990.
[12] Grzymala-Busse J, Tsatsoulis C, VanDyne M, and Woolery L. Multiple articles in progress.

61
Adapting the Nursing Informatics Pyramid to Implementation Monitoring

LAURA G. SPRANZO

1. Introduction

Advances in nursing informatics (NI) research will require the development and testing of conceptual models and frameworks that incorporate the unique attributes of this field. Attributes that reflect the combination of nursing science, information science, information technology and associated data-information-knowledge transformations are important model components [1]. Models depicting direction, interaction and purpose among components provide focus and guidance to research. Such models foster replication, refinement through comparative analyses and cumulative knowledge development in nursing informatics. The purpose of this paper is to describe and illustrate an example of adapting a existing research model into a framework for a systematic study of the process of implementation in NI. As a result of the development and application of this framework, several refinements and uses are recommended in the spirit of stimulating further study in the area of system implementation.

2. Background

Implementation monitoring is a tool used in evaluation studies involving a complex intervention such as the implementation of a computerized system. Its purpose is to assess the manner and extent of activities associated with an intervention in order to ascertain its construct validity, that is, to determine the relative strength of the intervention as an independent variable [2]. Implementation monitoring is often used to assess variations of an

Reprinted from *Nursing Informatics: An International Overview for Nursing in a Technological Era*, Grobe, S.J., Pluyter-Wenting, E.S.P. (Eds.). 1994, pp. 223–227, with kind permission from Elsevier Science—NL, Sara Burgerhartstraat 25, 1055 KV Amsterdam, The Netherlands.

intervention that may alter achievement of outcomes among experimental groups. This was the basis for its use in an evaluation study measuring the effects of a computerized nurse careplanning system (CNCP) on nursing practice, patient outcomes and nursing staff [3].

Recommended study methods for an implementation assessment include qualitative approaches, such as interviews with personnel, observation checklists, surveys and content analyses techniques. A categorical scheme or conceptual framework that illustrates the relevant aspects of the intervention facilitates a systematic approach to data collection and analysis. Such a scheme needs to reflect comprehensiveness, dynamic interaction between users and technology, and characteristics associated with implementation that influence the actual use of the system.

Research based literature addressing implementation in nursing or health care is scant and usually focused on selected aspects of implementation such as training, user involvement or user satisfaction [4]. Implementation monitoring applied to computerized systems generally only addresses system performance and not the implementation process itself [5]. Conceptualizing the process of implementation required expanding a more general, yet, flexible model.

3. Conceptual Framework for Implementation Monitoring

Schwirian's Pyramid Model for NI research was selected because of its relevance to nursing informatics and its applicability to a variety of research purposes [6]. Schwirian's triangular model depicts the three base elements of information, user context, and technology which interact to create nursing informatics activity. The apex of the model is considered as the goal toward which the three base elements are directed. This model displays bi-directional arrows to illustrate the interaction among the base elements and their relationship to the goal.

Adapting this model as a framework required expanding each of the base elements to include features reflecting the process of implementing CNCP within hospital nursing units. For example, the user context was the staff nurses on the nursing units where CNCP was implemented. Features selected to represent this element were training, implementation stress and user perceptions. The features within each element were conceptualized to be modified by certain characteristics. For example, training could be modified by the characteristic of how much time was available for training. The feature of implementation stress could be modified by the workload characteristics on the nursing units during implementation. And finally, the feature of user perceptions could be modified by nurse characteristics.

The goal toward which the base elements and features were directed was the production and actual use of the careplan by the nurse users of the system. This goal was selected to reflect the purpose of the framework as a guide to data collection and analysis on the nursing units receiving CNCP as a treatment variable. For this reason, the relationship of the elements, features and modifiers were depicted as an influence diagram. Bi-directional and straight arrows are used to indicate the interaction and direction among features of the elements and their relationship to the goal. Bent arrows are used to indicate the influence of modifiers.

Figure 1 illustrates the conceptual model applied to implementation monitoring. This adapted model differs from the Pyramid model in that it is more linear and temporal, a depiction that is consistent with implementation activities. However, the base elements are still considered interactive as illustrated by the dotted connecting lines. Following is a brief description of each element which includes suggested refinements based on findings from the application of this framework.

3.1 Information Element

The nurse care planning information, care planning data elements and the standards of care upon which care planning was based are considered as the information element. The feature of modification of CNCP was included to indicate its policy implications, in that, the information contained in the CNCP must be a reflection of the standards of care consistent with nursing as practiced in this setting. The amount of flexibility available to the users in modifying, adding and building the system to match their needs was considered essential to the successful use of the system. The data were analyzed to reflect themes related to the importance of information modification to match end users' needs, flexibility in modification and user involvement in this process.

Inclusion of these features proved appropriate given that, in actuality, significant modification of the CNCP had to take place in order for user involvement to take place. However, a recommended refinement is to include the modifier to user involvement that reflects the *value of the information* as a resource in patient care. In this case, nurses did not demonstrate a strong value of care planning information beyond the requirements of documentation. This finding tended to modify both the user involvement feature and user perceptions and consequently limit full use of the CNCP.

3.2 User Context Element

The user context element includes training, implementation stress and user perceptions. Training is modified by methods, frequency, personnel and time for preparing the nurses for use of the system. Kjerulff's conceptualization of the environmental factors to consider when studying the adoption of innovations contributed the characteristics for the user

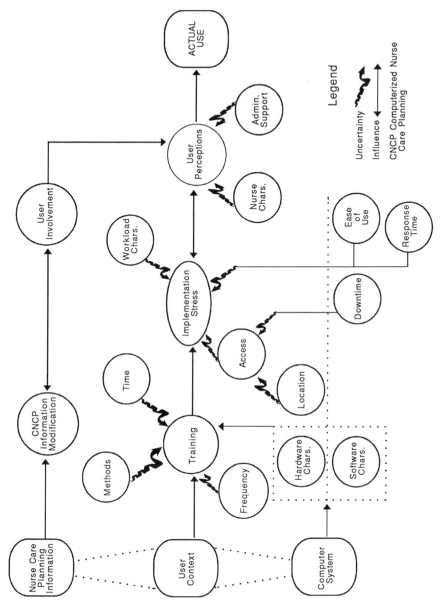

FIGURE 1. Conceptual model for implementation monitoring.

context element [7]. Workload characteristics such as staffing to patient ratios, patient intensity for nursing care time and census can increase the amount of implementation stress when incorporating a new technology. User perceptions can also relate to benefits to practice, changes in role expectations and expectations of continued use. Communication from management in support of technology incorporation influences the user's perceptions of the benefits of the technology to their practice.

A modifier that warrants inclusion and refinement is *leadership*. Characteristics of leadership in promoting the incorporation of a system into practice can be demonstrated by administration or staff. The relationship of leadership to successful implementations of systems is relatively under-investigated.

3.3 Technology Element

The element of technology or computer system included a description of the hardware and software and methods of input and output. Additionally, the location and accessibility of terminals and printers to the user group was assessed to determine variations in access. The characteristics of downtime, response time and ease of use were considered to influence the implementation and consequently user perceptions of the system. These features reflected the system's quality in terms of the service it provides.

A modifier which was not included in the framework but found to be influential was the *flexibility of the software* (*configurability*) in terms of its capacity to be modified to match the information needs of the user. A low level of software flexibility was found to limit the degree of user involvement and consequently alter user perceptions of the system.

4. Recommendations

The conceptual framework warrants further investigation and refinement. Future research could improve operationalization and measurement of the modifiers and examine their relationships to the goals of implementation. With this refinement the conceptual framework would become a tool with several uses. It can continue to be used to monitor the implementation process and provide ongoing feedback on the strengths and weaknesses of each element. It can also be used as a guide to retrospective analysis of implementation and offer predictions of elements and features that require additional resources to improve the effectiveness of implementation.

With further refinement, the conceptual model can provide the framework for studying the implementation process as an intervention in itself. Methods designed to strengthen selected aspects of the implementation could be developed and compared with conventional implementation methods. The results from such comparisons could provide feedback on the cost effectiveness of implementation methods in achieving successful use of computerized systems.

5. Conclusion

The application of the framework and use of qualitative methods for implementation monitoring provided several advantages to the evaluation of the effects of CNCP. First, the findings from the implementation monitoring were shared with the nursing information systems specialist who could then bolster the implementation and training as necessary. Second, the framework used as a guide to data collection was sufficiently comprehensive to assure that relevant aspects of the implementation process were addressed and provided insight to future areas of study. And finally, Schwirian's Pyramid model proved a valuable aid in conceptualizing the process of implementation as a dynamic interaction of user, information and technology.

References

[1] Graves J and Corcoran S. The study of nursing informatics. *Image* 1989, 21: 227–231.
[2] Mark M and Cook T. Design of randomized experiments and quasi-experiments. In Rutman L (ed). *Evaluation Research Methods*. Beverly Hills: Sage, 1984: 65–119.
[3] Keller-Spranzo L, McDermott S and Alt-White A. Effects of computerized nurse care planning on selected health care effectiveness measures. In: Clayton P (ed). SCAMC. New York: McGraw-Hill, 1991: 38–42.
[4] Bailey J and Rollier D. An empirical study of the factors which affect user satisfaction in hospitals. In: Greenes R A (ed). SCAMC. New York: IEEE Computer Society, 1988: 843–846
[5] Drazen E and Seidel J. Implementation monitoring: A critical step towards realizing benefits from hospital information systems. In: Cohen G (ed). SCAMC. Los Angeles: IEEE Computer Society, 1984: 148–151.
[6] Schwirian P. The NI Pyramid: A model for research in nursing informatics. *Comput Nurs* 1986, 4: 134–136.
[7] Kjerulff K. A theoretical framework for the study of nursing information systems. In: Greenes R A (ed). SCAMC. New York: IEEE Computer Society, 1988: 796–800.

62
Comparison of Computerized and Manually Generated Nursing Care Plans

WILLIAM L. HOLZEMER, SUZANNE B. HENRY, and VICKI KLEMM

Introduction

Although use of computer generated nursing care plans is increasing, little is known about the effect of computerized care planning on the quality of patient care delivered. Several authors have described the benefits of implementation of computerized care planning including structuring the diagnostic reasoning process, improving communication, and identifying creative care strategies (Albrecht & Lieske, 1985; Blaufuss, 1986; Hinson, Silva & Clapp, 1984; Murphy, 1988). Norris and associates (1990) demonstrated the superiority of a computerized protocol for care planning to traditional care planning on the quality of planned care for three hypothetical patients. Ferguson, Hildman, & Nichols (1987) studied three types of care plans and found no correlation between the type of care planing system used and patient outcome.

The purpose of this study was to examine differences in the number and type of activated patient problems and number of nursing interventions in computerized vs. manually generated care plans for HIV-infected patients hospitalized for Pneumocystis carinii pneumonia (PCP). Holzemer and Henry (in press) recently described lack of expert consensus about relevant patient problems and associated nursing interventions for patients with PCP. The analysis reported here is part of a larger study examining the relationship between activated patient problems, nursing interventions, and patient outcomes in AIDS patients with PCP (National Center for Nursing Research, NR2215, WL Holzemer, Principal Investigator).

Reprinted with permission from; *Nursing Informatics '91: Proceedings of the Fourth International Conference on Nursing Use of Computers and Information Science*; Hovenga, E.J.S., Hannah, K.J., McCormick, K.A. & Ronald, J.S. (Eds.). 1991, pp. 446–451. Heidelberg-Berlin, Germany: Springer-Verlag.

TABLE 1. Characteristics of the matched patient sample (n = 74)

	Manual (n = 37)		Computerized (n = 37)		Total (n = 74)	
	Freq	%	Freq	%	Freq	%
PCP admission						
First	23	62	23	62	46	62
Second	13	35	13	35	26	35
Third	1	3	1	3	2	3
Source of infection						
Sexual practice	34	92	34	92	68	92
IV drugs	1	3	1	3	2	3
Both	1	3	1	3	2	3
Unknown	1	3	1	3	2	3
	Mean	SD	Mean	SD	Mean	SD
Age	38.1	6.3	37.2	7.6	37.7	7.0

Methods

Sample

The sample consisted of 74 male patients admitted for HIV-related Pneumocystis carinii pneumonia (PCP). One half the sample was from an acute care hospital using manually generated care plans, while the remainder were admitted to a facility using care plans developed on a Technicon computerized system. The two groups of patients were matched on number of admissions for PCP and source of HIV infection (Table 1). The typical patient was a gay male experiencing his first admission for PCP.

Procedure

The nursing care plan data was collected from the patient chart during the hospitalization. The nursing care plans were transcribed by a trained research assistant into Ethnograph™. The activated patient problems were then categorized based on a coding scheme which was derived from standardized care plans from four San Francisco facilities providing care to patients with HIV infection and was validated by a panel of expert clinicians.

Results

Thirty-two percent of the patient sample had no care plan. There was no statistically significant difference between the number of completed computerized vs. manually generated care plans (Table 2). Computerized care

TABLE 2. Descriptive statistics on computerized vs. manually generated care plans

	Manual (n = 37)			Computerized (n = 37)			Chi square	p
	Freq			Freq				
Nursing care plans completed	28 (76%)			22 (60%)			1.54	0.21
Patient problems activated	57			70			NA	
Nursing interventions listed	195			349			NA	
	Mean	SD	Range	Mean	SD	Range	t	p
No. of problems per care plan	2.04	1.04	1–4	3.27	1.67	1–7	3.05	0.005
No. of interventions per care plan	6.89	3.91	1–19	15.77	11.13	2–42	3.57	0.002

TABLE 3. Problems identified in computerized vs. manually generated nursing care plans for AIDS patients with pneumocystis carinii pneumonia (PCP)

Overall rank	Problem	Manual (n = 28)			Computerized (n = 22)			Tests of significance[a]
		Freq	%	Rank	Freq	%	Rank	
								Chi-square p's
1	Altered nutritional/ fluid status	13	46	1	12	55	1	0.78
2	Impaired gas exchange	8	29	3	10	45	2.5	0.35
3.5	Well-being/anxiety	11	39	2	6	27	6	0.56
3.5	Potential for fever/ hyperthermia	7	25	4	10	45	2.5	0.22
								Fisher's exact p's
5	Altered bowel bladder/function	2	7	11.5	9	41	4.5	0.006
6	Potential increased risk of infection	1	4	13	9	41	4.5	0.001[b]
8.5	Alteration in comfort/pain	4	14	5	3	14	9	<1.00
8.5	Activity intolerance	3	11	7	3	14	9	<1.00
8.5	Alteration in skin integrity	3	11	7	3	14	9	<1.00
8.5	Grieving diagnosis and prognosis	2	7	9	4	18	7	0.380
11.5	Potential for injury/falls	3	11	7	1	5	11	0.630
11.5	Inadequate knowledge	4	14	10	0	0	12.5	0.120
13	Altered mental status	2	7	11.5	0	0	12.5	0.500

[a] Overall alpha = .05, alpha per comparison = .004 (.05/13).
[b] Statistically significant.

plans listed significantly more problems and interventions than the manually generated care plans.

Table 3 shows the problems identified in each care planning system. The top four ranked problems are reflective of the clinical presentation of acute PCP, however, it is of interest to note that only one third of these patients hospitalized for PCP had impaired air exchange as an activated patient problem. Chi square analysis and Fisher's exact test were used to examine differences in types of problems identified. Only one problem, potential for increased risk of infection, was activated more frequently in the computerized care plan. Future research is needed to examine the effect of computerized care planning on the quality of patient care delivered.

Discussion

Approximately one third of the patients in both care planning systems did not have a care plan. When comparing the profiles of problems from the two systems, the type of problems appear equivalent, however, the computerized care plans listed more activated problems and nursing interventions. It is not clear from this study if these differences translate to any difference in patient care outcomes. The presence of a plan of care is considered one criterion of quality patient care by the Joint Commission on Accreditation of Heath Care Organizations and the two systems were not significantly different on the number of care plans generated.

References

Albrecht, CA & Lieske, AM (1985). Automating patient care planning. *Nursing Management, 16*(7), 21–26.

Blaufuss, J (1986). Promoting the nursing process through computerization. *Proceedings of the Fifth Conference on Medical Informatics.* New York: North-Holland.

Ferguson, GH, Hildman, T, & Nichols, B (1987). The effect of nursing care planning systems on patient outcomes. *Journal of Nursing Administration, 17*, 30–37.

Hinson, T, Silva N, & Clapp, P (1984). An automated Kardex and care plan. *Nursing Management, 15*(7), 31–43.

Holzemer, WL & Henry, SB (in press). Nursing care plans for people with HIV/AIDS: Confusion of consensus? *Journal of Advanced Nursing.*

Murphy, J (1988). Developing the content and process for computerized nursing diagnosis-based standard care plans. *Proceedings of Nursing and Computers: Third International Symposium on Nursing Use of Computers and Information Science.* St. Louis: CV Mosby.

Norris, J, Cuddigan, J, Foyt, M, Leak, G, & Lazure, L (1990). Decision support and outcomes of nurses' care planning. *Computers in Nursing, 8*, 192–197.

63
Capturing Patients' Perceptions in the Computer-Based Patient Record: Essential Prerequisites to the Measurement of Health-Related Outcomes

WILLIAM L. HOLZEMER, CHERYL A. REILLY, SUZANNE B. HENRY, and C.J. PORTILLO

1. Introduction

The cost, quality, and outcomes of healthcare services have become the focus of national attention as providers, consumers, and payers of healthcare services grapple with healthcare reform in the United States. As policy makers and healthcare providers seek to enhance the effectiveness and efficiency of healthcare services, there is a critical need to understand the relationships between structure and process characteristics and client, provider, and setting outcomes. Given the importance of patient care data to the activities of all segments of the healthcare spectrum, the development and implementation of computer-based patient records (CPRs) has been recommended as CPRs have the potential to improve healthcare delivery, enhance outcomes research programs, and increase hospital efficiency [12]. The purpose of this paper is to advocate for the patient as an essential user of CPRs.

2. The Computer-Based Patient Record

Information technology is being considered as part of the infrastructure for the delivery and assessment of quality healthcare since the technology provides a means for examining the contributions of specific factors to variation in health-related outcomes. The emergence of information systems that gather clinical, financial, and administrative data provides a window into encounter-specific data on provider characteristics, patient characteristics, clinical factors, and other organizational factors. This data

Reprinted with permission from *MEDINFO '95: Proceedings of the Eighth World Congress on Medical Informatics*; Greenes, R.A., Peterson, H.E. & Protti, D.J. (Eds.). 1995, pp. 266–270. Edmonton, Alberta, Canada: Canadian Organization for the Advancement of Computers in Health (COACH).

can be used in the measurement and analysis of the relationships between structural characteristics, processes, and outcomes of healthcare services. The CPR has begun to be recognized as the central component of hospital information systems and is considered an essential technology for supporting the information needs of healthcare providers and other legitimate users of aggregated patient care data [12].

The CPR has been defined as an electronic patient record that resides in an information system specifically designed to support users by making available: complete and accurate data, practitioner reminders and alerts, clinical decision support systems, links to bodies of medical knowledge, and other aids [12]. Five objectives of CPRs have been identified and include the ability to: (1) support patient care and improve its quality; (2) enhance the productivity of healthcare professionals and reduce administrative costs; (3) support clinical and health services research; (4) accommodate future developments in healthcare technology, policy, management, and finance; and (5) ensure patient data confidentiality at all times [12]. In order to derive maximum benefits from CPRs, four user conditions must be fulfilled: users must have confidence in the data, users must use the record actively in the clinical process, users need to understand that the record is a resource which extends beyond the direct patient care encounter, and users must be proficient in the use of CPRs [12].

The value of CPRs rest solely on the ability of the CPR to capture relevant and accurate data and to represent that data in a uniform manner that allows for comparisons within and across a variety of institutions. The development of standards to facilitate the exchange of healthcare data is necessary in order for clinical data to be aggregated and analyzed for the purposes of improved decision making [12]. The standardization of healthcare vocabularies and the establishment of a composite data dictionary are necessary prerequisites for patient records of the future [12]. The Canon Group reports that the quality and effectiveness of healthcare depends on the efficient processing and interpreting of medical language and promotes a common, uniform, and comprehensive approach to the representation of medical information [5]. Health policy makers also recognize that the development of standard definitions, common formats, and methods for the linking of medical data are essential to medical effectiveness and health services research [16]. In addition to the standardization of healthcare data, health-related outcomes and factors that contribute to variation in outcomes need to be identified and captured in CPRs.

3. The Emergence of the Era of the Patient

Prior to the scientific revolution of the 17th century, the individual's experience of illness was the central focus of medical care. With the discovery and descriptions of diseases, Sydenham is credited with shifting the focus of medical attention from the particular manner in which an individual experienced illness, to the typical pattern of symptoms displayed by a population of patients with specific disease entities [17]. The pendulum has begun to swing once again as Western societies are experiencing a paradigm shift from a disease orientation to a focus on healthy functioning and well-being [7]. The perceptions, needs, preferences, values, experiences, outcomes, and expectations of healthcare services (from the eyes of the patient) have come to receive unprecedented national attention.

Reiser [17] proposed the emergence of a new era in healthcare called "The Era of the Patient"; this era engages the perspectives of patients in the transformation of healthcare. The modern medical ethics and the outcomes movement have been credited with the reemergence of the importance of the role and perspective of the patient as an active participant in the delivery of healthcare services [17]. Recent efforts to ensure the right of patients to learn about their illness and to participate in treatment-related decisions have enhanced the authority of patients in medical encounters and the authenticity of their views about their illness [17]. The modern outcomes movement posed the consequences of medical intervention to its recipient as a major criterion for determining its value; it also further enhanced the legitimacy and authority of the patient's perspective [12].

Driven by concerns over the variation in healthcare practice and the growing costs of healthcare, a new interest in outcomes measurement solidified the pivotal role of patient's perceptions in determining health-related outcomes [17]. The continuing escalation in healthcare costs in many counties necessitate the evaluation of new therapies not just in terms of their benefits, but also in terms of their cost-benefit ratio compared to that of the previously standard therapy for the same condition (Jenkins, 1992). As the ultimate aim of all healthcare interventions is to enhance the health-related quality of life, critical dimensions of the patient's quality of life must be taken into account when computing the benefit side of the cost-benefit ratio of specific health interventions. By capturing patients' experiences with illness and their evaluation of healthcare practices, healthcare will begin to reflect the individuality of the patient and return the patient's perspective to the center of medical attention [17].

This paradigm shift has prompted us to expand our thinking about the concept of health to encompass more than the absence of disease and the extension of the duration of life [7,17]. In addition to biologic homeostasis, the concept of a health-related quality of life includes functional status, psychological and social well-being, health perceptions, and disease- and treatment-related symptoms [11]. In order to incorporate these dimensions of health in the evaluation of the efficiency and effectiveness of healthcare interventions, significant energy, creativity, and resources have been invested in the construction of new measures of health-related quality of life [7]. The sole reliance on traditional measures of death, disease, and disability are no longer adequate in the measurement of health-related outcomes as they fail to incorporate other dimensions of health and they are not universally relevant to all patients with a given disease or problem [7]. CPRs must provide a structure for capturing these health-related outcomes in order to contribute to the measurement of health-related outcomes in a meaningful way.

4. The Patient: An Essential User of Computer-Based Patient Records

In order for the CPR to improve healthcare delivery, enhance outcomes research, and increase hospital efficiency, the patient must be considered an essential user of the CPR. As the role of the patient in determining the delivery and evaluation of healthcare services continues to expand, research and development of CPRs must ensure that the needs of patients are adequately addressed. Although the patient has been identified as a user of the CPR, the notion of patient access to the CPR is currently under debate [12]. Patient input into the process of care, patient reports of history and functional status, patient validation of data, and patient control and transport of pertinent parts of the medical record are some of the user activities currently under consideration, yet consensus on the need for and the role of the patient as a user of the CPR has not been achieved [12]. In an effort to demonstrate the need for the patient as an essential user of the CPR, the role of the patient in delineating and assessing her health problems, as an active contributor to processes which effect health outcomes, and as an evaluator of health-related outcomes will be considered.

Healthcare providers have traditionally relied on patients' reports of signs and symptoms for the purposes of the diagnosis and treatment of illness. Signs and symptoms provide clinical data about the patient and are the basic parameters on which medical diagnoses are made [3]. Signs are generally considered as objective measures of abnormal functioning [3]. Symptoms are subjective phenomena regarded by the individual as indicators of a condition departing from normal function, sensation, or appearance [3]. Symptoms can be considered as warning signals of impending threats to health, are the essential focus of healthcare [9], and have been referred to as "the iceberg of mortality" [20]. Comprehensive symptom management is considered a hallmark of quality healthcare as good disease control and superior symptom management constitute the most effective treatment healthcare providers can offer patients with chronic illnesses [20].

Symptom management begins with the assessment of the symptom experience from the patient's perspective [13]. As symptoms are phenomena experienced by a person and not directly observable by another, symptoms can only be identified through the report of the person being assessed [18]. Due to the subjective nature of symptoms, a basic principle in the measurement of symptoms is that symptomatology is what the pa-

484   W.L. Holzemer, et al.

tient says it is [6]. An expanding body of research has identified discrepancies between patients' and providers' perceptions of symptoms [4,8,10,11,14]. These studies support the assessment of symptoms from the perspective of the patient, as the sole reliance on providers' perceptions may potentially impede effective symptom management [14]. As patients are considered to be the best judge of symptoms, methods for patient self-evaluation of symptoms need to be incorporated in CPRs in order to provide valid data for the purposes of assessment, treatment, and evaluation of care.

Aside from the need to determine patient's preferences for certain healthcare interventions, the self-care processes of the patient also need to be considered as potential confounding variables in the measurement of health-related outcomes. Longo [15] has used the term "patient practice variation" to refer to domains of health, prevention, and illness and disease in which the influence of the patient may directly or indirectly impact on resource utilization and immediate or long-term outcomes. The concept of variation in patient practices raises questions about the role of patient perception, patient satisfaction, sick role and illness behavior in a life-style context, characteristics and dimensions of disease as experienced through the eyes of the patient, and the individual responsibility for one's lifestyle relative to health and prevention [15]. Patients who engage in poor health habits, who do not comply with treatment, and who do not respond to encouragement may have poorer health status than other patients, and this is independent of the quality of care delivered [7]. Aside from specific disease processes, patients' attitudes, beliefs, orientations, and preferences must also be considered for their effects on health outcomes. As useful as biological theories of diseases have been in the treatment of illness, there is a risk of overestimating the biological effects of the disease process and underestimating the biological and psychosocial interaction if patient characteristics are not considered [15]. To date, none of the variations literature has addressed the impact of patient practices [15]. The CPR needs to contain a method for assessing patient processes when examining individual health outcomes, as they may explain a large amount of variation in outcomes.

With the expanding definitions of health-related outcomes, the need for the patient's perceptions of outcomes is pivotal to the assessment of the efficiency and effectiveness of healthcare services. As the assessment of the health-related quality of life is essentially subjective in nature, the person whose quality of life is in question is the primary source of information [1]. There is current agreement that health-related quality of life measures should be obtained from patients themselves [11]. The weighting of items or dimensions also requires thoughtful consideration. Controversy exists as to whether or not preference-weighted or nonpreference-weighted scores should be used in the measurement of health status and quality-of-life measures [19]. With preference-weighting, states of health are weighted according to different rules and procedures such as paired comparisons, magnitude estimation, and category scaling. This approach allows the respondent to indicate preferences regarding areas of life and functioning that are most important to the individual, and weights are assigned according to preferences [19]. With nonpreference-weighting, Likert-type items are used to assign weights to items and scores are summed on the basis of ordinal ratings [19]. The patient's perspectives and preferences for health-related outcomes need to be assessed in order to tailor healthcare interventions to the individual. The CPR has the potential to enhance the assessment and delivery of individualized healthcare, provided the patient's perspective is incorporated in the patient record.

5. Conclusions

The current paradigm shift in healthcare requires the active involvement of the patient in the delivery and evaluation of care. The patient must be considered as an essential user of CPRs in order to exploit the benefits of information technology for the purposes of outcome assessment. In the measurement of outcomes, data needs to be obtained from the source that can provide the most valid assessment of the outcome under investigation. Often the most legitimate source of patient care data is the patient himself. Research and development of the future CPRs must incorporate the needs of the patient. Systems should be designed to meet these needs in order to capture the patient's perceptions in CPRs.

References

[1] Aaronson, N. K. "Quality of life research in oncology: Past achievements and future priorities." *Cancer* (1991) 67: 839–843.
[2] Institute of Medicine. *The computer-based patient record: An essential technology for healthcare.* Washington: National Academy Press (1991).
[3] Blacklow, R. S. Preface. In R. S. Blacklow (ed). *MacBryde's Signs and Symptoms.* Philadelphia: Lippincott (1983) p. xi.
[4] Camp, L. D. "A comparison of nurses' recorded assessments of pain with perceptions of pain as described by cancer patients." *Cancer Nursing* (1988) 11: 237–243.
[5] Evans D. A., Cimino J. J., Hersh W. R., Huff S. M., & Bell D. S. (for the Canon Group). "Toward a medical-concept representation language." *Journal of the American Medical Informatics Association* (1994) 1: 207–217.
[6] Fries J. F., & Spitz P. W. "The hierarchy of patient outcomes." In Spilker, B. (ed). *Quality of Life Assessments in Clinical Trials.* New York: Raven Press (1990) pp. 25–36.
[7] Greenfield S., & Nelson E. C. "Recent developments and future issues in the use of health status assessment measures in clinical settings." *Medical Care.* (1992) 30 (5 Supp.): MS23–MS41.

[8] Grossman S. A., Sheidler V. R., Swedeen K., Mucenski J., & Piantadosi S. "Correlation of patient and caregiver ratings of cancer pain." *Journal of Pain and Symptom Management* (1991) 6(2): 53–57.

[9] Hegyvary S. T. "Patient care outcomes related to management of symptoms." *Annual Review of Nursing Research* (1993).

[10] Holmes, S., & Eburn, E. "Patients' and nurses' perceptions of symptom distress in cancer." *Journal of Advanced Nursing* (1989) 14: 840–846.

[11] Holzemer W. L., Reilly C. A., & Slaughter R. E. *Patient and nurse reports of symptoms experienced by patients with AIDS.* Western Society for Nursing Research (in press).

[12] Institute of Medicine. *The computer-based patient record.* Washington, DC: National Academy Press (1991).

[13] Larson P. J., Carrieri V., Dodd M. J., Faucett JA., Froelicher E. S., Gortner S. R., Halliburton P., Janson-Bjerklie S., Lee K. A., Miaskowski C., Savedra M. C., Stotts N. A., Taylor D. L., & Underwood P. R. *A conceptual model of symptom management.* Image: The Journal of Nursing Scholarship (in press).

[14] Larson P. J., Viele C. S., Coleman S., Dibble S. L., & Cebulski C. "Comparison of perceived symptoms of patients undergoing bone marrow transplant and the nurses caring for them." *Oncology Nursing Forum* (1993) 20(1): 81–87.

[15] Longo D. R. "Patient practice variation: A call for research." *Medical Care.* (1993) 31(5 Suppl.): YS81–YS85.

[16] De Moor G. J. E. "Standardization in medical informatics." In. van Bemmel J. H, & McCray A. T. (eds). *Yearbook of Medical Informatics 1993*, pp. 61–66.

[17] Reiser S. J. "The era of the patient: Using the experience of illness in shaping the missions of healthcare." *JAMA* (1993) 269(8): 1012–1017.

[18] Rhodes, V.A. & Watson, P.M. "Symptom distress—the concept: Past and present." *Seminars in Oncology Nursing* (1987) 3(4): 242–247.

[19] Strickland O. L. Measures and instruments. In U.S. DHHS, U.S. Public Health Services, National Institutes of Health. *Patient Outcomes Research: Examining the Effectiveness of Nursing Practice* (1992) pp. 145–153.

[20] Verbrugge L. M., & Ascione F. J. "Exploring the iceberg: Common symptoms and how people care for them." *Medical Care* (1987) 25: 539–561.

[21] Vessey J. A., & Richardson B. L. "A holistic approach to symptom assessment and intervention." *Holistic Nursing Practice* (1993) 7(2): 13–21.

64
An International Nursing Library: Worldwide Access to Nursing Research Databases

CAROLE HUDGINGS

In today's rapidly changing environment, professional nurses face common dilemmas of producing a maximum of knowledge in a minimum of time, and maintaining knowledge of current advances within nursing and other healthcare disciplines. The explosion of scientific information makes it difficult for nurses to keep adequately informed. This problem is particularly acute for nurse researchers who must function as information specialists, yet often encounter difficulties in obtaining information about research in progress, and in establishing networks among other nurse researchers working in similar content areas. In addition, retrieval of relevant information is frequently hampered by lack of a universally accepted classification scheme to organize nursing's knowledge. Although thousands of nurses conduct research today, no library serves as a comprehensive focal point for nursing research. This paper describes efforts to establish an International Nursing Library (INL) to address these information needs for nurses worldwide.

Organizational Background

During 1979–1981 Sigma Theta Tau, the international Honor Society of Nursing, developed the Ten Year Plan, a strategic plan to guide the organization's activities during the 1980s. This plan provided a blueprint for the organization's expansion and served as a "focus for program priorities and financial decisions" (Rose, 1986, p. 6).

Consistent with the Society's overall mission (a commitment to improve the health of the people worldwide by increasing the scientific base of nursing practice), the Ten Year Plan identified three broad goals: knowl-

Reprinted with permission from; *Nursing Informatics '91: Proceedings of the Fourth International Conference on Nursing Use of Computers and Information Science*; Hovenga, E.J.S., Hannah, K.J., McCormick, K.A. & Ronald, J.S. (Eds.). 1991, pp. 780–784. Heidelberg-Berlin, Germany: Springer-Verlag.

edge development, knowledge dissemination, and knowledge utilization. An overriding premise was that nursing's knowledge base will be expanded through a global network of well-prepared nurses. Specific action strategies were identified for these three goals. The vision of the INL emerged from the primary action strategy "develop an efficient computerized storage and retrieval system for nursing research and nurse researchers" (Sigma Theta Tau, 1981). Momentum for continued INL development is contained in the organization's Actions for the 1990s, a strategic planning document that adds resource development as a fourth major goal (Sigma Theta Tau International, 1989).

International Nursing Library Planning

Work specifically targeted toward development of the INL began during 1987. A Survey of Interest and Needs for an Electronic Nursing Library and Resource Center was distributed to Sigma Theta Tau members and at various research conferences throughout the United States. This Survey requested nurses to rank the importance of various services in an ideal information service system, and to provide information about their current use of library and information technologies. Rankings from more than 1700 nurse respondents indicated the following five services as highest priority in an ideal information service system: literature searches, nursing instruments, research funding sources, nursing-related statistical sources, and research in progress. Potential services for the INL were prioritized into three clusters, with the cluster of highest priority containing the following information: research in progress, profiles of nurse researchers, and a calendar of professional events.

Results of the library needs survey were also used to structure the International Nursing Library and Resource Center Strategic Plan 1987–1989. This first plan for the INL contains objectives under three goals of knowledge development, knowledge dissemination, and knowledge utilization. The overall objective for the INL was "to increase information and improve information management for professionals and other consumers through the use and application of electronic technology" (Sigma Theta Tau International, 1987).

Services of the INL are designed to provide communication linkages between and among nurse researchers, nurses, and the public. The Library supports nurse researchers and practicing nurses in knowledge development, dissemination, and utilization; and provides the public with information about nursing and nursing research. Rather than duplicating information available through other traditional library resources, the INL is positioned to serve as a unique resource for the nursing research arena by creating on-line nursing databases and establishing links with existing library networks.

The INL expands on the traditional concept of "library" as a location for printed literary materials, to encompass recent technological advances for information management and communication. Present INL efforts seek to combine traditional library resources with state-of-the-art information systems and communications technology to:

- form electronic communication networks among nurse researchers worldwide,
- develop selected nursing databases useful to facilitate nursing research,
- provide a structured classification scheme to organize nursing information, and
- disseminate nursing research findings to the public.

Implementation of the International Nursing Library

Traditional library operations comprise one facet of the INL. A modest collection of books, journals, newsletters, audiotapes, and videotapes is maintained to facilitate internal activities of the organization, and to respond to requests for information and materials from members, nurses, and the general public. Staff utilize this collection, as well as on-line access to bibliographic databases and reciprocal borrowing agreements with health science libraries within the community, to respond to requests for diverse information about nursing.

Development of the electronic component of the International Nursing Library began in 1989 with acquisition of technology to support the development of electronic nursing research databases. Technological support is provided by a host computer, search software, and personal computer equipment. The host mini-computer stores the electronic databases of the INL, and provides access for individuals at remote locations using their personal computer, modem, and communications software.

A powerful and versatile full text management and retrieval software (BRS/SEARCH Software) is used as the database management program for storing, searching, and retrieving database information (Hudgings, 1990). Responding to members' identified needs for information about nurse researchers and research in progress, the premiere database of the INL describes nurse researchers and their current projects. This database is an on-line version of the recently published 1990 *Directory of Nurse Researchers*. Initially listing 2500 nurse researchers and their 3770 research projects, the on-line database of nurse researchers can be easily updated and modified to reflect the most recently available information.

A wide variety of databases are in the planning stages as future INL services. Projects approved for the next phase of development include:

- full text abstracts for projects in the nurse researchers database,
- full text abstracts for doctoral dissertations,
- bibliographic citations for clinically relevant topics,
- data reflecting international concerns,
- fugitive literature, and
- calendar of professional events.

Classification of Nursing Research

Sigma Theta Tau's classification scheme for nursing research identifies and categorizes terms that describe nursing's research activity, and represents the most extensive classification effort for nursing research today. This classification scheme serves as the infrastructure for the nurse researchers database, and seeks to facilitate networking and collaboration among the worldwide community of nurse researchers. Currently in its third version, this classification scheme was most recently revised in 1989 to serve as the data collection tool for the 1990 *Directory of Nurse Researchers*. The classification scheme identifies project specific information including demographics about the research project, e.g., subjects, data collection sites, funding, research design, statistics, and project descriptors, i.e., keywords that describe the content area of the research. The current classification scheme includes 637 discrete project descriptors which serve as access points for retrieving relevant information from the electronic nurse researchers database and other planned databases. The classification scheme is dynamic, changing as the body of knowledge evolves, and assists nurses with transforming data and information into structured knowledge, a major crisis facing knowledge workers today (Wurman, 1989).

Summary

In the current information age, the doubling of information every five years and the increasing specialization of knowledge make it imperative that nurses have access to the latest scientific information to assist in the delivery of high quality care. A variety of technological innovations have increased our access to information during the past two decades. Two of these technological innovations, the developing electronic databases of the INL and the Sigma Theta Tau International classification scheme for nursing research, can assist nurses in a variety of settings to have better access to information that supports scholarship. Nursing exists within dynamic environments for health care delivery, technological capabilities, and expansion of nursing knowledge. The INL serves as a unique resource for nursing scholarship, reflecting the organization's mission to increase the scientific base of nursing practice.

References

Hudgings, C.: Library on-line. *Reflections*, Summer 1990; 19.

Rose, M.: The ten year plan: A blueprint for excellence. *Reflections*, Winter 1986; 6–7.

Sigma Theta Tau: *Ten year plan*. Indianapolis, IN: Sigma Theta Tau, 1981.

Sigma Theta Tau International: *Actions for the 1990s*. Indianapolis, IN: Sigma Theta Tau International, 1989.

Sigma Theta Tau International: *International nursing library and resource center strategic plan 1987–1989*. Indianapolis, IN: Sigma Theta Tau International, 1987.

Wurman, RS: *Information Anxiety*. New York: Doubleday, 1989.

65
Data Management in Nursing Research

Steven M. Paul

As research carried out by nurses increases in its complexity of design and analytical strategies, so too has the need for an understanding of different computerized data management systems and techniques increased. Data management refers to coding and entry schemes, data cleaning, communication between different programs and systems, as well as statistical analysis.

This paper describes the development and content of a graduate level course in computer data management at the School of Nursing, University of California, San Francisco. Nurses are instructed in the advantages and disadvantages of working with microcomputer statistical packages and their mainframe alternatives. Considerations include cost, ease of use, type and complexity of statistical procedures, and clarity of output. Understanding the benefits and limitations of each system helps the nurse researcher to develop more efficient data collection instruments and questionnaires. Development of a well-planned research strategy before the start of data collection is a major emphasis of the course. Frequently no single package or system can accomplish everything the researcher needs. One package may have an excellent data entry system, while another may have an easier to use analysis of variance procedure. Different methods of transferring files between packages are presented so the researcher can operate in the most advantageous system at all times. Statistical knowledge is a vital research skill, but no less vital is the ability to manage the data in order to generate statistical results.

The course in data management at UCSF was instituted in 1988. It started as a formalization of a two-day workshop in the use of the CRUNCH (CRUNCH Software Corporation, 1987) microcomputer statistical package and has expanded to a full ten week course in the techniques of computerized data management.

Reprinted with permission from; *Nursing Informatics '91: Proceedings of the Fourth International Conference on Nursing Use of Computers and Information Science*; Hovenga, E.J.S., Hannah, K.J., McCormick, K.A. & Ronald, J.S. (Eds.). 1991, pp. 562–566. Heidelberg-Berlin, Germany: Springer-Verlag.

Students gain hands-on experience in the computer lab facility of the school and are presented with discussions of a full range of data management considerations.

The keys to efficient data management are advanced planning and flexibility. When questionnaires are developed or instruments are chosen to be used in a study, they should be viewed with an eye toward how the variables will be coded and entered into any computer system. A file code book including variable names, variable labels, value labels, and missing value indicators should be prepared before one even approaches the computer. It is at this point one may discover the pitfalls of asking questions such as "choose all that apply" or "check all medications that the patient was using." These are not simple questions to code, in fact each response is its own variable that must be coded "No" (0) or "Yes" (1). A file that one might have thought had ten questions in it may actually have to be represented by more than 100 variables.

The choice of statistical package is an important one. Although most packages available today can get the job done, a system that includes checks and balances in its data entry system and flexibility in its communication with other systems and programs is most advantageous. One should remember that all packages assume adequate statistical knowledge. They will perform whatever task they are asked to do, appropriate or not. Knowledge of statistical assumptions is the user's responsibility.

In the data management course at UCSF, students are familiarized with PC based and mainframe programs, specifically CRUNCH and SPSS/PC+ (SPSS, Inc., 1988) for microcomputers and SPSS-X (SPSS, Inc., 1988) on the mainframe. CRUNCH is a very simple interactive statistical package that is primarily menu driven. It is interactive in the sense that it provides options, the user picks one which branches off to other options, until the desired analysis is generated. As an example, to perform an independent groups t-test CRUNCH would prompt for the name of the dichotomous independent variable (e.g., SEX) then how the two groups were coded (Female = 1, Male = 2) and then a list of dependent variables to perform the test on.

Both SPSS packages on the other hand are essentially batch driven. A series of commands are written into a file and the file is submitted as a job to be run.

Both SPSS packages take more up front computer savvy on the part of the user, but the payoff may be in the power and sophistication of the statistical techniques available. CRUNCH, as of yet, does not perform advanced multivariate techniques (MANOVA, discriminant analysis, etc.) but the SPSS packages do.

Cost is a major consideration. There is no doubt that mainframe packages such as SPSS-X and its contemporaries such as SAS (SAS Institute, Inc., 1985) or BMDP (BMDP Statistical Software, Inc., 1988) are faster, more powerful, and include almost every statistical procedure a researcher would want to have available. They are also extremely expensive to use. Most major universities and institutions charge for basic mainframe access time and more charges are incurred when jobs are actually run and printouts generated. Their speed comes at a high price. Microcomputer packages although requiring an initial monetary investment, can in fact "pay for themselves" in the long run. That of course assumes one already has the microcomputer itself to work on.

One of the largest advantages of microcomputer packages are their accurate and easy to use data entry systems. One should never begin statistical analysis until the data files are error free. Perhaps the only way to be sure that data files are indeed "clean" is to employ a double entry strategy. The complete data file is actually entered twice and then all parallel entries are checked for perfect one-to-one correspondence. Perfect agreement is evidence of clean data. Double entry requires double the effort and sometimes double the cost.

The data entry components of both SPSS/PC+ and CRUNCH (in the new Version 4, now being beta tested) have the ability to set range checks that signal out of range values either during data entry itself or as a check after the file has been initially completed. For example, one could set the range check values for the variable AGE at "18 to 65." Values entered above or below this range would be flagged as errors. SPSS/PC+'s data entry system, Data Entry II (SPSS, Inc., 1988), can also utilize more elaborate checks called "cleaning rules" that specify logical relationships that should hold among the values of the variables. A cleaning rule might state "AGE < 20 IMPLIES INCOME < 25000." "Skip and fill rules" can be used when the values of some variables influence the values of others. This efficient technique enables the system to fill in dependent values of variables automatically.

For example, if the value of the variable "NUMBER OF CHILDREN" equals 0, the system can automatically fill in the "not applicable" value for variables concerning the sex or age of the nonexistent children.

It is not uncommon for a researcher to use one package for its data entry system and carry out the analysis on another. The laborious and time consuming data entry can be done on a microcomputer and the cleaned data file may be sent to the mainframe for fast and efficient statistical analysis. Some statistical procedures are easier to ask for or have clearer output in different packages. Repeated measures analysis of variance, for example, is cumbersome in SPSS-X, but quite straightforward in CRUNCH. The ability to transfer files between systems allows researchers to custom fit their management strategy to maximum advantage. After all, these programs are only tools to aid in the process. Knowing the best tool to fit the situation is a valuable skill.

How is the transferring of files accomplished? In some limited cases it is possible for one statistical package to directly read the files generated by another. SPSS, Inc. has made it relatively simple to create portable files that allow its mainframe package (SPSS-X) to communicate with is microcomputer package (SPSS/PC+). The IMPORT and EXPORT procedures of these packages create and read portable files. A modem connecting the microcomputer to the mainframe computer through telephone lines allows the transfer of files with the use of a standard communications protocol such as KERMIT (Columbia University) or Y-TERM (Yale University). It is important to consider the limitations of the package to which one is transferring data. SPSS/PC+ (Version 3.1) has a limit of 500 variables and one user defined missing value and one system missing value. SPSS-X is not restricted by these limitations and if they are not considered it can result in the loss or misrepresentation of data.

Quite often the microcomputer versions of statistical packages do not directly read or write files compatible with other systems. Compromises have been made in each of the packages. Some limit the researcher's ability to determine variable size in order to make the program easier to use. Others limit the number of variables that can be entered. Still others are written in completely different computer languages. Transferring of data between most different packages can be done but the process requires more preparation and effort (Turley, 1989).

Many statistical packages read and write ASCII files without much more effort than providing variable column locations. This enables the transfer of the raw data but unfortunately does not include transfer of the variable names, variable labels, value labels and the critical missing value indicators that have been painstakingly provided in the original file. Many data files can be transferred from one package to another using a file system based on one of the industry standard file structures. Examples of these standard file structures include: DATA INTERCHANGE FORMAT or "DIF", "DBF" from dBASE-III (Ashton-Tate, 1985), and "WKS" and "WK1" from Lotus 1-2-3 (Lotus Development Corporation, 1985). Each of these will at least transfer the variable names in addition to the raw data associated with that variable. Variable names and missing value indicators are essential to any file. Some researchers may consider variable and value labels as non-essential elements that only make for better looking output. But, if one has ever had to come back to a data set after any lengthy period of time, one will more than appreciate any labeling that has been done. Those cryptic eight character or less variable names often look like mysterious gibberish without their labels. However, reentering the variable names, labels, and missing value indicators into the new system is often a small price to pay for the advantages gained by using a different statistical package.

Students have found the data management course most useful when they are concurrently working on their own research projects. Practical problems and questions they have experienced with their questionnaires and instruments or with statistical packages can be shared and solved with benefits for the entire class. Accurate and efficient data management skills are essential elements of the research process.

References

Ashton-Tate: dBASE-III PLUS [Computer program]. Torrance, California, USA. 1985.

BMDP Statistical Software, Inc.: BMDP [Computer program]. Los Angeles, California, USA. 1988.

CRUNCH Software Corporation: CRUNCH [Computer program]. Oakland, California, USA. 1987, Version 3.13.

Lotus Development Corporation: LOTUS 1-2-3 [Computer Program]. Cambridge, Massachusetts, USA. 1985.

SAS Institute, Inc.: SAS [Computer Program]. Cary, North Carolina, USA. 1985, Version 5.

SPSS Inc.: SPSS-X Version 3, SPSS/PC+ Version 3.1, and DATA ENTRY II [Computer Programs]. Chicago, Illinois, USA. 1988.

Turley, JP: Transferring Data Files Between Microcomputer Statistical Packages. *Nursing Research* 1989;38:315–317.

66
The Use of a Relational Database Management System for the Categorization of Textual Data

Cheryl A. Reilly, William L. Holzemer, and Suzanne B. Henry

1. Background

As part of an ongoing research project examining the quality of nursing care of persons with AIDS, various data sources were utilized to describe patient problems and nursing activities at five points in time [1–4]. In order to prepare the textual data for analysis, a method for organizing and categorizing the data was necessary. This paper will first review the nature of the data generated and the tasks at hand. Secondly, the qualitative software programs the research team attempted to utilize to organize and categorize this data will be described. The usefulness and limitations of these programs for this particular data set will be presented. Ultimately the research team opted to utilize a relational database management system to prepare the data for analysis. The rationale for choosing a relational database management system will be discussed, and the advantages and limitations of the software program selected will also be addressed. In conclusion, the value of utilizing qualitative software programs and a relational database management system in the research process will be examined.

2. The Nature of the Data

Patients and nurses were interviewed by a nurse research assistant and asked to identify three or four major patient problems and the manner in which the nurse was helping the patient with his or her problems. The nurse research assistant also listened to the intershift nursing report and recorded patient problems and nursing activities identified by the nursing staff. Pa-

Reprinted from *Nursing Informatics: An International Overview for Nursing in a Technological Era*, Grobe, S.J., Pluyter-Wenting, E.S.P. (Eds.). 1994, pp. 515–520, with kind permission from Elsevier Science—NL, Sara Burgerhartstraat 25, 1055 KV Amsterdam, The Netherlands.

tient problems and nursing activities were also extracted from three additional sources in order to create a comprehensive view of patient problems and nursing activities. These sources included: the nursing care plan, the patient activity record, and the nursing kardex. The textual data derived from the patient interview, the nurse interview, and the intershift nursing report were in the form of short narrative responses. The data extracted from the nursing care plan, the patient activity record, and the nursing kardex were in the form of brief written statements. The data collected on 201 subjects resulted in a file with over 7,000 patient problems and over 21,000 nursing activities.

Once the data had been collected, a method for organizing and categorizing the data was required. The research team identified several fundamental criteria desired of a software program which were deemed necessary for preparing the data for analysis. First and foremost, a software program which provided a reliable data reduction method and allowed for the preservation of the original integrity of the data was necessary for the classification, the potential reclassification, and the subclassification of the data into contextual categories. It was important to maintain the integrity of the data in its original form, as the language people use to communicate their construction of reality [5]. The need to tabulate the number of patients identified as having a particular type of problem, and the number of problems and nursing activities reported within in a particular contextual category was also important. The research team also wanted to have the ability to sort the data by the hospital site, the point in time that the data had been collected, and the source of the data. In addition, the ability to search the data in a variety of ways was necessary to answer several of the research questions proposed in this study. The option of importing numerical data into a statistical analysis software package was also a desired feature. Lastly, a software program which was easy to learn and to use, and would provide the most efficient and effective method for organizing and analyzing this data were important requirements.

3. Qualitative Software Programs

In 1984, software programs specifically designed for the management of qualitative data became available. Qualitative analysis programs provide the researcher with an automated data reduction technique. The software permits the researcher to assign codes to unstructured text and to retrieve text segments according to similarly assigned codes, allowing for the eventual classification of text into a coding scheme [6]. All qualitative programs basically perform two major functions and differ in the available enhancement functions which include: automatic coding according to data structure, searching for co-occurring codes, selective searching, searching for a particular sequence of codes, and counting the frequency of the occurrence of codes in the data [7]. The majority of qualitative analysis programs are designed for descriptive analysis for research in which the main purpose is to achieve deeper insight, to search for commonalities across the study participants or sites, to explore uniqueness, and to interpret the meaning of patterns [6]. The major achievement of most current qualitative data analysis software has been the efficient coding of online data and the retrieval of coded segments [8].

Initially the research team decided to utilize The Ethnograph® software program [9]. The Ethnograph® is a qualitative software package which enables one to code, recode, and sort data files into contextual categories. The program allows the user to review text, mark text segments, and to display, sort, and print text segments in any order or sequence desired. Five steps are required in order to prepare a file for searching on code words. First the data must be transcribed on a word processor according to specific formatting instructions. Next the file must be converted to a standard ASCII file in order to import the file into the Ethnograph® program. Once the data has been imported, the user instructs the program to number the lines of the entire file. A printout of the file is utilized to manually record notes which will aid the researcher in developing a code mapping scheme. Once a code mapping scheme has been identified, the user must assign code words to various lines of text. Up to twelve code words can be used to define a segment of text and overlapping text lines can be contained in up to seven code words. A search is then conducted by entering specified code words. The lines of text associated with the code words are retrieved and the output can be sent to the screen, printer, or a disk. A template for face sheets can also be created which would allow the user to sort on both alphanumeric and numeric variables, such as sex and age, according to specified selection criteria.

The Ethnograph® program is useful for coding extensive text segments. Many lines of text can be attached to a single or multiple code words. In this study however, thousands of text segments were generated and individual text segments contained under 132 characters. The task of assigning thousands of line numbers to various code words seemed very labor intensive, considering the fact that the program does not tabulate the number of text segments retrieved. By utilizing the face sheet function, the ability to sort the data by the additional variables of interest was possible, yet once again manual tabulation was necessary once the data had been sorted. The option of importing numerical data into a statistical analysis software package is not a feature of this program. The Ethnograph® program is relatively easy to learn and use and the manual provides clear instructions. In the final analysis, the Ethnograph® program did not seem to provide the research team with an efficient and effective method for organizing and analyzing this data set.

After considering the limitations of the Ethnograph® program for the purposes of this study, the research team explored the possibility of utilizing a recently developed qualitative software program, MARTIN® [10]. MARTIN® was designed to allow for maximum flexibility in facilitating qualitative analyses. The program uses the Microsoft Windows' graphical environment and is essentially a Windows application which operates in accordance with the conventions of the Windows environment. MARTIN® is designed to make the process of reading text, extracting and organizing significant passages, and developing observations related to the text as efficient and flexible as possible. A MARTIN® project generates numerous icons in the course of the analysis and each icon is represented by its own window. Icons include texts, cards, folders, and groups. Texts are the original documents imported into the program. Marginal notes can be added to texts. Cards are electronic similes of index cards on which you copy passages. Key codes can be attached to cards for searching purposes. Folders are electronic similes of files in which you can arrange and store cards with related themes or content. Cards may only be placed in one file. Groups are larger files which store related folders. Groups themselves can be categorized into related, larger groups. Detailed summaries can be attached to various cards, folders, and groups. The number of icons you can create and display is primarily limited by the availability of computer resources within the Windows environment. The printing of cards, folders, groups, and summaries can occur at any time.

MARTIN® did allow for the preservation of the original integrity of the data and provided a method for categorizing the data into contextual categories, yet the program did not provide a mechanism for subcategorizing major categories, while still retaining the broader categories. Since a card can only appear in one folder it was impossible to include text segments in two categories. Additionally, the maximum amount of text to be imported into MARTIN® is approximately 12.5 pages per project which severely limits the ability to work with a vast amount of text without partitioning the data. The program did not offer a means for tabulating the text segments or importing the numerical data into a statistical software package. The ability to sort the data by the other variables did not seem possible with this program. MARTIN® contains an online help menu and the manual provided dependable support for using the program. The generated output of this program did not seem to warrant the tremendous resources required to utilize this program.

Although the decision to utilize a qualitative software package had been previously made, the research team began to question the usefulness and expediency of utilizing a qualitative software package for coding short answer textual data. The ultimate purpose of any data management scheme is to facilitate a systematic process of data analysis that can be communicated to others [11]. These qualitative software programs may have facilitated the process of determining contextual categories, yet due to the enormous data set, the programs were of limited use for the purposes of this study.

4. A Relational Database Management System

Prior to the mid 1980s, researchers utilized word processing and database programs to aid in the organization and analysis of textual data. Database management programs allow the researcher the ability to create, store, search, sort, and group phenomenologically valid units of data [12]. Several disadvantages of utilizing a database management program for organizing and categorizing qualitative data have been identified. Historically, powerful database programs have been difficult to learn and use. Pfaffenberger [12] noted that most database management programs do not permit changes in the structure of the database once the data has been entered. Those that do allow changes place limits on the scope of reorganization that is possible. Tesch [6] reported that when using database managers, the data must be structured before entry or the boundaries of the text passages are not indicated in the retrieved material, resulting in segments which consist of entire paragraphs or a specified number of lines or words instead of representing the meaning unit.

Due to the nature of the data which emerged in this study, a database management program seemed to offer a feasible alternative to utilizing a qualitative software package. As text segments to be coded and organized were in the form of short answer responses or fairly brief statements, an entire text segment could be contained in one field. Paradox® [13], a full-featured relational database management system, was chosen for this project. All information in Paradox® is arranged in tables. Each table is comprised of fields designated by the user. Fields are defined by entering a field name, defining the field type, and indicating whether or not it is a key field. Field types include: alphanumeric, numeric, currency, short number, and date fields. A table can always be redesigned as fields can be modified, inserted, or deleted at any time. The user can work with data in a table or on a form, and changes in one are immediately reflected in the other.

Paradox® query ability is the heart and soul of the program. The user can create queries to find or select information from a table, combine information from more than one table, perform calculations on the data, insert new or delete old data, change selected values, and define groups and sets of information on which to perform calculations and comparisons. The user can query up to 24 concurrently open tables provided the tables contain identical key fields. In constructing query statements, one enters an example in a field, essentially telling the program to display only those records that have certain values in one or more fields. Paradox® provides 41 query operators which aid in the process of sorting the data by set conditions. Queries can be constructed according to any single parameter or by any desired combination or sequence of characters. Other fields are then selected to appear in the answer table by inserting a check make via a function key.

TABLE 1. An example of a Paradox® table with coded data

Problems	PTID	Time	Source	Type	Subtype
I can't breathe	1	1	1	1	1
Respiratory status	1	1	2	1	1
Diarrhea	1	1	2	2	
Activity intolerance	1	1	3	1	2
O2 Saturations down	1	1	3	1	1
Potential for hypothermia	1	1	4	1	3
Activity intolerance: ADLs	1	1	4	1	2
Potential for injury; safety	1	1	5	1	12
Disturbances of emotional well-being	1	1	5	3	
Impaired gas exchange	1	1	6	1	1
Potential for hypothermia	1	1	6	1	3

For the purposes of this study, Paradox® provided a reliable data reduction method and allowed for the preservation of the original integrity of the data. The program accommodated the need for the classification of broader contextual categories, the subclassification of these categories, and the inclusion of additional variables of interest (Table 1). Paradox® provided a mechanism for tabulating data and importing numerical data into a statistical software package. The powerful query function allows for the retrieval of data in a variety of ways. Paradox® is simple to utilize and is designed for computer users with all levels of experience. Paradox® is highly visual and is a menu driven system. Context sensitive online help is available and the manual is well written and easy to use. In short, Paradox® provides novice and expert users with significant versatility and the power to perform complex functions. Paradox® appeared to be the most efficient and effective software program for organizing and analyzing this data.

5. Conclusion

As Knafl and Webster [11] suggested, the purposes of a study and the research questions proposed dictate the manner in which data is organized and categorized for eventual analysis. In a descriptive study, coding is more refined and is a means to the researcher's ultimate intent of identifying and delineating major descriptive themes. Likewise, the intent of coding and the specifics of coding techniques vary according to the purposes of a study. If the purpose it to collect qualitative data for illustrating quantitative results of various categories, the coding scheme is derived from variables or constructs measured in the larger study. For the purposes of instrument development, the aim of the coding scheme is to classify the range of subjects' responses so they can be translated into structured questions or scales.

Therefore the appropriate class of software programs to be utilized for the purposes of organizing and categorizing data is dependent upon the purposes of the study and the research questions to be examined. In studies where lengthy segments of textual data need to be preserved in their original form, a qualitative software package appears to be most appropriate. For studies where the nature of the data is in short narrative responses or fairly brief written statements, a relational database management system offers the researcher additional functions and versatility.

A relational database management system appears to be an ideal software program for the purposes of instrument development. The responses to open ended questions can be entered into the program and then responses can be coded and tabulated. A relational database manager also holds great promise for examining the reliability of a coding scheme. The reliability of the coding scheme can be assessed in two ways. Interrater reliability and intrarater reliability can be determined by computing correlations on individual ratings. Querying on the particular derived categories and listing the associated textual data allows for a team of experts to review the data that has been assigned to a particular category. This method would also enhance the validity of a particular coding scheme. Paradox® provides the researcher with a powerful tool for coding analyzing short answer open ended responses while maintaining the original integrity of the data. Differences among individuals and or groups of individuals can be easily identified by performing a simple query. Once the coding has been completed, the data can easily be exported to a statistical package for additional analyses.

Acknowledgments. This study was supported by "Quality of Nursing Care of Persons with AIDS," NIH-NCNR-R01NR02215, W.L. Holzemer, Principal Investigator. We thank the members of the Quality of AIDS care team and our clinical collaborators for their continued support.

References

[1] Holzemer WL and Henry SB. Computer-supported versus manually generated nursing care plans: A comparison of problems, nursing interventions, and patient outcomes. *Comput Nurs* 1992, 10:19–24.
[2] Holzemer WL and Henry SB. Nursing care plans for people with HIV/AIDS: Confusing or consensus? *J Adv Nurs* 1991, 16:257–261.
[3] Henry SB, Holzemer WL, and Reilly C. Nurses' perceptions of the problems of hospitalized PCP patients: Implications for the development of a nursing taxonomy. In: *Proceedings of the Fifteenth Annual Symposium on Computer Applications in Medical Care*, 1991. Los Alamitos, CA: IEEE Computer Society Press.
[4] Janson-Bjerkile S, Holzemer WL, and Henry SB. Patients' perceptions of problems and nursing interventions during hospitalization for *Pneumocystis carinii* pneumonia. *Am J Criti Care* 1992, 1:114–121.

[5] Leonard VW. Heideggerian phenomenologic perspective on the concept of the person. *ANS Adv Nurs Sci* 1989, 11:40–55.

[6] Tesch R. Computer programs that assist in the analysis of qualitative data: An overview. *Qual Health Res* 1991, 1:309–325.

[7] Tesch R. Software for qulitative researchers: Analysis needs and program capablities. In: *Using Computers in Qualitative Research.* NG Fielding and RM Lee (eds). Newbury Park, CA: Sage 199:16–37.

[8] Richards L and Richards T. Computing in qualitative analysis: A healthy development? *Qual Health Res* 1991, 1:234–262.

[9] Seidel JV, Kjolseth R, and Seymour E. *The Ethnograph®: A User's Guide (Version 3.0).* Littleton, Colorado: Qualis Research Associates 1988.

[10] Diekelmann NL, Lam S, and Schuster RM. *MARTIN® (Version 2.0).* Madison, Wisconsin: School of Nursing, University of Wisconsin-Madison 1991.

[11] Knafl KA and Webster DC. Managing and analyzing qualitative data: A description of tasks, techniques, and materials. *West J Nurs Res* 1988, 10:195–218.

[12] Pfaffenberger B. *Microcomputer applications in qualitative research.* Newbury Park, CA: Sage Publications 1988.

[13] Borland International. *Paradox® (Version 3.5).* Scotts Valley, CA: Author 1990.

67
The Development of a System for Computer Aided Research in Nursing (CARIN)

Betty L. Chang and Stephan Gilbert

Introduction

The purpose of this paper is to report on a portable system for the collection of patient interview and examination data. This system will automatically abstract the information for interfacing with commercial statistical packages such as SAS and BMD-P. Traditionally, nurse researchers have recorded patient questionnaire and physical examination data on paper forms. According to this method, the completed forms had to be coded, a code book developed, and the coded numerical data then entered into the computer in either 80-column or free-form formats for statistical analysis. The coding had to be verified carefully for errors, and "cleaned" prior to being used for statistical analysis. This procedure was extremely labor intensive and expensive.

Background

Although some clinical research software (e.g., Clinical Research System, 1983/84)[1] are available, they include only a limited ability to answer queries, and to perform standard descriptive procedures. However, these queries and procedures are much too limited for the types of analysis used by nurse researchers. Systems have been reported on audit systems for ambulatory care in medicine.[2] These audit systems address quite a different database than databases of concern to nurse researchers.

The interview questions for the present system were based on an extensive nursing assessment guide developed by faculty members at the University of California, Los Angeles (UCLA).[3] This guide also has been

Reprinted with permission from *Proceedings: Twelfth Annual Symposium on Computer Applications in Medical Care*, Greenes, R.A. (Ed.). 1988, pp. 801–803. © 1987, American Medical Informatics Association (formerly SCAMC): Bethesda, MD.

subsequently refined based on a number of reliability and validity studies.[4] The guide has been used as a basis for a separate and quite different system for nursing diagnosis and intervention reported in detail elsewhere.[5]

The prototype for Computer-Aided Research in Nursing (CARIN) has been developed primarily for use by nurse researchers. It is being tested at the UCLA Medical Center, and we hope to have it prepared for nation-wide beta-site testing in the near future.

User Considerations in Design

Major considerations in the design of the CARIN software were that: (a) there must be minimal data entry time; the patient interview and physical examination data be entered easily with a minimum of time spent at the computer, (b) there must be user modifiability for future changes in assessment data, for example, in the event of a change in nomenclature for nursing diagnosis, or for use in specialized patient-care units, (c) the data output and abstraction in numerical code format must be automatic so as to avoid having to "punch-in" the data at the end of a study.

Minimizing Data Entry Time: User Interface

Anticipating that the Clinical Nurse Specialist (CNS) will enter the data while interviewing and examining the patient, the data entry time must be minimal. The design and layout of the user interface should not only allow the user to operate the program with ease, but also allow the researcher to quickly move along within the assessment guide. Time consuming keystroke repetitions, unnecessary screen-crowding, and long pauses while executing had to be avoided. The assessment guide was programmed as a series of questions with fixed choice and write-in answers. If the answer was of the simple type "yes/no," a "no" answer was entered as a default value recorded simply by pressing "return." In case of a complex answer, the researcher typed in the keywords directly to display the available list of keywords from which she/he can choose.

The program responded by displaying the answer, and proceeding to the next question. The researcher can also open a "note pad" to describe the findings in her/his own words. A set of menus is also available to return to a previous question or suspend the assessment.

User Modifiability

Constant modifications and/or additions to the assessment guide dictated an engine architecture whereby all relevant information is directly linked to each individual question. The assessment processing "engine" requires a fixed set of tokens and a rigid data format thus implementing a standardization of the questions and patient answer data set. By following simple instructions, the researcher can update the questions without the need of a system analyst or programmer. Whenever the assessment guide is edited, a compiler will be invoked to translate the guide to the appropriate data base format.

Data Output and Abstraction

After completing an assessment, the researcher may print out a summary of the abnormal findings for the patient records and for CNS information in formulating care plans. The program also adds the normal as well as abnormal findings to the statistical data file (standard ASCII text file) upon request. This standard file will allow further processing by any well-known statistics program package such as SAS, SPSS, and BMD. Several support functions enable the researcher to translate files from older to newer versions of the assessment guide and to print out an alphabetical list of the variables within their respective categories. It is anticipated that the format of the output file(s) generated during a session can be readily used to construct a knowledge base for a diagnosis and intervention expert system in the future.

Program Implementation

The hardware selected was a portable computer that can be taken to the bedside. The rationale for this was based on the principle that the data should be entered as close to the source as possible. This procedure eliminated the duplication of labor that would be required if the interview data had to be recorded on paper at the bedside and transcribed to a centrally located computer.

The program was written to run on IBM AT compatible lap top computers such as Toshiba 3100. The modules and interfaces were written in a combination of languages (Prolog, C) using a set of previously written support functions. The program runs in a window environment. A help screen is available to refresh the researcher's memory in determining the various levels according to prespecified definitions (e.g., levels of independence in self-care).

An example of the dialogue developed from the assessment guide can be seen in Figure 1.

1) Have thare been any major changes in your life in the last year or two? Yes

> Move
> Marriage
> School (graduate or starting)
> new job
> hospitalization
> children
> illness
> [other]*

2) What were the changes?

> Nota Pad: Please type-in

3) When you face a problem or change, how often do you use the following ways to cope with stress?

> 1 never
> [2 occasionally   ]*
> 3 half the time
> 4 often
> 5 always

> a. Think through different ways of solving the problem.
> [b. Find out more about the situation.]*
> c. Put the problem out of mind/Think of something else.
> d. Get mad, worry, cry, take off by yourself.
> e. Pray, put trust in God/Daydream fantasize.
> f. Accept situation as it is/Resign yourself do nothing and hope situation will improve.
> g. Sleep, meditate, exercise/eat, smoke, drink alcohol, take drugs.
> h. Seek comfort or help from Family/friends.
> i. Other

* Highlighted areas are answers selected by user.

FIGURE 1. Example of a dialogue.

Summary

We have reported on a prototype system for Computer-Aided Research in Nursing (CARIN), designed to facilitate the coding and retrieval of data in a cumulative fashion for future statistical analysis. This prototype is being field tested at UCLA at the present time. The patients and staff nurses have been very accepting of the system. The nurse researchers are able to directly enter the data from the patients' charts, then proceed to the patient's bedside for the interview and physical examination. All data are automatically entered in an ASCII file format for statistical analysis eliminating the need to re-enter and clean the data.

This system has resulted in a considerable savings of time. Total data collection for each patient takes approximately 45 minutes to one hour. In the past, the coding of this information took approximately 4 hours for each patient. In addition, a second research assistant spent approximately 2 to 3 hours for verification and "cleaning up" of the data. In CARIN, the coding is automatic such that 6 to 7 hours of time is saved from the coding time frame for each patient. This software has substantially reduced the cost of data coding for statistical analysis, as well as the tedious chore of entering hundreds and thousands of numerical codes per patients.

References

[1.] Shideman, J.R. (1983/4). *Clinical Research System CRS*; International Medical Products Corporation, 4503 Moorland Avenue, Minneapolis, Minnesota, 55424, USA.

[2.] McCoy, M.J., Dunn, E.V., Borgiel, A.E. (1987). A Portable Computer System for Auditing Quality of Ambulatory Care. W.W. Stead (Ed.). *Proceedings of the 11th Annual Symposium on Computer Applications in Medical Care*, Nov. 1–4, Washington, D.C. IEEE, Computer Society Press, pp. 655–658.

[3.] Chang, B.L., Eisz, M., McAuliffe, M. Development of a tool for research on nursing diagnosis. (1985). *Summary of Presentations of the Meeting of the Council of Nurse Researchers: Nursing Research: Integration, into the Social Structure*, San Diego, CA.

[4.] Chang, B.L., Gonzales, E., Caswell, D. (1988). Reliability and Validity of an Assessment Guide for Nursing Diagnosis. *Australian Journal of Advanced Nursing*, Dec.–Feb., 5(2), 16–22.

[5.] Chang, B.L., Roth, K., Gonzales, E., Caswell, D., DiStefano, J. (1988). CANDI: A Knowledge-Based System for Nursing Diagnosis. *Computers in Nursing*, Jan.–Feb., 6(1), 13–21.

68
High Performance Computing for Nursing Research

S.L. MEINTZ

1. Introduction

From the validation of supercomputing for nursing and health data research in 1991 to supercomputers powering nursing research discoveries in 1992, research efforts continue to maximize the utilization of supercomputers for data research in nursing, health science, and associated disciplines. A window of opportunity was opened for nurse researchers through the UNLV/ CRAY Project for Nursing and Health Data Research (PNHDR) of the University of Nevada, Las Vegas, USA, to determine the viability of supercomputing for analyzing huge datasets of health data archived by government and nongovernment sources (Meintz, 1992). Analysis of such large samples of population could support or nullify the current theories supporting nursing practice and the foundations of health care. Although supercomputers seem necessary to analyze huge datasets of archived health data, the use of the supercomputer by nursing researchers demanded a break from traditional methodologies.

Nurse researchers typically use classical analysis to formulate theories—that is, they reduce data to a manageable size and form generalizations for larger populations and broader theories. Frequently the sample size is barely large enough to be statistically significant; however, the research results are added to the body of scientific nursing knowledge, and nursing practice is based on this theory without the benefit of validation from huge samples.

With a Cray Research grant to PNHDR, the supercomputer application was able to open new directions for analysis. For the first time, nursing science entered the high performance computing environment to confirm,

Reprinted from *Nursing Informatics: An International Overview for Nursing in a Technological Era*, Grobe, S.J., Pluyter-Wenting, E.S.P. (Eds.). 1994, pp. 448–451, with kind permission from Elsevier Science—NL, Sara Burgerhartstraat 25, 1055 KV Amsterdam, The Netherlands.

nullify, and/or deduce new parameters in nursing and health science with the ultimate goal of providing better prescriptive and preventative health care within controlled economic boundaries. Parameters of health previously established with a sample size of 1,000 could now be evaluated with a sample size of 25,000 to 50,000 to 10 million.

2. Research and Development (R&D) Methodology

The PNHDR's R&D project involves seven phases of research and development. The phases include: (1) Conceptualization of complex problem resolution, (2) Design of product and/or process, (3) Development of product and/or process, (4) Dissemination of preliminary results and/or prototypes, (5) Alpha site application for testing and debugging, (6) Beta site application for refinement and further debugging, and (7) Dissemination of product and/or process through software, manuals, educational programs, publications, and/or presentations. The phases are independent and interrelated resulting in a multilevel approach for supercomputing application to establishing the foundational parameters of health through mega/tera data base analysis.

To facilitate the R&D effort, a framework for application of supercomputing to nursing and health data research was developed as a means to clarify the input, throughput, output, and outcome of R&D phase one. Pioneer efforts by nursing scientists to enter the high performance computing environment with application of the CRAY Y-MP 2/216 Supercomputer were successful in validation of the supercomputer application. The validation Case Study utilized a manageable data base of 17,000 cases and analyses with the Statistical Package for Social Scientists (SPSS) using computer platforms including personal computer, Sun, and the Cray supercomputer. Needless to say, the personal computer was unable to process the analysis and the Sun was slower than the CRAY Y-MP which completed the analysis in approximately 127 seconds.

3. Research Progress

Although nursing professionals are relative latecomers to the high performance computing and communication environment, this path to discovery is well worth the effort. Through the use of the Cray Research system, databases with millions to trillions of bytes can be analyzed in seconds instead of hours or days. Critical elements related to humans and the nursing meta paradigm are available in many diverse databases—databases whose size demands the capabilities of supercomputing for analysis.

While the supercomputing solution seems like the only current option, barriers to this application also exist. Most nursing researchers need new skills to facilitate supercomputing applications, even with the assistance of engineers and computer scientists. Supercomputing standards, while generally familiar to traditional users, are not familiar to nursing professionals who are accustomed to a personal computer interface. Additionally, many of the available statistical software packages for high performance computing require programming, a skill not currently taught in nursing curricula, and very few nurse scientists understand the components or architecture of supercomputers. Although they may be skilled in the use of a personal computer and its role in secondary data analysis on small datasets, they need further knowledge to analyze large datasets with supercomputers.

Nurse researchers also are limited by existing tools. Because their personal computers are constrained by performance and lack of connection to important networks, nurse researchers using supercomputers often must "borrow" the workstation of a scientist or engineer, run the program, and print out the results which often consist of reams of paper for a relatively simple analysis in order to share these results with other researchers. Traditional users of supercomputers have ready access to a networked workstation and can often view results in graphical form and share them easily with others via an electronic connection.

The application of supercomputing in the nursing profession has generated a new branch of nursing science called *Nurmetrics* which incorporates the two specialties of Computational Nursing and Nursing Informatics (Meintz, 1992). Each is defined:

Nurmetrics, the branch of nursing science applying mathematical form and statistical techniques to the testing, estimation, and quantifying of nursing theories and solutions of nursing problems.

Computational Nursing, the branch of Nurmetrics using mathematical/computer models and simulation systems for the application of existing theory and numerical methods to new solutions for nursing problems or the development of new computational methods.

Nursing Informatics, the branch of Nurmetrics applying the principles of computer science and informatics to understanding the interplay of the architecture of information form (data, text, audio, visual) with information function (generating, processing, storing, and transmitting) for the solving of problems in nursing administration, nursing education, nursing practice, and/or nursing research.

Nurmetrics with computational nursing and nursing informatics represents a new specialty area within Computational Health Sciences. Nursing has been identified as an appropriate alternative to expensive health care costs; therefore, nurse researchers utilizing the principles of nurmetrics can be expected to impact significantly the future of health care.

These new directions in nursing will form the foundation for new discoveries powered by supercomputing. The framework for application of supercomputing to nursing and health data research illustrates the components involved in the conceptualization of complex problem resolution for supercomputer application. A paradigm shift in statistical analysis to Global Analysis Tera Exploratory Statistics (GATES) has occurred. GATES provided the direction for development of a prototype software and the conceptualization of VuSTAT, a graphic user interface linking GATES with computer model simulations emphasizing trends.

Although there are many barriers to analyzing datasets with supercomputers, it is the only current resource that can support this nursing and health application. The PHNDR's goal is to address the outstanding issues, making the supercomputing solution easily accessible to nursing researchers. As identified by current PNHDR research, ease of access will not be possible until: (1) a new statistical program is created to analyze trends in massive datasets, (2) all interfaces required by nursing researchers are transparent and include a visual postprocessing package, (3) current social science statistical software packages are modified for mega datasets, and (4) nursing researchers are teamed with the traditional users of supercomputers—engineers, computer scientists, and computational scientists.

4. Importance of the Research

Nursing research utilizing mega/tera data bases typically applies one of two analysis pathways—either (1) to confirm or nullify what is existing or (2) to establish new relationships (or parameters) not previously discerned. To confirm or nullify what is existing can be accomplished by modifying current statistical analysis methodologies to run on the CRAY Supercomputer and by addressing technical problems related to handling the mega/tera data sets. However, to established new relationships not previously discovered involved the development of a technical presentation of data in a visual format allowing the nursing scientist to see the new relationship. The primary importance of this phase of the PNHDR project was to conceptualize the path and design the tools necessary to result in a paradigm shift from models identifying specifics toward the general to models that present mega/tera data in a format allowing the nursing scientist to visualize new relationships. The paradigm shift in statistical analysis has resulted in the design of Global Analysis Tera Exploratory Statistics (GATES). The software prototype for GATES was designed using 249 megabytes of data from the Hispanic Health and Nutrition Examination Survey obtained from the National Center for Health Statistics. The prototype was a joint design effort with Vance Faber, Ph.D., Group Leader, Computer Research and Applications Group, Los Alamos National Laboratory. The application of GATES and other new methodologies will lead to the establishment of a scientific foundational baseline for the parameters of health across the life span through analysis of mega/tera databases. Without establishing a foundational baseline, difficulty is experienced in monitoring trends, predicting intervention impacts, or controlling allocation of scarce resources—both human and fiscal. From the scientific foundation for parameters of health emerge the mechanisms for monitoring health trends, determining health cost control methods, identifying impacts on global health care, coordinating environmental data with health data, and providing the scientific information for the future biotech revolution.

Currently, approximately 250 gigabytes of nursing and health data exist in the United States alone. The supercomputer would allow for perusal of this data in about 10 hours. Because researchers benefit from the ability to access and analyze the mega/tera data sets, a Data Analysis Network Initiative (DANI) with a Health Interactive-Data Analysis Network (HI-DAN) is proposed. The DANI would provide a communication link from the researcher's location to the high performance computing capability with an interactive nursing and health data archive for access and analysis.

5. Summary

Nursing research has found a new source of power in the high performance computing and communication environment with the application of the CRAY Y-MP 2/216 supercomputer. The paradigm shift in statistical analysis to Global Analysis Tera Exploratory Statistics (GATES) redefines the statistical methodology for analysis of mega/tera databases using data visualization as a supercomputer completes computations in seconds or minutes. The avenue for including graphic user interfaces to link GATES with computer model simulations and data analysis networks provides for future directions. In the future, after establishing the foundational parameters of health, new applications may lead to a formula for predicting effects of nursing action and intervention on health trends, or application of virtual reality techniques for educating both laypersons and professionals about health parameters, or a means for analysis of acute care data as the data are being collected. The possibilities for discovery and advancement in Nurmetrics, Computational Nursing, and Nursing Informatics are significant when the high performance computing and communication environment is explored with a CRAY Y-MP supercomputer for analyses of mega/tera datasets in nursing and health.

Acknowledgements. This research is supported by Cray Research, Inc., National Supercomputing Center for Energy and Environment, National Center for Health Statistics, Advance Computing Laboratories, Los Alamos National Laboratory, and Silicon Graphics, Inc.

References

[1] Meintz S. Supercomputers Open Window of Opportunity for Nursing. *Computers in Nursing* in press for May 1993.

[2] Meintz S. Supercomputer Application to Nursing and Health Data Research. In *Communicating Nursing Research Vol. 25:489*. Boulder: Western Institute of Nursing.

[3] Meintz S. Supercomputer Application to Nursing Data Research. Podium Presentation: *First Japanese International Research Conference* Japan: Tokyo, 1992.

[4] Meintz S. Supercomputers Power Discoveries in Nursing. *Cray Channels* 1992, 14:20–21.

69
Computer Support for Power Analysis in Nursing Research

Steven M. Paul

1. Introduction

One of the most frequently asked questions during the planning stages of any research study is how large a sample is needed. The basis for such a decision must take into account a power analysis. That is, the systematic determination of the probability that the statistical tests proposed for the study will lead to the rejection of stated null hypotheses. The sometimes tedious calculations necessary to perform statistical power analyses have been dramatically simplified with the advent of computer applications that assist the researcher in manipulating the components of the process in an interactive fashion. This paper describes the use of computer assisted power analysis.

The power of a statistical test can be thought of as its likelihood of detecting a significant effect, if one indeed exists. A well-designed and thoughtfully planned research study should have a good chance of detecting clinically relevant and meaningful relationships or perhaps of detecting differences between contrasting treatments. The ability to generalize sample results to the population that a study sample is intended to represent is often based on statistical hypothesis testing procedures. Achieving statistical significance is a common criteria by which the merit of many research projects are judged. Although many other factors must be considered, it is vital that research in nursing be carried out with a full understanding of the power of statistical tests to detect significant findings.

Power analyses have become mandatory requirements for any research proposals that compete for funding at a federal, state, or local institutional level. A grant proposal that does not include considerations of statistical

Reprinted from *Nursing Informatics: An International Overview for Nursing in a Technological Era*, Grobe, S.J., Pluyter-Wenting, E.S.P. (Eds.). 1994, pp. 491–494, with kind permission from Elsevier Science—NL, Sara Burgerhartstraat 25, 1055 KV Amsterdam, The Netherlands.

power when attempting to justify the proposed project's sample size will most likely be dismissed as incomplete. Funding agencies need to know that their money will be well spent. They want to be assured that there is a reasonable chance that the project will be able to detect what it is intended to find.

2. Hypothesis Testing and the Parameters of Power

To understand how computers have become invaluable aids to the researcher concerned with power estimations. a brief description of hypothesis testing procedures and the parameters involved in power calculations is required.

A null hypothesis is "the hypothesis that the phenomenon to be demonstrated is in fact absent [1]." One does not hope to support this hypothesis. In fact, typically the researcher hopes to reject this hypothesis in favor of the alternative that the phenomenon in question is in fact present [2]. Results from a random sample drawn from a population will only approximate the characteristics of the population. Consequently, even if the null hypothesis is, in fact, true, a given sample result is not expected to mirror this fact exactly. The researcher must consequently set appropriate probability standards, i.e., significance criteria, for research results which provide a basis for rejection of the null hypothesis. The significance level is selected before the sample data are gathered. The researcher selects an appropriately small criterion value, such as the typical .05, so that the following statement may be made. If the null hypothesis is true, the probability of the obtained sample result is no more than 5%, a statistically significant result. The idea being that the probability of the sample result is so low as to bring the truth of the null hypothesis into question. The null hypothesis is rejected at the stated probability significance level, also referred to as the alpha (α) level or Type I error rate. If the probability of the sample result is greater than the stated alpha level, the researcher has failed to reject the null hypothesis at that particular significance level. The alpha level is the risk of mistakenly rejecting the null hypothesis when it is true, that is, drawing a spuriously positive conclusion (Type I error). The beta (β) value is the probability of failing to reject the null hypothesis when it is false (Type II error).

Any given statistical test of a null hypothesis can be viewed as a complex relationship among the following four parameters [3]:

1. The power of the test, defined as $1-\beta$ (the probability of rejecting the null hypothesis).
2. The region of rejection of the null hypothesis as determined by the α level and whether the test is one tailed or two tailed. As α increases, power increases.

3. The sample size, n. As n increases, power increases.
4. The magnitude of the effect in the population, or the degree of departure from the null hypothesis. The larger the effect size the greater the power.

These four parameters are so related that when any three of them are fixed, the fourth is completely determined. Consequently, when a researcher decides for a particular research scenario, the α level, estimated effect size, and desired level of power, the sample size is determined. The most common level of desired power found in nursing research is .80. The investigator would like to have an 80% chance of detecting a statistically significant effect. Unfortunately, the power analysis process is most typically hindered by the fact that the researcher does not know the magnitude of the effect size in the population. Without this restriction, power analyses would not be too much more than a series of straightforward mathematical calculations.

Jacob Cohen, the authority on power analyses for the behavioral sciences, suggests three general strategies for determining the size of the population effect that a researcher is trying to detect:

1. Previous research. Pilot work by the current researcher or studies that others have conducted involving the variables and relationships closely related to the study being planned can reflect the magnitude of effect that can be expected. Review of relevant literature or perhaps a meta-analysis of the issue can help suggest a reasonable range of expected values.

2. Practical significance. Conceptually different from statistical significance, in some research areas the investigator may be aware of some minimum population effect that would have either practical or theoretical significance. As an example, a nurse researcher may decide that the effect of a new procedure for reducing blood pressure in adolescents facing surgery would have to show an effect of at least 10 points before she would be willing to suggest changing current policy.

3. Conventional definitions. One can use certain suggested, conventional definitions of small, medium, and large effects provided by Cohen in his classic text on power analysis [2]. These conventional effect size values may be used by choosing one or by determining power for all three population effect sizes. The researcher could then make revisions in the research plan based on his estimates of the various effect sizes to the particular problem at hand.

Although previous research and practical significance are preferred methods for estimating population effect sizes. The availability of computerized power programs enables an investigator almost unlimited options in calculating the power and sample size requirement for dozens of potential effect size estimates and research scenarios.

3. Procedures Available in Power Programs

Two power analysis computer programs that are currently available are *Statistical Power Analysis: A Computer Program* by Michael Borenstein and Jacob Cohen [4] and *SOLO Statistical System Power Analysis* by Jerry Hintze [5]. The Cohen and Borenstein program provides power calculations for t-tests for the difference between two means, correlations, the difference between proportions, one-way and factorial analysis of variance (ANOVA), and multiple regression and correlation. It does not, however, deal specifically with repeated measures analyses. Hintze's SOLO program includes all of the statistical procedures mentioned above and in addition includes the nonparametric analogues to the independent samples t-test (Mann-Whitney) and matched paired t-test (Wilcoxin), repeated measures ANOVA, the difference between two correlations, log-rank survival tests, logistic regression, matched case-control, and bioequivalence for means or for proportions. The Borenstein and Cohen program can generate Monte Carlo simulations. These simulations enable the researcher to run a study on the computer and determine whether or not the findings are likely to be significant, before gathering data on the actual subjects. In the simulations procedure the researcher uses the program to create populations that mirror the intended hypothesis. Both programs have the capability of producing graphic plots that show values of power for various alpha levels and sample sizes at specific effect size estimations.

4. An Example

The most commonly used statistical test is the two-sample t-test. There are several variations of the t-test. The standard deviations of the two groups may be known or unknown, equal or unequal. The sample sizes of the two groups may be equal or unequal. The underlying distribution of the data may or may not be normal. The following example, based on a scenario presented by Cohen and Borenstein [4], will illustrate the use and flexibility of computer assisted power analysis.

A researcher plans to run a study in which patients suffering from muscle spasms will be treated with either Drug-A or placebo. After a month of treatment the level of spasms, defined as the rating on a 40-point scale, will be compared in the two groups. The analysis is initiated by providing the following estimates and values: Drug-A mean = 20, Placebo mean = 24; standard deviation for both groups = 10, sample size for both groups = 20. The test will be done at a two-tailed alpha of .05. Because the drug carries the risk of serious side effects, its use would be appropriate only if it could effect a clear and substantive improvement, that is a large effect. Cohen [2] defines the effect size, d, for the two-sample t-test as the difference between the two population means divided by the population standard deviation. He gives guidelines that suggest that a small d is .20, a medium d is .50, and a large d is .80. The power program would indicate that for the initial estimates the effect size is only, .40, which is somewhere between small and medium. The researcher can elect to modify the population estimates. She decides to lower the estimate of the Drug-A mean from 20 to 18. She also decides that her initial estimate of the population standard deviations were too high and lowers them from 10 to 8. The program would indicate that the new estimated effect size is .75, which is just below large. The researcher may now decide that the effect is now large enough to be substantively important.

The program would indicate that the power for the current status of the parameters would be .64. The researcher desires the power to be at least .80. She changes the sample size estimates upward and watches as the program indicates the change in power that corresponds with the changes in sample size. When the sample size for both groups reaches 30, the power equals .81. When the sample size reaches 38 per group, the power equals .90. The sample size would have to equal 47 per group for the power to be .95. The researcher can then decide what sample size best fits with her needs, expectations, time constraints, and other factors that impact on the research process.

5. Practical Applications

The advantage of an interactive power analysis program is that one can see instantly what the effect of changing one parameter has on any of the other parameters. This is often most easy to see when one uses either the table presentation or graphic plot options of the programs. Often many different scenarios are investigated before a reasonable compromise between desired power and needed sample size may be reached. The ease and speed with which the computer can make the necessary calculations makes this intensive but necessary process feasible. Power calculations should be examined for every statistical test that will be performed in a study. With knowledge of the sample size requirements for each specific analysis, the sample requirements for the entire study can be efficiently determined.

Although the experience of many investigators is one in which their power analysis indicates that the sample size necessary to provide them with a reasonable chance of detecting what they are after is larger than they might have hoped for, it is also quite possible that the sample size requirements derived from a thorough power analysis may be much less than what was originally thought to be necessary.

If the sample size for a particular research study cannot be increased, due perhaps to the limited availability of subjects that meet the study's entry requirements, a power analysis is still a worthwhile endeavor. Why would one go to the time and expense of conducting a study that has only a 50%

chance of finding significance when significance actually exists and it is of practical importance? It would be better to know what the limitations of the study are at the outset of the process and cancel the project if need be, than to find out too late. Perhaps by considering alternative recruitment strategies or increasing the value of alpha, e.g., from .01 to .05, one could increase the likelihood of finding significance to an acceptable level.

While the most common use of power analysis is to determine sample size during the design phase of a study, it is also legitimate to conduct a post hoc power analysis after a study is concluded. Questions that can be answered include: What sample size would have been needed to detect a difference (or relationship) of the magnitude observed in the study with alpha = .05 and power = .80? What is the smallest difference (effect size) that could be detected with this sample size, at certain values of alpha and power?

Consider a researcher whose intent is not to reject the null hypothesis. In situations where an investigator would like to show that there are no differences between two treatments, for example, simply not rejecting the null hypothesis of no difference is not enough. Any critic of the study could claim that a significant difference does actually exist in the population in question, but that the study did not have the adequate power to detect it. If the researcher could determine the magnitude of the difference between the treatments that would be of practical importance, it would be possible to determine if the study could have detected this treatment effect. If the conclusion of the study is not to reject the null hypothesis, the researcher can be confident that no real important difference exists between the treatments.

Statistical power is only one of the many considerations that are part of developing the scientific merit of a research project. Researchers must also pull from their extensive clinical and practical experiences and the research of others when developing a study. The necessary power calculations, which can give a research proposal the justification that it deserves, have become easy and accessible through the use of computerized power programs.

References

[1] Fisher, R.A. *The Design of Experiments*. New York: Hafner, 1949.
[2] Cohen, J. *Statistical Power Analysis for the Behavioral Sciences*, Second Edition. Hillsdale, New Jersey: Lawrence Erlbaum, 1988.
[3] Cohen, J. and Cohen, P. *Applied Multiple Regression/Correlation Analysis for the Behavioral Sciences*, Second Edition. Hillsdale, New Jersey: Lawrence Erlbaum, 1983.
[4] Borenstein, M. and Cohen, J. *Statistical Power Analysis: A Computer Program*. Hillsdale, New Jersey: Lawrence Erlsbaum, 1988.
[5] Hintze, J. *SOLO Statistical System Power Analysis*. Los Angeles: BMDP Statistical Software, Inc., 1991.

Part V
Nursing Education

The opportunities for nurse educators to utilize computers, not only as teaching tools, but also as the focus point in the development of nursing informatics curricula, have taken a quantum leap during the past twenty years. In addition, students who use the computer as a learning tool now have a myriad of technology selections and content areas available. Section V provides a veritable treasure of selected articles for nurses interested in utilizing computers as a teaching tool and in preparing nurses and students to function with computer technology in the education and clinical environments.

The first article by Ronald looks at the relationship between the computer's use in the practice and education environments and the administration that nurse educators need to think "in totally different, if not revolutionary ways, in light of the challenges and opportunities provided to us by the computer." This is a good first article to read in preparation for the more specific ones in this section of the anthology. It sets the tone for nurse educators who are interested in computer technology. The remaining articles can be grouped into five broad categories: curriculum, computer-assisted instruction (CAI), clinical decision making, distance learning, and competence/attitudes of users.

If one accepts the premise that a sound curriculum is the basic requirement for successful nursing informatics programs, the first category of articles should be of interest. Ronald's second article provides educators with a succinct overview of her school's (State University of New York at Buffalo) preparation of students in nursing informatics from the undergraduate through the graduate level. At the doctoral level, she describes a collaborative model that combines expertise from a School of Nursing and a School of Management. Romano and Heller follow with a comprehensive description of a prototype graduate education curriculum in Nursing Informatics at the University of Maryland. They also discuss the major duties, knowledge required, and resulting interactions related to the nursing informatics role. Aarts provides the reader with an interesting comparison to Romano and Heller's article by describing a postgraduate program in nursing informatics at the Hagenshool Midden Nederland in the Netherlands, which was initiated one year after the University of Maryland's program. Both programs stress the necessity of collaboration with other health care institutions for field experience and practice.

Sinclair's article on "Database Instruction for Nursing Students" complements the above articles on nursing informatics curricula models, because it addresses a specific content area, that is, databases. As databases support every aspect of information processing, this article should be reviewed and kept in mind when nursing curricula are being developed and evaluated by faculty.

Perciful's article moves the reader from the more generic topic of the curriculum to the specifics of implementation methodology, that is, the use of computer-assisted instruction (CAI) within the clinical component of one course in a baccalaureate nursing program. The reader is provided with some interesting questions with respect to curriculum planning and integrating simulations within nursing education. Hodson et al. take CAI another step, as she and her coauthors describe the design, development, and implementation of a simulated HIS for the laboratory experiences of undergraduate nursing students. This article shows the innovation that can take place as faculty become more involved and enthusiastic about computers in the education setting.

The article "Evaluating Computer-Assisted Instruction should be familiar to nurse educators before they pursue CAI as a teaching methodology. Bolwell explains why a computer is a unique delivery system and the attributes that make a CAI program suitable for such delivery. McGuiness' article takes the reader beyond Bolwell's evaluation of CAI programs to the actual implementation of computer-assisted learning (CAL) and computer-managed learning (CML) systems. It includes discussion concoming selecting software, hardware configuration, and location of computers in the learning environment. This information provides a foundation for the nurse educator who is beginning to use computers.

A slightly different approach with CAI is taken by Pogue and Pogue, as they look at CAI through the continuing education and in-service training arenas. The authors conclude that "CAI developed for the practice setting must be different from CAI developed for the academic setting." Devney et al. take CAI another step by describing the use of television as an interactive component of CAI, which is referred to as computer-based interactive video instruction (CBIVI). Especially unique is their experience with and advocacy of error detection as a strategy for teaching the preparation of subcutaneous injections.

The third set of articles address clinical decision making, a major step up from CAI. It is the expert nursing systems that address the clinical decision making that will expand the availability of the expertise of sophisticated clinicians to their colleagues and students. Larson's article first provides readers with an overview of expert systems and nursing practice and then goes on to delineate the process of the development of an expert system to assist nurses caring for AIDS patients. Engberg and White and Hovenga and Whymark's articles offer educators an opportunity to compare the approach of the University of Pittsburg with the approach of the Central Queensland University in Australia in developing and utilizing the computer as a teaching tool for decision making. These programs can provide a blueprint that others can emulate.

The fourth group of articles addresses electronic distance learning through the computer, as approached by different schools. Hodson et al. describe a plan designed to provide technological access for registered nurses enrolled in six televised nursing courses located in a number of strategic geographic areas in a midwestern state. Mikan et al. describe a totally different focus for distance learning in which three geographically distant universities in the United States are connected by electronic communication networking, so that graduate students can interact within and between graduate nursing education programs.

It is fitting that the final two articles address the computer competence and attitudes of computer users. Armstong presents the results of her study of computer competencies for nurse educators in basic and continuing education environments. She warns that "attempting to integrate computer technology into nursing education is certainly more than the placement of equipment and programs." Harsanyi and Kelsey provide the results of a descriptive study of nursing and medical educators' attitudes toward computer technology. It has been expressed by many and confirmed by these authors that competence and attitude can impact mission and proliferation of technological innovations in the education and clinical environments.

All the articles in this section contribute proof to the fact that nursing has come a long way in its sophistication in the use of computer technology. However, there is much more in the future awaiting the innovative, knowledgeable, and risk-taking nurse. The challenge is there and needs to be embraced by the profession and its individual members.

70
The Computer as a Partner in Nursing Practice: Implications for Curriculum Change

Judith S. Ronald

Introduction

Nursing education literature is replete with suggestions for improving the curriculum. Changes in the curriculum development paradigm have been suggested (Bevis & Watson, 1989) as well as specific content changes in response to shifting demographics, changing health care systems and the evolving nursing role. In addition to curriculum issues related to content and process, using the computer for both teaching and testing has been described in the literature.

The most common use of the computer in the nursing curriculum has been as a teaching tool. Its primary purpose has been to modify patterns of access to knowledge by altering the place and time at which knowledge can be accessed. Computer-assisted instruction and interactive video provide remediation, enrichment, practice in clinical decision-making using simulations, and can be used in place of, or in conjunction with, selected classroom and clinical experiences. In addition, the computer is being used in some schools to provide students with experience in automated documentation of patient care using a simulated computerized hospital information system (Hodson, Hansen, & Brougham, 1988). These uses of the computer in education serve to enhance the curriculum as it currently exists as well as to provide students with hands-on experience in using the computer to support the current practice environment. However, such uses do not fully recognize the computer's ability to access, manage and process information in totally different ways not only in the educational environment, but more importantly in the practice environment (Ronald, 1985).

Reprinted with permission from *Nursing Informatics '91: Proceedings of the Post Conference on Health Care Information Technology: Implications for Change*; Marr, P.B., Axford, R.L. & Newbold, S.K. (Eds.). 1991, pp. 149–153. Heidelberg-Berlin, Germany: Springer-Verlag.

The Computer in Nursing Practice

Most nursing education curricula do not take into account the ubiquitous nature of the computer in the health care system and society. It is highly likely that by the year 2000, if not before, most practitioners and students will have their own computer or work station available to them. They will have point of care access to a multi-disciplinary electronic nursing knowledge base. Such a knowledge base has yet to be developed, but initial efforts have been described by Ozbolt and Swain (1990), Evans (1990) and Graves (1987). Students can access the same multi-disciplinary electronic knowledge base used by the practicing nurse, but in different ways and for different purposes. The availability and active use of such a database in the curriculum could dramatically change the current approach to nursing education.

Technology exists that allows nurses to organize, manage and retrieve information from the knowledge base in much the same way they do in their minds—by association. They can create individual pathways that are best suited to their own learning needs. Users can use intuitive approaches in the search for knowledge and choose from learning environments that include text, graphics, sound, video or animation (Skiba and Ronald, 1989).

In addition to using the computer to access a knowledge base, nurses will use it to retrieve patient information and record assessment, planning, implementation and evaluation activities. Decision support systems will assist in the analysis of patient data in relation to the knowledge base to help determine the most appropriate interventions. Nurses will select from a variety of possibilities or generate others not suggested. They will do this through their knowledge of the whole and their ability to integrate and synthesize information provided by the computer and their own knowledge of the patient and his family.

Not only will health care professionals have access to information, but patients too will be able to retrieve information about themselves and their condition using computers in health care facilities, individual homes, doctors offices, libraries, drug stores and other places. They will be informed, knowledgeable members of the health care system and will be full partners in decisions about their care.

Curriculum Implications

The changing practice of nursing in response to collaboration with the computer raises many questions for educators. What different skills will be required of the practicing nurse to function effectively in partnership with the computer? How will the computer influence the way in which people learn and think about it? How can the computer support the new educative-caring paradigm being set forth by Bevis and Watson (1989)? How can the goals of the new paradigm support the nurse's ability to work effectively with the computer?

Both Medicine and Dentistry have begun to examine some of these issues. Weed (1989) has explored changing medical practice in an information age and its related impact on medical education. It is his belief that the present premises and tools of medical education and medical care do not support or allow the evolution of health care. "Much of the frustration felt by so many hard-working people in the medical profession has its roots in flawed premises and inadequate tools" (p. 209). According to Weed, the primary flaws in the premises under which we now function are the current reliance on memory both in practice and education and the organization of knowledge into discrete academic packages or courses.

Eisner (1991) has also written of his concerns with the relevancy of the dental curriculum for current and future practice. He states ". . . in almost every North American dental school, today's professional degree curriculum reflects yesterdays realities. . . ." He describes the curriculum as lecture-based using the traditional overhead and/or slide projector with evaluation of student knowledge being done primarily through multiple choice examinations. The curriculum, according to Eisner, can be characterized as fact-based and passive. In addition to methods used for teaching and testing, Eisner also comments on the students perception of the lack of relevancy of prerequisite courses. He believes that learning should be problem-based using a multi-disciplinary dental database.

Both Weed's and Eisner's observations could equally well be made of most nursing curriculums. Nursing programs are, for the most part, teaching as they always have. They use the lecture method, rely heavily on memory and use multiple choice testing. The computer has been introduced primarily to provide computer literacy and as an alternative instructional method to support the traditional behaviorist model of education.

In an age of a rapidly expanding knowledge base, it is not possible for learners to remember the myriad of facts they are taught during their educational programs. In addition, knowledge is expanding so rapidly that whatever is learned is quickly outdated. With the advent of the computer and its almost universal availability, there is no reason to require students to memorize extensive amounts of information. The reality of nursing practice in the very near future is that there will be little need for students or practitioners to rely on their memories. It may actually be dangerous for them to do so.

Current and future nursing practice will use electronic extensions of both human memory and analytic ability of the mind. It is within this context that educators need to examine what it will mean to provide nursing care in partnership with the computer.

Nurses will have access to current knowledge and patient information wherever they are, at the bedside, in the home or at school. The skills needed will be to identify what information is needed and when and how to access that information. With the assistance of the computer, nurses will analyze the information and apply it to meet the unique needs of individual patients and their families.

Without the tyranny of teaching information to be recited back at a later time, the classroom can be as envisioned by Bevis and Watson (1991), an opportunity for interaction, with the teacher serving as the "metastrategist who establishes a climate of sorority and fraternity, of equality, of scholarly seeking; who raises questions and issues and dialogues with students so that they become partners in education, not objects of education"(p. 254)

The teacher and student will be partners in the learning process in the same way that the nurse and the patient are partners in health care. As patients become increasingly knowledgeable, nurses will no longer be information givers, but instead will have to assist patients in interpreting and applying their knowledge to their own lives. Such a role requires sophisticated educative and caring skills. Nurses are often uncomfortable caring for health care professionals. They are unsure what to teach, if anything, and exactly how to interact with them. In the information age, all patients will be closer to the professional in their knowledge level.

It is not the relatively few characteristics that patients with a given disease have in common that determine the best intervention for them, but rather the myriad of things they do not have in common (Weed, 1988). Human response to illness characterizes the practice of nursing. The individualization of care plans and interventions based on scores of patient and family factors is what requires professional knowledge and skill, not being able to write down the standard care plan for specific nursing diagnoses.

Computers provide information about care plans, drugs, treatments, selected patient data and so forth. Only the nurse looks at the whole and can provide an interpersonal caring relationship with the patient and family. Even in a setting in which computerized care plan are not available, students can be given standardized plans and focus on modification based on individual client needs. Testing techniques can be changed from multiple choice to open book. Most students do not like open book exams. Faculty do not give them very often. Why? Perhaps because an open book exam requires students to access information and apply it, rather than repeat what is already in the book. Perhaps because faculty are unsure how to devise tests within this context. Open book testing assesses very different skills from multiple choice examinations. It also gives a much different message to students, i.e memorizing information is not important; knowing what information to retrieve, how to retrieve it and using it to solve patient problems is important.

The challenges for nursing practice and nursing education are great. Computers provide us with the tools to develop a multi-disciplinary electronic knowledge base and to extend our memories and analytic skills. If we can use this tool appropriately, it will free us to focus on curriculum goals to help learners become critical thinkers, more responsive to societal needs, more caring and compassionate, and have increased insight into ethical and moral issues (Bevis & Watson, 1989, p. 348).

Nursing educators have to begin thinking about nursing education in totally different, if not revolutionary, ways. All of us need to consciously break habits of thinking about nursing practice and education as we know it. The field of nursing and the learning process in nursing need to be carefully examined and reconceptualized in light of the challenges and opportunities provided to us by the computer.

References

Bevis, E. O. & Watson, J. (1989). *Toward a caring curriculum: A new pedagogy for nursing.* New York: National League for Nursing.

Eisner, J. (1990). Unpublished paper. State University of New York at Buffalo School of Dentistry. Buffalo, New York.

Evans, S. (1990). The COMMES nursing consultant system. In J.G. Ozbolt, D. Vandewal & K.J. Hannah (Eds.), *Decision support systems in nursing*, pp. 97–119. St. Louis: C. V. Mosby.

Graves, J. R. (1987). A knowledge base for pain management. *Nurse Educators Microworld, 2* (5), 1,3.

Hodson, K. E., Hansen, A. C. & Brougham, C. J. (1988). Integration of computerized assessment screens into psychomotor skill modules at a school of nursing. *Computers in Nursing, 6* (3), 103–107.

Ozbolt, J. G. & Swain, M. A. P. (1990). Representing a nursing knowledge base for a decision support system in Prolog. In J. G. Ozbolt, D. Vandewal & K. J. Hannah (Eds.), *Decision support systems in nursing*, pp. 139–163. St. Louis: C. V. Mosby.

Ronald, J. S. (1985). Nursing education: computer as catalyst. In K.J. Hannah, E.J. Guilemin & D.N. Conklin (Eds.), *Nursing uses of computers and information science.* Amsterdam: Elsevier Science Publishers B.V.

Ryan, S. (1985). An expert system for nursing practice: Clinical decision support. *Computers in Nursing, 3* (2), 77–84.

Skiba, D. J. & Ronald, J. S. (1989). Hypermedia: creating learning pathways. *Nursing Educators Microworld, 4* (1). 1,3.

Weed, L. L. .(1989). New premises and new tools for medical care and medical education. *Methods of Information in Medicine, 28*, 207–214.

71
A Collaborative Model for Specialization in Nursing Informatics

JUDITH S. RONALD

Nursing Informatics has been defined by Graves and Corcoran (1989) as "a combination of computer science, information science and nursing science designed to assist in the management and processing of nursing data, information and knowledge to support the practice of nursing and the delivery of nursing care." It is an emerging area of specialization that is rapidly becoming an essential component of educational programs at all levels, in response to the pervasive use of the computer in the health care system. Graves and Corcoran's definition acknowledges the necessity of using a multidisciplinary approach to fully utilize the potential of the computer in nursing. More importantly, it provides direction for education by placing the computer in its proper perspective and focusing on it as a tool for managing and processing healthcare information.

The State University of New York at Buffalo School of Nursing currently integrates basic concepts of nursing informatics into curricula of its graduate and undergraduate programs. In addition, it provides opportunities for specialization in nursing informatics at the graduate level through collaborative efforts with the School of Management.

Historical Background

The School of Nursing at State University of New York at Buffalo has included content about computers and their application to nursing in its curriculum since 1976. The first course was an elective entitled "The Impact of the Computer on Nursing" and included fundamental computer concepts, basic principles of systems analysis and design, and nursing applications (Ronald, 1979). There was minimal hands-on experience at that time.

Reprinted with permission from; *Nursing Informatics '91: Proceedings of the Fourth International Conference on Nursing Use of Computers and Information Science*; Hovenga, E.J.S., Hannah, K.J., McCormick, K.A. & Ronald, J.S. (Eds.). 1991, pp. 662–666. Heidelberg-Berlin, Germany: Springer-Verlag.

Both graduate and undergraduate students took essentially the same course.

In the late 1970's and early 1980's, more hands-on experience was added with emphasis on learning editing systems and BASIC programming. The large University Mainframe systems were used. Through the use of an editing system, students were able to learn how to individualize standardized nursing care plans. Students benefited from using a time sharing system, developing an understanding of telecommunication and the potential that it had for the healthcare system. In order to add programming elements to the course, algorithm development for simple computer programs replaced content related to basic concepts of systems analysis and design. This emphasis on programming as an essential component of computer literacy was congruent with the definition of "computer literacy" that was developing outside of nursing (Skiba and Ronald, 1988).

Hands-on experience was provided in large computer laboratories and classrooms run by the Department of Computer Science and shared by the whole university. The School of Nursing had only two terminals connected to the mainframe. They were used primarily by faculty for research and data analysis.

The 1980s brought a changing definition of computer literacy throughout the educational system. With the increased availability of the microcomputer, hands-on experience increased and the use of generic application software became an important component of the course. Programming was deleted as a requirement and information science concepts were reemphasized. Students were asked to look at nursing as an information intensive profession and to analyze nursing information needs and information flow in clinical situations with which they were familiar. They developed algorithms and flow charts to describe their analyses. This application of basic information processing concepts to nursing required a level of thinking and depth of knowledge in nursing that precluded the same course being offered to graduate and undergraduate students. As a result, in 1986 two separate courses were developed. Undergraduate students were exposed to basic information processing concepts while the graduate students were expected to apply these concepts at a beginning level. In addition, a second graduate level course, "Microcomputers in Nursing Administration" was developed at this time.

The availability of computing power within the school of nursing expanded dramatically in the 1980s and made it possible to provide extensive hands-on experience. Between 1980 and 1986, the School of Nursing expanded its computing laboratory from two to eight terminals and added a microcomputing classroom with 20 PCs. In 1988, the PC classroom was upgraded to a NOVELL network for 16 of the PCs and in 1989 eight additional terminals to the mainframe, along with a high speed printer, were added to the data analysis laboratory. Most importantly, a half-time computer laboratory director with a PhD degree was hired. He has six teaching assistants who staff the lab six days a week. The growth of the computer facility was funded partially from grant funds and partly by the University based on the documentation of exponentially increasing use of the facility. Interactive video will be added in 1990. All of the computer facilities, both instructional and research are housed in several different rooms on one floor of the School of Nursing to facilitate staffing and security.

Current Status of Nursing Informatics in the Curriculum

In 1988, the School of Nursing Faculty decided that all students graduating from the undergraduate program after June 1993 would have basic concepts and skills in nursing informatics. Students will use the computer as a tool in their educational program as well as in their practice. Students graduating from the masters and doctoral programs are currently required to use the computer for data analysis. In addition, all nursing administration graduates use word processing, database management systems and spreadsheets to help solve nursing information management problems. Graduate programs in the clinical areas do not require any informatics competencies, beyond those of data analysis, for graduation.

To achieve the undergraduate program goals, students are required to successfully complete a one semester computer science course prior to entry into the School of Nursing. The class entering in Fall, 1990 was the first class to meet this requirement. In this course, students learn basic computer concepts, use of an integrated package, algorithm development and simple programming. In the School of Nursing, they are expected to use the word processor for their papers and care plans. In addition, they are assigned activities such as: (1) developing a database of their patient care experiences, (2) using spreadsheet software to keep track of their courses and grade point averages, (3) using on-line literature searches, and other appropriate applications. In addition, nursing courses use computer-assisted instruction, a simulated hospital information system and other appropriate software. Selected courses include content related to automated management of nursing information. Curriculum development is continuing in this area.

At the graduate level, all students are required to take a one credit laboratory course in data analysis using the computer, as part of their research sequence. The elective course in nursing informatics is strongly recommended for all students. Students entering the masters program in Nursing Administration are encouraged to acquire basic computer skills prior to entry into the program. However, this is not yet required for admission. Nursing Administration students are required to take a course entitled "Microcomputers in Nursing Administration" that includes the principles and practice of word processing, database management and spreadsheets for nursing management information systems. In addition, informatics content is incorporated into Nursing Administration I and II, as well as the course on Planning, Budgeting and Forecasting. Plans are being made for additional integration.

Collaborative Informatics Program for Doctoral Students

An increasing number of doctoral students have indicated a need for indepth preparation in nursing informatics, along with a desire to do research in this area. Nursing administration students, particularly, are seeking a strong foundation in management information systems as they relate to the role of the nurse executive. Although there are two graduate programs in Nursing Informatics in the United States—one at the University of Maryland (Heller, 1985), the other at the University of Utah—many students cannot attend one of these programs. Thus, different educational models need to be explored to meet the learning needs of students interested in informatics.

The School of Nursing at State University of New York at Buffalo has developed a collaborative model with the School of Management to provide selected doctoral students in nursing administration with an opportunity to specialize in management information systems. The School of Management has a six course sequence in Management Information Systems. One Management faculty member specializes in healthcare information systems and has done considerable research in this area.

Since nursing doctoral students are required to take a minimum of fifteen credits in a cognate area to support their dissertation, those interested in informatics fulfill this requirement by taking the sequence in Management Information Systems. They are admitted to the management sequence based on recommendation from the Faculty of the School of Nursing and interviews by faculty in Management Information Systems. Depending on an individual student's background, one or more of the required management courses may be waived. The courses in the Management Information Systems sequence include: Information Technology (1.5 Cr), Introduction to Information Systems (3 Cr), Management Information Systems I (COBOL and Database Management Systems) (3 Cr), Management Information Systems II (Systems Analysis and Design) (3 Cr), Decision Support Systems (3 Cr) and Seminar in Management Information Systems (3 Cr). The courses include major projects that students can do in the healthcare environment. There are frequent meetings between nursing faculty and students to facilitate the students' application of concepts and methods learned in the management courses to nursing and healthcare.

To date, two doctoral students have taken advantage of this option. The first student had considerable background in computer and information science courses before entering the doctoral program. Thus, she took only three management information systems courses: Management Information Systems II, Decision Support Systems and Seminar in Management Information Systems. In addition, she took Introduction to Nursing Informatics and did an independent study in Nursing Decision Support Systems with a nurse researcher who specializes in decision support systems. She also served as a teaching assistant in the Nursing Computer Laboratory for two years. She is currently at dissertation stage. Her committee is chaired by a School of Nursing faculty member and includes a member from The School of Management.

The second student in this area has just begun his doctoral program. He graduated from the School of Nursing Masters Program in Nursing Administration in 1990. While in the masters program, he took a course in nursing informatics, did both an internship (role related) and a practicum (project related) in nursing informatics and served as a teaching assistant in the computer laboratory for two years. He has been accepted into the Management Information Systems sequence and has decided to take the whole sequence, even though he could have had at least one course waived. Students have found that interaction and collaboration with faculty and students in the School of Management are invaluable in providing them not only with new concepts and methods, but also with a different perspective on the healthcare system.

Conclusion

The study of nursing informatics is central to understanding nursing as an information intensive profession. Because of this, nursing's full potential to contribute to the health care system will not be realized until theoretical, practice and evaluation models for nursing informatics have been developed. This can only be accomplished if nursing informatics becomes an integral part of nursing education at all levels and nursing informatics specialists are developed at the graduate level. Different models for nurses to achieve advanced preparation in informatics at the doctoral level need to be explored. This paper has presented one such alternative using a collaborative design that combines expertise from a School of Nursing and School of Management. Thus far it appears to be a viable alternative.

References

Graves JR, Corcoran S: The study of nursing informatics. *Image* Winter 1989;21(4):227–231.

Heller B et al.: Graduate specialization in nursing informatics. *Computers in Nursing* September/October 1989;7(5):209–213.

Ronald JS: Computers and undergraduate nursing education: A report on an experimental introductory course. *Journal of Nursing Education* 18(9):4–9.

Skiba DJ, Ronald JS: *A journey through the computer paradigm.* Paper presented at Third International Conference on Nursing Informatics, Dublin, Ireland, June 1988.

72
A Curriculum Model for Graduate Specialization in Nursing Informatics

Carol A. Romano and Barbara R. Heller

Introduction

As the utilization of computers and information technology in health care has expanded, so also have the applications of such technology in nursing proliferated. Computers applied to clinical practice, education, research, and nursing administration have already begun to revolutionize the management of patient care and health care systems. These technologies must be reliable, easy to learn and use, and adaptable to the changes in nursing, in organizations, and in the health care environment. Nursing experts have already asserted that leadership from nursing in the design, implementation, and management of information technology must be developed [1,2,6, & 8].

Unfortunately, the need for knowledge in this field of nursing remains a void yet to be filled. Information in and of itself had become a vital commodity of a technological society and has been recognized as a phenomenon for scholarly study. The assertion of an educational program, then, is merely an acknowledgement of the need for trained information system specialists and for scholars. These individuals need to explore the synergism which is evolving among the computer/information systems and the health care professional.

The purpose of this paper is to describe the emerging role of the nurse as an Information Systems Specialist and to present a graduate master's level nursing curriculum designed to prepare nurses to function in such a role.

Role Description

Stevens [7] notes that for some roles in nursing, any description is bound to be an oversimplification because it may have too broad a scope for meaningful summarization. The role of the nursing information systems

Reprinted with permission from *Proceedings: Twelfth Annual Symposium on Computer Applications in Medical Care*, Greenes, R.A. (Ed.). 1988, pp. 343–349. © 1987, American Medical Informatics Association (formerly SCAMC): Bethesda, MD.

specialist is one such role. A multifaceted approach was used by these authors to clarify this emerging role in relation to the knowledge and abilities required, the tasks and functions performed, and the nurse's relationship to individuals and groups in the environment. A review and analysis of the activities of nurses currently employed in this pioneer role were conducted. Position descriptions across agencies were compared and contrasted, nurses were interviewed, recruitment materials for employment opportunities were collected, and current and potential employers were querried as to the role expectations of the nursing information systems specialist.

Major Duties Performed

Naisbitt [4] asserts that the work of health care professionals is information intensive, particularly for nurses who serve as the primary link between the patient and the health care system. Major duties of the nursing information systems specialist include but are not limited to the following activities. First, the identification of the properties, structure, use, and flow of clinical and management information from the patient (health care consumer), to the health care provider, and subsequently throughout the health care organization is considered basic to the function of this role. Next, the assessment of real and potential problems related to the communication, accessibility, availability, and use of information for clinical and administrative decision-making is also required. Analysis of the cause and scope of information type problems and the determination of priorities for investigation is needed. The delineation of alternative methods of information handling and of system design options which consider subtle differences and the need for a high degree of flexibility to accommodate growth is noted as a major responsibility of the nurse in this role. In addition, the orchestration of change is recognized as one of the most challenging duties of the nursing information systems specialist, as it demands directing the technology transfer in environments usually laden with dated, traditional methodologies. Finally, evaluation of the cost/risks in relation to the benefits or effectiveness of information technologies are also encompassed by this role.

Knowledge Required

Knowledge required by the nurse functioning as an information systems specialist includes an understanding of nursing, information science, and systems theory in clinical and managerial decision-making. Expertise in organizational and group dynamics and its impact upon the delivery of nursing and health care services is also required. Knowledge of the social and human aspects of information systems and their impact on nursing practice is also needed. This knowledge base allows the nurse to develop new structures, work processes, and/or information handling systems that influence the delivery, communication, and documentation of nursing care. These systems facilitate how nursing interrelates with other professionals and health agencies in its pivotal role of health care coordinator. Finally, a comprehensive understanding of the interrelationship between people, organizations, information, technology, nursing, and health care delivery is identified as a critical component of the role.

Interaction

In an environment where communciation and information technology and nursing are evolving at a rapid pace, the nursing information systems specialist needs to interface simultaneously with a variety of individuals and groups on many different organizational levels. Personal work contacts can foster collaboration, supply advice, help interpret, and seek support for new work methods and resulting policies. Many times the implementation and maintenance of a clinical and management information systems program involves coordination of the activities of several disciplines and the negotiation of controversial political as well as technological issues [5]. A great deal of explanation and tact is required in achieving satisfactory solutions and compromises in problem solving.

Educational Specialization in Nursing Informatics

The ultimate goal of an educational program in Nursing Informatics is to prepare nurses for the role described above. Graduates need to be prepared to manage the challenges of modern health care with the new tools of this era and to take advantage of the growing opportunities provided by the appropriate administration of information technology. An educational program in Nursing Informatics is designed to provide the skills and knowledge necessary for the effective and efficient development and management of information technologies in nursing and health care. Those completing such a program would be able to:

1. Analyze nursing information requirements for clinical and management information systems.
2. Analyze information needs and technological issues related to productivity and quality assurance programs in nursing.
3. Develop strategies to manage technological and organizational change and innovation.

4. Apply management and nursing theories and information science to the planning, development, implementation, and administration of nursing information systems.
5. Evaluate the effectiveness of nursing information systems in patient care delivery.
6. Define methodologies related to technology and engineering planning for information systems in health care and nursing.
7. Apply concepts of budget, staffing, and financial management to the design of management information systems.
8. Apply concepts of nursing theory and research to the design of health care clinical information systems.
9. Develop and implement user training programs to support the utilization of clinical and management information systems.
10. Analyze the contribution of information technology to nursing education, administration, clinical practice, and research.
11. Examine the political, social, ethical, and influential forces in health care as they relate to the use of information technology and management.
12. Evaluate hardware, software, and vendor support for information technologies that underpin clinical and management decisions in nursing.
13. Examine data base management principles in relation to nursing information system file structures.
14. Apply concepts of programming logic to the analysis of a simple computer program.

Educational Prototype

In response to the need for such educational preparation of nurses and in accord with the stated objectives of the role requirements, the University of Maryland School of Nursing decided to expand its existing Master's program concentration in Nursing Administration to include a new specialty track in Nursing Informatics and to enroll students by September 1988. This decision was based on the availability of resources and the findings of a feasibility study and needs assessment [3].

The resources and facilities of the University of Maryland available to support Nursing Informatics include well-established graduate programs in Computer Science, Information Systems Management, and General Administration that facilitate an interdisciplinary approach to the curriculum. A dynamic and qualified faculty with curriculum and research expertise as well as experience in computer applications contributes to assuring a high quality program of study in Nursing Informatics. In addition, more than 60 community and health care agencies cooperate with the graduate programs of the School of Nursing in providing sites for field experience and practice.

Primary sites for practical and field experience in Nursing Informatics include the University of Maryland Medical Systems Hospital; the Clinical Center, National Institutes of Health; and the Johns Hopkins Hospital. The Clinical Center, National Institutes of Health is recognized as a national model for the integration of computerization with nursing practice.

Curriculum

The curriculum consists of 42 credit hours. Coursework uses an interdisciplinary approach combining detailed study of the discipline of nursing with theoretical and practical foundations of management and information science. Courses offered by the Department of Information Systems Management and the Graduate Program in General Administration of the University of Maryland support those in Nursing Informatics. The program can be completed in three semesters of full-time study (see Figure 1 for typical curriculum pattern configuration). Opportunities for part-time study are also available.

The track in Nursing Informatics is consistent with the general curriculum design of the Graduate Program, University of Maryland, School of Nursing which contains six components: core courses, major (specialization) courses, support courses, elective courses, thesis/non-thesis option, and a comprehensive examination as described below:

• Core—There is an essential core of advanced nursing knowledge needed in all clinical specialties and roles. Therefore, all graduate nursing students, regardless of their area of concentration, are required to take 15 credits of core courses. These focus on the clinical, philosophical, and theoretical bases for advanced nursing practice (NURS 601 and NURS 602); organizational behavior and the societal forces that influence health care delivery and professional practice (NURS 606); and six credits of theoretical and applied research courses which introduce students to research methods and design, statistical interpretation, and the use of computer programs (NURS 701 and NURS 702).

• Major (Specialization) Courses—In these courses, the student is introduced to the area of concentration. Topics include theories of organization and management in nursing (NURS 691), applications of computerization and information science in nursing and health care (NURS 706), and principles and practices of nursing informatics (NURS 707). A practicum experience (NURS 708) in selected agencies provides opportunity for students to develop the skills needed for implementation and evaluation of clinical and management information systems in nursing and health care.

• Support Courses—Support courses are intended to add breadth or depth to the area of concentration and may be taken in departments or schools other than nursing. This component requires at least three areas of study in information science: a foundational course in operations analysis,

Full-Time Plan of Study

Semester I		Credits
Intro to Advanced Clinical Nursing Practice	NURS 601	3
Critical Approaches to Nursing Theories	NURS 602	3
Nursing Research Designs & Analysis I	NURS 701	3
Applications of Computers and Information Science in Nursing & Health Care	NURS 706	3
Information Systems Theory	IFSM 600	3
		15

Semester II		Credits
Influential Forces in Nursing & Health Care	NURS 606	3
Organizational Theories: Applications to Nursing Management	NURS 691	3
Nursing Research Designs & Analysis II	NURS 702	3
Concepts in Nursing Informatics	NURS 707	2
Foundations of Operations Analysis	IFSM 601	3
		14

Semester III		Credits
Modeling & Simulation	IFSM 605	3
Practicum in Nursing Informatics	NURS 708	4
Elective		3
Elective		3
		13

	TOTAL CREDITS	42

FIGURE 1. Curriculum Pattern. Nursing Informatics.

theories of information systems, and modeling and simulation. These courses are offered through the Department of Information Systems Management.

Elective Courses—Students may select from courses in the areas of nursing, management, or information science available on any of the University of Maryland campuses.

- Thesis/Non-Thesis Option—Depending on career goals, students may select a thesis or non-thesis option. Thesis students design, implement, evaluate, and orally defend a research project (equivalent to six graduate credits). Those pursuing the non-thesis option take six elective credits in courses related to individual interests, and produce a scholarly paper or project.
- Comprehensive Examination—All students electing the non-thesis option take a written comprehensive examination.

Admission Requirements

Requirements for admission include:

- Baccalaureate degree with an upper division nursing major from an NLN-accredited program.
- Photocopy of current Maryland registered nurse licensure.
- Official scores on the Graduate Record Examination (Aptitude Test).
- G.P.A. of 3.0 on a 4.0 point scale on undergraduate record. If G.P.A. is between 2.75 and 3.0, provisional acceptance may be considered if candidate can demonstrate graduate potential via other means.
- Successful completion of a course in elementary statistics.
- Evidence of personal and professional qualifications via three professional references. Two of these must be from nurses.
- At least two years of professional nursing experience.
- Personal interviews are encouraged.

Impact

Program completion will provide career opportunities as Nursing Information Systems specialists in every commercial, governmental, and service organization that employs computer-based information services related to health care. The program provides instruction in those competencies needed for entry as well as for acquiring increased responsibility in a very wide range of occupations in both the private and public sectors.

Within the past few years, there has been a significant increase in the numbers of graduate students wishing to pursue advanced study in nursing informatics. Currently no other school of nursing either in the United States or abroad offers such specialized education. Consequently, students have had no way to fulfill their goals. The University of Maryland has designed and implemented the first Master's level program of study for role preparation of the NIS specialist. This curriculum will serve as a model for the development of other Nursing Informatics programs in the future.

The ultimate impact of such an educational program will be to improve the quality of nursing services through the preparation of NIS specialists who are qualified and competent to practice in acute care, long-term care, or community-based health care delivery settings. A more immediate visible contribution is the increased availability of appropriately prepared specialists in nursing informatics. The lack of such specialists is viewed as a basic impediment to strengthening the organization and management of nursing services within the health care system.

Because of their familiarity and interaction with almost all aspects of operation and systems design, graduates of such a specialized program of study can contribute to management decisions that affect issues beyond nursing services. Enhanced collaborative efforts in research and in nursing administration and informatics, along with improved dissemination of research findings, are anticipated as outcomes of the program.

References

[1] Ball, M.J. & Hannah, K.S. (1984). *Using Computers in Nursing*. Reston, VA: Reston Publishing.
[2] Heller, B., Romano, C., Damrosch, S., Parks, P. (1985). Computer applications in nursing: Implications for the curriculum. *Computers in Nursing, 3*(1), 14–21.
[3] Heller, B., Romano, C., Damrosch, S., McCarthy, M. (1988). The need for an educational program in nursing informatics. In Ball, M., Hannah K., Gerdin-Jelger, *Nursing Informatics: Where Caring & Technology Meet*. New York: Springer-Verlag.
[4] Naisbitt, J. (1982). *Megatrends*. New York: Warner Books, Inc.
[5] Romano, C. (1984). Computer technology and emergency roles. *Computers in Nursing, 2*(3), 80–84.
[6] Saba, V. & McCormick, K. (1986). *Essentials of Computers for Nurses*. Philadelphia, PA: J.B. Lippincott Company.
[7] Stevens, B.J. (1975). *The Nurse as Executive*. Wakefield, Mass., Contemporary Publishing.
[8] Zielstorff, R.D. (Ed.). (1980). *Computers In Nursing*. Wakefield, Mass: Nursing Resources.

73
A Postgraduate Program in Nursing Informatics

JOS AARTS

1. Introduction and Rationale

In 1988 the Hogeschool Midden Nederland decided to create a new postgraduate program in nursing informatics as a part of the postgraduate educational programs for health care professionals, which also include management, professional innovation, clinical specialization and research methods. The program builds on the established nursing informatics courses in the various nursing programs of the Institute for Higher Health Care Education of the Hogeschool [1].

The reason for this initiative is twofold. A survey conducted under the auspices of the Dutch Ministry of Health showed that further development of information systems supporting care is hindered by a lack of education about information technology of the health care professional [2]. In June 1987 Working Group 8 (Nursing) of the International Medical Informatics Association established knowledge and competency levels for various groups of nurses and identified the need for a special program to educate nurses who can provide leadership in the development of (computerized) information systems to support health care delivery [3].

The rationale can be found in the fact that the health care professional is more and more made answerable for the quality of patient care and for the issue of balancing benefits and costs of health care delivery. This development is prompted by the need for professionalization which means that the delivery of care is based on scientific knowledge, but also external factors play an all important role. The general public is more demanding than ever and does not take "no" (or "yes") for an answer. In Europe the governments are setting standards for the quality and costs of care and gradually the European Community becomes more influential in determining these

Reprinted with permission from *Proceedings: Thirteenth Annual Symposium on Computer Applications in Medical Care*, Kingsland, L.C. (Ed.). 1989, pp. 773–775. © 1989, American Medical Informatics Association (formerly SCAMC): Bethesda, MD.

standards. In the Netherlands a major revision of the health care delivery and financing system is taking place which allows the private carrier to be influential in terms of costs and quality of care. All these changes require data to be explicit and the amount of data is expected to increase enormously. It is only the use of automated information systems that can cope with these demands and developments.

Dutch health care information systems will develop into health care support information systems but the involvement of the health care professional is crucial for a successful change.

2. Program Contents and Organization

The postgraduate program in nursing informatics has adopted a conceptual model of medical information processing developed by Van Bemmel [4] as a philosophy for the course contents. We feel that this model is not only valid for nursing information processing but also endorses the humanistic approach in the use of computers.

The program consists of 420 hours of theoretical education and 420 hours of practical work in a health care institution. Essentially the program is part-time and can be completed in one year. However, it is expected that the completion of the theoretical part will require more time of the students and therefore the contents of the program has been organized into a modular structure with well-defined courses.

Upon completion of the program the student will essentially be able to analyze nursing information needs, use professional nursing knowledge to design nursing applications of information technology, compare and evaluate vendor products, identify user learning needs and implement training programs and assess and evaluate the effectiveness of clinical and/or management information systems to support the delivery of care.

The student completes the theoretical part of the program by written exams of each course and the practical part by a thesis which he defends before an examination board. The theoretical part starts with an introductory set of courses which are shared by all above mentioned postgraduate programs, followed by the main track of the informatics program. Table 1 is an outline of the theoretical part of the program including the introductory courses. In the practical period the student applies his knowledge of nursing and informatics to the development and/or design of nursing applications, preferably in the institution where he holds his job. On a modest scale the Hogeschool can provide for projects. Our policy for this approach is to make the gained knowledge and skills as soon as possible available for the institution and to enhance its responsibility for the learning process of the student.

The student will be able to choose a differentiation in the field of nursing care or nursing management. Therefore he can select courses from the post-

TABLE 1. The curriculum of the nursing informatics program (outline)

Introductory courses
duration 100 hours
themes
— principles of care, quality and organization of health care delivery in the Netherlands
— health care policies and management
— methods of research, including statistics
— introductory health care informatics

Main track

Module 1: *Management, administration and research*
Module 1.1.: **Organization and information policy**
duration 30 hours
contents
— management, decision making and information
— administrative organization
— information policy and planning

Module 2: *Professional innovation*
duration 72 hours
contents
— data collection in nursing
— reporting and records in nursing
— "unified nursing language system": standardization of nursing concepts
— clinical decision making
— protocols and quality assurance in nursing
— protocols and specialization in nursing
— nursing audit
— the DRG concept and the minimal nursing data set

Module 3: *Informatics*
Module 3.1.: **Computer science**
duration 36 hours
contents
— representation of data
— architecture and principles of computers
— peripheral devices
— operating systems
— data communication
— data collections and storage structures
— programming languages
Module 3.2.: **Elementary information science**
duration 39 hours
contents
— information handling in an organization
— data analysis and data structuring
— developments in informatics
Module 3.3.: **Databases**
duration 30 hours
contents
— database principles
— hierarchical, network and relational DBMS
— development of nursing "data dictionary"
Module 3.4.: **Systems analysis**
duration 39 hours

TABLE 1. (*Continued*)

---

contents
— objectives and methods
— project organization
— methods and techniques (SDM, ISAC, SISP etc.)
— design, realization and introduction
— role of 4 GL tools

Module 3.5.: **Informatics and health care**
duration 36 hours
contents
— health care information systems
— departmental applications
— principles of decision support systems
— applications in nursing management
— national health care information systems

Module 4: *Societal and ethical issues of information technology*
duration 24 hours
contents
— information technology and professional responsibility
— job innovation
— data protection
— responsibilities with respect to the management of health care data
— rights of patients
— legal issues

Module 5: *Social skills*
duration 24 hours
contents
— negotiating, presenting and conflict handling techniques
— methods of supervision

---

graduate programs in clinical care nursing, professional innovation and/or management. The modular structure of our educational system facilitates possible choices. Also, this structure allows the faculty to grant exemptions from the program if the student shows adequate knowledge in a particular subject. The student can complete the program within a year when he can devote 50% of a nominal working week to attend the courses and do the practical work while at least another 10 hours per week is required for self-study. We expect that most students will choose to complete the program in 1.5 to 2 years.

3. Student Pool and Faculty

It is our policy to select the students from applicants who work in an institution for health care (hospitals, community health care institutions, etc.) because we hold the opinion that primarily the institution should profit from the education offered. This is made visible by the requirement that the practical work should be carried out at the place where the student is employed. We will however consider applications from students who are not employed and seek a career in health care informatics.

The prerequisite for this program is a baccalaureate or master's degree in nursing or equivalent to the judgment of the admission board. Also the student needs to have a working experience of at least two years.

A survey held among hospitals in the Utrecht area showed interest in our initiative but some hesitation about the prospect of having well-defined jobs in the area information technology and nursing. Most hospitals reacted very positively to the intention to relate the contents of the program to the health care profession, instead of offering another computer science course. A few hospitals were very positive to send students to our program and will charge them with duties in the field of nursing information processing. It is our expectation however that the number of jobs will increase, because there are quite a few senior nurses who have duties in the area of information systems as a part their current job description. These duties are expected to grow into new functions as the impact of information technology grows. We now estimate a steady yearly enrollment of about 20 students who will come from all over the Netherlands. For the 1989/1990 academic year 11 students have enrolled into the program; table 2 sketches a profile of this student pool.

Faculty for the program is mainly derived from the existing staff of the Hogeschool while for specific subjects specialists are hired from hospitals and other health care institutions, software houses and colleague universities. We believe that introducing specialists from practice as teachers in our program strengthens the involvement of health care in education.

TABLE 2. Profile of student pool, academic year 1989/1990

Number of students: 11
3 female, 8 male, all professional nurses (RNs)

Provenance:
General Hospital: 3
Psychiatric Hospital: 2
Mental Health Institution: 3
Community (extramural) Health Care: 2
Other: 1

Places of provenance:
Amsterdam: 2
Utrecht:
Utrecht area (50 km radius circle): 4
Arnhem (East of Netherlands): 1
Vught (South of Netherlands): 1
Leeuwarden (North of Netherlands): 1

4. International Cooperation

Our program is unique in its contents and duration in Europe. From the start we have strived towards international cooperation because we are convinced that an advanced program should be supported in an international network. It is not coincidental that we have established contacts with the University of Maryland, Campus for the Professions, at Baltimore where the School of Nursing in 1988 has started a master's degree program in nursing informatics [5,6]. This program has set an example for us [7].

The Hogeschool strives towards cooperation with universities and colleges in the European Community, advanced programs like our postgraduate program in nursing informatics are instrumental to achieve this in the field of education and research. This cooperation reflects the opportunity graduates have to work all over the EC and the fact that boundaries for them are vanishing. The magic year 1992 casts its shadow over our activities.

The Hogeschool has established formal links among others with the University of Wales at Cardiff, Brighton Polytechnic and the City University of London in Great Britain in the field of nursing and paramedic education.

5. Conclusion

The program finds its roots in the development of the nursing profession and the issues of quality of care and bears relationship to the development of new health care information systems.

We were able to start this program because its builds on the informatics nurses which have been established in all our educational nursing programs. This approach reflects our philosophy that informatics should be considered as a tool for the health care professional.

The program is expected to attract 20 students per year; the number might increase as the impact of information technology on health care delivery becomes more visible.

The fact that this program is unique for Europe opens the way for international cooperation in and outside Europe; also it can stimulate research in the field of health care delivery and informatics.

Acknowledgment. We acknowledge the generous financial support of the Dutch Ministry of Health by grant DGVgz/GBO/OZ 515406.

References

[1] Aarts, J.E.C.M., A curriculum in nursing informatics, in: Salamon, R. et al. (eds.), *Medical informatics and education*, Victoria: School of Health Information Science, University of Victoria, 1989: 381–383.

[2] Ouwerkerk, W., Iersel, F.M.M. van, Op Hey, J.G.L.M.M., Towards future hospital information systems: a government strategy, in: Bakker, A.R. et al. (eds.), *Towards new hospital information systems*, Amsterdam: North Holland, 1988: 303–307.

[3] Peterson, H.E. and Gerdin-Jelger, U. (eds.), *Preparing nurses for using information systems: recommended informatics competencies*, New York: National League for Nursing, 1988.

[4] Bemmel, J.H. van, A comprehensive model for medical information processing, *Meth. Inform. Med.* 1983; 22: 124–130.

[5] Heller, B.R. et al., Education for specialization in nursing informatics, in: Daly, N. and Hannah, K.J. (eds.), *Proceedings of third international symposium on nursing use of computers and information science*, St. Louis: C.V. Mosby, 1988.

[6] Heller, B.R., et al., A needs assessment for graduate specialization in nursing informatics, in: Greenes, R.A. (ed.), *Proceedings of twelfth annual symposium on computer applications in medical care*, New York, IEEE Computer Society Press, 1988: 337–342.

[7] Romano, C.A. and B.R. Heller, A curriculum model for graduate specialization in nursing informatics, in: Greenes, R.A., *Proceedings of twelfth annual symposium on computer applications in medical care*, New York, IEEE Computer Society Press, 1988: 343–349.

74
Database Instruction for Nursing Students

Vaughn G. Sinclair

Introduction

Our nursing school graduates are entering health care settings that are increasingly saturated with computer applications. Due to curricular compression, very little time in core curricula is usually allotted to informatics content. If opportunities for teaching computer applications are limited, databases may be the most useful instructional focus area among all the generic computer applications. Other computer applications may be useful for certain nursing specialties (such as spreadsheets for nurse administrators), but every specialty can benefit from exposure to database management concepts. Databases are a particularly useful application for nursing students to assimilate since databases illustrate the computer's ability to sift through enormous quantities of data and compile that unorganized data into relevant information. Since an enormous portion of our time is relegated to information handling, the computer's time savings in this area may ultimately transform our roles.

Support for Information Processing

A conceptual model of information processing functions (Griffiths & King, 1986), adapted for nursing, may resemble the model in Figure 1. Databases support the genesis of information (creation and composition) by facilitating the organization of data into patterns. Databases provide for efficient data storage, transfer, and access, thereby facilitating the analysis and evaluation of information. In addition, databases promote the appropriate application of knowledge by facilitating identification of significant

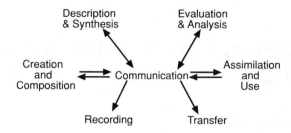

FIGURE 1. Information processing functions of nursing.

patterns and trends, which may clarify therapeutic directions for nurses. Databases therefore support every aspect of the information processing model.

According to Matheson and Cooper (1982), two major goals for managing information include:

a)   filtering in relevant useful information from external sources;
b)   organizing internal files needed to manage the organization.

Appropriate use of databases can address both categories of information management problems.

Filtering Information from External Sources

To filter in relevant external information, large professional databases may be tapped for access to literature citations, full-text journal articles, or networking resources (Armstrong, 1985; Loepprich & Smith, 1983–84). Benefits attributed to computerized literature searching include rapid retrieval of relevant information from one source, ability to search for information by categories other than author's name and topic (such as journal name and title words) and, most importantly, the ability to link several concepts to sharply define useful subsets of information. Ongoing advances in telecommunications technology insure decreased costs coupled with improved quality of communications in the future (Howitt & Weinberger, 1984). Furthermore, current attempts to facilitate professional database access (with standardized command languages, specialized software such as Grateful Med, and eventually nature language) will steadily improve ease of access. These trends indicate that access to professional databases will soon become more appealing to nurses (Sinclair, 1987).

Accessing Reference Databases

To illustrate the computer's potential to filter pertinent information for the nursing professional, nursing students may be taught to select and combine subsets of data, access MEDLINE and perform a simple search, utilizing only a few commands. Accessing a reference database such as MEDLINE also illustrates the components of databases so that students may quickly learn the fundamentals of database terminology and structure from the records of citations they obtain. Special classroom instruction accounts may be obtained from the DIALOG system in Palo Alto, California, so that students may search at reduced rates.

Reviewing the literature with the help of a large reference database can be a very positive experience for students since they successfully obtain highly relevant information from a fascinating machine which sifts throught millions of records in seconds. The relevance of the experience is greatly enhanced if students conduct a search for information needed for an assigned class project or paper. Students appreciate the unique advantages of computerized literature searching when it saves them considerable amounts of time on a project.

Educational Goals

For every interactive computer experience, educators must balance goals related to three areas of learning:

1. cognitive—recall through evaluation of didactic material;
2. affective—overcoming "computerphobia," which blocks effective computer utilization (Koch, 1984); and
3. psychomotor—achieving facility with computer skills.

The author emphasizes the cognitive domain, so that students learn concepts and principles related to computer utilization which may be transferred and applied to a variety of situations. Positive changes in the affective domain, however, are extremely important to enhance the transfer of learning and readiness to use the computer. The literature search provides a nonthreatening introduction to the computer. A successful search can positively affect student attitudes toward computers while reinforcing didactic content about the diversity and benefits of professional online information (Grobe, 1984).

Organizing Internal Files

Nurses utilize database technology in information systems in various settings. In addition to greatly enhancing nursing's communication and documentation in hospitals, database technology in hospital information systems can improve the quality of care delivered by sorting and summarizing health care information, coordinating care, and identifying potential problems. The capability of searching fields related to nursing care simplifies the nurse researcher's attempts to ascertain the effectiveness of nursing interventions. For nurses practicing in community settings, the database technology in information systems allows for rapid retrieval of data identifying high-risk patients or patients who missed appointments, or any other group of patients in need of special support. These database capabilities, which can help nurses improve the quality of health care, should be identified for students so that they can encourage computer use in their practice settings (Kline, 1986).

"Hands-on" Experience with Database Files

The capability of databses to retrieve and format useful information can be demonstrated in one or two sessions of "hands-on" experience. The information to be inserted and formatted in the database may be clinical or administrative in nature (Skiba, 1985). For example, students could be given a list of frequently occurring health care problems, and asked to think about the *input* needed for the computer to produce the desired output. Using software that is simple to use, students can construct a limited database (actually a file) with sufficient fields for gathering data related to some prescribed questions. For a sample of questions pertinent to an administrative file (for nursing administration students), refer to Figure 2. The database exercise may be customized for students according to their specialty to enhance relevance. Nurse practitioner students, for example, may construct a file of clinical data on fictional patients and address plausible questions, perhaps related to the recall of an antihypertensive drug or a need to identify groups of high-risk patients.

The author has discovered that simple software with limited options is more useful than sophisticated database packages requiring complex interactions. For example, software which requires users to specify the category and length of fields in constructing the database form require far more instructional time than software allowing variable length fields, and attending to these details distracts from the main purposes of the exercise. It is also advantageous for the software's selection criteria (needed for running reports) to be as logical and simple to use as possible.

Providing students with a list of the sequence of instructions they will use to accomplish the project spares them from reading the documentation, which would require too much time. After setting up the database form or template, a small number of records (usually fictional records) may be inserted and, depending upon software, merged with the files of other students to quickly enlarge the number of records. The students therefore have the advantage of acquiring a large file for running reports without a

Students will create and run six reports from their database which address the following administrative questions related to your nursing staff:

1. Who needs to update their CPR certification and safety certification by this November?

2. You have heard concerns expressed about excessive absenteeism on the unit. Who, if anyone, has exceeded their authorized amount of sick leave?

3. Which RNs are currently enrolled in school?

4. You would like the computer to print out your staff's names sorted as RNs or LPNs.

5. You would like to keep a "seniority report" on file with important credentials for individual staff members listed. Your are interested in how long the employee has been with the unit, if they are full- or part-time, their level of licensure and education, and the degree of interest they have demonstrated in continuing education. You would like the report sorted by employment date with the employees with the most seniority listed first.

6. Your are interested in an educational profile of your staff and would like to obtain graphical reports with a bar graph and a pie chart indicating the percent of your RN staff with diplomas, associate degrees, and baccalaureate degrees.

FIGURE 2. Sample Administrative Database Project.

great deal of tedious data entry. Students may then be taught to design and run reports related to the assigned information problems.

Educational Objectives

Although databases used by students in their clinical practice will vary, certain principles of database management remain standard across different software packages. Constructing relevant reports on any database requires that the information seeker answer two fundamental questions:

1. Which categories (fields) are pertinent for answering the information questions at hand? (data format)
2. Which records are needed to answer the question? (selection format)

In addition to conveying the concepts of data and selection formats, the exercise can teach students the usefulness of databases for managing information overload. The experience can familiarize students with the:

— precise and rigid syntax required for interaction with the present generation of computers.
— the ease with which the computer sorts and reorganizes information.
— importance of structuring databases with thorough consideration of output in mind.
— capability of databases to organize reports related to patterns and trends which can improve quality and cost-effectiveness of health care.
— exposure to a particular database software package illustrates certain aspects of selection criteria, primarily range of options available and ease of use.

Conclusion

Successful completion of a database exercise similar to that described in Figure 2 results in a more positive attitude toward the computer. In addition to promoting changes in the affective domain and teaching some psychomotor skills, interaction with a database which addresses concrete nursing information problems achieves cognitive goals. Students comprehend the capabilities and limitations of databases as managers of clinical, research, and administrative information. Furthermore, students can conceptually apply database technology to address clinical information problems, such as the identification of a set of high-risk patients in a clinic (McAllister & Corey, 1986). Comprehending that input determines output, students can attempt to analyze the type of database support that would effectively address information problems, whether they be in risk management, quality assurance, or clinical research. Experiences with databases help close an "imagination gap" for students so that they are able to take full advantage of automation capabilities in their practice settings.

References

Armstrong, M. L. (1985). Techniques of networking in the computer world. *Nursing Clinics of North America, 20*(3), 517–527.

Griffiths, J. M. & King, D. W. (1986). *New directions in library and information science education.* White Plains, NY: Knowledge Industry Publication, Inc., 63–65.

Grobe, S. J. (1984). Conquering computer cowardice. *J. Nurs. Educ., 23*, 232–239.

Howitt, D. & Weinberger, M. I. (1984). *Databasics: Your guide to online business information.* New York: Garland Publishing, Inc., 455–468.

Kline, N. W. (1986). Principles of computerized database management: Considerations for the nurse administrator. *Computers in Nursing, 4(2)*, 73–81.

Koch, P. B. (1984). The missing component in computer education: The affective domain. In G. S. Cohen (Ed.), *Proceedings of the eighth annual symposium on computer applications and medical care* (pp. 676–678). New York: Institute of Electrical & Electronics Engineers.

Loepprich, J. C., & Smith, J. L. (1983–1984). Can computers solve nursing's information overload? *Imprint, 30*(5), 49–55.

Matheson, N. W., & Cooper, J. A. D. (1982). Academic information in the health sciences center. *Journal of Medical Education, 57*(10: Pt. 2), 11–25.

McAlister, N. H., & Corey, P. (1986). Teaching medical computing to medical students. In R. Salamon, B. Blum, & M. Jorgensen (Eds.), *MEDINFO 86* (pp. 912–916). New York: North-Holland Publishing Co.

Sinclair, V. (1987). Literature searches by computer. *Image, 19*(1), 35–37.

Skiba, D. J. (1985). Interactive computer experiences: The missing ingredient. *Nursing Clinics of North America, 20*, 577–584.

75
Curriculum Planning and Computer-Assisted Instruction (CAI) Within Clinical Nursing Education

Eileen Grow Perciful

Introduction

The potential benefits of computer-assisted instruction (CAI) within nursing education have been reiterated in the literature. There have been many studies that have attempted to validate these benefits by measuring the effectiveness of CAI on a variety of variables, such as, student learning. Some educators have voiced a concern that if studies measuring the effectiveness of CAI within higher education have not been based upon a planned approach to the implementation, then the results of these studies may be suspect [1, 2].

Hales [3] and Hannah [4] have stated that the integration of the computer within nursing education needs to be planned. Hales also stated that there was a need for a body of knowledge that describes the planning and implementing of CAI. This literature would formulate a knowledge base for the effective and efficient use of CAI for not only classroom teaching, but also clinical teaching.

The use of CAI within nursing education continues to grow. Between 1983 and 1990, the use of CAI within nursing education increased from 38% to 79% [5]. While literature focusing on the use of CAI within the classroom component of the nursing curriculum is readily available, there is a paucity of literature addressing the planning, implementation, and evaluation of CAI within clinical nursing education. A recent study [6] revealed that there is a strong relationship between the degree of planning used to implement CAI and the degree of its successful implementation ($r = .86$, $p < .05$). If the integration of CAI within nursing education is to be successful, then a knowledge base concerning the planning, implementation, and evaluation needs to be developed and shared.

Reprinted with *Permission from Proceedings: Sixteenth Annual Symposium on Computer Applications in Medical Care*: Supporting Collaboration, Frisse, M.E. (Ed.). 1992, pp. 414–418. © 1993, American Medical Informatics Association: Bethesda, MD. * Supported in part by a University of Utah Research Grant.

The purpose of this paper is to add to a knowledge base for the successful implementation of CAI. The information in this paper is based upon a two year study of the use of CAI within the clinical component of one course within a baccalaureate nursing program in a small liberal arts private college in Pennsylvania [7]. A description of the plan, implementation, and evaluation of this approach to clinical nursing education is provided.

The Initial Plan

Preassessment of Needs

Administrative support during the planning phase has been shown to be a major factor in predicting successful implementation of CAI [6]. The initial planning for CAI use had administrative support at both the college and department levels. In the spring of 1988 the college sent out a call for grant applications for funds specific to hardware and software purchase. Heermann's [8] book, *Teaching with Computers*, was an excellent resource for both developing the initial plan and completing the grant application. Planning started with a preassessment of needs with respect to resources and curriculum. Resource needs include: hardware, software, people, and money. Curriculum needs focus primarily upon learner needs and teaching style.

Resources included two computers and no software specific to the content area (psychiatric nursing), adequate resource people, and grant money specifically for computer needs. Assessment of the curriculum showed that learners' needs within clinical education were for integration and application of psychiatric nursing concepts. After examining the curriculum, it was decided that simulations were the appropriate form of CAI for the learning task. The teaching style necessitated by the learners' needs was that of facilitator. The initial curriculum plan for integrating CAI use within one component of clinical nursing education addressed: content, students, faculty, hardware, and software.

Content areas that needed to be integrated and applied in the clinical settings were identified. The assessment revealed that twelve students and two faculty would need to use these simulations throughout the semester. It was decided that 4 computers within the department would be sufficient for this initial phase of CAI integration. Several software vendors were contacted for information and eventual preview of selected simulations. Eight simulations were identified for purchase. The grant was funded and enabled the department to have the desired 4 computers and 8 computer simulations.

Use of Simulations as a Supplement

The next step in developing the plan was to determine how the simulations would be used. Davis [9] suggested that nurse educators examine the effectiveness of CAI use within clinical nursing education as either a supplement to, or a replacement for, some actual clinical experiences. Since this was the first time that CAI would be integrated into the curriculum there was no support for CAI to replace actual clinical experiences. The simulations would be used as a supplement to actual patient care in the acute inpatient psychiatric setting. Guidelines for using the simulations were developed. The guidelines provided basic information about the use of the computer and simulations, a reading list for completing each of the simulations, and learning objectives specific to each of the simulations.

Evaluation Criteria

The final planning step was to establish evaluation criteria. Learning outcome would be the major criterion for evaluation. Learning outcome was to be measured by students' clinical grades that included the psychiatric clinical rotation and scores on the National League for Nursing's Psychiatric Nursing Examination. Finally, the students' scores would be compared with those of the previous year's students who did not have simulations included in their clinical nursing education.

Implementation of the Initial Plan

Computer simulations were integrated into clinical nursing education with the junior level nursing students during the fall of 1988. The purchased simulations were commercially prepared by Medical Examination Publishing Company (MEPC), now known as Medi-Sims. The simulations included the following 8 patient care scenarios: an adolescent with an eating disorder, a patient with an acute schizophrenic episode, a patient with a history of substance abuse, a patient with a major affective disorder, a suicidal adolescent, a patient with psychosis and mania, a patient with pain and anxiety, and a chronic patient.

Each patient assignment sheet identified a simulation that best reflected the actual patient care situation. The day before the clinical experience each student was required to complete the required readings relevant to the assigned patient and the assigned simulation. Students had to independently complete the assigned simulation on their own time. They were informed that the purpose of the simulation was not to teach, but rather to assist with integrating and applying the learned concepts of psychiatric nursing.

In order to assure that the simulation was completed, students were required to register their name and ID number at the beginning of the simulation and submit a printout of their scores for that simulation to their clinical instructor. Students also were told that while scores would be retrieved from the simulation for purposes of verification, they would not be used in the calculation of their clinical grades. Students had to complete a simulation each time there was an assigned patient exhibiting a different behavioral pattern. Every student completed at least 2 simulations, and some students completed as many as 4.

Evaluation of the Initial Plan

A lack of adequate resources and faculty support were reflected in the problems encountered during the implementation. A lack of adequate resources and faculty support during the implementation phase have been identified as significant predictors of successful implementation of CAI [6]. Problems encountered during the implementation included: not enough copies of simulations, difficulty getting students to adequately prepare for the simulations, and initial resistance from the other clinical faculty involved with the simulation use.

At the end of the semester students were asked for feedback concerning the simulation use as well as suggestions for its future use (see Table 1). Not every student provided feedback and those students who made negative comments tended to make more than one comment. Negative feedback came from five students. The negative student feedback is believed to be related to the time commitment required to prepare for and complete the simulations and the initial resistance of their clinical instructor.

Learning Outcomes

Learning outcomes (see Table 2) are understood better after a brief description of the two classes. Both classes ranged in age from 19 to 39 years of age with the majority of students from both classes being between 19 and 22 years of age. In both classes 50% of the students expressed some level of fear as well as some level of interest in the specialty of psychiatric nursing, before their psychiatric nursing clinical experience. It is interesting to note that the class that completed the simulations had higher scores on the

TABLE 1. Using simulations as a supplement (N = 12)

Valuable experience	58% (7)
Questionable learning experience	33% (4)
"Hassle" to complete simulations	25% (3)
Suggestions for future use:	
Give students clinical time to complete simulation	33% (4)
Do not use for testing	25% (3)
Provide adequate reading list to complete simulation	25% (3)

TABLE 2. Comparison of learning outcomes (N = 24)

Learning outcomes	No simulations (N = 12)	Simulations (N = 12)
Clinical grade	$\bar{X} = 91$	$\bar{X} = 85$
N.L.N. psychiatric nursing examination scores		
Theory	$\bar{X} = 44$	$\bar{X} = 63$
Interventions	$\bar{X} = 50$	$\bar{X} = 64$

standardized evaluation criterion, the NLN Psychiatric Exam, than the class that did not complete the simulations. At present there is no clear explanation for why the students who completed the simulations had lower clinical grades than those students who did not complete the simulations.

The Revised Plan

The initial plan for integrating CAI simulations into clinical education was revised according to the feedback obtained from the evaluation criteria. The revised plan included use of 10 simulations. Two additional simulations were received from Nurs Comps. It was decided that these simulations would be used in order to offer a greater variety of patient care scenarios. One of these simulations related to care of a patient with anxiety, and the other a patient with bipolar disorder.

Using Simulations to Replace Some Clinical Experiences

Some actual clinical experiences would be replaced by simulations. Students would receive sixteen hours of clinical time for preparation and completion of 8 simulations. Simulations would be completed in groups. Structured pre- and post-simulation activities were developed. The purpose of the pre-simulation activity was to determine who would work together and in which order the 2 required simulations would be completed. Post-simulation activities would resemble post-conferences in which students would share their experience with the simulations and compare these with their experiences with actual patients.

Other changes reflected in the revised plan were to focus more on a theory or conceptual approach to clinical education. This change involved greater attempts to correlate clinical learning experiences with the theory being taught in the classroom. The 10 simulations were divided into 4 broad behavioral themes to correlate with the theory being taught within the classroom. The themes were: anxiety, depression, withdrawal, and dependence. New guidelines were developed for student use of the simulations.

The 10 available simulations were divided among the behavioral themes to reflect the patient care scenario. The guidelines had operating instructions for both the computers and the simulations, more thorough reading lists to better prepare the students to complete the simulations, and the learning objectives identified with each of the simulations.

Implementation of the Revised Plan

Students were required to complete 2 simulations for that week's theme prior to their actual clinical experience. Since there were 10 simulations, there were a couple of weeks when students were able to choose 2 of 3 simulations. All students completed 8 simulations. The students met with the clinical instructor for the brief pre-simulation activity. Students completed the simulations in groups of 2 or 3. After the simulations were completed the clinical group and the instructor met for the post-simulation activities. Later that day or the next clinical day, students worked with their assigned patients. Attempts were made to correlate patient assignments with the weekly theme.

Evaluation of the Revised Plan

The practical problems that were encountered reflect a need for a more detailed plan. Structured post-simulation activities were difficult to complete as a group. Some students completed the simulations in less than an hour while others took almost 2 hours for the same activity. Individual differences in time to complete the simulations together with increased experimentation when simulations were completed in groups seem to be the reasons for these problems. The correlation between the class theory, behavioral theme for clinical, and actual patient assignments was not always readily apparent to students.

At the end of the semester students were asked what they liked most and least about using the simulations (see Table 3). The Nurs Comps' simula-

TABLE 3. Using simulations as a replacement (N = 12)

Positive:	
Increased confidence &/or decreased anxiety	50% (6)
Reinforced class theory	41.5% (5)
Negative:	
Not enough feedback from the simulations	58.1% (7)
Choices for simulations were not always good	25% (3)
Some simulations were too slow	16.6% (2)

tions were the stimulus for the negative feedback. These simulations were used even though they were not previewed. The sole criterion for their use was the fact that they were free which is not adequate rationale. Student comments supported Farabaugh's [10] suggestion that well designed simulations which provide feedback are needed to maintain student interest in CAI.

Additional single comments were provided by students. These comments included: simulations were a nice change in teaching strategy, they helped increase experience with computers, and they aided in identifying patient needs and establishing priorities in patient care.

Learning Outcomes

Learning outcomes for the three classes (see Table 4) are more accurately interpreted when the classes are compared with respect to major variables. The class that used simulations to replace some clinical experiences was slightly younger than either of the two preceding classes. These students ranged in age from 19 to 29 years of age. The three classes reported that 50% of the students expressed some level of fear associated with the psychiatric nursing clinical experience. However, only 16.7% of the students from the class that completed simulations as a replacement for some clinical experiences expressed any level of interest in psychiatric nursing before their actual clinical experience compared with 50% of the students from both preceding classes.

Both classes that utilized simulations within their clinical education scored higher on the standardized measure for learning outcome, the NLN Exam. The class that used simulations to replace some clinical experiences scored lower on the theory component of the NLN Exam than the class that completed simulations as a supplement to their clinical experience. Plausible explanations for this finding would be this class' low level of expressed interest in psychiatric nursing prior to the clinical experience, completing simulations in groups, the conceptual approach to the classroom theory, and their younger age.

TABLE 4. Comparison of learning outcomes (N = 36)

Learning outcomes	No simulations (N = 12)	Supplementing w/simulations (N = 12)	Replacing w/simulations (N = 12)
Clinical grade	$\bar{X} = 91$	$\bar{X} = 85$	$\bar{X} = 85$
N.L.N. psychiatric nursing examination scores			
Theory	$\bar{X} = 44$	$\bar{X} = 63$	$\bar{X} = 54$
Interventions	$\bar{X} = 50$	$\bar{X} = 64$	$\bar{X} = 64$

Conclusion

Several questions are raised with respect to curriculum planning and integrating simulations within clinical nursing education.

Should simulations be used to supplement other teaching strategies within clinical nursing education or should they be utilized to replace some actual patient care clinical experiences?

Should simulations be completed as an individual and independent learning experience or as group learning experiences?

When integrating simulations into clinical nursing education, should the scenarios in simulations correlate with class theory being taught or with actual patient experiences?

How many simulations provide the most effective and efficient learning experience?

In conclusion, the importance of assisting students to feel as comfortable and confident as possible with actual patient care experiences cannot be over emphasized. The use of simulations within clinical nursing education helps students to increase their confidence and comfort as they start new clinical experiences. Simulations offer students a safe way to get acquainted with some clinical situations prior to the real clinical experience. Learning can be enhanced with the appropriate use of simulations within clinical nursing education.

The questions raised in this paper support Hales' [3] recommendation that nursing education needs studies that focus on the implementation process. Nurse educators must have a knowledge base concerning teaching strategies for the appropriate use of simulations. As the use of all forms of CAI increases, nurse educators are charged with the responsibility to make educationally sound decisions about which CAI they will choose to use, where to use it, and how it will be used. Nursing education is preparing today's nursing student to work in an increasingly complex society that is inundated with computer technology. Our students must be ready to assume their place in this changing society.

References

1. Belfry, M., & Winne, P. 1988. A review of the effectiveness of computer-assisted instruction in nursing education. *Computers in Nursing*, 6, 77–85.
2. Clark, R. 1985. Evidence for confounding in computer-based instruction studies: Analyzing the meta-analysis. *Educational Communication Technology Journal*, 33, 249–262.
3. Hales, G. 1985. Current research on computer use in nursing. In National League for Nursing (N.L.N.), *Perspectives in Nursing- Based on Presentations at the Seventeenth N.L.N. Biennial Convention*, pp. 43–50. New York: N.L.N.
4. Hannah, K. 1988. Using computers to educate nurses. In M. Ball, K. Hannah, U. Jegler, & H. Peterson (Eds.). *Nursing Informatics: Where Caring and Technology Meet*, pp. 289–300. New York: Springer-Verlag.

5. 1990: 91% of US Schools of Nursing have microcomputers. 1991, April/May. *Nursing Educators' Microworld*, 5(4), p. 3.
6. Perciful, E. G. 1992. The relationship between planned change and successful implementation of CAI. *Computers in Nursing*, 10, 85–90.
7. Perciful, E. G. February, 1992. CAI simulations as a clinical teaching strategy. Paper presented at the Annual Meeting of the Council for Nursing Informatics, San Francisco, California.
8. Heermann, B. 1988. *Teaching and Learning with Computers*. San Francisco: Jossey-Bass.
9. Davis, G. C. 1987. Keeping the focus on nursing. Nursing Outlook, 35, 285–287.
10. Farabaugh, N. 1990. Maintaining student interest in CAI. *Computers in Nursing*, 8, 249–253.

76
Design and Development of a Simulated H.I.S. for a School of Nursing

KAY E. HODSON, ANN C. HANSON, CAROLE BRIGHAM, and WILLIAM VERBRUGGE

Introduction

Since 1985 sophomore baccalaureate nursing students have been using case studies in their simulation laboratory experiences for both practice and evaluation of basic care-giving and clinical skills (Hodson, Brigham, Hanson, & Armstrong, 1988). In addition, the administration and faculty at Ball State University have been committed to a major computer literacy program, fostered and funded at all educational levels by the state of Indiana. Nursing has been very active in the computer literacy efforts receiving its share of internal and external grant monies for purchase of hardware and software. Nursing faculty believe that computer literacy for the practicing nurse is no longer an option, but a necessity. Recent literature supports computer literacy efforts in nursing education (Heller, Romano, Damrosch, & Parks, 1985; Newbern, 1985; Soja & Lentz, 1987; Ziemer, 1984).

Discipline-specific computer literacy is the emphasis at this university. The sophomore level nursing faculty, in congruence with this belief, has focused computer integration on nursing applications. Obviously, one of the main computer uses in nursing is and will continue to be the management of client information. Case studies already in use in our simulation laboratory provided a made-to-order situation for a computerized data base. The client records had been developed for each case study in the form of the traditional paper "charts." When the students prepared for their first day in a clinical agency, they used the multi-media module to learn how to find information in the client chart. When they reported to the simulation laboratory for final performance evaluation, they similarly used the client chart to prepare for their care-giving routine. It was a relatively small step

Reprinted from *Nursing Informatics: An International Overview for Nursing in a Technological Era*, Grobe, S.J., Pluyter-Wenting, E.S.P. (Eds.). 1994, pp. 567–569, with kind permission from Elsevier Science—NL, Sara Burgerhartstaat 25, 1055 KV Amsterdam, The Netherlands.

to move the client information to a computerized format from the already-existing paper chart.

Planning Phase

There would be two major components of a simulated hospital information system (H.I.S.). The first would be the physical equipment necessary: computer terminals and printers, tables and chairs, electrical outlets. The second would be the computer program itself. Various options were considered. A grant proposal to the Helene Fuld Health Trust was funded to support the purchase of the necessary physical equipment. The portion of the proposal that was not supported by the Helene Fuld Health Trust was funded by Ball State University, thus making it possible for eight computer stations to be placed in the simulation laboratory as a simulated nursing station.

It was believed that time and energy should not be spent developing a computer program if there was already something produced commercially that might be made available for use. Some of the commercial producers of hospital and medical information systems as listed by Saba and McCormick (1986) were contacted regarding their interest in collaborating with an educational institution. Although there was considerable interest from many vendors, it became evident that this was not a viable option. Factors of time, cost, program complexity, personnel training, equipment compatibility, and mainframe disk space would not be overcome easily. Computer consultants from the University Computing Services had been involved in the investigation from its beginning, and they began to recognize the possibility of developing and programming a simulated information system on the University's large mainframe system. With the assurance of technical support and a major commitment of time from computer analyst/consultants, the nursing content area specialists decided to proceed.

The decision to plan and implement the simulated hospital information system was based on the above factors and also the fact that considerable computer resources are available on the Ball State campus. The H.I.S. was crated on a VAX 11/785 Digital Equipment Corporation (DEC) computer running under the VMS operating system (16MG). The foundation of the H.I.S. is a commercial relational data base management system (RDBMS) developed by ORACLE Corporation, Belmont, California, U.S.A. The RDBMS is available on most mini and mainframe computing systems (e.g. Apollo DOMAIN, VAX/ULRIX, VAX/AT&T, UNIX System V, IBM VM/SP, Data General ADS/VS, etc.). The central ORACLE product is the ORACLE RDBMS. It includes the kernel data base manager and several other subsystems to assist data base administrators in maintaining, monitoring, and manipulating data. ORACLE includes a complete implementation of Standard Query Language (SQL). Using FORTRAN,

Screen management, and the ORACLE database, the simulated hospital information system consists of the following:

14 Database Tables
14 Application Form Programs
60 Main and Subprograms
80 Screen Designs

Design

The first objective of the project was to transfer the case study information from the traditional paper "chart" to the computerized database. Two flow charts were developed, one by the nursing content specialists and one of the computer analyst/consultants. It would be necessary to understand information flow through the simulated hospital information system, through the computerized client "chart" and through the nursing component of the client "chart." Two priorities were established: 1) the program would be easy to use, and 2) elements of good screen design would be utilized.

Examples of existing nursing and/or hospital information systems were reviewed (Clinical Center Nursing Department, 1984; Romano & McNeely, 1982; Romano, Ryan, Harris, Boykin & Power, 1985; St. Lawrence, 1985). MacArthur and Sampson's (1985) ideas on screen design were studied. Site visits to agencies with both mainframe and micro-based systems were completed.

The major design task involved the format in which the case study client information was to be presented. The School of Nursing conceptual framework is Putt's (1978) General Systems Theory, therefore a systems format was used. Since the primary users in the first phase would be sophomore-level nursing students learning basic assessment and clinical skills, the nursing content specialists began by developing a format for client assessment. Screen design was kept simple with the use of "windows" to present only the necessary information for completing each segment of the assessment. The information system presently includes 11 parts. Seven parts are Fortran programs that provide a number of options or menus. The remaining four parts accept information for entry into the ORACLE database table. Screens are similar to patient chart forms with which students are already familiar.

Development

The development phase encompassed approximately nine months of weekly work sessions and meetings between nursing faculty and computing services consultants. As each client assessment component was designed, it was presented to the computer consultants for programming. Any questions or problems from the previous week's work were discussed. As the content specialists worked on the format for the nursing assessment information, it became evident that these screens could be used as a learning tool by themselves, apart from the presentation of the case study data. Physiological systems, psychosocial systems, and nursing concerns; such as, safety, education and coordination of care were given an organization framework. The result was that phase one of the project was redefined. Entry of the case study information was moved to phase two, and phase one became the introduction of the blank assessment screens with each assessment learning module.

For example, one of the earliest units for sophomore nursing students is the assessment of the integumentary system (skin, hair, teeth, and nails). The students must learn what constitutes a complete assessment and what terminology to use in describing or documenting their assessments. As designed, the assessment screens for the simulated H.I.S. provide the components of the assessment: Skin: Color, texture, temperature. At each point of data entry, a "window" appears on the screen which provides the choices relative to the element being assessed: Skin: color: 1. WNL, 2. pale, 3. cyanotic, 4. jaundiced, etc. Responses are indicated by the typing of the appropriate numeral. The program causes the appropriate word to appear on the screen; such as: Skin: color: pale. It was hypothesized that learning the content and correct terminology for assessment of each biopsychosocial system would be enhanced with use of the computer screens.

Implementation

The simulated H.I.S. currently consists of two parts: the blank assessment screens and the case study data base. Both programs have been presented to the user as one H.I.S., and at entry the user chooses whether to review the case study data or to access blank screens for data entry. Data entered onto the blank screens does not become part of the database. Students simply print the screen before advancing to the next screen. The printed screens are used for a variety of purposes. Students submit screens as assigned for each module, use them in actual client assessment at the clinical agency, and also use the screens to practice case study simulations.

The computerized case studies are reviewed as part of the multi-media module. The pilot study group of students also used the computerized case study data base when preparing for their final performance evaluation in the simulation laboratory. Informal evaluation revealed no additional preparation time and no unusual difficulty with this transfer from the traditional chart to an automated chart form. Data is being collected for a research study to compare the written documentation of students who have used this computer application with the documentation of students who had not used it. Data from this study will be analyzed during the early academic year 1988–89.

Future Plans

Interaction of the assessment database with other components of the system has begun. For example, computer consultants are working to allow students to indicate whether data is positive (evolutionary) or negative (entropic). Positive and negative data will be transferred via the computer to a "problem list" in each student's assigned computer space for generation of a nursing care plan. Other possible applications being considered include computer analysis of entered data with computer-suggested nursing diagnoses and interventions.

References

Clinical Center Nursing Department. (1984). *National Institutes Health Warren Grant Magnuson Clinical Center Medical Information System (M.I.S.) Computerized Printouts*. Bethesda, MD: National Institutes of Health.

Heller, B. R., Romano, C. A., Damrosch, S., & Parks, P. (1985). Computer applications in nursing: implications for the curriculum. *Computers in Nursing, 3*(1), 14–21.

Hodson, K. E., Brigham, C. J., Hanson, A. C., & Armstrong, K. (1988). Multi-media simulation of a clinical day. *Nurse Educator* (In press).

MacArthur, A. M., & Sampson, M. R. (1985). Screen design of a hospital information system. *Nursing Clinics of North America, 20*(3), 471–486.

Newbern, V. B. (1985). Computer literacy in nursing education. *Nursing Clinics of North America, 20*(3), 549–556.

Putt, A. M. (1978). *General Systems Theory Applied to Nursing*. Boston: Little, Brown & Company.

Romano, C., and McNeely, L. D. (1982). Nursing documentation: a model for a computerized data base. *Advances in Nursing Science, 4*(2), 43–56.

Romano, C., Ryan, L., Harris, J., Boykin, P., & Poer, M. (1985). A decade of decisions: four perspectives of computerization in nursing practice. *Computers in Nursing, 3*(2), 64–76.

Saba, V. K., & McCormick, K. A. (1986). *Essentials of Computers for Nurses*. Philadelphia: Lippincott.

St. Lawrence, K. (1985). *Computerized Clinical Nursing Reference Information System*. Washington, DC: Oryn Publications, Inc.

Soja, M. E., & Lentz, K. E. (1987). Development of a hospital-based computer users' course for student nurses. *Computers in Nursing, 5*(1), 15–19.

Ziemer, M. M. (1984). Issues of computer literacy in nursing education. *Nursing and Health Care, 5*(10), 537–541.

77
Evaluating Computer-Assisted Instruction

CHRISTINE BOLWELL

Computer-assisted instruction (CAI) is nothing more than instruction delivered by a computer (Ball & Hannah, 1984). Nurse educators have been capably evaluating instructional programs delivered by other methods for many years. They have expertise in evaluating instructional materials delivered by lecture, textbook, group discussion, and videotape to name a few. Educators evaluate the instruction delivered by these systems for accuracy and currency of content, too much or too little information, instructional sequence, audience level, and likelihood of achieving a stated learning outcome, among other personal and institutional criteria and values (Billings, 1984).

Suitability of the delivery system for the educator's intended purpose is also weighed. While the above criteria are applied to the evaluation of the instructional aspects of CAI, additional criteria must be considered (Grobe, 1984). What is new to educators are the criteria by which to judge the suitability of instruction delivered by the microcomputer. This paper describes the attributes of a computer that make it unique as an instructional delivery system and the concomitant attributes that should be found in a CAI program making it suitable for delivery by a computer.

Attributes of Other Delivery Systems

Educators know that instruction delivered by lecture is suitable for conveying the same information to a large group simultaneously. A textbook conveys the same information to many individuals but adds student control. A student can pick up and put down a textbook, refer to pages previously read, check the glossary, mark important passages, and know how much

---

Reprinted with permission from *Proceedings of Nursing and Computers: The Third International Symposium on Nursing Use of Computers and Information Science*; pp. 825–830. Daly, N. & Hannah, K.J. (Eds.). 1988. St. Louis: The C.V. Mosby Company.

and what kind of material lies ahead. Group discussion is selected when instruction is enhanced by interactivity, information exchange, and immediate feedback and when reinforcement is desired. Videotape is selected for its ability to present realistic action video and sound (Hannum & Briggs, 1982, deTornyay & Thompson, 1987).

Attributes of a Computer

What, then, are the attributes that make instruction delivered by a computer suitable? The computer, as a machine, performs several tasks admirably: calculation, repetitive tasks, information storage, information manipulation, presentation of graphics, animated graphics, and sound (Saba & McCormick, 1986).

The original computers were designed to perform rapid calculations. Since the computer only understands ones and zeros, all calculation is accomplished by repetition ... performing the same task over and over. The computer stores information in both its internal memory and in peripheral storage media such as floppy disks. Written coded instructions direct the computer to sort through information stored in its memory, compare one piece of data with another using an "if ... then" process, and then display specific messages on the screen (Saba & McCormick, 1986). Instructions also direct the computer to respond to commands from the keyboard to manipulate text or objects on the screen, draw a picture, or simulate a sound.

The computer is the medium of doing (Hawkins, 1987), a tool designed to perform for the person using it. In order to perform there is on-going interaction, a continuous cycle of input and output, Input from the user, output from the computer. However, whether the computer is asked to calculate the speed and trajectory of a rocket, or to present instruction, it can do no more for its user than to follow coded instructions in a program written by a human.

Attributes of a CAI Program

While evaluation of instructional characteristics that are common to all educational programs designed for any method of delivery is essential, a CAI program is suitable only when the author's instructional design maximizes the attributes of the microcomputer. The true test of the suitability of a CAI program is to ask the questions: Could this program be delivered as well or better using another method of delivery? Has the author exploited the computer's inherent attributes to deliver an instructional program?

The specific criteria for evaluating the suitability of instruction by computer include identification of the program's type and frequency of interactivity with the student, and the employment of the computer's ability to store, sort, compare, and display individualized feedback, to calculate, and to produce graphics, animation, and sound (Bolwell, 1988). What follows are examples of strategies that should be found in the design of a CAI program indicating its suitability for use on the computer as an educational delivery system.

Interactivity

The hallmark of computer-assisted instruction is interactivity. The computer is a *doing* machine. This concept is easily demonstrated when using a word processor or an electronic spreadsheet. The user issues a command, the computer responds, the user evaluates the response, makes changes or additions, and the computer responds. The reciprocal action continues until the task is completed.

The interactivity that is possible when using a CAI program can vary from simple to complex for both student and computer. Responses from the student may be as simple as typing a number, letter, a "Y" or "N" to answer "yes" or "no" to a question, or pressing the return/enter key as a signal to continue the program.

In response, the computer compares the student's entry with the entries expected by the program's author. The author, who has considered the spectrum of potential student entries, has listed a variety of appropriate feedback statements, which are stored in the computer's memory. The computer compares the student's entry with the author's expectations, and displays the matching response on the screen.

Interactivity between the student and the computer can be more complex. The student may be required to type original thoughts, or solve problems by manipulating objects, text, or icons on the screen. In response to the student's actions, the computer may be programmed to compare the correct spelling or synonyms of the student's entry, or display a complex three-dimensional graphic that can be manipulated by the student.

The degree of interactivity is also judged by its frequency. Reputable CAI instructional designers suggest that an interaction should occur at least every 15 seconds (Bork, 1985). It soon becomes evident to the educator evaluating CAI that the attributes of a computer have not been exploited when a student is required to read pages of text from the screen, and when the only interaction is to press the return key to "turn the page." The best indication of a well-designed CAI program is observed when a student is totally captured by the activity and is enthusiastically involved in the interactive learning environment.

Individualized Feedback

Individualized feedback is possible in a CAI program because of the computer's ability to store information and to compare student entries with the program author's expectations. When a student makes an entry, there are many possible individualized responses. The response may be a simple declaration of correctness and reinforcement. The program can be written to assess the student's level of understanding and then compare that level with instructions from the author to display a distinctively congruent response. The response may be to offer the student a different depth of information, questions with a different level of difficulty, additional explanatory examples, the opportunity to review previous material, or the program may branch to another section.

Individualized feedback that is specific for each student's needs and learning style, coupled with the student's ability to set his or her own pace of learning and to repeat the program as needed, encourages mastery learning for every student (deTornyay & Thompson, 1987).

Rapid Calculation

This computer attribute can be maximized in many ways to enhance learning. Immediate scoring is one asset. Score analysis and a printed report for the instructor is another. Calculation of numbers as well as elapsed time can be incorporated in the design to achieve learning objectives.

Computerized scoring, while typically summative, can be both formative and summative. As the student moves through a program, all responses are stored in the computer's memory. The program's author may choose to display running scores, scores after completion of a set of questions or, upon completion of the program, the accumulated scores. These scores can be presented as total scores or divided into significant categories, converted to percentages, and compared to preselected performance ranges.

Faculty understanding of class progress is enhanced by having a computer analysis of individual student performance or the class as a whole. The total scores, scored categories, and other data tracked through the program for each student can be stored on the program's disk. The computer analyzes the accumulated scores for each student and the class, and then formats and prints out a report.

Computer calculation can be incorporated into the instructional design. In a drug calculation program, for example, the student is given a clinical calculation problem and enters the formula that will solve the problem. If the formula is judged to be correct, the computer calculates the formula, and the student assesses the product for accuracy.

Physiological modeling programs use rapid calculations to simulate changes in physiological parameters in response to acute patient problems or chronic disease, as well as therapeutic interventions such as drugs and stress reduction, or compensatory responses to such normal activities as exercise. The program's author constructs algorithms that, when calculated by the computer, demonstrate the expected physiologic change in selected parameters. For example, a student, experimenting with the relationship between amounts of blood loss and the range of hemodynamic compensation observed in heart rate and vascular changes can select the number of cc's lost by a hemorrhaging patient and observe the concomitant physiological adaptations.

The computer's ability to calculate elapsed time can be used in several different ways. A simulated digital clock displayed on the screen documents the passage of time, or it can generate a sense of urgency. The measurement of elapsed time between display of a problem and the student's response indicates the level of student understanding or confusion.

Creative us of the computer's ability to perform rapid calculations can result in motivation and enhanced understanding of nursing concepts.

Graphics, Animation, and Sound

"When sound and motion are added to pictures, their usefulness as a teaching aid is multiplied by both learning retention and transfer, because more senses are brought into play by the student" (deTornyay & Thompson, 1987, pg. 108). The computer can be programmed to supply these aides. The clip-art type of pictures are most appropriate for computer programs. Simple line drawings, caricatures, and symbols can be used to clarify concepts, act as memory hooks, attract attention, or become part of the interactive environment within which the student manipulates objects. While some exotic and detailed pictures have been drawn on the computer screen, such pictures rarely contribute to the achievement of a CAI program's learning objectives.

An animated sequence can be explanatory and illuminating. Animation that is controlled by the student promotes involvement and understanding.

Sound can be used as motivation, to direct attention, to surprise, or simulate life-like sounds such as heart and breath sounds.

While all components of a CAI program ought to directly contribute to the achievement of the stated learning objectives, it is especially important that graphics, animation and sound be used judiciously (Armstrong & deWit, 1985). A student whose progress is thwarted by a non-contributory display of pictures or animation will become frustrated. A student given negative feedback with sound will become embarrassed.

Cost-Effectiveness

In this day of tight budgets, it is important to evaluate the cost-effectiveness of a CAI program. The cost of software and microcomputer hardware is high. If a CAI program does not exploit the unique attributes of its delivery system, it is probably not worth paying any price. There are less expensive methods to deliver instruction. For example, a program that consists of pages of text would not only be less expensive on paper, it would be easier for a student to read. Research has demonstrated it takes 20 to 30 percent longer to read text from a computer screen than to read the same text on paper (Mills & Weldon, 1987).

Cost-effective considerations include the number of student hours that a CAI program can be used and the time saved by students and faculty.

The cost per student hour is significantly reduced when one student can benefit from using the same program more than once. It is also reduced when many students use the same program.

The research literature has demonstrated that, when CAI is used, learning time is significantly reduced over traditional methods (Chang, 1986, Robler, 1985). This factor is especially important when a salaried nurse is taking time off the job for continuing education.

The research literature also indicates that faculty time is expensive and is often in excess of $10.00 per student hour (Larson, 1981, Kearsley, 1982). If a CAI program can free nursing instructors from repetitive types of instruction, their time can be better allocated to educationally creative and facilitative activities.

Summary

While nursing educators have a great deal of experience evaluating instructional materials, judging the suitability of instructional materials for use on the computer requires additional expertise. As with all instruction delivery, the unique attributes of the method of delivery selected should be exploited to enhance learning. The lecture, textbook, group discussion, and videotape all have unique attributes. Educators select the media that is suitable for achieving their teaching goals.

When evaluating CAI, instruction delivered by a computer, identifying the presence or absence of the unique attributes of this medium is important. If the attributes are absent, the instruction would be better accomplished using another method. Attributes that should be present in a CAI program include: frequent and varied types of interactivity, employment of the computer's ability to store, compare, and display individualized feedback and to calculate, and the judicious use of graphics, animation and sound.

The educator who finds these attributes incorporated in a CAI program, and is pleased with the instructional value, will have a teaching tool that offers an entirely different method of instruction delivery, one that can save student and faculty time, and provide an interactive environment in which the student is actively involved in learning.

References

Armstrong, M. L. & deWit, S. C. (1985). Choosing software: The importance of instructional design, *Nurse Educator*, *10*(4), 13–17.

Ball, M. J. & Hannah, K. J. (1984). *Using Computers in Nursing*. Reston, VA: Reston Publishing Co.

Billings, D. M. (1984). Evaluating computer assisted instruction, *Nursing Outlook*, *32*(1), 50–53.

Bolwell, C. M. (1988). *The 1988 Director of Educational Software for Nursing*. New York: National League for Nursing.

Bork, A. (1985). *Personal Computers for Education*. New York: Harper & Row, Publishers. Hannum, W. H. & Briggs, L. J. (1982). Systems design differ from traditional instruction?, *Educational Technology*, January, 1982, 9–14.

Chang, B. (1986). Computer-aided instruction in nursing education. In H. H. Werley, J. J. Fitzpatrick & R. L. Taunton (Eds.), *Annual Review of Nursing Research* (Vol. 4), 217–233.

deTornyay, R. & Thompson, M. A. (1987). *Strategies for Teaching Nursing*. New York: John Wiley & Sons.

Grobe, S. J. (1984). *Computer Primer & Resource Guide for Nurses*. Philadelphia: J. B. Lippincott, Co.,

Hawkins, W. M. (1987). The medium of doing, *Personal Computing*, October, 1987, 304.

Kearsley, G. (1982). *Costs, Benefits, and Productivity in Training Systems*. Reading, MA: Addison-Wesley.

Larson, D. E. (1981). Is it worth it? Determining the cost-effectiveness of using computer-assisted instruction in nursing education. *Proceedings of the Association for the Development of Computer-Based Instructional System*. Bellingham, WA: ADCIS. Western Washington University, 76–80.

Mills, C. B. & Weldon, L. J. (1987), (submitted for publication). Reading text from computer screens.

Robler, M. D. (1985). *Measuring the Impact of Computers in Instruction*. Washington, DC: The Association of Educational Data Systems.

Saba, V. K. & McCormick, K. A. (1986). *Essentials of Computers for Nurses*. Philadelphia: J. B. Lippincott Co.

78
Using Computers in Nurse Education, Staff Development, and Patient Education

BILL MCGUINESS

Introduction

Imagine that you are living during the cave man era. You are sitting at home carving some notes onto your favorite piece of bed rock when a salesperson enters your cave and demonstrates a "marvellous new product called Paper." You select a piece and examine it. It seems to flimsy too be of any use but, being inquisitive by nature, you buy a ream and begin to experiment with it. Before long you find it has several advantages. You can carry much more information at any one time because it is lighter. There are associated cost savings because it is cheaper to buy and can be reused, and by drawing lines on it you are able to provide much neater presentations. Before long the stone axe you used for scribing has been discarded in preference for pencils, pens, typewriters, photocopiers and fax machines.

To some extent the relationship between the nurse educator and computers is like that between the cave man and paper. At first glance nurses have been skeptical about the advantages a machine has to offer a nurturing, caring profession such as nursing. Now, little by little, nurse educators are beginning to experiment with this teaching tool.

The purpose of this paper is to describe the advantages and disadvantages that have been identified, to date, in order to provide a foundation for the nurse educator who is beginning to use computers. The term "nurse educator" will refer to the undergraduate and post graduate college or university teacher, the staff development officer, and the patient educator.

In true nursing tradition this paper will begin by defining some common abbreviations. Although there can be a range of abbreviations (eg: CBT Computer-based training, CAI computer-assisted instruction) most fall into one of two categories. Computer-Assisted Learning (**CAL**) uses the com-

Reprinted with permission from *Nursing Informatics '91: Pre-Conference Proceedings*; Turley, J.P. & Newbold, S.K. (Eds.). 1991, pp. 43–50. Heidelberg-Berlin, Germany: Springer-Verlag.

puter for the purposes of instruction or teaching. This includes most of the software used in nursing education, and can include drill and practice, tutorial or simulation type software. Computer-Managed Learning (**CML**) means using computers for more than instruction. The computer is used to manage the learning environment, either by controlling a variety of media (eg video or compact disc players) and/or keeping records of student results, for the generation of reports regarding student use, and performance trends, both on an individual or group basis.

Why Use Computers in Nurse Education?

To answer this question it is best to examine what currently happens in nursing and patient education. Presenting information to a student or patient is often limited to one or more sessions. The success of each session is dependent on a variety of factors, including the emotional status of teacher and student, the time of day, the environment, and the material being taught. Problems such as teacher or student fatigue, boredom, inactivity, and a distracting environment will all help to decrease the effectiveness of any educational experience. This can be further complicated by the time teacher or student are forced to wait for performance feedback. Items such as tests, assignments, and examinations are often the only evaluation tool available, and are conducted at a time that frequently prevents any identified deficits being addressed. Computers can help overcome some of these problems.

Computers do not get fatigued. When a computer presents material to students, it is consistent to every student. This helps eliminate the possible disadvantage to students that can arise from a fatigued or disinterested lecturer.

Computers do not sleep, which means that students are free to access material at their optimum learning time, rather than attending a scheduled lecture time when they may be fatigued or disinterested. We all have a preferred learning time. I prefer eight to twelve at night, a time prohibitive to most lectures, but convenient for a computer. This feature is also particularly beneficial for nursing staff who may wish to access information during an evening or night duty, or a patient that may wish to learn at a time when staff are busy or the clinical nurse specialist is off duty.

Computers do not have time constraints. Student are able to work at their own pace. They are no longer restricted by the scheduling of lectures or tutorials. If they require a break due to fatigue or illness they are able to do so and pick up where they left off. It also enables students to access information more than once.

Computers are able to assess student as they perform. This instant feedback allows students to review material while their motivation to do so is high. They are also able to repeat the assessment. This is particularly suited to clinical decision making where mistakes can be made without the patient consequences. Finally, computers can access a variety of media. Students can see video images, hear sounds, or watch animation, all of which encourage the students to become interested, or engaged, in the material.

Evaluation of CAL to date reveals that students learn faster using computers and that retention times are longer. This differs with content and student anxiety regarding computer use (Bitzer & Bourdreax 1969; Koch, Guice, & Ellis 1988).

For the teacher, CAL and CML offers the following: a range of media, earlier assessment of student understanding, and more opportunities to have didactic material reinforced. At present nurse educators are forced at times to rely on painting mental images. By using the computer as a "control panel" for a variety of media, the teacher is able to present information using a range of student senses, either during a lecture or in a CAL environment. Computers can also be used as early warning devices for the teacher. By recording and storing student performance on CAL teachers are able to detect possible trends. Any deficiencies are detected early enough for the teacher to instigate the appropriate remedial strategies.

It would be remiss to finish this analysis without identifying potential cost benefits. Computer technology is not a cheap option but over time cost savings can be realized. For nursing schools, costs may be reduced by using computers to teach students the initial principles (eg: how to draw up injections, perform aseptic dressings or prime an intravenous giving set). The equipment needed, and hence the cost, to repeatedly perform these tasks will be reduced. Further cost reductions can be made by using CML to reduce the quantity of marking and the time needed to mark, especially if sessional markers are used. The latter will also provide the teacher with more time for the preparation of higher quality teaching thus reducing the costs of remedial or follow up mechanisms.

Hospitals may be able to reduce the cost of staff development by having a computer rather than an educator present selected content during evening or night shifts. Staff would also be able to access information form their ward unit thus reducing the time lost by having to meet in a central venue for educational purposes such as lectures.

Finally cost savings can be realized in patient education. By using computers to teach patients the basic information, nurses will be able to devote time to information specific to the patient's needs. This in turn can reduce the potential for return visits resulting from of a lack of understanding. Computer-assisted instruction for patients would also increase the access for all patients, regardless of staff availability. This would assist in health awareness and help decreases non-essential of health care agencies. Of course any cost savings will initially be offset by the costs of computer equipment but, over time the savings described above may be realized.

Implementing CAL and CML Systems

There are four fundamental areas to consider when implementing a computer learning environment. Which content will the computer teach? What is the most appropriate software? What hardware configurations will be needed? How much staff time is available for development? And, what are the attitudes towards computer-assisted learning?

The latter is the most important area. Regardless of the "courseware," software or hardware used, if staff and students have a negative attitude towards the medium it will not reach its potential. Nurse educators have been criticized for their reluctance to use computers. Factors such as a lack of opportunity to learn, computer anxiety, little or no release time, or the exclusion of computer development from promotional criteria are often cited as reasons (Jacobson, Holder, & Dearner 1989, Christensen & Murphy, 1990). Computers, like other educational tools, require special skills to use. It is therefore essential that any move towards the use of computers is supported by appropriate time allocations and non-threatening familiarization processes.

Locating a computer in a common room with "fun" activities (computer games) may encourage their use. Later, provide a selection of frequently used information, for example, educational time tables for teachers, exam results for students, leave entitlements for registered nurses, and meal menus for patients. By keeping the access to this information simple, people will be encouraged to use it and at the same time, the computer. Next, invite some suppliers to demonstrate their range of software and hardware. Finally, conduct programming classes, as Volckell and Rivers (1984, p. 1) state "one of the best ways to teach educators how to use computers for instruction is to teach them how to write actual programs". Authoring systems (described later) will provide the easiest entry into this skill level.

Once an interest has been generated, form a small development group. If you attempt to go it alone you may find that you expend large amounts of energy with little return. This group should be responsible for: 1) identifying strategies to free up staff from other commitments (eg reducing services or employing sessional staff), 2) choosing the most appropriate content to be presented by CAL, 3) selecting the appropriate software and hardware configurations, and 4) establishing quality assurance and evaluation mechanisms.

Content that is suitable for CAL is really up to the imagination, but difficult concepts that students will have to access a number of times, content that is repeated several times to small groups of students, and content that is difficult to present in an interesting manner using didactic methods are all suitable. It is also a good time to determine the structure and purpose of any CML. Will the CAL results contribute to the overall grade of the unit or will they be for student feed back only? Who will have access to student results? Will audio and video images be needed?

These are important questions when the selection of software and hardware are to be made, specifically the latter. If audio and video are to be used, the purchase cost of both software and hardware will be substantially higher.

When selecting software, two major choices are available. The first is commercially prepared software that is purchased intact and runs on the available hardware. The second is to develop software within the school either by contracting a programmer or using available teaching staff.

Commercially prepared software is usually developed using large budgets. As a consequence, the presentation quality is usually high, as it is prepared using advice from expert nurses, and the product will have been through a series of quality assurance tests before being placed on the market. Also, it is sold with instructions. All that the teacher need do is select the desired software from a catalogue (eg Directory of Educational Software Computers in Nursing, local suppliers) and make it available to students.

Problems with commercial software may arise from its contextual bias, operating system, ability to preview (at least in Australia), and costs. Within Australia the development of nursing software is in its infancy. This means software needs to be selected from either the United Kingdom or the United States. These packages may contain content not applicable to the Australian context. Having to explain to students that some content is not applicable (eg drug names, nursing practices) reduces the validity of the product in their eyes and may reduce its effectiveness.

Commercial software is available for one of two environments: Apple or IBM based. Unless the educator is fortunate enough to have both options available, the selection of software will be limited by hardware. Fortunately this is becoming less of a problem as more and more software is now being made available for both systems.

Obtaining software for preview may also cause problems. Suppliers are reluctant to carry stock as it is expensive and easily damaged. Experience has taught them that lending software on approval can result in it being copied or rendered unsaleable because of damage of breakage of licensing agreement seals. The result is that nurse educators, within Australia, may be forced to buy before they try, an option that is not viable either from an educational or cost containment standpoint. This is resolving, however, as the demand for nursing software within Australia increases. Finally, high quality commercial software is costly to produce, which means that it can be costly to purchase. The market for nursing software is not as great as for, for example, a word processing package, thus the cost per unit will be higher. This makes evaluation of software imperative to ensure that dollars are spent most effectively.

One solution to these problems is to develop the software within the school of nursing. By developing your own software it is possible to present content that is specific to either your curriculum, context, or philosophical leanings. Three options are open to the software developer. Using programming languages (eg BASIC, Pascal or C), authoring languages (e.g., Hypertalk), or authoring systems (eg Hypercard, Supercard, Macromind director, Authorware) (Christensen & Murphy 1990). Programming languages provide the maximum flexibility but require detailed knowledge of the language. Authoring languages are easier to use because of their plain language but still require extensive learning times. Authoring systems are the easiest to use because they are semi-programmed. The user is able to design software by simply selecting the features he or she would like and the computer constructs the finished article.

The disadvantage of "in house" development is the time and the hardware needed to produce software of acceptable standard. Even with authoring systems, time is needed to learn how to drive the software, and then to develop the CAL. In my experience, forty to fifty hours can be spent developing a package of thirty minutes duration. Also, specialized hardware is sometimes required for development. Authoring systems can require large amounts of random access memory, which in turn requires the purchase of more expensive hardware for both development of the software and, in some instances, delivery to the student.

Hardware configuration is the next decision to be made. The basic configuration would be a microcomputer with one megabyte of random access memory and potential for expansion, monitor (monochrome), and keyboard. To enhance the presentation, items such as a color monitor, compact disc drive, and video disc players can be added. To enhance access and retrieval, items such as a mouse, bar code reader, touch screen monitor and modem can be added. For large student numbers, computer laboratories will need to be established which house multiple computer stations, and can either stand alone or be connected to a computer network. Hardware configurations will be primarily determined by the content to be presented, number of students and the available budget. Generally the better the presentation, the higher the cost.

When choosing hardware it is important to note that hardware selection can restrict software selection. The problems of Apple verses IBM have already been explained, selecting either will to some extent determine the availability of software. Also, at present, selecting either video disc or compact disc players will restrict software purchases. As many aspects of nursing are audio-visual, it is easy to be lured into the interactive video disc of compact disc hardware configurations. However, it is important to remember that it is not possible to record video or audio to these media outside of the factory. Prohibitive costs of in-house development in this area, will often restricts the selection of software to commercial packages. On a brighter note, advances are taking place in this area, known as WORM (Write Once Read Many). In the future, in-house development of both compact and video disc storage may be possible.

Conclusion

To some extent this paper presents a picture of problems and frustrations for the nurse educator who is interested in using computers. But the problems presented here are for the purpose of awareness only—not to generate further fear. Computers offer several established advantages for nurse education, staff development, and patient education.

Allowing students access to information several times over, at their own pace, during a preferred time will enhance their opportunity to learn. By allowing the teacher access to performance trends, multimedia teaching environments, and the facilities to develop software specific to their curriculum and contextual needs, will enable maximum use of this resource. The provision of inservice education during all modes of shift work will mean that practitioners find it easier to keep up to date. They will also benefit from being able to identify the efforts they make in continuing education, for promotional and personal reasons. Finally computers provide health education to a larger population than any nursing staff could hope to educate. This should increase patient understanding and thereby reduce complications and unnecessary use of health care services.

Like all change, computers have their disadvantages. The technology is costly and its implications not fully explored. But by prudent use and evaluation of this medium, nurses should be able to capitalise on the advantages and minimise the disadvantages. After all, where would we be now if the cave man had placed "paper" in the "too hard basket" and returned to his stone tablet.

Reference

Bitzer MD, Boudreaux MC: Using a computer to teach nursing, *Nursing Forum* 1969 (8) 235–254.

Bolwell C: *Directory of Educational Software in Nursing*, New York: National League for Nursing, 1988.

Christensen MN, Murphy MA: Authoring systems finding the right tool for your courseware development project *Computers in Nursing* March/April 1990, 73–79.

Jacobson CF, Holder ME, Dearner JF: Computer anxiety among nursing students, educators, staff, and administrators *Computers in Nursing* November/December 1989; 266–272.

Koch B, Guice R, Ellis M: The Nursing Uses of Computer Assisted Learning (CAL) in *Electrocardiogram Identification and Interpretation*. Not Published 1988.

Vockell EL, River HR: *Instructional Computing for Today's Teachers*. New York: Macmillan Publishing Company, Inc.

79
Integrating Computer-Assisted Instruction into Continuing Education and Inservice Training in the Practice Setting

Lucille M. Pogue and Richard E. Pogue

Introduction

The following perspectives are based on over eight years as a nurse educator and three as director of a staff development department in a major teaching hospital, and a collective 22 years experience in instructional computing. For the last five years the senior author has also directed the implementation of primary nursing throughout the department of nursing, is currently coordinating a research project to evaluate the viability of using a primary partnership between RNs and non-professional staff as the mode for organizing the delivery of nursing care within critical care units, and thus has direct involvement in nursing practice within the hospital.

The nursing practice setting should be fertile ground for the use of computer-assisted instruction (CAI), perhaps even more so than the academic setting. To this time, however, the potential for CAI in this setting has been mostly overlooked, both by those interested in use of computers in the practice setting and those interested in the use of CAI in the academic setting.

There are undoubtedly many reasons for this neglect of focus, including the following: (1) Much of nursing CAI development has been grant-supported, with an academic rather than practice focus. (2) There are typically only a few educators in most health care institutions, they tend to function independently of those in other organizations, and they have thus not formed strong professional organizations similar to those established by academic nursing. (3) The focus of nurse educators in the practice setting is usually on using available educational resources, not on the development of new resources. (4) For these reasons, the case for use of CAI in the practice setting has not been made to nursing administration or funding sources. (5)

Reprinted with permission from *Proceedings of Nursing and Computers: The Third International Symposium on Nursing Use of Computers and Information Science*; pp. 657–663. Daly, N. & Hannah, K.J. (Eds.). 1988. St. Louis: The C.V. Mosby Company.

Many educational departments in the practice setting concentrate on initial staff orientation and inservice needs, i.e. the focus is to meet immediate needs rather than the professional development of staff after they are employed. (6) Historically, the practice setting has met special instructional needs of nursing staff by sending selected staff members to continuing education workshops, an expensive approach which benefits only a few.

Objectives of Practice Education

What should be the focus of instruction in the practice setting? To state it concisely, the objective should be to provide appropriate and effective instruction when and where it is needed. The "when needed" is the time at which a practicing nurse needs instruction in how to provide effective care to patients under her care at that time. The "where needed" is within the unit setting where the nurse is working, i.e. within the institutional setting rather than at some location remote from the workplace. Preferably this would be at the nursing unit, but might also be at some other location within the institution for certain types of instruction. The instruction itself must (1) be appropriate to the practice situation, (2) be specific to the immediate learning needs of the individual nurse, (3) be concise and specific to the point on which she needs immediate help, and (4) provide the opportunity for in-depth study when time permits.

Why CAI in the Practice Setting

Where does CAI fit into this picture? The strengths of properly developed CAI are its ability to provide an interactive and individualized learning experience specific to each nurse's learning needs. Moreover, CAI can be delivered within the practice setting where the nurse is working, and be available upon demand, i.e. immediately when needed by the nurse. It can be competency based, so that the nurse knows when she has learned the material, and the institution can automatically obtain records of competencies achieved by each nurse if needed. CAI can also be used to provide high quality specialized training which may not otherwise be available within the institution. CAI may also be the most cost-effective approach to many aspects of staff education, an important factor in the practice setting. Finally, it does not require the direct involvement of an instructor, allowing nurse educators to spend more time on instructional activities which do require their active participation.

These advantages are of little value unless CAI provides an effective learning experience. Research in CAI generally shows that students learn at least as well as with other instructional media, and generally take less time to achieve the same level of learning. However, much of this research is increasingly being questioned because of difficulties in providing comparable learning experiences, and such comparisons may thus not be valid

(Hagler & Knowlton, 1987). Moreover, much of the research compares CAI with lecture, which is not a readily available option within the practice setting.

Another way of assessing the potential of CAI as an instructional medium is to evaluate whether it can be used to develop lessons which employ the principles of learning theory (Gagne, 1985, Reigeluth, 1987). Based on such analysis, it seems clear that CAI which uses instructional design approaches solidly based on learning theory can provide instruction which is superior to any other instructional approach except for a one-to-one high quality instructor–student interaction. The shortcomings of lecture are well known, but it is nonetheless widely used because it is an effective use of an instructor's time. From the student's standpoint, lecture is impersonal and not individualized, nor does it provide a student with an assessment of his or her understanding of content as it is being presented. CAI is also much more appropriate for teaching problem solving techniques because the student can be provided the opportunity for practice, with immediate feedback on performance. Other instructional media suffer from many of the unidirectional characteristics of the lecture. Paper-based programmed instruction can be cumbersome to use unless the content is simplified to some subset of a larger topic, and can be boring and tedious to use. As a result, many students eventually begin reading the material rather than following the question-answer-evaluation scenarios built into the materials. Moreover the modes of interaction possible with programmed instruction are much more limited than the rich interaction which can be provided with CAI.

Experience with CAI in the Practice Setting

The Staff Development Department at the Medical College of Georgia is responsible for initial orientation and the continuing educational needs of the nursing staff in a 525-bed teaching hospital within a health sciences university. The department has established professional development tracks that include clinical preceptorships in Adult Nursing, Adult Critical Care, and Maternal-Child Nursing. These tracks span a two-year period for new graduates, while experienced nurses enter the tracks at the appropriate level. In addition, externship programs that have been developed jointly with the School of Nursing are available to rising seniors in pediatric and obstetrical nursing. A nine-week refresher program for nurses who have been out of practice for several years is offered annually.

In addition, nurse educators are active on most hospital committees, and have had a major role in helping implement primary nursing. All educators make use of the computer in various ways to assist them in record keeping, document writing, and other uses. Instructional approaches used within the program include lecture, paper-based self-instructional packets, videotape and CAI.

Use of CAI

Use of CAI was implemented in 1981 when the senior author began developing a 17-lesson pharmacology series with support from a computer grant from the Apple Education Foundation. The series was recently published by a major nursing publisher (Pogue, L., 1987). The motivation for choosing this topic, and for developing a series covering all major drug categories, was to resolve problems relating to the hospital requirement that all new nursing employees pass a comprehensive test on the major drug categories before being allowed to administer drugs. An investigation into the need for such a project showed that considerable time had been lost during the previous year by staff who had failed to complete the drug test in a timely manner (Pogue, L., 1982). The pharmacology series has been used since 1982 to provide instruction during orientation to nurses who fail one or more parts of the drug test. As a result of the use of CAI, every nurse is now able to complete the test successfully by the end of the first week of orientation, even when orientation classes contain over 60 new employees. When classes are large, computers in the central library learning laboratory are used to supplement the seven Apple IIe/GS microcomputers used for instructional purposes within the department.

In addition, the pharmacology series is used by staff nurses to prepare for the five-year drug recertification test which is part of the hospital requirement. A pilot project has also been carried out in which a nursing unit with its own microcomputer uses the pharmacology series for pharmacology review. A second nursing unit is in process of obtaining a microcomputer, with the intention of doing the same thing. The refresher students also use the pharmacology series as the sole means of instruction in pharmacology.

We have also obtained a fetal monitoring CAI lesson which is being used successfully to provide an intermediate-level learning resource for L&D nurses. New L&D nurses will soon be using an entry level learning packet currently under evaluation, and we intend to develop a short CAI lesson on drugs used in L&D. We are currently reviewing other CAI packages on the market for their suitability for other practice learning needs, including an EGK program which we hope to use for unit-based review on telemetry units and to assess knowledge of dysrhythmia interpretation of experienced nurses going to critical care units.

A major frustration in attempting to expand our use of CAI is the relatively few CAI lessons which we find suitable to the practice setting. As a result, we are in the process of developing plans for further CAI development using the clinical expertise of nurse educators and staff on the units. We also intend to use the CAI currently under development by the authors in conjunction with the American Nephrology Nurses Association.

Evaluation of Our Use of CAI

Our use of CAI has been demonstrably successful in most situations. As mentioned earlier, the initial objectives of the pharmacology project have been met in full, and all new nursing employees complete the drug test successfully by the end of the first week of employment. CAI has been well received by the nursing staff, as reflected by both an early evaluation study and continuing anecdotal evidence obtained as a routine part of the evaluation of all our offerings. It has been particularly successful in orientation with both RNs and LPNs, where it is frequently cited as one of the best parts of orientation. Another indication of its acceptance is that orientees will ask to take lessons on drug categories for which they passed the test, but nonetheless feel uncomfortable with their knowledge. It has also been well received by most of the staff preparing for the five-year recertification exam, although we are beginning to conclude that the lessons contain more instruction than this group really needs. It has been interesting to observe that experienced nurses may take less than $^1/_2$ hour to complete lessons on content with which they are familiar, whereas those with minimal background on a category may take as much as two hours for the same lesson.

Students find that using CAI is very energy consuming because they are involved in a highly interactive mode of learning. Sufficient time and a quiet environment are required to make the learning experience a successful one.

Academic Versus Practice CAI

One conclusion which is coming out of the experience is that CAI for the practice setting must be different from CAI developed for the academic setting, i.e. we hypothesize that there are two types of nursing CAI, "Academic CAI" and "Practice CAI." We observe that attitudes toward learning are gradually changing as the level of professionalism within nursing becomes greater. Nurses in the practice setting are increasingly assuming responsibility for their own learning, and are truly becoming "adult learners." As adult learners, they know that it is that they do not know, and want to assume greater control over their CAI and other learning experiences. Some, of course, are finding this change painful because it is new to their previous experience.

Appropriate Use of Technology

A concern which also follows from this experience is the belief that an inappropriate emphasis has been placed on the technology of computers rather than on the educational reasons for using computers as an instructional medium, with a detrimental effect on the entire nursing CAI effort (Pogue, R., 1988). Renewed emphasis needs to be placed on educational outcomes, and in providing timely, appropriate and effective instruction specific to each practitioner's learning needs.

Our success with text-based CAI has demonstrated to our satisfaction that a great amount of effective instruction can be provided without using fancy graphics, videotape, or videodisc. Our development philosophy is to use graphics, videotape, or videodisc. Our development philosophy is to use graphics and other interactive media only when the content cannot be presented effectively in any other way. This not only save development time, because developing effective graphics can add considerable time to courseware development, but also saves the cost of equipment which may be used with only a small number of lessons. Recent research appears to support our concern about uses of graphics not directly related to the needs of the content (Surber & Leeder, 1988). However, as computers become increasingly graphics-based and as software tools for creating graphics continue to improve, we fully expect to make increasing use of graphics in our courseware. We have likewise found that current instructional design techniques are adequate for a great number of learning needs, and that we do not need to use artificial intelligence techniques to provide effective learning environments. While the technology mentioned above has its place, we need not delay our CAI efforts until these technologies become affordable and widely available.

Developing CAI

Developing effective CAI lessons is a time-consuming process which should not be undertaken without considerable thought and planning (Pogue, L., 1988). Entering lessons into the computer and editing them is not a barrier because we use a powerful CAI authoring system designed for that purpose (Pogue, R., 1984–85. 1985. Pogue & Pogue, 1985). The fundamental difficulty is that creating highly interactive instructional materials is very different from creating self-instructional materials which "tell." As a result, we are placing renewed emphasis on providing training in interactive design techniques for new authors, and on the design and development of entire lessons on paper before they are entered into the computer.

The Future and What Is Needed

The future of CAI in the practice setting offers tremendous potential for increasing the professional competencies of nurses in practice, for improving the quality of nursing care, and for doing so in a cost effective manner. It also seems worth pointing out that the potential audience for CAI may be larger in the practice setting than the academic setting because there are more practicing nurses than there are nursing students.

The scenarios which we find most exciting, and likely to be most effective, involve the integration of instruction as an integral part of clinical computer applications used to support direct nursing care. Our hypothesis is that each nursing unit will have its own "Clinical Nursing Support System" based on microcomputers which can communicate with other computer systems within the organizational setting. An example of what we visualize is based on the use by one of our clinical units of a computer application for generating nursing care plans. In the future, this type of application will allow each unit to develop care plans specific to unit needs, with instruction built in to help nurses use these care plans effectively. The first level of instruction would provide immediately available "help" giving concise explanations of the whys and wherefores of each element of a plan, i.e. information as instruction. A second level would provide a series of in-depth reviews, tutorials, and practice problems appropriate to each plan. The nurse would most likely use the immediate help level at the time of direct patient care, and the in-depth level of instruction for study when time permitted. This example is one which we intend to explore over the next few years.

What is needed to realize the potential value of CAI in the practice setting? Obviously, two integrated resources are needed: courseware appropriate to the practice setting, and computer hardware on which the courseware can be utilized. The continuing drop in computer prices, which is projected to continue at least for the next few years, suggests that hardware availability and costs is not really the problem. In fact, computers with the power to deliver courseware can be obtained, at least in the U.S., for about the price of a video tape player and monitor. The crux of the matter is the lack of suitable courseware, a problem which plagues academic nursing education as well as the practice setting. Until major efforts are devoted to producing such courseware, which will require a major commitment of funding support by appropriate agencies, it is unlikely that a dramatic increase in use of CAI will occur in the near future. One advantage which the practice setting may have over the academic setting is that all agencies involved in delivering health care—local, regional and national—have a vested monetary interest in good nursing care. Cost figures can be placed on the consequences which less than optimum nursing care may have on nursing capacity and patient safety, and on alternative modes of instruction, because training time is money in this environment.

Unfortunately, we see relatively few efforts to demonstrate the potential and make the case for CAI in the practice setting, and to provide the leadership necessary to convince practice agencies of the potential of this approach as a solution to some of the problems within the health practice setting. Is there a better time to begin than now?

References

Gagne, R. M. (1985). *The Conditions of Learning and Theory of Instruction*. Holt, Rinehart and Winston, New York, NY.

Hagler, P. & Knowlton, J. (1987). Invalid implicit assumption in CBI comparison research. *Journal of Computer-Based Instruction, 14*(3), 84–88.

Pogue, L. (1982). Computer-assisted instruction in the continuing education process. Topics in *Clinical Nursing*, 4:3.

Pogue, L. (1987). *Pharmacology in Nursing CAI*. Mosbysystems, The C. V. Mosby Company, St. Louis, MO.

Pogue, L. (1988). Courseware development: emphasis on practical outcomes. In *Shaping the Directional of Computer Use to Meet Nursing Education Teaching and Learning Needs*. Southern Regional Education Board. Atlanta, GA.

Pogue, R. (1984–85). Authoring systems: the key to lesson development. *Journal of Educational Technology System*, Vol 13(2).

Pogue, R. & Pogue, L. (1985). Authoring systems: a key to efficient production of computer-based nursing learning materials. In *Nursing Uses of Computers and Information Science*, Hannah, K. J., Guillemin, E. J., & Conklin, D. N., Ed. North-Holland: Elsevier Science Publishers. Amsterdam, The Netherlands.

Pogue, R. (1985). *Microinstructor: The CAI Authoring System*. Mosby-systems, The C. V. Mosby Company, St. Louis, MO.

Pogue, R. (1988). Guest Viewpoint: Computers in nursing education: where is the educational perspective? *Computers in Nursing*. (In press).

Reigeluth, C. J., ed. (1987). *Instructional Theories in Action*. Lawrence Erlbaum Associates, Hillsdale, NJ.

Surber, J. R. & Leeder, J. A. (1988). The effect of graphic feedback on student motivation. *Journal of Computer-Based Instruction, 15*(1), 15–17.

80
Detecting Procedural Errors: A Strategy for Designing Interactive Video Instruction for Nursing Procedures

ANNE M. DEVNEY, BROCKENBROUGH S. ALLEN, and DAVID M. SHARPE

Film, video or live demonstrations of procedures in an instructional setting rarely present the learner with examples of incorrect techniques. It has been thought that this would result in errorful learning. Computer-based interactive video instruction (CBIVI) however, permits explicit demonstration of procedures with greater assurances that appropriate feedback will be given the learner to reinforce the correct technique and avoid future real-life performance errors. A CBIVI program was designed to teach preparation of subcutaneous injections using an error detection strategy. The learner is shown the correct procedure, given the option to practice and review the steps, and then asked to watch several trials of the procedure and identify those which contain errors. The learner is given feedback relevant to his/her responses. This paper will present the instructional design algorithm used to develop this interactive videodisc lesson (see Figure 1).

Computer-based interactive video instruction (CBIVI) is an efficient way to teach and assess procedural knowledge. It permits exposition of both correct and incorrect examples of procedures and definition of the proper sequence of steps. The additional control provided by the CBIVI technology allows the use of instructional technologies which require the learners to detect instances of errors and overtly indicate such recognition. Measurement of the learner's responses can then be used to direct the system to select appropriate remediation strategies when necessary. An emphasis is placed on learner acquisition of the correct chaining of procedural steps. Learner detection of errors is used for reinforcement in the transfer of correct techniques to actual practice and the avoidance of errors in future performance.

This program presents a simple procedure essentially as a concept, i.e., the correct procedure is (1) defined by the presence of critical attributes (steps,

Reprinted with permission from *Proceedings of Nursing and Computers: The Third International Symposium on Nursing Use of Computers and Information Science*; pp. 606–608. Daly, N. & Hannah, K.J. (Eds.). 1988. St. Louis: The C.V. Mosby Company.

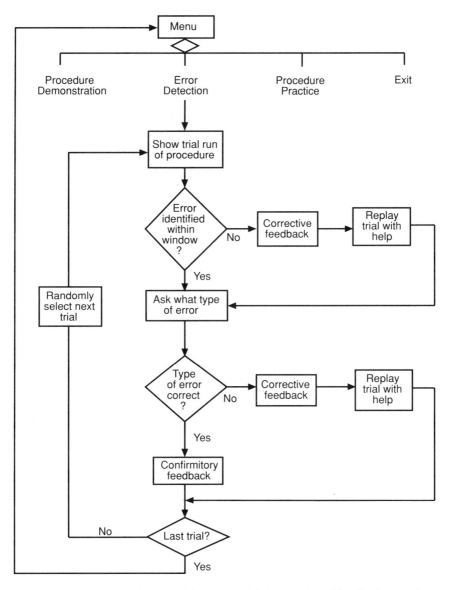

FIGURE 1. Error Detection algorithm used with interactive videodisc instruction.

sequence of steps, decisions, etc.) and (2) the absence of certain clearly defined errors. Often the practitioner is expected not only to perform the procedures correctly but also to identify errors in another's performance, e.g., contamination of instruments or a wound during aseptic technique. Failure of recognition of serious errors can result in actual harm committed by the practitioner, either of one's own performance or an observed performance.

The algorithm used to organize the instructional content for this presentation has four basic paths: (1) correct demonstration of this procedure, (2) guided practice, (3) error detection with trial examples of the procedure, and (4) exit from the program. The learner is permitted to reselect any option without penalty.

The learner is given an introduction, directions, and the program menu for module selection. The error detection module is composed of six randomly selected trial runs of the procedure, four of which contain errors. The lesson used for this program is the preparation of subcutaneous injections with an emphasis on correct medication checks and aseptic technique. The learner is instructed to view the procedure and press the spacebar at the moment he/she observes an error. The system compares the flagged frame number with the designated acceptable range ("response window"). The learner is given feedback by the system based on the timing and accuracy of his/her response. After error identification, the learner is asked what type of error was displayed. Corrective or confirmatory feedback follows and the system moves onto the next trial. False identification and failure of detection are treated as incorrect responses. A second incorrect response is followed by a repeat of the video with overlaid text or narration describing the nature of the error and any principles it violates. The video frame is frozen on the error and an audible beep may sound during the explanation. If the learner falsely detects an error, he/she is informed there was no error and shown the segment again.

Guided procedure practice is learner controlled. Steps may be repeated as necessary using keyboard commands. Emphasis is placed on correct sequencing and chaining of procedural steps.

It is felt that the use of error detection exercises, together with guided practice, may enhance a student's abilities to internalize, conceptualize, and skillfully perform the steps of a procedure.

81
Development of a Microcomputer-Based Expert System to Provide Support for Nurses Caring for AIDS Patients

Donna E. Larson

Introduction

One problem related to the nursing care of patients with AIDS (acquired immune deficiency syndrome) in the United States is that nursing expertise is currently clustered in specific geographic areas. In other words, many nurses practicing in AIDS-intensive areas such as New York and San Francisco have developed considerable expertise in caring for patients with AIDS. However, nurses in non-AIDS-intensive areas have not had the opportunity to develop expertise needed to care for AIDS patients, even though the AIDS population is evident in these areas, albeit in relatively small numbers.

Through the use of computer technology (a microcomputer-based expert system specific to the nursing care of AIDS patients), the expertise of clinical nurse specialists in AIDS care could be captured and distributed in an easy, cost-effective, and timely manner to nurses and students who are less then expert, but who so desperately need the consultation and decision-support of AIDS nursing experts.

With internal funding from Grand Valley State University, work has proceeded since summer of 1987 on the design of an expert system to the nursing care of AIDS patients. This paper discusses expert system development in general and specifically describes the design of the AIDS nursing expert system.

Reprinted with permission from *Proceedings of Nursing and Computers: The Third International Symposium on Nursing Use of Computers and Information Science*; pp. 682–690. Daly, N. Hannah, K.J. (Eds.). 1988. St. Louis: The C.V. Mosby Company.

Expert Systems and Nursing Practice

What Are Expert Systems?

Artificial intelligence, a melding of computer science and cognitive psychology, uses computers to perform tasks that require human reasoning. Expert systems, one component of artificial intelligence technologies, emulate the problem solving processes of human experts (Van Horn, 1986; Feigenbaum & McCorduck, 1983). Expert systems have built into them the knowledge of human experts; the system draws upon the knowledge base to assist humans in making decisions and solving problems (Bloom, Leigner, & Solano, 1987).

Expert systems are comprised of three major components. The first component is the artificial intelligence or programmed intellectual functions, the "inference engine," whereby the computer is programmed to "think"—to simulate human reasoning. The second component is the knowledge base which is supplied by experts in a particular discipline. The third component is the user interface, that part of the expert system that facilitates the interaction between the end user and the system (Laborde, 1984; Ryan, 1985).

Expert Systems in Nursing

The great benefit of expert systems is that they can capture, replicate, and distribute expertise—a much needed benefit to nursing (Ryan, 1985). Nursing expert systems can make available to nurses and students with varying levels of education and experience the expertise of highly sophisticated clinicians.

Whereas considerable progress has been made in the development of medical expert systems, little has been accomplished to date in nursing (Holzemer, 1983; Ozbolt, 1986). Four groups that have been working in the United States to apply artificial intelligence to nursing are: (1) the University of Michigan nursing expert system group, under the direction of Judy Ozbolt, Ivo Abraham, and Sam Schultz; (2) the Creighton University nursing expert system group, COMMES (Creighton On-Line Multiple Medical Expert System), under the direction of Sheila Ryan and Steve Evans; (3) the Case Western Reserve University nursing expert system group, under the direction of Pat Brennan and Ivo Abraham; and (4) the University of California, Los Angeles, expert system project, under the direction of Betty Chang.

The Creighton University expert system, COMMES, has been under development for over seven years and is currently being test-marketed in a variety of acute care hospital sites and schools of nursing. COMMES, a very large and complex system, uses a semantic network (Evans, 1985; Ryan, 1985, 1985, 1983). COMMES is an entire health care system based on patient signs and symptoms; its most apparent application to nursing is as an extensive information resource (Holzemer, 1984).

Another pioneering expert system development project was at the University of Michigan. This project focused on the development of an expert system for nursing practice in the area of elimination needs of elderly persons (Abraham et al, 1986, 1984; Ozbolt, 1986, 1982; Ozbolt et al, 1985, 1984).

A new expert system for nursing is now under development at Case Western Reserve University. External funding has recently been granted to support the design and development of an expert system to support clinical nursing decisions in adult critical care areas of hospital nursing practice.

Another new expert system for nursing, CANDI (Computer-Aided Nursing Diagnosis and Intervention) is currently under development at the University of California at Los Angeles. This project focuses upon integrating a nursing expert system into a large hospital information system (Chang, 1988).

To date, no nursing expert system focuses upon the specific nursing care needs of AIDS patients.

Why an AIDS Expert System?

The scope of the AIDS problem continues to increase. At this time, the number of AIDS victims in the United States doubles each years. By the end of 1990, it is estimated that the cumulative total of persons who have died of AIDS will be greater than a quarter of a million in the United States alone (Koop, 1987).

Because of the epidemiology of AIDS, there is a clustering effect that causes the highest incidence to occur in specific geographic areas. Due to their repeated experience with the needs of AIDS patients, nurses in AIDS-intensive areas have developed considerable expertise in planning and providing quality care for the many AIDS patients with whom they work. However, nurses and students in non-AIDS-intensive areas have not been able to develop the clinical expertise necessary to provide high quality care.

Projections are for a rapid growth in the AIDS population in almost all geographic areas, regardless of the current AIDS-intensity of the region. For example, *AIDS Update*, a bi-monthly publication of the Michigan Department of Public Health, reported that a total of 518 AIDS cases had been reported among Michigan residents by January 1, 1988. However, it is estimated that 2,300 to 3,600 Michigan residents will have developed AIDS by the end of 1991—this represents a startling 595% increase in just three years (Michigan Department of Public Health, January 12, 1988). It is evident that nurses in all geographic areas (including those that are currently non-AIDS-intensive) need access to timely, efficient, inexpensive, and accurate AIDS nursing knowledge and care strategies.

An AIDS nursing expert system will provide access to that clustered nursing expertise—an accessible, usable, consistent, accurate expert AIDS nurse consultant at every nurses' shoulder. An expert system of which each nurse and student could ask questions such as "What is happening with this patient," "What do you suggest I do now," "What are the most 'on target' nursing diagnoses for this particular AIDS patient?," What is the suggested plan of care for this particular AIDS patient?," and "What is the rationale for the suggestion?"

Not only would an AIDS expert system capture and disseminate the knowledge and decision-making strategies of expert nurses to students and nurses who are "less than expert" in AIDS care, but the system would also serve as an instructor, so that the users learn to be more expert themselves as they interact with the system. A characteristic of the newest generation of expert systems is that they can be queried by users. In other words, users can ask the system and receive answers to such questions as "Why are you asking for that particular patient information?," "How did you arrive at that diagnosis?," and "Why are you suggesting this particular plan of care for my patients?"

Through the use of an expert system, all nurses and students can have their own personal AIDS nursing expert consultant by their sides. They can ask the rationale for the suggestions and receive "real English" answers to their questions. By interacting with the system in such a way, users are able to learn not only the "what" but also the "why" of the expert consultant's knowledge base and clinical judgment. In such a way, an expert system assists users to become more expert themselves.

AIDS Nursing Expert System Development

With the support of Grand Valley State University, work began in the summer of 1987 on the development of a microcomputer-based expert system to provide decision support for nurses and students caring for AIDS patients.

Expert system development can be viewed as five highly interdependent and overlapping phases: (1) identification, (2) conceptualization, (3) formalization, (4) implementation, and (5) testing (Waterman, 1986).

Phase One: Problem Identification

During phase one of expert system development, the important features of the problem are determined. This includes identification of the problem itself, the human experts needed for the development, and the required resources (time, computing facilities, money, etc.) (Waterman, 1986; Citrenbaum, Geissman, & Schultz, 1987; Geissman & Schultz, 1988).

For the AIDS nursing expert system project, phase one activities have already been accomplished through work that began in summer, 1987. Specific activities related to phase one are detailed below:

Identification of the Problem

Throughout the summer and fall months, professional literature and clinical practice settings related to the nursing car needs of AIDS patient were researched. An up-to-date annotated bibliography on the topic was developed. Through content analysis of the literature, the most frequently used nursing diagnostic statements applied to AIDS patients were identified. Sixteen "AIDS-appropriate" nursing diagnostic statements were identified; they are being used as the beginning framework for the AIDS nursing expert system knowledge base:

1. Ineffective breathing pattern related to chronic tissue hypoxia, respiratory muscle fatigue, or impaired respiratory mechanism.
2. Ineffective airway clearance related to increased viscosity of secretions and/or pharyngeal pain secondary to candida infection.
3. Impaired gas exchange related to hyperpnea, hyperventilation, altered oxygen supply, or alveolar hypoventilation.
4. Anxiety related to unfamiliar environment or prognosis.
5. Alteration in nutrition: less than body requirements related to decreased oral intake or increased utilization of nutrients.
6. Alteration in comfort: chills and excessive diaphoresis related to persistent or recurrent fever associated with opportunistic infection.
7. Alteration in oral mucous membranes related to stomatitis, pharyngitis, or esophagitis secondary to candida infection.
8. Activity intolerance related to exhaustion associated with a disturbance in usual sleep pattern, increased basal metabolic rate, malnutrition, or tissue hypoxia secondary to impaired alveolar gas exchange due to infection.
9. Self-care deficit related to activity intolerance or activity restrictions imposed by the treatment plan.
10. Sleep pattern disturbance related to fear, anxiety, frequent assessments and treatments, chills, excessive diaphoresis, dyspnea, decreased physical activity, or unfamiliar environment.
11. Potential for injury related to increased susceptibility to infection secondary to decreased immunocompetence.
12. Sexual dysfunction related to alteration in usual sexual activities, decreased libido, or impotence.
13. Ineffective individual coping related to depression, fear, anxiety, drug withdrawal, or inadequate support system.
14. Grieving related to changes in body functioning, lifestyle, roles, or probably premature death.

15. Social isolation related to others' fears of contracting AIDS, precautions necessary to prevent spread to disease, or client's fear of contracting an infection from others.
16. Knowledge deficit related to follow-up care.

Human Experts Needed for Development

In addition to identifying the problem focus, another task in phase one of expert system development is to identify the human experts needed for the projects: the knowledge engineer, programmer, and content experts.

A knowledge engineer is critical to the development of an expert system. The knowledge engineer helps the content experts to express and clarify their thoughts so that the knowledge base can be built. Typically, the knowledge engineer will intensively talk with and observe the clinical practice of the experts. The knowledge engineer will then ask for clarification of thought processing to derive axioms that embody the key knowledge (Van Horn, 1986). According to Hancock (1987), essential skills for knowledge engineers include:

1. Expertise in knowledge representation, thought processing, and knowledge acquisition
2. Knowledge of the psychological implications of decision making and problem resolution
3. Extensive experience in interviewing and interpretation
4. A pleasant and persistent personality, oriented toward listening.

The knowledge engineer for the AIDS expert system development project, a cognitive psychologist whose expertise is in problem solving and decision making, possesses all of these identified skills.

Content experts, sometimes referred to as domain experts, provide the essence of any expert system (the knowledge, the expertise, the decision-making strategies). It is the expertise of the content experts that is attempted to be captured and replicated in the expert system. To accomplish this, the content experts and knowledge engineer work very closely together. According to Hancock (1987), an expert:

1. Can solve a particular type of problem that most people cannot solve efficiently and effectively.
2. Is an authority in the top 10–20 percent of a given subject.
3. Knows how to search his/her own knowledge base swiftly and arrive at reasonable and accurate conclusions.
4. Has acquired a superior knowledge base of materials related to his/her field of expertise.
5. Possesses both surface knowledge of many related items and deep knowledge of his/her area of expertise.

The six content experts for the AIDS nursing expert system are masters prepared clinical nurse specialists in AIDS nursing, all practicing in New

York, an AIDS-intensive geographic area. Each of the six is a specialist in a particular area of AIDS nursing: (1) AIDS in homosexual and bisexual men, (2) AIDS in intravenous drug users, (3) AIDS among minorities, (4) AIDS in children, (5) AIDS in pregnant women and newborns, and (6) home care of AIDS patients.

A programmer for the AIDS nursing expert system has not as yet been identified. Because an expert system shell (authoring system) development tool will be used for this project, it is anticipated that the programming needs will not be intensive. However, some customization will undoubtedly be necessary.

Required Resources

Resources required for the AIDS expert system development project include computer software and hardware, identification of human resources, and development of a budget for anticipated financial requirements.

A number of software products designed for the development of expert systems were evaluated for this project. With the advent of commercially available "expert system shells" (authoring systems) in mid-1986, it no longer is necessary to be in a programmer- and artificial intelligence-intensive environment in order to develop expert systems. Rather through the use of an expert system shell, along with some programming support, it is now possible for small groups working in small to medium sized universities and other settings to develop sophisticated and functional expert systems that provide decision support for specific applications. As a result, artificial intelligence has come out of the large research institutions and is now spreading into smaller, instruction-focused settings.

After evaluating a number of expert system shells, it was decided that Personal Consultant Plus offered the best possible match with the requirements of this AIDS expert system development project. Personal Consultant Plus is an inexpensive expert system development tool (shell) produced by the Texas Instruments Corporation, U.S.A.

The reasons for selecting Personal Consultant Plus were many. Personal Consultant Plus is a rule-based system, the most widely-used and proven framework for expert system development. The product also provides "hooks" to external programs (such as databases, graphics libraries, interactive video). This ability to incorporate other software greatly increases an expert system's power of presentation and performance. Personal Consultant Plus allows both backward and forward chaining, a strength when constructing expert systems which will be used in clinical situations. Personal Consultant Plus also allows the user to query the system at any time during the consultation. Another strength is the user interface; the screens are attractive, functional. and well-designed, and the interactions between the user and the system are easy to understand. Texas Instruments, the producer of Personal Consultant Plus, encourages the development of expert systems that can be widely distributed; the licensing agreement allows for widespread distribution (at no additional cost) of any expert systems developed with the product. Finally, Texas Instruments provides quality product support (training, "hot line" consultation, no cost updates, 40% educational institutional discounts, etc.) to the users of Personal Consultant Plus.

While expert system development software was being evaluated for potential use in the project, computer hardware was also evaluated to determine the configuration that would provide the power and flexibility required for expert system development. After evaluating a number of computers, it was determined that the IBM PS/2 Model 80 microcomputer would provide the best development platform for the AIDS expert system project. Because of the new generation of integrated circuits used in the PS/2 Model 80, it was felt that this particular computer would offer the most speed. dependability, flexibility, and graphics capability with the widest technology horizon for the project at the lowest cost.

Another aspect of determining resource requirements was the determination of the financial support needed to continue and complete development of the project. Since the financial needs of such a project were clearly beyond what could be provided internally by Grand Valley State University, a grant proposal was developed to seek outside funding.

Phase Two: Conceptualization

During conceptualization, decisions are made about what concepts, relations, and control mechanisms are needed to describe problem solving in the particular domain (Waterman, 1986). The analysis of decisions and the resultant development of decision-making flow charts is an essential step in developing an expert system.

To determine the feasibility of designing an expert system based upon a nursing diagnostic framework, three closely based upon a nursing diagnostic framework, three closely related nursing diagnoses (from the sixteen previously identified "AIDS-appropriate" diagnostic statements) were identified:

1. Ineffective breathing pattern
2. Ineffective airway clearance
3. Impaired gas exchange

A clinical judgement matrix and decision tree (flow chart) were then developed to illustrate the clinical decision making process as a nurse differentiates between the three diagnoses. A "mini" knowledge base was built using Personal Consultant Easy, the prototyping version of Personal Consultant Plus, the selected expert system shell. This prototyping effort resulted in a much clearer conceptualization of the scope and structure of the intended expert system.

Phase Three: Formalization

"Formalization involves expressing the key concepts and relations in some formal way, usually within a framework suggested by an expert system building language" (Waterman, 1986, p. 137). When determining resource requirements in phase one, it was decided that a commercially available expert system shell, Personal Consultant Plus, would be used for the AIDS expert system development project. Therefore, knowledge engineering efforts to capture the knowledge and expertise of the AIDS nursing content experts will be conducted within the framework already established by this specific software development tool. Since Personal Consultant Plus is a rule-based system development tool, the knowledge and decision-making strategies of the AIDS nursing content experts will be represented by IF-THEN rules. The sixteen previously identified "AIDS-appropriate" nursing diagnostic statements, along with identified etiologies and defining characteristics, will serve as the initial framework, later to be augmented by specific nursing care planning knowledge.

Phase Four: Implementation

During implementation, the formalized knowledge is transformed into a working computer program (Water, 1986). Through use of the selected expert system shell, the knowledge base of the AIDS nursing content experts which now represented by IF-THEN rules is transferred into the computer so that the knowledge and decision-making strategies of the experts can be replicated. Expert system development requires prototypes to ensure that the system will perform as required (Hancock, 1987). It is anticipated that a number of working prototypes, each building upon the other, will be developed as this project progresses.

Phase Five: Testing

Testing involves evaluating the performance and utility of the prototype program and revising it as necessary (Waterman, 1986). This phase involves the critical review of the system by the experts as well as invited outside expert and users. An extensive formative and summative evaluation plan has been developed for the AIDS nursing expert system. In addition to extensive formation evaluation which will take place throughout the development and initial field testing of the AIDS expert system, a full-scale summative evaluation will also be conducted. The following aspects will be tested:

1. Accuracy/Precision
2. Adequacy
3. Appeal/Acceptance/Usefulness
4. Breadth/Depth/Wholeness

5. Validity
6. Reliability

If any expert system is to be used, it must be appealing and credible to the end-users (Marcot, 1987). Since it is intended that the AIDS nursing expert system will be deliverable and usable, the entire design and development process will be conducted with the end-user in mind. The end user is critical in the testing of the system.

Impact of an AIDS Nursing Expert System

By using the AIDS expert system, nurses and students who are "less than expert" in their care of AIDS patients will benefit from the timely, available, and consistent computer-mediated consultation from nurses who are truly expert in this area of nursing. No longer will AIDS clinical nursing expertise be clustered in specific geographic areas. Now all nurses and students, wherever located, can have access to expert clinical decision support. Through the technology of portable computers, there is the potential for constant availability of expert AIDS nurse consultants at the fingertips of every nurse and nursing student!

Not only will the expert system help nurses and students make accurate and timely clinical judgments, but the end users' clinical judgement skills may be enhanced by the ready availability and modeling of the decision-making heuristic of clinical nurse specialists. It is anticipated that the AIDS nursing expert system will positively impact both the delivery of nursing care and the education of nurses and students.

Another impact of this project concerns research. According to the pioneering work conducted by Benner and her associates, it currently requires five to seven years for a novice nurse to progress to the level of exert clinician (Benner, 1984). The obvious research question that will result from this project is: If the knowledge base and clinical decision-making skills of expert clinical nurse specialists were consistently provided through a expert system to students and novice nurses, is it possible to decrease the amount of time necessary to develop along the continuum, from novice to expert? If so, the implications for health care and society are tremendous. This area of research will be pursued following the development of the AIDS nursing expert system.

Reference

Abraham, I., & Schultz, S. (1986). Knowledge representation in clinical inference in nursing: Structures and their application to information systems. In *Proceedings of the Fifth World Congress on Medical Informatics (MEDINFO 86)*. Amsterdam: Elsevier Science Publishers (North-Holland), 194–198.

Abraham, I., Schultz, S., Ozbolt, J., & Swain, M. (1984). A multivariate mathematical algorithm for diagnostic information systems: Procedures for clinical inference. In *Proceedings of the Eighth Symposium on Computer Applications in Medical Care.* Silver Spring, MD: IEEE Computer Society Press, 107–111.

Benner, P. (1984). *From novice to expert: Excellence and power in clinical nursing practice.* Menlo Park, CA: Addison-Wesley.

Citrenbaum, R., Geissman, J., & Schultz, R. (1987 September). Selecting a shell. *AI Expert, 2* (9), 30–39.

Chang, B., Roth, K., Gonzales, E., Caswell, D. & DiStefano, J. (1988 January/February). CANDI: A knowledge-based system for nursing diagnosis. *Computers in Nursing, 6* (1), 13–21.

Evans, S. (1985). Clinical and academic uses of COMMES: An implemented AI expert system. In *Proceedings of the Ninth Symposium on Computer Applications in Medical Care.* Silver Spring, MD: IEEE Computer Society Press, 337.

Feigenbaum, E., & McCorduck, P. (1983). *The fifth generation, artificial intelligence, and Japan's computer challenge to the world.* Menlo Park, CA: Addison-Wesley.

Geissman, J., & Schultz, R. (1988 February). Verification & validation of expert systems. *AI Expert, 3* (2), 26–33.

Hancock, B. (1987 May). Expert systems. *DEC Professional, 6* (5), 40–48.

Holzemer, W. (1983). Computer-assisted decision making in the nursing process. In *Perspectives in nursing.* NLN Publication #41–1985. NY: National League for Nursing, 51–62.

Koop, G. (1987). Surgeon General's Report on Acquired Immune Deficiency Syndrome, Washington, D.C.

Laborde, J. (1984 July/August). Expert systems for nursing? Computers in Nursing, 2 (4), 130–135.

Marcot, B. (1987 July). Testing your knowledge base. *AI Expert 2* (8), 42–47.

Michigan Department of Public Health (1988 February 9). *AIDS Update, 3* (3).

Ozbolt, J. (1986). Developing decision support systems for nursing: Issues of knowledge representation. In *Proceedings of the Fifth World Congress on Medical Informatics (MEDINFO 86).* Amsterdam: Elsevier Science Publishers (North-Holland), 186–189,

Ozbolt, J. (1982). A prototype information system to aid nursing decisions. In *Proceedings of the Sixth Symposium on Computer Applications in Medical Care.* Silver Spring, MD: IEEE Computer Society Press, 653–657.

Ozbolt, J., Schultz, S., Swain, M., & Abraham, I. (1985). A proposed expert system for nursing practice: A springboard to nursing science. *Journal of Medical System, 9* (1/2), 57–68.

Ozbolt, J., Schultz, S., Swain, M., Abraham, I., & Farchaus-Stein, K. (1984). Developing an expert system for nursing practice. In *Proceedings of the Eighth Symposium on Computer Applications in Medical Care.* Silver Spring, MD: IEEE Computer Society Press, 654–657.

Ryan, S. (1985). An expert system for nursing practice: Clinical decision support. *Journal of Medical Systems, 9* (1/2), 29–41.

Ryan, S. (1985 March/April). An expert system for nursing practice: Clinical decision support. *Computers in Nursing, 3* (2), 77–84.

Ryan, S. (1983). Applications of a nursing knowledge based system for nursing practice, inservice, continuing education, and standards of care. In *Proceedings of the Seventh Symposium on Computer Applications in Medical Care*. Silver Spring, MD: IEEE Computer Society Press, 491–494.

Van Horn, M. (1986). *Understanding expert systems.* NY: Bantam Computer Books.

Waterman, D. (1986). *A guide to expert systems.* Reading, MA: Addison-Wesley.

82
Can Computers Help Us Teach Clinical Decision Making to Advanced Nursing Specialists

Sandra J. Engberg and Joyce E. White

Using the Computer to Teach Decision Making

The ability to make sound clinical decisions is an essential component of nursing practice. It becomes even more critical as nurses move into advanced clinical practice where they work with increasing autonomy. While the decision making process can be taught, development of real expertise in decision making requires grounding in the nursing specialty content, guided clinical practice, and feedback.

Our teaching and evaluation of clinical decision making is based on Carnevali's diagnostic reasoning model (Carnevali, 1984). According to this model, successful decision making is dependent on the nurse's ability to identify and cluster relevant cues and to generate accurate hypotheses early in the diagnostic task. These early hypotheses guide subsequent data collection and evaluation. The nurse continues to collect data to rule in or out the hypotheses until, finally, one is accepted.

Use of the diagnostic process is influenced by the expertise of the individual clinician, the nature of the diagnostic task, and the setting in which the diagnosis is occurring. Clinical expertise influences cue selection and clustering and the effectiveness of early hypothesis generation and evaluation. Thus, it has a major influence on diagnostic accuracy.

In our didactic sessions on clinical decision making, we present this model to the student. Using the computer simulations, we structure our program to allow the student's opportunities to practice effective clinical decision making. We evaluate students' ability to effectively select clinical cues, to generate hypotheses early in the clinical encounter, and to evaluate those hypotheses, as well as to measure their diagnostic accuracy. In past years, we have used a variety of methods to teach clinical decision making, but for

Reprinted with permission from; *Nursing Informatics '91: Proceedings of the Fourth International Conference on Nursing Use of Computers and Information Science*; Hovenga, E.J.S., Hannah, K.J., McCormick, K.A. & Ronald, J.S. (Eds.). 1991, pp. 672–675. Heidelberg-Berlin, Germany: Springer-Verlag.

the past three years faculty-developed computer simulations have played a major role in teaching and evaluating clinical decision making.

Our interest in computer simulations grew out of our conviction that the most effective way to learn clinical decision making was within the context of actual clinical problems. We are committed to the concept of problem-based learning. At the same time, we want to be sure that all students are exposed to patients of similar complexity (McDowell, Nardini, Negley, White, 1984). Initially we used simulated patients, actors who portrayed patients, to teach and evaluate this content, but found that the costs were prohibitive.

As we became convinced that computer simulations were a viable alternative, we searched for commercially available ones. We wanted a non-menu driven system that permitted a natural language interface and allowed the students the same degree of flexibility in collecting clinical data that characterized most clinical situations.

We were unable to find commercially available simulations that met our needs and turned to looking for a way to develop our own. We selected the authoring system, Precept, developed by Dr. Abdulla Abdulla, a cardiologist and John Henke, an engineer (Abdulla & Henke, 1987). This system was designed specifically for the development of clinical simulations.

The computer simulations that we develop are based on patients from our clinical practices. Using Precept, we write a program to "put the patient into the computer" so that the student can query the computer in much the same way that she would interview an actual patient. The addition of interactive video allows the demonstration of non-verbal cues and tests the student's ability to identify abnormal physical findings.

When the student types in certain questions, she actually sees the patient responding or sees the findings on examination of the requested system.

We have a work station in our Learning Resource Center where students can complete the simulations at their convenience. Students use the keyboard to query the simulated patient about his/her current problem, past medical history, family history, and review of system as well as to gather patient profile information. They can also request various parts of the physical examination and a variety of diagnostic tests. In keeping with an actual clinical encounter, the amount of diagnostic data immediately available is limited. Students might be told, for example, that the results of a particular diagnostic test won't be available for 48 hours. The system is not menu-driven. Students must ask specifically for each piece of information. The program allows students to collect data using a process driven by student hypotheses rather than in linear fashion. Students can move back and forth between the history and physical examination. The program also provides feedback and remediation to the students.

We have used these computer simulations in a variety of our courses. One of the early courses in our program is a health promotion course. One of the content areas of this course deals with the identification and evaluation of health risk factors. After this didactic content is presented, students are assigned to complete a computer simulation which allows them to practice these skills. In our physical diagnoses course, we use a computer simulation to teach and evaluate history taking. We also use a simulation in teaching students how to approach clinical decision making situations. In our adult management courses, we use a clinical simulation to teach decision making around the prescription of oral contraceptives and to evaluate the students' ability to effectively use the decision making process in diagnosing and managing a common episodic illness.

We have evaluated the effectiveness of our computer simulations in a number of ways. We used one of our simulations in a research study designed to compare novice and expert clinical decision making. As part of the study, we asked participants to evaluate the credibility of the simulations. The evaluation was overwhelmingly positive.

We also compared student learning of content taught within the context of simulation to the same content taught by traditional methods. Students learned the content equally well from the simulation. We are currently conducting a study designed to examine the criterion-related validity of the simulations by comparing performance on the simulations to that in actual clinical practice.

References

Abdulla, A.M., Henke, J., Watkins, L. (1987). Computer-aided learning: Experienced, perspectives and promises. *Journal of the American College of Cardiology*, *9*(3), 678–683.

Carnevali, D.L. (1984). The diagnostic reasoning process. In D.L. Carnevali, P.H. Mitchell, N.F. Woods, & C.A. Tanner (Eds). *Diagnostic reasoning in nursing* (pp. 25–56). New York: J. B. Lippincott Company.

McDowell, B.J., Nardini, D.L., Negley, S.A. & White, J.E. (1984). Evaluating clinical performance using simulated patients. *Journal of Nursing Education*, *23*(1), 37–39.

83
Educating Clinicians to Use Casemix Data for Decision Making

EVELYN J.S. HOVENGA and GREGORY K. WHYMARK

1. Introduction

The Australian Government's aim has been to contain health expenditure. In 1990–91, the amount expended was 8.1% of gross domestic product (GDP), which represented a slight increase from previous years, but was considered to be of much the same magnitude as that expended during the 1980s. The proportion spent on hospitals has declined slightly [1]. The private insurance task force (1993) estimated that for 1992/93, public patient admissions accounted for 53% of all hospital admissions. Total health outlays provided for in the 1993/94 budget by the Commonwealth government amounted to 14% of the total budget. Public hospital services accounted for 32.6% of the health budget. Real growth in hospital services for 1993/94 is expected to be 7.5% [4]. There is continued pressure to find efficiency improvements.

State Governments are primarily responsible for the equitable distribution of available funds for the delivery of most health services to the community. Funds are also allocated to individual health agencies and to services under the direct control of Government departments. There exists an increasing demand for health service delivery, shorter lengths of stay in acute hospital settings, and a shift of care from institutions to community settings. Funds are allocated to promote continued efficiency gains in public hospitals, including "$7.5 m for the continued development of cost-based casemix systems to allow more informed resource management in the hospital system and assist meaningful comparisons of hospital performance" [4].

The Victorian government was the first to introduce output based funding (in July 1993) and now considers itself to be paying for services provided

Reprinted with permission from *MEDINFO '95: Proceedings of the Eighth World Congress on Medical Informatics*; Greenes, R.A., Peterson, H.E. & Protti, D.J. (Eds.). 1995, pp. 1247–1250. Edmonton, Alberta, Canada: Canadian Organization for the Advancement of Computers in Health (COACH).

to hospital patients, instead of providing hospital funds. Hospitals will receive a fixed annual grant plus a payment based on the hospital's casemix as defined by diagnosis related groups (DRG). Additional grant allocations are made for extra costs associated with teaching staff and for aspects of hospital care, for which current DRGs do not apply. New accountability processes were introduced through the Health Service Agreements between the Victorian government and hospitals [5].

2. Australian DRG Development

The first national conference on DRGs in Australia was held in 1985. Interest in a variety of casemix applications had become evident from State health authorities, public and private hospitals, and health insurers. Proposed applications included health care resource usage and allocation, planning, quality assurance activities, and utilization reviews. A proposal by the Commonwealth Department of Community Services and Health to the Australian Health Ministers Advisory Council (AHMAC) in early 1990 led to the endorsement of the establishment of a national standard casemix classification. Another Commonwealth initiative was the National Health Strategy Review, an important component of which was to assess the use of casemix for funding purposes. At least two Australian State health departments were using casemix as a factor in determining public hospital budgets. At the first consensus conference the following recommendations were agreed to:

1. A version similar to the New York system should be selected as the national standard. It was recognized that this would need to be modified for Australian clinical practice.
2. A version similar to the Refined DRG system, with inclusion of desirable features of the New York version, should be developed for use in support of studies where greater clinical detail is desirable.
3. Research should be initiated to determine whether a single combined version might eventually serve all purposes.

An interim clinician steering group, now the Australian Casemix Clinical Committee (ACCC), was established to coordinate the development of a standard inpatient classification method for use in Australia. The ACCC is of the view that "a more clinically precise classification and one reflecting Australian Health Care will be more effective for use in funding and in clinical management" [9]. Other casemix working groups were responsible for formulating all project requirements, including education, cost weights, finance design, documentation standards and conventions, and information technology. Changes needed to be consistent to ensure that Australian Commonwealth policy objectives were met.

Major difficulties identified affecting the empirical data analysis, where: (1) the absence of a "single authoritative sample of Australian patient discharge data that uniformly represents the practices of Australian health care providers"; (2) "resource measures throughout Australia do not consistently include the cost of services rendered"; and (3) "standards and conventions for documenting DRG data elements differ across the States" [6]. Notwithstanding these difficulties, the AN-DRGs released in 1992 are said to be "a synthesis of state-of-the-art US DRGs with clinical modifications that better characterize the organization of acute care in Australia" [6].

In Australia, a number of potential applications for DRGs have been identified, including casemix based funding, the comparison of lengths of stay, resource use for individual DRGs between hospitals or States, and enhanced hospital management within individual hospitals to improve both the quality and efficiency of hospital services. The Casemix Development Program funded by the Commonwealth commenced in Australia in 1989. This program included funding improvements in the infrastructure such that the data needed for classification purposes is now available from every medical record in every hospital. The Casemix Strategic Plan 1993–98 provides a formal strategy for the implementation of casemix over the next five years.

3. Subject Objectives

As part of Commonwealth's Casemix Development Program, the authors were funded to develop and implement education modules for use at the postgraduate level and for in-service training. The modules that resulted aim to improve the students knowledge of casemix funding and reporting, information system evaluation and selection, and how casemix could support decision makers in both the clinical and administration environments. In particular, on successful completion the student would be able to:

- Identify critical casemix information needs that are hospital or discipline specific.
- Establish hospital specific IT needs.
- Evaluate existing software in the light of these needs.
- Analyze the many relationships between data processed by existing hospital and casemix based information systems.
- Define and discuss issues associated with the use of casemix data for various purposes.
- Identify uses of this information to improve the efficiency of hospital processes in concert with effectiveness improvement.
- Establish the decision support information system requirements of a (student defined) decision maker using casemix related data.

4. Subject Content

Prior to developing the educational modules, there was a need to establish the type of decisions being made and the type of information needed to make them. Our objectives for data collection were to answer the questions: "How is casemix applied and how would hospital staff like to use casemix data?" Data gathering consisted of: hospital visits where various staff were interviewed, collection of system specifications detailing functional requirements, and system descriptions gained from vendors and hospitals.

Objectives for the hospital visits were to:

- familiarize ourselves with the information needs of practicing managers and clinicians and the type of decisions required of them;
- collect information on the type of casemix data in use;
- determine the casemix data that they would like to have available in the longer term;
- identify sources of information.

A subject outline was developed to establish the framework for the module development. Two prerequisite subjects were also identified. These are Management of Health Services and Information System Development, both of which are scheduled to be offered via the Professional and Graduate Education Consortium (PAGE) and SBS broadcast television network. The authors plan to present the subjects described here through this medium in 1996.

It was considered that, for clinicians and managers to successfully use casemix data for decision making, a number of topics needed to be covered in the teaching program. The first section includes an overview of hospital processes used to produce its output (casemix and DRGs). Included in this section are casemix development and usage in Australia, the relationship between revenue, costs, labor resource usage, efficiency, effectiveness, and quality, the meaning and use of relative value units and service weights, the tracking of inputs throughout the length of stay by patient, and the associated issues, such as critical path and case management.

Secondly, it was considered that students required knowledge regarding analytical and problem solving techniques, including an introduction to work study, operations research and quantitative methods, risk, and value analysis. The third section includes an overview of existing casemix and hospital information systems in use in Australia and covers issues such as establishing and using information system requirements for system evaluation and selection, an overview of possible data structures, standards and outcome measures, relationships between system architecture, database structures, and the ability to obtain required information.

The fourth and final section focuses on decision making. It includes decision analysis, decision support systems, and executive information systems and draws on the extensive amount of theory and teaching material available in the information systems discipline [7,8]. This allows the course material to provide highly relevant succinct but complete coverage of how decision making can be improved by utilizing casemix data and modern information systems.

The course material is not prescriptive, but has the objective of showing the student the potential as well as providing the means. As no one suitable textbook is available for this, subject development has involved a considerable amount of writing as well as utilization of a variety of additional resource materials.

5. Proposal for Teaching

The subject is presented by the Health Science and the Business Faculties as a joint offering. It will be available in a wide number of programs at CQU, including as an elective in the Graduate Diploma Health Administration and Information Systems, the Master of Health Administration and Information Systems, the Master of Health Science (Midwifery), the Master of Health Science (Primary Health Care), the Master of Health Science (Advanced Nursing), the Master of Business Administration, and the Master of Information Systems.

All graduate programs in both faculties (Health Science and Business) are available for part time and distance (or open learning) education. Each of the programs mentioned here is strongly supported by external part-time enrollments, as it is particularly attractive to health professionals in full-time employment. It has also been proposed to make this unit available as part of a four subject program called a Graduate Certificate in Health Informatics (CASEMIX).

6. Conclusion

The role of education and training is important not only for the professional development of the individual, but also for the development of the health system itself [3]. Modern management requires participation for a successful organization, just as information systems development requires knowledgeable users to participate in the development if the system is to be effective. Both are necessary if the changes in health system funding being sought by Australian legislators are to succeed.

The curriculum developed and described in this paper will assist in educating health professionals and making them more aware of the gains to be achieved by using management support facilities utilizing casemix data. Our purpose is to foster clarity and understanding, and to make clinicians and administrators better equipped to work in a casemix funding environment. The new modules will be available in postgraduate programs in 1995.

Acknowledgments. The authors acknowledge the finanical support provided by the Australian Government for this project.

References

[1] Australian Institute of Health and Welfare *Australia's Health*. The Third Biennial Report of the AIH&W. AGPS Canberra (1992).

[2] Commonwealth Department of Health, Housing, Local Government and Community Services. *Casemix Development Program Consultancy Brief*. Canberra (May 1993).

[3] Chong Yok Ching. *Design of a National Management Information System for Hospital Use*. PhD Thesis, University of Malaya (1994).

[4] Department of Health, Housing, Local Government and Community Services 1993 *Budget Papers*. AGPS Canberra.

[5] Health and Community Services (H&CS). *Casemix Funding for Public Hospitals Victoria's Policy*. Acute Health Services Division, Melbourne (1993).

[6] McGuire T. "Australian Acute Patient Classification Project—Evaluation and Refinement Final Report." In *Proceedings of the Fourth National Casemix Conference, Gold Coast*. CDHH&CS (August 1992).

[7] Turban E. *Decision Support and Intelligent Systems: Management Support Systems*. New York: Macmillan (1993).

[8] Sprague and Watson. *Decision Support Systems: Putting Theory into Practice*. Sydney: Prentice Hall (1994).

[9] Verco C. *Development of the Australian Inpatient Casemix Classification Standard*. Australian Casemix Clinical Committee (ACCC), Adelaide, SA. (1991).

84
Development of Technological Access for RN Degree-Completion Students at Distant Learning Sites

Kay Hodson, Ann C. Hanson and C. Brigham

1. Introduction

The growth of national electronic networks for education and research will significantly impact the nursing profession [1]. Increased electronic connectivity will improve the ability of the end-user researcher and educator to access data processing capabilities and other researchers/faculty electronically to advance scholarship and educational activities [2,3,4]. The significance of the trend can be a reconceptualization of the research and educational process. It is, therefore, critical that nursing students and nurse clinicians become knowledgeable users of electronic networks which focus on quality health care delivery.

2. Problem Statement

It is critically important that the practicing professional, such as the registered nurse, be prepared to plan and deliver client services which utilize all the capabilities of our increasingly technological age. Improving technological access for students at the distance learning sites who, for the most part, received their basic education in a precomputer era is critical to enabling these students to retain their current positions of leadership in their profession and to become active participants in a world increasingly networked through communication channels.

Reprinted from *MEDINFO '92: Proceedings of the Seventh World Congress on Medical Informatics*, Lun, K.C., Degoulet, P., Piemme, T.E. & Rienhoff, O. (Eds.). 1992, pp. 560–564, with kind permission from Elsevier Science—NL, Sara Burgerhartstraat 25, 1055 KV Amsterdam, The Netherlands.

3. Background

Ball State University is a major provider of distance education programs to the State of Indiana, offering full degree programs and numerous general studies and in-service courses by one-way television and two-way audio. The Indiana Higher Education Telecommunications System (IHETS) has been the primary carrier of distance education services in the state and has been successful in delivering higher education directly to the employment site or to an educational site near the student's home.

The distance learning program of the School of Nursing illustrates the effect of this television/audio transmission of coursework on the lives of professional nurses across the state. With a total enrollment of approximately 500 students, the BS in Nursing completion program serves about eighty registered nurses each semester. The majority of people enrolled in these televised degree programs are in their late twenties to early forties, have family and home responsibilities, and still need to complete their degrees for professional growth and job security. The opportunity for televised courses has been a most effective and efficient method for the transmission of didactic content.

The University has adopted as a general goal that distance learning students should have, through electronic media, a learning environment that is comparable to the on-campus technological environment. They should have electronic access to services, resources, faculty, and other students, including at least the following: library card catalog and indexes, state and national databases, electronic mail and bulletin boards to communicate with other students, instructors, advisors, administrators; on-line access to instructional software; assistance with software and hardware questions; and on-line access to administrative procedures, including advising, registration, and career counseling.

4. Project Description

A proposed solution to the delivery of computing and networking services to this distance learning student will be pilot tested in the Spring semester, 1993–94 with Nursing 309, the first of five courses in the RN-Completion program. Each of the approximately 30 students in the course will be provided with a suitable laptop computer fully configured with all necessary storage, applications software, instructional software, and communications capabilities. They would be able to do much of their course-related computing communication in a stand-alone environment. However, for data communication two approaches will be considered. First, the student laptops will be equipped with data-compression, error-checking modems that permit baud rates of up to about 40,000, compared to the 2,400 to 9,600 commonly available now. Ball State will provide 800 numbers and networked modems so that students can dial into university computer systems as needed. Second, where greater network speed is needed, other institutions could, at very low cost, provide a small number of ethernet ports, in a library, for example, where distance learning students could simply attach their laptop computers and log into Ball State networks over Internet and the IHETS Data Network. Most of Indiana's higher education institutions are equipped to make such network access available at moderate cost to the institution.

5. Projected Outcomes

The project has a direct effect on improving the classroom learning environment for students. Implementation of this project will create a futuristic reconceptualization of the classroom learning environment for the distance learning student. They will have unprecedented electronic access to services, resources, faculty, and other students, including at least the following: library card catalog and indexes, state and national databases; electronic mail and bulletin boards to communicate with other students, instructors, advisors, administrators; on-line access to instructional software; assistance with software and hardware questions; and on-line access to administrative procedures including advising, registration, and career counseling. The improved technological access for students at the distance learning sites who, for the most part, received their basic education in a pre-computer era will enable them to become active participants in a world increasingly networked through communication channels.

The project is an innovative approach to deal with an existing problem or issue. Nurse educators must address the issue of technological access for the distance learning student [5,6]. Currently, Ball State University broadcasts classes to ninety-seven different locations throughout Indiana and Kentucky. Ball State currently reaches 38% of the 253 sites in Indiana that are set up to receive classes via the state's educational television system. The potential for growth in the area is evident from these figures. In fact, the office of Continuing Education reported enrollments for the 1990–91 year to be 678 full time equivalents (FTEs). Continuing Education plans to increase enrollments by ten percent each year to reach 1499 FTE by the academic year 2001–02.

The proposed model for computer and information resource access at the distance learning sites eliminates most of the site support problems experienced in the past and reduces considerably the costs for computing support at the remote sites. Successful completion of the pilot project would establish protocols for technological access sharing across the state of Indiana. It is an innovative approach in line with university, state and federal incentives. Information processing skills will become an integral component of the student's approach to learning.

The project involves collaboration among faculty. This project is the culmination of work completed by a university-wide, multi-disciplinary committee. Faculty members from the two disciplines with a large number of distance education students, College of Business and the School of Nursing, will work collaboratively with personnel from University Computing Services to successfully implement the pilot phase of the project during 1993–94. The pilot project will then establish the framework for further implementation of the university-wide plan to other disciplines involved with distance education learning.

The project has potential for initiating long-term change. For example, implementation of the pilot project will facilitate student access to the State University Library Automation Network. It will foster complete development of computer aided instruction software to instruct students how to access on-campus computers. The pilot project will establish the framework for the university to provide distance learners with adequate computing resources without requiring a trip to campus.

References

[1] Gore A. The Information Infrastructure and Technology Act. *EDUCOM Rev* 1992, September–October, 27–29.
[2] Krumenaker L. Electronic Universities: Learning on your time. *PCToday* 1991, October, 57–60.
[3] Carr CWN. On the Leading Edge. *OUTPUT* 1992, 12:9–13.
[4] Sholes W and Edwards V. Distance Learning: Innovative Applications of Tele-communication Technology. *J Med Technol* 1992, 3:28–30.
[5] Twigg CA and Brennan, PF. Distance Learning and Support through Computers. *Nurs Educ Microworld* 1991, 5:9,11.

85
Intercollegiate Electronic Networking among Nursing Graduate Students

Kathleen J. Mikan, Kay Hodson, and Linda Q. Thede

1. Background

Many opportunities for networking among professional colleagues are now possible with the recent advances in computer technology. Electronic communication networking is a rapidly growing field that provides opportunities for scholarly interactions [1]. A major advantage of electronic communication is its ability to facilitate interaction between individuals who have similar interests but who are geographically separated. Advances in technology and participation in networks by academic institutions in the United States have made it possible for academicians to have free-access to wide-area (even global-area) networks [2–3]. While these electronic resources are now available in most academic institutions, electronic networking among professional nurses is in its infancy [4–5]. Uses of electronic communication by nurses on a regular basis for scholarly purposes have just started. The reasons for this are many, but the net results are that very few nurses in the United States use electronic communication for scholarly interactions.

2. Purpose

The purpose of this exploratory research project was to initiate and evaluate the use of electronic communication networking among nursing graduate students located at three geographically distant universities in the United States. The three universities that participated in this study were

Reprinted from *Nursing Informatics: An International Overview for Nursing in a Technological Era*, Grobe, S.J., Pluyter-Wenting, E.S.P. (Eds.). 1994, pp. 574–578, with kind permission from Elsevier Science—NL, Sara Burgerhartstraat 25, 1055 KV Amsterdam, The Netherlands.

Ball State University at Muncie, Indiana; Kent State University at Kent, Ohio; and University of Alabama at Birmingham in Birmingham, Alabama. Collectively, the researchers wanted to (a) explore the use of electronic communication networking; (2) provide intercollegiate sharing of information between graduate students; (3) identify uses, problems, and issues associated with intercollegiate student exchange of electronic information; and (4) identify ways to promote intercollegiate graduate student electronic communication in the future.

3. Participants

Three nursing professors, each located at a different school of nursing in a different state, were responsible for teaching a graduate course on the use of computers in nursing at their respective institutions. Part of the "course" expectations was for students to learn to communicate electronically. It was hoped that once graduate students learned how to use electronic communication as students, they would continue to use it as graduates.

Each of the academic institutions participating in this study had access to Internet, a worldwide electronic communication system that is available 24 hours a day, 365 days a year. Thus, Internet became the electronic linkage between and among the three groups of graduate students. Because of the vast public distribution (in the United States) of microcomputers, modems, and Internet, students at all three schools were encouraged to access Internet from their home, work, or school—wherever and whenever they wished. Designated terminals were available within each institution for students who did not have an Internet access outside of the academic institution.

4. Methodology

Subjects for this study were graduate nursing students enrolled in an introductory computer course offered at each of the three participating institutions by three different nursing professors. All three institutions, beginning in 1993, included content and hands-on learning exercises on the use of electronic communication in their respective computer course. At two of the sites, the course was an elective while it was a required course at the third institution. Data reported in this paper were collected from subjects enrolled in the nursing computer course offered at one of three participating institutions between January and September 1993.

All students who enrolled in the computer course were expected to communicate via electronic mail (E-mail). Students' and instructors' E-mail addresses were shared among the participating institutions and students.

Students were taught to send, receive, save, and delete electronic messages as well as how to upload, download, and perform "housekeeping" tasks with their files. The graduate students were encouraged to communicate with their student colleagues electronically.

In addition to personal E-mail communication, all students were expected to use electronic communication networking to access two different on-line databases: Sigma Theta Tau International Nursing Library whose purpose is to make nursing research available to the nursing community, and ETNet, a national conference network which is a part of the National Library of Medicine in Washington, DC. Additionally, one of the professors created, using the ListServ software, a private on-line discussion group for practicing nurses. Although other ListServ electronic nursing interest groups did exist, none of them focused on situations encountered by practicing nurses.

5. Data Collection

Data were collected using researcher-developed instruments which focused on the uses, problems, and issues of electronic communication by graduate students. A questionnaire was administered to all subjects at the beginning of the course. This instrument (Electronic Networking Technologies) collected data about the subjects' use and knowledge of electronic networking technologies and their ideas about electronic communication purposes and applications. Another questionnaire was administered at the end of the course.

The second data collection instrument was the Electronic Communication Access Record which the students were asked to complete whenever they accessed the electronic network. This log identified the type of networking activity they engaged in during each network access. Depending on which network the student accessed, additional data were collected about the nature of the type of information exchanged. For example, if they accessed an on-line database, graduate students were asked to indicate if, during that interaction, they sought information (read only), gave information (answered a question), posed a problem (opinion), or shared a solution to a problem (solution). Students could check multiple activities per network interaction.

At the conclusion of each network interaction, students were asked to indicate if they were able to complete their interaction without having electronic difficulties, if they were able to "sign off" without difficulties, and the amount of time spent on the computer during each interaction. Students were also asked to identify any problems they had encountered during the electronic interaction and what they gained from their interaction. These data were collected immediately following the students' electronic communication network interactions.

6. Data Analysis

Data collected at all three sites were combined for purposes of data analysis. Between January and September, 1993, a computer "course" for graduate students which contained a section on electronic communication was offered a total of five times at the three participating institutions. The total graduate student enrollment during the five times the "course" was offered was 43. Due to differences in length of the computer "course" at each of the participating institutions, no between institutional comparisons were made with the data.

Analysis of the pre-course questionnaire data revealed that a high percentage of the nursing graduate students had no prior experience in using electronic communication, but they had had experience in using computers for clinical practice, self-instruction, word processing, library searches, and statistical analysis. A few students reported prior use of a computer to communicate with friends or family (E-mail) using a commercial service while even a fewer number of students reported any prior experience with E-mail with professional colleagues, electronic document/file transfer, electronic conferences, or discussion groups. A few students reported using electronic resources such as the local on-line library. None of the students reported prior experience in searching off-campus libraries or accessing electronic publications or journals. Only a few indicated they had every used Internet/BITNET before. None of them had ever accessed ETNET, Sigma Theta Tau, or ListServ prior to taking the course. The pre-course questionnaire indicated that students were able to identify uses for electronic communication within their individual health care institutions. The post-course questionnaire revealed that the learning experiences provided in the graduate computer course expanded the students' understanding of electronic communication to include information available outside their health care institution and provided them with beginning skills in how to access this information. Additionally, the course strengthened the students' beliefs in the value of electronic communication within an institution and created a desire to have the ability to access informational resources beyond those available at their local institution.

The forty-three graduate students accessed electronic communication a total number of 232 times during the course. Data analysis of the Electronic Communication Access Record revealed that the most frequent use of electronic communication was for E-mail. Reading personal messages was the most frequent activity followed by sending messages to known colleagues. Reading messages sent by the ListServ groups to which they subscribed was the next most frequent activity.

Most students were able to complete their interaction without any electronic difficulties and were able to sign off. The average amount of time spend on the computer during a session was 53.86 minutes ($SD = 52.064$). The length of time students accessed the network ranged from 5 minutes to 360 minutes. The averaged number of reported uses of electronic communication by students was 4.3 and ranged from 1 to 15 ($SD = 2.2882$).

7. Findings

The findings indicated that a high percentage of the nursing graduate students had no prior experience in using electronic communication, encountered technical problems (after they were once on Internet) infrequently, accessed a variety of information items on the network, and generated numerous potential uses for electronic communication within nursing.

The types of problems students encountered during the networking sessions related to learning the mechanical operation of the communication software and computer/modem at the local level, the slowness of the computer response time (baud rate of transmission plus slow mainframe response time), and information anxiety [6], i.e., understanding the structure of information in different databases, comprehending the vast amounts of information systems already available, and being orientated to where the student was in the electronic information universe. Students also had difficulty relating the available electronic information networks and resources to the practice area of nursing, i.e., most electronic information sources did not directly relate to nursing practice. Overall, the types of problems students encountered were user, not technical, problems.

As novice users of on-line electronic communication databases, students found electronic sources of information to be "unfriendly," i.e., on-line "help" was either not available or the user directions were unclear. The students reported gaining insight into the variety of electronic information sources available, being pleased to learn that they could communicate electronically, and being able to engage in collaborative scholarship with other nurses.

Incidental findings during the study were that students who lived and worked at some distance from the participating institutions were enthusiastic about the possibilities of electronic communication being a help in meeting some of their personal and professional communication needs. Those who could access the network using a home computer used electronic communication more than those who did not have network access from their homes. Nevertheless, all students saw electronic communication as a means to contact other nurses, decrease their feelings of isolation, and solve nursing problems. Students were positively motivated toward the use of electronic communication and became aware of the wealth of information available with the touch of a key. Students seem to appreciate the fact that their professors were nurses who were able to translate the world of electronic networking into something that was relevant to the professional practice of nursing.

During the initiation and evaluation of the electronic communication learning experiences, the professors identified some problems and issues that needed to be addressed when teaching graduate students the use of electronic communication systems in the future. The professors found that students needed (1) assistance in arranging for access to Internet off-campus without having to pay for long distance phone calls (i.e., many of the graduate students lived at a distance from campus), (2) a comprehensive orientation to electronic communication, (3) to be supported during their initial interactions on the networks, and (4) to be encouraged to share questions, concerns, items of interest, or problems with others whom they did not know personally. Detailed handouts (often in the form of manuals) were needed for each of the networks the student were expected to access. Frequently the guides supplied by the "Network" agencies were confusing and had to be rewritten for local use. The professors found that students who had some familiarity with word processing, although beneficial, had to switch to line, rather than text, editing when using many network systems. Participation in on-line conferences was not done as frequently as the instructors wished; there seemed to be a reluctance on the part of the graduate students to either offer advice or ask questions of others on the network. Also, because it is difficult for students to absorb so many new things that are so different, students needed learning and processing time. To become comfortable with the concepts, methods, processes, and usages of electronic communication takes time. The professors learned that electronic communication can not be accomplished in one or two class sessions.

From an intercollegiate standpoint, minimum difficulties were encountered outside of differences in course scheduling (two institutions offered the computer course on a semester basis and one institution offered the computer course on a quarter basis). This meant that some graduate students only had ten weeks in which to interact with the network while the majority of the students were able to interact with it over a 16-week time span. However, in the future, as more nurses become comfortable with networking, electronic interactions by nurses will not be confined to the length of a "academic computer" course, but rather they will be on-going discussions of nursing situations that all nurses can use as they wish 24-hours a day. Now that nurses can communicate electronically worldwide, it is hoped that graduate nurses (and students) will consider requesting and offering help to colleagues all over the world.

Another incidental outcome of this exploratory research study was that once the electronic communication activities of the students became known to other graduate nursing programs in the United States, the authors received requests from other schools of nursing to allow their graduate students to also participate on GRADNRSE. As a result of this project and the interest of nurses both in education and practice, the GRADNRSE discussion group has been made public.

Other issues that the professors found that needed to be addressed when developing an intercollegiate electronic communication course were: (1) socializing students into the use of electronic communication for scholarly interactions, (2) teaching electronic communication etiquette [7], and (3) helping students get access to Internet after the course was completed so that they could continue to use the knowledge and skills learned and apply them in nursing practice.

8. Summary

Electronic communication offers many opportunities for nurses to share scholarly information worldwide. The technology is in place. The information sources are available. What is missing are nurses who are knowledgeable users of electronic communication. Based on the researchers' successful preparation of a cadre of knowledgeable electronic communication users at each of their respective institutions, it is hoped that the findings of this study will inspire other nursing programs worldwide to consider the initiation and integration of electronic communication within and between nursing education programs. Then and only then will nursing have a true worldwide electronic network of scholars.

References

[1] Harrison TM and Stephen T. On-line Disciplines: Computer-Mediate Scholarship in the Humanities and Social Sciences. *Computer Hu* 1992, 26:13–25.
[2] Krol E. *The Whole Internet User's Guide & Catalog.* Sebastopol, CA: O'Reilly & Associates, Inc. 1992.
[3] Lynch DC and Rose MT. *Internet System Handbook.* Reading, MA: Addison-Wesley Publishing Company, 1993.
[4] Schneider D. Internet: Linking Nurses, Scholars, Libraries. *Reflections* (Sigma Theta Tau International Newsletter, Spring, 1993) 19:9.
[5] Skiba, D. Collaborative Tools. *Reflections* (Sigma Theta Tau International Newsletter, Spring, 1993) 19:10–12.
[6] Wurman RS. *Information Anxiety.* New York: Doubleday, 1989.
[7] Kehoe BP. *Zen and the Art of the Internet A Beginner's Guide.* Englewood Cliffs, NJ: Prentice Hall, 1993.

86
Before Instructional Information Systems Must Come Computer Competent Nurse Educators

MYRNA L. ARMSTRONG

Determining professional role expectations regarding computer technology can guide nursing faculty as they plan and implement instructional information systems. Computer competencies were identified, critiqued, and ranked for nurse educators. Forty-five present-day and 44 future (1990) competencies were judged to be of high importance. Faculty assessment of the important computer competencies can aid in conducting applicable workshops and conferences.

The nurse educator must be knowledgable in computer technology in order to guide nursing's future decision makers in this information-based society. A measure of the nurse educator's competency is data which describes to what extent schools of nursing are incorporating computers and providing technological information. Surveys, unfortunately, continue to identify a small group of nursing schools which either provide computer courses, or require computer prerequisites. If there are going to be future curriculum changes to accomodate computer technology health care issues and incorporate instructional information systems, there must be computer competent nurse educators to forge ahead with the ideas for implementation of these programs.

One suggested method of meeting that challenge is by determining guidelines for performance in meeting professional role expectations of a particular activity with the development of competencies.[1] Identification of these competencies, critiqued through the judgment of nurse experts, can be an effective strategy in refining educational needs.

Reprinted with permission from *Proceedings: Eleventh Annual Symposium on Computer Applications in Medical Care*, Stead, W.W. (Ed.). 1987, pp. 421–424. © 1987, American Medical Informatics Association (formerly SCAMC): Bethesda, MD.

Computer Competencies

This study identified, critiqued, and ranked present and future (1990) computer competencies for nurse educators in basic and continuing education. From a ten-year review of related nursing literature, information was found relevant to the profession for the formation of 68 present computer competencies. Sixty-four future computer competencies were created from projections of representatives from health-related hardware manufacturers, software producer/distributers, and nurse researchers. Computer statements were grouped into 9 categories and developed around psychomotor, cognitive, and affective issues surrounding use of the computer, and its related technology, with nursing. They were related to the profession in four prominent areas: practice, education, administration, and research. Categories surrounding these major areas included documentation, patient monitoring, patient education, nursing role/issues, instruction by computer, computer instruction, instructional support, nursing administration, and nursing research.

The Delphi technique was used as a method of collecting and organizing judgments in an effort to reach agreement on present needs and projections of future ideas. The evaluation panel was comprised of nurse educators knowledgeable about computer technology from associate and baccalaureate degree schools of nursing, hospital staff development departments, university continuing nursing education faculty, and those employed with nursing organizations and nurse consultants. Fifty-six participated, from 28 states, during round one and 55 continued for the second round of review.

A median and interquartile range (IQR), commonly used with the Delphi technique, was computed for each computer competency following round one. Panel members were sent results of the group's median and IQR illustrating the preliminary trend of group consensus, then asked to compare and revise their opinions, as they desired. A Delphi consensus occurred in this study with decreased IQRs and stability of the median rating.

The evaluation panel singled out forty-five present competency statements as listed in Table 1. Forty-four future competency statements, as found in Table 2, were found to be of high importance. Ten present and ten future computer competencies were judged to be in the very high range of this rating. A total of 39 competency items (30%) received between 80% to 98% agreement, within the IQR, for the designated importance ranking. Three present competency statements were rated as low importance. These related to knowledge of: (a) programming language, (b) differentiation of digital/analog computers, and (c) various brands of computer hardware.

TABLE 1.* Elements of present computer competencies rated of high importance and high IQR agreement**

	Median* (N = 55)	IQR #	IQR %
Clinical Practice			
Documentation:			
Emphasize nursing process with computerized charting & care plans.	4.8	0.7	
Discuss problems of confidentiality with information systems.	4.6	1.0	95
Describe use of information systems.	4.0	0.8	
Distinguish traditional and computerized medication procedures.	3.7	1.1	85
Patient monitoring:			
Determine nursing responses after analysis of monitoring data.	4.3	1.0	
Patient education:			
Address computerized multidisciplinary discharge planning.	3.7	1.2	82
Nursing role/issues:			
Describe protection of patient rights when using computerized systems.	4.7	0.9	
Identify computer training needs of nurses.	4.6	1.0	95
Discuss nursing involvement with implementation of information systems.	4.5	1.2	
Evaluate impact of change when considering computer technology in nursing.	4.2	0.9	
Assess nurses role when using computers.	4.2	1.0	
Discuss dehumanization vs personalization aspects when using computers in nursing.	4.2	1.0	
Project health care computing trends in nursing.	4.1	0.8	
Discuss machine dependence vs independence.	3.7	1.2	84
Discuss increase vs decrease job availability using computers in health care.	3.6	1.1	91
Analyze consumer benefits/limitations of computer technology.	3.6	1.2	85
Nursing Administration			
Discuss the impact of the computer on the manager's role.	4.6	1.1	95
Describe an information system to enter MD orders and develop acuity/care plans.	4.1	0.7	
Explain computerized data to analyze and assist with delivery of care.	4.1	0.7	
Discuss programs with staffing, budget, and patient need identification.	4.1	0.8	
Nursing Research			
Support research to examine impact of computer technology in nursing.	4.3	1.0	
Manipulate data using statistical analysis software.	4.0	0.9	
Nursing Education			
Instructional support:			
Operate a word processing program.	4.4	1.1	
Identify learner needs by means of a computerized assessment system.	4.0	0.9	

TABLE 1.* *(Continued.)*

	Median* (N = 55)	IQR #	%
Nursing Education (cont.)			
Describe use of a spreadsheet program.	3.7	1.1	87
Instruction by computer:			
Assess CAI objectives for learners' needs.	4.6	1.0	98
Discuss CAI-related material with lecture, clinicals, and skills labs.	4.6	1.1	93
Explore CAI and other creative methods to deliver nursing content.	4.6	1.1	96
Encourage development of CAI for integration into curriculum.	4.5	1.1	95
Substantiate cost effectiveness and usefulness of software.	4.4	1.1	95
Encourage CAI development with faculty rewards for scholarly pursuit.	4.4	1.1	
Encourage CAI development with release time for faculty.	4.4	1.2	87
Differentiate various ACI formats to meet instructional objectives.	4.3	1.1	
Establish information about computer applications in curriculum.	4.2	0.9	
Encourage CAI development with content expertise.	4.2	1.0	
Encourage CAI development by determining learner characteristics.	4.2	1.0	
Determine levels of computer education needed by nurses.	4.2	1.0	
Encourage CAI development using instructional design principles.	4.2	1.1	
Monitor progress of learners using CAI.	4.1	0.8	
Evaluate facilitator, consultant role of the educator when using CAI.	4.1	0.8	
Describe assistance to meet learning needs when using computers in education.	4.0	0.7	
Communicate resources in educational computing.	4.0	0.7	
Computer instruction:			
Establish faculty development time to explore computer capabilities.	4.6	1.0	95
Evaluate courseware for interactive, self-paced instruction.	4.6	1.1	89
Discuss copyright laws related to computing.	4.4	1.1	
Discuss the computer as an object of instruction, an instructional medium, and a problem-solving tool.	4.3	0.9	
Analyze software documentation.	4.2	0.8	
Communicate, using computer terminology.	4.1	0.8	
Load and run a variety of software.	4.1	0.8	
Use terminal and menu-driven programs for instruction and reports.	4.0	0.7	
Investigate CAI for instructional design principles.	4.0	0.7	
Explain modem/communication software.	3.6	1.1	93
Identify, describe, and demonstrate components of computer and peripherals.	3.6	1.2	82

* Importance: 1 = No, 2 = Low, 3 = Medium, 4 = High, 5 = Extreme.
** Reprinted with Permission: *IMAGE:* The Journal of Nursing Scholarship Vol. 18, No. 4 Winter 1986, pp. 155–160.

TABLE 2.* Elements of future computer competencies rated of high importance and high IQR agreement**

	Median* (N = 55)	IQR #	IQR %
Clinical Practice			
Documentation:			
Discuss confidentiality while using voice synthesis terminals.	4.9	0.6	82
Explain nursing process/diagnosis proficiency using information systems.	4.7	0.9	
Demonstrate pocket-size computers.	4.6	1.0	96
Evaluate on-line computer systems that provide greater speed and conciseness.	4.3	1.0	
Analyze use of artificial intelligence programs for patient care activities.	4.1	0.7	
Discuss changes when MD enters own orders.	4.1	0.7	
Explain medication monitoring systems to track pharmaceutical supplies.	3.6	1.2	82
Patient monitoring:			
Discuss closed loop infusion systems to monitor/diffuse meds.	4.1	0.6	
Describe bedside computer systems.	4.1	0.7	
Identify client data transmitted from infusion devices with modem ports.	4.0	0.6	84
Patient education:			
Encourage client use of CAI for health education.	4.3	1.0	
Identify client concerns experiencing	4.1	0.7	
CAT scan imagery:			
Design teaching plans for clients using infusion pumps.	4.1	0.7	
Instruct clients to their "mini-charts" containing pertinent medical data.	4.1	0.8	
Describe sonar detector terminals that contain client education on health.	3.4	1.1	91
Nursing role/issues:			
Join nursing association computer networks.	4.8	0.9	
Discuss impact of legislation, research, and economics on health care/technology.	4.5	1.0	98
Analyze nursing when actions of each health discipline are documented.	4.3	0.9	
Evaluate reality of third-party payment as a result of computerized documentation.	4.3	1.0	
Project future jobs for nursing, i.e. space program.	3.6	1.2	86
Nursing Research			
Analyze research on impact of computerization on nursing practice.	4.7	0.9	
Discuss research of humans interacting with machines more than people.	4.6	1.0	96
Support research regarding computerization, nursing education, and adult education principles.	4.3	1.1	
Support research to explore learner self-esteem levels while using CAI.	4.2	0.9	
Use minimum core nursing data bases to facilitate nursing research.	4.2	1.0	

TABLE 2.* (*Continued.*)

	Median* (N = 55)	IQR #	%
Nursing Research (cont.)			
Support research to explore need of sophisticated branching in CAI.	4.1	0.7	
Support research to investigate need for learner tracking systems in CAI.	4.1	0.7	
Encourage participation in a manufacturer users' group.	4.1	0.8	
Nursing Administration			
Describe on-going evaluation/revision regarding information systems.	4.6	1.0	98
Project proactive role needed by nurse manager as part of health team.	4.3	1.0	
Nursing Education			
Instruction by computers:			
Describe criteria for software evaluation and instructional design principles.	4.6	1.0	98
Describe criteria for software evaluation and continuing education programs.	4.6	1.0	96
Prepare all nurses at basic level of "information specialist."	4.6	1.1	93
Discuss preparation of the graduate level "systems specialist."	4.3	0.9	
Include computerized nursing care plans disk as part of learning activities.	4.3	0.9	
Describe criteria for software evaluation with other instructional methodologies.	4.3	0.9	
Assist learners with their portable computers.	4.3	1.0	
Implement CAI/CAIV systems for educational experiences.	4.3	1.0	
Identify directories when using networks.	4.1	0.7	
Use computerized multidisciplinary self-assessment/learning centers.	4.1	0.7	
Share guidelines with learners for rental and/or purchase of CAI.	4.0	0.8	
Employ an authoring language to develop CAI.	4.0	0.9	
Describe criteria for software evaluation and Informatics.	3.9	0.6	80
Computer instruction:			
Encourage problem-solving and logic exercises in curriculum.	4.5	1.1	95
Discuss the new code of ethics for CAI security.	4.3	1.0	
Differentiate between CAI/CAIV capabilities to meet learning objectives.	3.7	1.2	82
Describe a high-level, human-like computer language.	3.4	1.2	80
Instructional support:			
Identify health care publishers of CAI continuing education programs.	4.2	0.8	
Access data bases and software libraries for "store for use" material for class.	4.1	0.6	80
Identify national registeries to access health/medical/drug data.	4.1	0.7	

TABLE 2.* (*Continued.*)

Nursing Education (cont.)	Median* (N = 55)	IQR #	%
Describe a learner's life-long educational record, airmail stamp size.	3.6	1.2	80
Discuss telematics, made possible by laser/optical fiber advances.	3.5	1.1	89
Produce color computer graphics.	3.5	1.1	89

* Importance: 1 = No, 2 = Low, 3 = Medium, 4 = High, 5 = Extreme.
** Reprinted with Permission: *IMAGE:* The Journal of Nursing Scholarship Vol. 18, No. 4 Winter 1986, pp. 155–160.

Implications for Nursing

Upon review of the major categories containing the present competencies judged to be high of importance, it appears that an emphasis for the nurse educator teaching in basic and continuing nursing education, should be on: (a) how to use the computer as an instructional tool, (b) knowledge about computer technology, (c) recognition of the nurses role and issues with the computer in health care, and (d) use of the nursing process in the development of computerized charting and care plans. Evaluation of the major categories with the most statements judged to be of high importance for the future computer competency statements, indicate that emphasis should be on: (a) use of the computer as an instructional, documentation, and research tool, (b) evaluation of the effects of computerization in nursing, and (c) involvement of computers with client health education. The instruction by computer category received the highest number of rated high importance statements, both on the present and future computer competency questionnaires. It was concluded that this area of computer technology whould be a high knowledge priority for the nurse educator, both for the present, and in the future.

Knowledge of important present computer competencies and projections for important future trends could be a method of assessing what the present level of education is for that specific competency category, and what a panel of colleagues judge to be important. The more succinctly nurse educators identify these discrepancies, the better they will be able to assess their education needs. This assessment could then be a motivator for the nurse educator to seek further educational activities designed around the necessary computer competencies and could produce more satisfaction because real-life tasks and problems are addressed.

Attempting to integrate computer technology into nursing education is certainly more than the placement of equipment and programs. Effective implementation and use comes when the faculty understand and work with the idea. An excellent opportunity now exists for the nurse educator to assess her personal level of knowledge with regard to each critiqued computer competency. Once knowledgeable with the agreed upon areas of computer proficiency in their profession they can begin to take an active part in the evolution and development of instructional information systems which can certainly add another dimension to nursing education.

References

1. Knowles, M.S. *The modern practice of adult education: From andragogy to pedagogy*, 1980, Chicago: Association Press.

87
Attitudes Toward Computer Technology between Nursing and Medical Educators

Bennie E. Harsanyi and Clyde E. Kelsey, Jr.

Introduction

Technological innovations have revolutionized educational and clinical practice environments. Although the availability of biomedical technology is escalating at an unprecedented pace, a belief exists that biomedical technological innovations are being diffused at a slow rate among health care professionals [1,2,3,4]. The literature on technological innovations emphasizes the significance of attitudes regarding the human-machine interface in influencing the diffusion process [5,6]. An understanding of health care professionals' attitudes toward technological innovations can contribute to an understanding of the biomedical innovation diffusion process. The medical and nursing educators' mission is to prepare professionals to function competently in health care educational and clinical environments. Medical and nursing educators, however, are slowly adopting and implementing the technological advances available for educational and health care delivery environments. Nursing and medical educators' attitudes toward the human-machine interface can impact this mission and the diffusion process.

Attitudinal Literature Regarding Health Care Professionals

Previous research has not specifically contrasted the attitudes toward computer technology between nursing and medical educators. Scores on questionnaires from previous studies regarding attitudes toward computer technology: (a) predicted adopters' adaptation to the subsequent phase of

Reprinted with permission from *Proceedings: Thirteenth Annual Symposium on Computer Applications in Medical Care*, Kingsland, L.C. (Ed.). 1989, pp. 802–809. © 1989, American Medical Informatics Association (formerly SCAMC): Bethesda, MD.

implementation; (b) identified groups with negative and positive attitudes; (c) identified the basic components of attitudes for attitudinal change strategies; (d) impacted employee retention and job satisfaction; (e) impacted professional role function, values, culture, and practice; (f) impacted user educational and training designs; and (g) measured attitudinal change over time.

The most favorable attitudes among physicians were exhibited toward technology which enhanced patient care delivery. In contrast, the least favorable attitudes were exhibited toward technology which infringed on the physicians' management role or threatened traditional clinical practice, professional role, and professional status [7,8,9,10]. Results revealed that physicians' attitudes can facilitate or impede the diffusion process [11,12]. Physicians' attitudes could also be successfully predicted and constructively altered over time [13,14]. Social network analysis used to explore factors affecting physician utilization of technological systems revealed that physicians rely heavily upon peers regarding decision making and information concerning practice innovations [15].

Results regarding nurses' attitudes toward computer technology revealed conflicting results [16,17,18,19]. Studies regarding technological innovations in nursing education have focused primarily on nursing educators' and students' attitudes, knowledge, usage, effectiveness, and experience regarding technologically-based instructional methodology [20,21]. Although acceptance of technological innovations as efficient, necessary, and unavoidable was evident among nursing educators, adoption and implementation of technological innovations were minimal. In addition, computer literacy among nursing faculty and administrators was uncommon [22,23,24,25,26].

Education, age, cognitive style, previous exposure, experience, and knowledge were the most frequently cited influencing variables [27,28]. Attitudes toward technological innovations were also impacted by nursing culture, values, and clinical practice [29,30].

The purpose of this descriptive study was to assess and compare the attitudes toward computer technology in general between nursing and medical educators. The study investigated: (a) the effect of demographic characteristics on positive or negative attitudes, (b) the effect of previous experience and education regarding computer technology on attitudes, and (c) the effect of the usage of computer technology in the educational and clinical environments on attitudes.

Methods

A comparative, correlational survey design using stratified random sampling technique was used. The subjects were full-time or part-time nursing and medical educators teaching in a school of nursing, offering a baccalaureate degree in nursing, or in a school of medicine in the State of Texas. Survey packets were mailed to 486 medical faculty subjects and 62 nursing faculty subjects. Anonymity of subjects' responses was assured, and a self-addressed, stamped envelope was included for response returns. 131 medical faculty and 46 nursing faculty returned the survey packets for an overall 32.3 percent return rate. All responses were used in the data analysis.

The "Attitudes Toward Computers in General" questionnaire, a 20-bipolar semantic differential type rating scale, was used to measure attitudes toward the general concept of computer technology [31]. The cue, "computers are, in general," was used to elicit subject response. Seven-point rating scales were used, and a total score for each subject was derived by reversing the negative items and summing over the 20 items. A score of 80 indicated a neutral point. The range of scores could be 20, indicating an extremely negative attitude, to 140, indicating an extremely positive attitude. The items selected were chosen on the basis of face validity, and the Cronbach's Alpha for the instrument was .85.

Subjects also completed the "Computer Attitude Profile" to obtain information regarding demographic variables, previous experience and education regarding computer technology, and the usage of computer technology in educational and clinical environments [32]. Demographic variables included age, sex, highest level of education, profession, position title, years as an educator, years as a physician or nurse, and area of clinical specialty and practice. Previous experience included personal use and professional use in education and/or clinical practice environments. Previous education included the number of contract hours of instruction and actual hands-on education regarding computer technology. The usage of computer technology in educational and clinical environments included the type and frequency of usage.

Data Analysis and Results

Data collected from the "Computer Attitude Profile" was used to describe the characteristics of the respondent population. It was comprised of 177 subjects, 131 (74.0%) Texas medical and 46 (26.0%) nursing educators. The disproportion of medical educators to nursing educators was reflective of the actual proportions of medical educators to nursing educators in Texas. The majority of the respondents was between the age of 31 to 55 (83.6%) with a mean age of 41 to 45 (24.9%). The respondent population included 62 (35%) females and 114 (64.4%) males. In regard to years as an educator, 82.5 percent of the respondents had 20 years or less years of experience as an educator with a mean of 11 to 15 years. The highest percentage of physicians (27.9%) had been in practice 11 to 15 years. The highest percentage of nurses (33.3%) had been in practice 16 to 20 years.

TABLE 1. Differences between nursing educators' and medical educators' attitudes

Variable	x̄	t	Df	Prob
Group 1 (Nursing educators)	102.26	1.34	173	0.182
Group 2 (Medical educators)	98.78			

As shown in Table 1, the results of the t-test indicated no significant difference ($p < 0.05$) between nursing and medical educators' attitudes. Both groups possessed a slightly positive attitude. The mean scores, however, indicated that nursing educators were slightly more positive than medical educators. Stepwise regression analysis was used to determine the effect of previous experience and education regarding computer technology, the usage of computer technology in educational and clinical environments, and demographic characteristics. As shown in Table 2 with an accepted correlation coefficient of .250 or above, previous experience with computer technology was significant but negatively correlated; whereas, education regarding computer technology was not significant. Demographic variables were not significant. Usages of computer technology in educational and clinical practice environments also were not significant. Although negatively correlated, record keeping and word processing, in that order, were the only two significant education variables to impact educators' attitudes. In the clinical environment, diagnosing was positively correlated whereas patient assessment and network systems were negatively correlated with attitudes toward computer technology.

Discussion

The findings contribute to an understanding of nursing and medical educator's attitudes toward computer technology and to the slow diffusion of technological innovation in educational and clinical environments. The

TABLE 2. Correlation Matrix: Previous experience and education regarding computer technology

	CPT	CTH	CONPROHR	CONHANHR	ATCIG
Computer technology for personal use	1.00	.156	−.058	−.134	−.268
Computer technology for professional use, health care delivery, or education		1.00	−.058	−.147	−.326
Contact hours of instruction			1.00	.439	.130
Contact hours of hands-on education				1.00	.130
Attitude toward computers in general					1.00

findings lend support to previous, although conflicting results, regarding the existence of favorable attitudes toward computer technology among physicians and nurses. The findings also lend support to previous studies regarding the existence of favorable attitudes toward technology which enhances patient care delivery. The finding that computers were viewed as good, efficient, and useful also supports previous research. Although significant, the negative correlation of previous experience with current attitudes could illustrate a frustration among educators regarding the lack of availability of integrated software and technologically based systems for educational and health care delivery environments. The quality and quantity of the previous experience could also explain this negative correlation. Results regarding previous education, which showed nonparticipation in continuing education activities over the past year, could indicate, when compared to the years of previous experience in using computers, a moderately high level of comfort with the use of computer technology for personal and professional use in education and health care delivery environments. Although negatively correlated, record keeping and word processing, in that order, were the only two significant education variables to impact educators' attitudes. These variables enhance the traditional faculty role especially in regard to research and publication expectations. Results indicated, however, that educators were not using computer technology as a tool for instructional purposes. The finding regarding the significance but negative correlation for patient assessment and networking and the positive correlation of diagnosing, appears to indicate a desire to use computer technology for these activities, but it also could indicate a disappointment in the results achieved when using technology in clinical practice environments.

Summary

Further research is needed regarding nursing and medical educators' attitudes toward specific technological innovations which are perceived as enhancing or threatening traditional professional roles in educational and clinical practice environments. Longitudinal studies are needed regarding nursing and medical educators' attitudes toward technological innovations. The significance of professional peer influence and the educators' role in professional networks on attitudes toward technological innovations in educational and clinical practice environments are other areas for investigation. It is recommended that attitude assessment data be used in the design of continuing education, faculty development, training, and attitude modification programs. It is the challenge of health care professionals to use technological innovations to creatively meet society's health care needs. It is the responsibility, accountability, and authority of nursing and medical educators to prepare the present and future generation of health care professionals to accept this challenge.

References

[1] Anderson, J. G., and Jay, S. J. (Eds.). (1987). *Use and impact of computers in clinical medicine.* New York: Springer-Verlag.

[2] Cox, H., Harsanyi, B., and Dean, L. (1987). *Computers and nursing: Application to practice, education and research.* East Norwalk Ct: Appleton and Lange.

[3] Dowling, A. F. (1980). Do hospital staff interfere with computer system implementation? *Health Care Management Review, 5*(4), 23–32.

[4] Grann, R. P. (1984). Attitudes and effective use of computers among hospital personnel. In G. S. Cohen (Ed.), *Proceedings of the Eighth Annual Symposium on Computer Applications in Medical Care, 8,* 543–547.

[5] Kaplan, B. (1986). Impact of a clinical laboratory computer system: Users' Perceptions. In R. Salamon, B. Blum, M. Jorgensen (Eds.), *Medinfo 86* (pp. 1057–1061). Amsterdam: North Holland, Elsevier Science Publishers.

[6] Kjerulff, K. H., Counte, M. A., Salloway, J. C., and Campbell, B. C. (1983). Measuring adaptation to medical technology. *Hospital and Health Services Administration, 28,* 30–40.

[7] Melhorn, J. M., Legler, W. K., and Clark, G. M. (1979). Current attitudes of medical personnel toward computers. *Computers and Biomedical Research, 12,* 327–334.

[8] Singer, J., Sacks, H. S., Lucente, F., and Chalmers, T. C. (1983). Physician attitude toward applications of computer data base systems. *Journal of the American Medical Association, 249,* 1610–1614.

[9] Startsman, T. S. and Robinson, R. E. (1972). The attitudes of medical and paramedial personnel toward computers. *Computers and Biomedical Research, 5*(3), 218–227.

[10] Teach, R. L., and Shortliffe, E. H. (1981). An analysis of physician attitudes regarding computer-based clinical consultation systems. *Computers and Biomedical Research, 14,* 542–558.

[11] Friedman, R. B., and Gustafson, D. H. (1977). Guest Editorial: Computers in medicine: A critical review. *Computers and Biomedical Research, 10*(3), 199–204.

[12] Hudson, D. L. and Cohen, M. E. (1985). The role of user interface in a medical expert system. In M. J. Ackerman (Ed.), *Proceedings of the Ninth Annual Symposium on Computer Applications in Medical Care, 9,* 232–236.

[13] Kjerulff, K. H., Counte, M. A., and Salloway, J. C. (1986). Attitudes toward computers and employee turnover during implementation of a pharmacy information system. In R. Salamon, B. Blum, and M. Jorgensen (Eds.) *Medinfo 86* (pp. 1046–1051). Amsterdam: North Holland, Elsevier Science Publishers.

[14] Kjerulff, K. H., Counte, M. A., Salloway, J. C., Campbell, B. C., and Noskin, D. E. (1984). Medical information system training: An analysis of the reactions of hospital employees. *Computers and Biomedical Research, 17,* 303–310.

[15] Anderson, J. G., and Jay, S. J. (Eds.). (1987). *Use and Impact of Computers in Clinical Medicine.* New York: Springer-Verlag.

[16] Brodt, A. and Stronge, J. H. (1986). Nurses' attitudes toward computerization in a Midwestern community hospital. *Computers in Nursing, 4,* 82–86.

[17] Merrow, S. L. (1984). Nursing educators' and nursing service personnel's knowledge of and attitudes toward computer use in nursing practice. *Dissertation Abstracts International, 45*/09B, 2870. (University Microfilms No. 84-25987).

[18] Ronald, J. S. (1982). Attitudes and learning needs of nursing educators with respect to computers: Implications for curriculum planning. *Dissertation Abstracts International, 43*/09A, 2879. (University Microfilms No. 83-03098).

[19] Theis, J. B. (1975, Winter). Hospital personnel and computer-based systems: A study of attitudes and perception. *Hospital Administration*, 17–25.

[20] Cleveland, L. M. (1985). Computer utilization within nursing curriculum. *Dissertation Abstracts International, 46*/10A, 2902. (University Microfilms No. 85-26856).

[21] Delaney, C. J. (1986). Administrator and faculty acceptance of the computer as a technological innovation in baccalaureate nursing programs in independent colleges in the Midwest. *Dissertation Abstracts International, 47*/07A, 2388. (University Microfilms No. 86-22760).

[22] Armstrong, M. L. (1983). Paving the way for more effective computer usage. *Nursing and Health Care, 4*, 557–560.

[23] Goethler, A. N. (1985). Nursing education update: Computer technology. *Nursing and Health Care, 6*, 509–510.

[24] Johnson, B. M. (1983). *Microcomputers in the Nursing Dean's Office.* Washington, DC: American Association of Colleges of Nursing.

[25] Murphy, M. A. (1984). Computer-based education in nursing—Factors influencing its utilization. *Computers in Nursing, 2*(6), 218–223.

[26] Thomas, B. S. (1985). A survey study of computers in nursing education. *Computers in Nursing, 3*, 173–179.

[27] Aydin, C. E. (1988). *Social Information Processing and Individual Differences in Information System Attitudes and Use.* Unpublished manuscript. University of Southern California, Annenberg School of Communications, Los Angeles, Ca.

[28] Morin, P. J. (1982). A comparative study of attitudes toward computer assisted instruction and learning styles of nursing students. *Dissertation Abstracts International, 43*/03A, 653. (University Microfilms No. 82-17547).

[29] Kadner, K. (1984). Change: Introducing computer-assisted instruction (CAI) to a college of nursing faculty. *Journal of Nursing Education, 23*(8), 349–350.

[30] Murphy, M. A. (1984). Computer-based education in nursing—Factors influencing its utilization. *Computers in Nursing, 2*(6), 218–222.

[31] Kjerulff, K. H., and Counte, M. A. (1984a). Measuring attitudes towards computers: Two approaches. In G. S. Cohen (Ed.), *Proceedings of the Eighth Annual Symposium on Computer Applications in Medical Care, 8*, 529–535.

[32] Harsanyi, B. (1987). *Computer Attitude Profile.* Unpublished profile.

Index

grant to study linkages between health care and academic centers, 395–400

KERMIT communications protocol, 495

Key codes, in MARTIN, 500

Key concepts, identifying for knowledge acquisition systems, 164

Key interventions, focus on, in clinical path development, 319

Knowbots, search for connectivities by, 84–85

Knowing
  incorporating in knowledge systems, 408
  for nursing practice, 408–409

Knowledge
  acquisition of, 163–165
  adequacy of, evaluating an artificial intelligence system, 315, 317
  database for an artificial intelligence system, 312–318
  defined, 409, 429
  for developing expert systems for nursing, 158–167
  for the nurse information systems specialist, 539–540
  nursing, 4, 162–163
    access through computers, 528
    base for expert systems, 307–308
    about statistics, for using software, 493
    structures for, 162
    supplemental information to build, 433–434
    transformational effects of, 3
    See also Information

Knowledge base, of expert systems, 600

Knowledge-Based Systems, 10

Knowledge engineer, for AIDS expert system development, 604–606

Knowledgement II (database management system), 432

Knowledge test, for a study of clinical decision making, 452

Korner Report, 438

L

Laboratory data, downloading to bedside workstations, 288–289

Languages
  of experts interfacing with users, 160
  natural, focus on, 33
  non-Latin, use of computer with, 12
  official, of the International Council of Nurses, 43
  of respondents, integrity of, 498
  standardized
    for interfacing components of integrated systems, 272
    for nursing, 246
  See also Nursing Minimum Data Set; Standardization; Vocabularies

Laptop computer, for a distance learning program, 621–622

Learner, process for using computer-aided instruction, 598

Learning, opportunities for in computer assisted instruction, 587

Learning Resource Center, for simulation systems, 612

Learning theory, developing lessons that employ the principles of, 590

Learning time, in computer-aided instruction, 579

Legal issues
  in expert system decision making, 308–309
  in medical practice with informatics support, 12
  in ownership of information stored in computers, 99
  in recording procedures, 128

Legal protection, for medical record privacy, 109

Legibility, of computerized records, versus handwritten records, 384

Length of stay (LOS)
  for a casetype, 319, 320–321
  as a proxy for cost, 395
  relating to diagnosis related group, 390

LERS software, 467

Computers and Medicine *(continued from page ii)*

Knowledge Engineering in Health Informatics
Homer R. Warner, Dean K. Sorenson, and Omar Bouhaddou

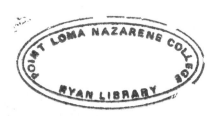

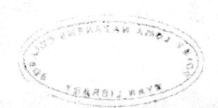